W9-CCC-953

6th EDITION

Modules for Basic Nursing Skills

VOLUME I

© 1996 by Lippincott-Raven Publishers

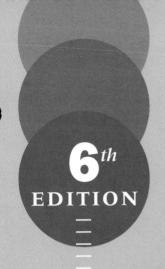

6th EDITION

Modules for Basic Nursing Skills

Janice Rider Ellis, RN, PhD

Elizabeth Ann Nowlis, RN, EdD

Patricia M. Bentz, RN, MSN

Shoreline Community College • Seattle, Washington

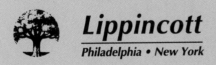

Lippincott

Philadelphia • New York

Sponsoring Editor: Mary P. Gyetvan, RN, MSN
Coordinating Editorial Assistant: Susan M. Keneally
Project Editor: Erika Kors
Design Coordinator: Melissa Olson
Production Manager: Helen Ewan
Production Coordinator: Nannette Winski
Indexer: Anne Cope

6th Edition

Copyright © 1996, by Lippincott-Raven Publishers.

Copyright © 1992, by J. B. Lippincott Company. © 1988 by
Houghton Mifflin Company. All rights reserved. This book is
protected by copyright. No part of it may be reproduced, stored
in a retrieval system, or transmitted, in any form or by any
means—electronic, mechanical, photocopy, recording, or otherwise—without the prior written permission of the publisher,
except for brief quotations embodied in critical articles and reviews. Printed in the United States of America. For information
write Lippincott-Raven Publishers, 227 East Washington
Square, Philadelphia, PA 19106.

Library of Congress Cataloging in Publication Data

Ellis, Janice Rider.
    Modules for basic nursing skills / Janice Rider Ellis,
Elizabeth Ann Nowlis, Patricia M. Bentz. — 6th ed.
        p.   cm.
    Includes bibliographical references and indexes.
    ISBN 0-397-55171-1 (v. 1 : alk. paper). — ISBN 0-397-
55170-3 (v. 2 : alk. paper)
    1. Nursing—Outlines, syllabi, etc.   2. Nursing—
Problems, exercises, etc.   I. Nowlis, Elizabeth Ann.
II. Bentz, Patricia M.   III. Title.
    [DNLM: 1. Nursing—programmed instruction.
WY 18.2 E47n 1996]
RT52.E44   1996
610.73'076—dc20
DNLM/DLC
for Library of Congress   95-37176
                                          CIP   9 8 7 6 5 4 3

The material contained in this volume was submitted as previously unpublished material, except in the instances in which
credit has been given to the source from which some of the il-
lustrative material was derived.

Any procedure or practice described in this book should be applied by the health-care practitioner under appropriate supervision in accordance with professional standards of care used
with regard to the unique circumstances that apply in each
practice situation. Care has been taken to confirm the accuracy
of information presented and to describe generally accepted
practices. However, the authors, editors, and publisher cannot
accept any responsibility for errors or omissions or for any consequences from application of the information in this book and
make no warranty, express or implied, with respect to the contents of the book.

The authors and publisher have exerted every effort to ensure
that drug selection and dosage set forth in this text are in accordance with current recommendations and practice at the time
of publication. However, in view of ongoing research, changes
in government regulations, and the constant flow of information relating to drug therapy and drug reactions, the reader is
urged to check the package insert for each drug for any change
in indications and dosage and for added warnings and precautions. This is particularly important when the recommended
agent is a new or infrequently employed drug.

Materials appearing in this book prepared by individuals as part
of their official duties as U.S. Government employees are not
covered by the above-mentioned copyright.

CONTENTS

List of Skills   *vii*
To the Instructor   *xi*
To the Student   *xv*

Unit I
FOUNDATION SKILLS   *1*

1   *An Approach to Nursing Skills*   *3*
2   *Basic Infection Control*   *15*
3   *Safety*   *31*
4   *Basic Body Mechanics*   *59*
5   *Documentation*   *71*

Unit II
ASSESSMENT SKILLS   *103*

6   *Introduction to Assessment Skills*   *105*
7   *Temperature, Pulse, and Respiration*   *123*
8   *Blood Pressure*   *141*
9   *The Nursing Physical Assessment*   *155*
10   *Intake and Output*   *193*
11   *Collecting Specimens and Performing Common Laboratory Tests*   *211*
12   *Assisting with Diagnostic and Therapeutic Procedures*   *249*
13   *Admission, Transfer, and Discharge*   *277*

Unit III
FUNDAMENTAL PERSONAL CARE SKILLS   *299*

14   *Bedmaking*   *301*
15   *Moving the Patient in Bed and Positioning*   *325*
16   *Feeding Adult Patients*   *357*
17   *Assisting with Elimination and Perineal Care*   *371*
18   *Hygiene*   *391*
19   *Basic Infant Care*   *431*

Unit IV
ASSISTING WITH ACTIVITY AND REST   *455*

20   *Transfer*   *457*
21   *Ambulation: Simple Assisted and Using Cane, Walker, or Crutches*   *489*

© 1996 by Lippincott-Raven Publishers

22   *Range-of-Motion Exercises*   *521*
23   *Caring for Patients with Casts and Braces*   *545*
24   *Applying and Maintaining Traction*   *575*
25   *Special Mattresses and Therapeutic Frames and Beds*   *597*

Unit V

PROVIDING FOR COMFORT, ELIMINATION, AND NUTRITION   *617*

26   *Applying Bandages and Binders*   *619*
27   *Applying Heat and Cold*   *653*
28   *Administering Enemas*   *679*
29   *Tube Feeding*   *701*

Unit VI

PROCEDURES FOR SPECIAL SITUATIONS   *717*

30   *Emergency Resuscitation Procedures*   *719*
31   *Postmortem Care*   *743*

Glossary   *765*
Answers to Quizzes   *779*
Index   *I-1*

© 1996 by Lippincott-Raven Publishers

LIST OF SKILLS

The following skills are included in this volume. For easy reference, a module number and a page number are provided for each skill.

Skill	Module	Page
Admission	13	282
Air-Fluidized bed	25	605
Airway obstruction, clearing foreign body (Heimlich maneuver)	30	729
Alternating pressure mattress	25	602
Ambulation	21	492
Auscultation		
Bowel sounds	9	167
Heart	9	161
Lungs	9	164
Back rub	18	401
Bandaging		
Circular	26	624
Figure-8	26	626
Recurrent fold	26	627
Reverse spiral	26	626
Spiral	26	624
Stump wrapping	26	630
Wrapping ankle and lower leg	26	627
Bathing		
Bedbath, complete	18	396
Bedbath, partial	18	399
Bedbath, self-	18	399
Infant	19	438
Shower	18	400
Tub bath	18	399
Bedmaking		
Occupied bed	14	311
Postoperative bed	14	310
Unoccupied bed	14	306
Bedpan, assisting with	17	377
Binders, applying	26	623
Blood, occult in feces	11	230
Blood pressure	8	144
Body mechanics, basic	4	62
Bone marrow aspiration/biopsy, assisting with	12	261
Bottle-feeding an infant	19	439
Braces, applying	23	562
Cane, using	21	494
Cardiopulmonary resuscitation		
Infants and small children	30	727
One-rescuer	30	723
Two-rescuer	30	727
Casts, assisting with application of		
Fiberglass	23	551
Plaster of Paris	23	553
Casts, bivalving and windowing	23	554
Casts, caring for patients in		
Immediate	23	556
Ongoing	23	557
Circle (CircOlectric) bed	25	603
Clinitron bed (*See* Air-Fluidized bed)		
Cold, applying		
Cooling sponge bath	27	665
Disposable instant cold pack	27	662
Gel filled cold pack	27	662
Hypothermia blanket	27	662
Ice cap	27	661
Ice collar	27	661
Thermal blanket (cooling)	27	662
Collecting specimens	11	215
Contact lens care	18	407
Crutchwalking	21	496
Cultures		
Dry	11	231
Urine	11	232
Wet	11	231
Data gathering	6	113

© 1996 by Lippincott-Raven Publishers

Skill	Module	Page
Diapering	19	435
Disaster plans	3	49
Discharge	13	289
Documentation		
Charting by exception	5	91
Flow sheets	5	76
Focus charting	5	91
Mechanics	5	77
Narrative charting	5	83
Problem-oriented records/SOAP format	5	83
Dorsal recumbent position	15	339
Enema administration		
Cleansing	28	683
Cooling	28	684
Oil-retention	28	684
Pediatric	28	689
Return-flow	28	684
Feeding patients		
Adults	16	360
Infants		
Solids	19	441
Bottle	19	439
Fire plans	3	48
Foam rubber mattresses	25	601
Fowler's position	15	338
Hair care	18	405
Handwashing	2	23
Hearing aid care	18	409
Heat, applying		
Diathermy	27	660
Disposable instant hot packs	27	659
Electric heating pad	27	660
Gel filled hot pack	27	660
Heat cradle	27	660
Heat lamp	27	660
Hot water bags (bottles)	27	660
Hypothermia blanket	27	662
Sitz bath	27	664
Soaks	27	663
Thermal blanket (warming)	27	660
Warm moist compresses	27	663
Water-flow heating pad	27	659
Heimlich maneuver (*See* Airway obstruction)		
Inflatable mattresses	25	602
Inspection		
Abdomen	9	167
Breasts	9	166
Capillary refill time	9	170
Hand vein emptying time	9	171
Neck veins	9	171
Pupils	9	160
Intake	10	198
Knee-chest position	15	340
Lithotomy position	15	339
Liver biopsy, assisting with	12	259
Low air loss bed	25	604
Lumbar puncture, assisting with	12	258
Mediscus bed (*See* Low air loss bed)		
Moving the patient in bed		
Closer to one side of the bed	15	330
Up in bed: One-person assist	15	330
Up in bed: Two-person assist	15	331
Oral care		
Conscious patient	18	402
Dentures	18	404
Flossing	18	403
Toothbrushing	18	402
Unconscious patient	18	403
Orthopneic position	15	339
Output	10	198
Palpation		
Abdomen	9	167
Breasts	9	166
Rectum for fecal impaction	9	168
Paracentesis, assisting with	12	256
Percussion		
Abdomen	9	167
Chest	6	112
Perineal care		
Catheterized patient	17	381
Nonsurgical patient	17	381
Postpartum or postsurgical patient	17	381
Physical examination, nursing	9	171
Positioning a patient		
In a chair	15	338
Prone	15	337
Side-lying	15	336
Supine	15	335
Postmortem care	31	746
Pulse		
Apical	7	132
Apical/radial	7	132
Doppler	7	135
Peripheral	7	130

© 1996 by Lippincott-Raven Publishers

Skill	*Module*	*Page*
Range-of-motion exercises		
Ankle	22	531
Elbow	22	529
Fingers and thumb	22	531
Hip and knee	22	531
Neck	22	528
Shoulder	22	529
Toes	22	533
Wrist	22	529
Recording (*See* Documentation)		
Respiration	7	132
Restraints		
Belt	3	43
Crib nets and domes	19	443
Elbow or knee	3	44
Jacket	3	43
Mitt	3	44
Mummying	19	443
Vest	3	43
Wrist or ankle	3	44
Roto-Rest kinetic bed	25	606
Safety		
For the child	3	42
For the dependent patient	3	41
In patient rooms	3	40
In working spaces and halls	3	38
Shampoo	18	406
Sigmoidoscopy, proctoscopy, and colonoscopy, assisting with	12	262
Sims's position	15	340
Slings	26	633
Specimen collection		
Ascitic fluid	12	256
Blood	11	220
Cerebrospinal fluid (CSF)	12	258
Pleural cavity fluid	12	253
Sputum	11	220
Stool	11	220
Stool for occult blood	11	230
Urine	11	215
Stryker frame	25	603
Stump wrapping	26	630
Temperature		
Axillary	7	126
Electronic thermometer	7	128
Oral	7	127
Rectal	7	127
Thoracentesis, assisting with	12	253
Traction, applying		
Skeletal		
Balanced suspension	24	586
Skull tongs	24	587
Skin		
Bryant's	24	583
Buck's	24	581
Cervical halter	24	584
Humerus	24	581
Pelvic	24	583
Pelvic sling	24	584
Russell's	24	582
Traction, maintaining	24	588
Transfer (to another unit or facility)	13	285
Transferring a patient		
Bed to chair: Hydraulic lift	20	467
Bed to chair: One-person maximal assist	20	462
Bed to chair: One-person minimal assist	20	463
Bed to chair: Two-person lift	20	465
Bed to chair: Two-person maximal assist	20	463
Chair to chair: Two-person lift	20	464
Horizontal lift: Two- or three-person	20	470
Slider board	20	469
Trendelenburg position	15	340
Tube feeding		
Infants	29	704
Prefilled sets	29	709
Reservoir	29	708
Turning a patient		
Back to abdomen	15	333
Back to side	15	332
Logrolling	15	334
Urine testing		
Blood	11	228
Glucose	11	224
Ketones	11	227
pH	11	228
Specific gravity	11	223
Walker, using	21	495

© 1996 by Lippincott-Raven Publishers

TO THE INSTRUCTOR

The sixth edition of *Modules for Basic Nursing Skills* continues to provide a resource for students to learn basic skills and procedures. We have used the same nursing-process-oriented, self-instructional approach that has proven valuable in previous editions, while improving visual appeal through the use of two colors.

In preparing this edition, we have tried to look at our instructions and directions from a student's standpoint. We have tried to clarify the new language of healthcare that students are learning at the same time they are mastering skills. We recognize that the formal, official terms used for equipment and skills are not always the same as the "short-hand" that students will hear in a clinical setting. Therefore, we have provided both sets of terms in many instances.

As more students enter the college setting with varied educational backgrounds, language and reading levels become ever more important. In a skills text, perhaps more than anywhere else, the focus must be on clear, straightforward language. We are grateful for the responses of our students in helping us with this task.

COMPREHENSIVE SKILLS COVERAGE

There are now 58 modules in two volumes. Volume 1 contains the most basic skills and is appropriate by itself for some courses enrolling nursing assistants. Volumes 1 and 2 together are most useful in programs for LPN/LVN and RN students although the LPN/LVN will not use all of them. Because programs vary considerably from state to state and from institution to institution, we have tried to make the two volumes as adaptable as possible to many different programs by offering comprehensive coverage of nursing skills.

ORGANIZATION

The modules are organized into units that reflect broad concepts of nursing care. This structured presentation will help the student understand how individual skills relate to particular human needs and to the nursing process. The first unit focuses on skills that students must master in order to deal safely and effectively with patients. As in the previous edition, throughout the two volumes skills are arranged in a progression from simple to complex, but each module is self-contained so that skills can be omitted or reordered according to the needs of particular programs.

SELF-INSTRUCTIONAL FORMAT

By consistently emphasizing the nursing process and appropriately highlighting rationale, the format of the modules focuses on the student's practice and mastery of skills and procedures. The elaborate program of features is designed to encourage understanding, independent learning, and self-instruction.

Module Contents

An outline of the module contents helps the student identify the information and specific skills that are included in the module.

Prerequisites

The list of prerequisites lets the student know what other modules and significant material are essential to successful completion of the particular module. This information is especially helpful when the order of modules is adjusted to meet the needs of individual nursing programs. It can also be used advantageously by the student who wishes to prepare for a particular patient-care situation.

Overall Objective

A general statement of the overall objective concisely describes what the student can expect to learn in the module.

Specific Learning Objectives

Arranged in tabular form, the outline of learning objectives previews the important steps in the skill and indicates what basic knowledge and application of

© 1996 by Lippincott-Raven Publishers

knowledge are required in addition to psychomotor skills.

Learning Activities

The learning activities provide additional guidance to the student about what steps to take in order to accomplish the desired objectives. Note that each module directs the student to prepare as if planning to *teach* the skill to others. Because teaching is so integral to the nursing role, we believe students should consider that from the start.

Vocabulary

A list of key terms for each skill is provided. These terms are defined in the glossary at the back of each volume.

MODULE CORE

The discussion of each procedure includes necessary background information and step-by-step instructions, with carefully chosen photographs and technically precise illustrations.

Instructions are presented in a nursing process format when the skill is one that is used with patients and when the nursing process is appropriate to the skill. The steps in the process—Assessment, Planning, Implementation, and Evaluation—are clearly delineated by headings. This emphasis reinforces for students the fact that nursing process is relevant to practice. Nursing diagnoses are not included in the procedure itself. Where appropriate, the nursing diagnoses for which the particular skill might be used are presented in a separate display.

Documentation is included with every skill. The increasing emphasis on documentation for both evaluative and legal reasons makes the learning of correct documentation essential. Our premise is that although systems differ in *how* documentation is done, *what* needs to be documented is fairly standard. We have included specific examples of flow sheets and progress notes (in narrative, SOAP, and focus formats) to help students make the transition to the record system they will be asked to use.

Rationale for the use of each skill is explained at the beginning of every module. Rationale for the specific actions that are part of the procedure is emphasized throughout the discussion by the use of italic type.

Because the approach to many skills is the same, whenever possible a general procedure for a group of specific procedures has been identified. The purpose of this is to facilitate the student's ability to transfer basic principles from one situation to another. We have tried to do this in a way that does not create confusion and that can be followed when practicing the skill.

Illustrations were carefully chosen to help the students as they work through the module independently. We have expanded the examples of charting and have placed the examples of nursing progress notes on chart facsimiles to help the student transfer knowledge to the actual clinical setting.

A glove icon, new in the sixth edition, reminds the nursing student to wear gloves for procedures requiring Standard Precautions. To provide consistency and easy readability, we use this icon for the appropriate procedures that are formatted according to the nursing process. This does not imply that gloves are not required in other situations mentioned in the book.

Critical Thinking Exercises

Skill development for the nurse must constantly be framed within the context of the individual patient. In order to focus on this important concept, we have added critical thinking exercises to each module. These exercises assist the student in placing the skills into the context of providing nursing care for each unique patient. Students are asked to consider a patient situation that has problematic aspects and to determine needs, priorities, or approaches that would be appropriate for the particular patient. There are no "right" answers to these situations. They might form the basis for a discussion, for a written paper, or for personal thoughtful study.

References

The references given are to research data regarding the skill or the recommendations of an authoritative agency such as the Centers For Disease Control and Prevention (CDC). The most recent research is cited. In the case of skills, this research may be older than expected. For example, the many excellent studies on the procedure and timing used for taking temperatures were done 10 years ago, but remain the basis for current recommendations. The CDC change their recommendations only when their decision-making bodies determine that the data warrant a change.

Unfortunately, there is little research data to support many of the nursing techniques used. Therefore, you will also note an emphasis within the mod-

© 1996 by Lippincott-Raven Publishers

ules on consulting policy and procedure manuals in institutions. These are generally established by groups of nurses working together with legal as well as healthcare goals in mind. Learning to use the official policy and procedure manual will be an asset both to the student and to the practicing nurse.

Performance Checklist

The performance checklist follows the nursing process approach and can be used for quick review and for evaluation of the student's performance in terms of psychomotor skills. To facilitate review and evaluation, all steps of each procedure, including those that are first presented as part of a general procedure, are outlined in the performance checklist. In the sixth edition, the format of the performance checklist has been modified to allow more space for feedback.

Quiz

A self-test is provided at the end of each module to allow students to test their mastery of the material in the module. The quizzes may also be used by instructors for evaluation purposes.

Glossary

The terms in the vocabulary lists are defined in the glossary at the back of each volume. The glossaries are a convenient reference source for students.

The glossary defines terms within the context in which they are used in nursing and healthcare. This is particularly useful for the beginning student who often finds that words have special connotations in nursing and healthcare that are not included in the traditional dictionary definition.

Answers to Quizzes

Answers to quizzes are given at the end of each volume.

Index

An index is provided at the back of each volume.

CONVENIENT PACKAGING

The pages of both volumes are three-hole punched and perforated, so students can either tear them out and hand them in or keep them in notebooks.

TESTING SUPPLEMENT

A test bank accompanying Volumes 1 and 2 includes multiple-choice questions for all the skills that are covered.

Modules for Basic Nursing Skills, Volume 1 and 2, Sixth Edition, can be used in conjunction with the text by Ellis and Nowlis, *Nursing: A Human Needs Approach*, Fifth Edition, which treats the theory behind nursing practice. However, the two volumes of modules are designed to stand alone and can be used by themselves in a course addressing nursing skills. *Modules for Basic Nursing Skills* can also be used in conjunction with any other text covering nursing theory or fundamentals.

ACKNOWLEDGMENTS

We would like to thank the following individuals for their reviews of the manuscript at various stages and for their many useful suggestions:

Suzanna Johnson, MSN, ARNP
Skills Laboratory Coordinator
Shoreline Community College
Seattle, WA

Janet T. Barrett, PhD, RN
Director, BSN Program
Deaconess College of Nursing
St. Louis, MO

Marty Carlson, RN, MSN, MEd
Instructor
Life Sciences Division
Parkland College
Champaign, IL

Vicki Christenson, RNC, MN
Pediatric Nursing Faculty
Intercollegiate Nursing Center
Spokane, WA

Judy Davy, RN, BSN, FNP
Professor of Nursing
Department of Nursing
Humboldt State University
Arcata, CA

Marilyn Deig, RN, MSN
Instructor
Indiana Vocational Technical College—Evansville
Evansville, IN

© 1996 by Lippincott-Raven Publishers

Latrell Fowler, RN, PhD
Instructor
Medical University of South Carolina Satellite
at Francis Marion University
Florence, SC

Gay Greaves, RN, BNSc, MEd, EdD
Assistant Professor
Queens University School of Nursing
Kingston, Ontario

Karen Halbasch, RN, EdD
Associate Professor
Department of Nursing
Community College of Philadelphia
Philadelphia, PA

Joyce Ann Harney, RNC, CNA, MSN
Director of Health & Human Services
Ivy Tech State College
Columbus, IN

Genevieve A. Harris, RN, MSN
Assistant Professor of Nursing
Richard J. Daley College
Chicago, IL

Elizabeth Krekorian, PhD, RN
President/CEO
Deaconess College of Nursing
St. Louis, MO

Mary C. Shoemaker, PhD, RN
Associate Professor, Level I Coordinator
Saint Francis Medical Center
College of Nursing
Peoria, IL

Barbara Taylor, RN, MSN
ADN Instructor
Chipola Junior College
Marianna, FL

Bonnie Young, RN, BSN
Lead Instructor
Sharon Regional Health System
School of Nursing
Sharon, PA

We are especially grateful to all our students and colleagues who used the modules as they were originally written, worked through the changes made for the first five editions, and assisted in the planning of this revision. Their constant feedback has been essential to us.

J.R.E.
E.A.N.
P.M.B.

© 1996 by Lippincott-Raven Publishers

TO THE STUDENT

The modules in these two volumes are designed to enable you to learn the procedures that are basic to your role as a healthcare provider. Each module contains the following parts, unless they are not applicable to a particular skill:

Module Contents

The outline of the module contents provides you with an overview of all the information and specific skills contained in the module. Often a module contains several skills, and these will all be listed in the contents.

Prerequisites

The list of prerequisites describes the specific skills or abilities needed to master the new skill and indicates other modules that contain information necessary to an understanding of the skill.

Overall Objective

A general statement of the overall objective describes the basic skill that is taught in the module.

Specific Learning Objectives

A table of specific learning objectives breaks down the basic skill you are studying into specific subskills on which you can test yourself after completing the module.

Learning Activities

The learning activities are designed to help you progress safely and gradually into performing the new skill. Practice, in whatever setting is available, is essential to skillful performance. The amount of practice needed by each student will differ, depending on manual dexterity and previous experience. If your school provides audiovisual aids to use with the module, view them after reading the module but before actually practicing the skill. Do not hesitate to contact your instructor if you encounter difficul-

ties. Note that you are asked to study as if planning to *teach* the skill. Teaching others to provide care for self, family, and others is an integral part of the nursing role.

Vocabulary

The vocabulary list gives key terms used in the module. A glossary at the back of each volume gives the definitions of these terms, though some are best understood in the context of the module itself.

Module Core

The discussion of each procedure includes necessary background information and step-by-step instructions, with carefully chosen photographs and technically precise illustrations.

Instructions are presented in a nursing process format when the skill is one that is used with patients and when the nursing process is appropriate to the skill. The steps in the process—Assessment, Planning, Implementation, and Evaluation—are clearly delineated by headings. This emphasis reinforces for students the fact that nursing process is relevant to practice. Nursing diagnoses are not included in the procedure itself. Where appropriate, the nursing diagnoses for which the particular skill might be used are presented in a separate display.

Documentation is included with every skill. The increasing emphasis on documentation for both evaluative and legal reasons makes the learning of correct documentation essential. Our premise is that although systems differ in *how* documentation is done, *what* needs to be documented is fairly standard. We have included specific examples of flow sheets and progress notes (in narrative, SOAP, and focus formats) to help students make the transition to the record system they will be asked to use.

Rationale for the use of each skill is explained at the beginning of every module. Rationale for the specific actions that are part of the procedure is emphasized throughout the discussion by the use of italic type.

Because the approach to many skills is the same,

© 1996 by Lippincott-Raven Publishers

whenever possible a general procedure for a group of specific procedures has been identified. The purpose of this is to facilitate the student's ability to transfer basic principles from one situation to another. We have tried to do this in a way that does not create confusion and that can be followed when practicing the skill.

A glove icon, new in the sixth edition, reminds the nursing student to wear gloves for procedures requiring Standard Precautions. To provide consistency and easy readability, we use this icon for the appropriate procedures that are formatted according to the nursing process. This does not imply that gloves are not required in other situations mentioned in the book.

An increasing number of people are being cared for at home who were previously cared for in the acute care hospital. Therefore, in the sixth edition, we have expanded our discussion of how you would integrate the information on a particular skill into your planning for home care. Another area of increasing importance in healthcare is long-term care. In long-term care, adaptations of procedures and techniques may also be needed. We have added references to these changes and adaptations where appropriate. Unique icons make Home Care and Long-Term Care instantly recognizable.

Critical Thinking Exercises

Skill development for the nurse must constantly be framed within the context of the individual patient. In order to focus on this important concept, we have added critical thinking exercises to each module. These exercises will assist you in placing the skills into the context of providing nursing care for each unique patient. In the critical thinking exercises, you are asked to consider a patient situation that has problematic aspects and to determine needs, priorities, or approaches that would be appropriate for the particular patient. There are no "right" answers to these situations. They might form the basis for a discussion, for a written paper, or for personal thoughtful study.

References

The references given are to research data regarding the skill or the recommendations of an authoritative agency such as the Centers For Disease Control and Prevention (CDC). The most recent research is cited. In the case of skills, this research may be older than expected. For example, the many excellent studies on the procedures and timing used for taking temperatures were done 10 years ago, but remain the basis for current recommendations. The CDC change their recommendations only when their decision-making bodies determine that the data warrant a change.

Unfortunately, there is little research data to support many of the nursing techniques used. Therefore, you will also note an emphasis within the modules on consulting policy and procedure manuals in institutions. These are generally established by groups of nurses working together with legal as well as health care goals in mind. Learning to use the official policy and procedure manual will be an asset both to the student and to the practicing nurse.

Performance Checklist

The performance checklist is used as a guide for practicing the skill and judging your performance of it.

Quiz

The quiz is a brief review for self-testing.

Glossary

The glossary at the back of each volume provides definitions for the key vocabulary terms.

Answers to Quizzes

The answer key at the end of each volume allows you to score yourself on the quizzes.

Index

An index is provided at the back of each volume.

We hope you will find gaining these essential skills to be a satisfying endeavor, and we wish you our best as you begin your studies.

J.R.E.
E.A.N.
P.M.B.

© 1996 by Lippincott-Raven Publishers

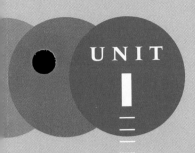

Foundation Skills

MODULE 1
An Approach to Nursing Skills

MODULE 2
Basic Infection Control

MODULE 3
Safety

MODULE 4
Basic Body Mechanics

MODULE 5
Documentation

1

AN APPROACH TO NURSING SKILLS

MODULE CONTENTS

RATIONALE FOR THE USE OF THIS
    INFORMATION
PATIENT RIGHTS
Rights Supported by Law
  Right to Self-Determination/Consent
  Right to Information on Which to Base
    Decisions
  Right to Privacy/Confidentiality
  Right to Safe Care
Rights Supported by Ethics
  Right to Personal Dignity
  Right to Individualized Care
  Right to Assistance Toward Independence
  Right to Evaluate and Obtain Changes
    in Care
RESEARCH BASE FOR NURSING
    PRACTICE
THE NURSING PROCESS

Assessment
Analysis/Nursing Diagnosis
Planning
Implementation
Evaluation
Documentation
TECHNICAL COMPETENCE
Appropriate Technique
Organization
Dexterity
Speed
METHODS FOR DEVELOPING
    TECHNICAL COMPETENCE
Reading the Module
Mental Practice
Physical Practice
CRITICAL THINKING EXERCISES

© 1996 by Lippincott-Raven Publishers

OVERALL OBJECTIVE

To understand how patients' rights and the nursing process relate to performing nursing skills with technical competence and safety.

SPECIFIC LEARNING OBJECTIVES

Know Facts and Principles	Apply Facts and Principles	Demonstrate Ability	Evaluate Performance
1. Patient rights			
List patient rights in eight major areas that are of special concern to nurses.	Give an example of a nursing behavior that supports each right listed.	Consistently strive, in contacts with patients, to maintain patient rights.	Evaluate with instructor.
2. Nursing process			
List the major steps of the nursing process. Define each step of the nursing process.	Give an example of a nursing behavior that demonstrates each step of the nursing process.	Write an outline of the nursing process you used in relation to an uncomplicated patient problem.	Evaluate your process with your instructor.
3. Technical competence			
List four components of technical competence. Identify which component is most critical. Identify three techniques to assist in developing technical competence.	Give an example of behavior you can use to enhance your ability in each component of technical competence. Identify a way to increase your technical competence in each skill approached.	Demonstrate increased technical competence in each skill practiced.	Evaluate your technical competence with your instructor.

© 1996 by Lippincott-Raven Publishers

LEARNING ACTIVITIES

1. Review the Specific Learning Objectives.
2. Look up the module vocabulary terms in the glossary.
3. Read the material on patient rights, the nursing process, the nursing role, and direct care skills in Ellis and Nowlis, *Nursing: A Human Needs Approach,* or comparable material in another text.
4. Read through the module as though you were preparing to teach the content to another person.
5. Check the policy manual of the facility where you will practice for information on:
   Confidentiality/privacy
   Patient rights
   Consent
   Patient criticism/concerns
6. Arrange to go to a nursing unit as an observer. Make observations in the following three categories:
   a. Patient rights
      Identify and record staff actions that support any of the patient rights emphasized in the module.

      Identify and record any behaviors that appear to interfere with patients' rights.
   b. Nursing process
      Write down examples of nurses carrying out various steps of the nursing process.
   c. Technical competence
      Observe two different staff members perform an uncomplicated procedure (such as bed making). Obtain their consent before observing.
      Time each person doing the task.
      Identify the factors that contributed to or interfered with rapid completion of the task.
      Compare the dexterity of the two staff members.
      Compare the organization of the two staff members.
7. In a discussion group with other students, share your observations.

VOCABULARY

advocate	ethical	nursing process	sanction
assessment	evaluation	objective	self-care
confidentiality	healthcare system	ombudsman	self-determination
consent	health status	organization	subjective
data	implementation	physical practice	technical competence
dexterity	mental practice	planning	
dignity	nursing diagnosis	privacy	

© 1996 by Lippincott-Raven Publishers

An Approach to Nursing Skills

Rationale for the Use of This Information

The patient in the healthcare system has ethical and legal rights. Failure to recognize these rights can result in ethical sanctions and even legal action against the care provider and the institution. The nursing student, therefore, must approach every patient with these rights in mind. Nursing is more than just performing skills. The nursing process provides a framework for the total role of the nurse and for all nursing activities. A concern for patient rights and the nursing process should be part of your approach to any nursing skill. Technical competence is important, but it must be situated within the broad context of the nursing role.

Although each nursing skill is presented separately for learning purposes, no single nursing skill exists outside the context of the individual patient and the specific situation. Nursing skills are most valuable when the rights of the patient, the framework of the nursing process, and the value of technical competence are kept in mind.[1]

PATIENT RIGHTS

Patient rights include rights that are supported by law and would be upheld in court and ethical rights that the healthcare community recognizes as important to the patient's well-being. Various groups, such as the American Hospital Association, individual healthcare agencies, and state nurses' associations, have adopted statements related to their view of patient rights. These statements differ slightly because each focuses on the healthcare services provided by a particular agency or group. This module presents some general concepts usually included in discussions of patient rights and focuses on how you can support these in your nursing practice.

Rights Supported by Law

These rights either are specifically stated in the laws of a particular state or jurisdiction or have consistently been supported in court.

Right to Self-Determination/Consent

The patient has the right to make personal decisions regarding healthcare. This is often called the right to consent. *All adults older than 18 years (21 years in some states) have the right to make their own decisions about healthcare. Only those who have been declared incompetent by a court (and who therefore have a court-appointed guardian) and those who are unconscious do not have this personal right.* Advanced age is never a valid reason for ignoring the right to self-determination. *For children, parents exercise these rights. Even young children, however, are often included in the decision-making process. This enhances their ability to participate in care, even though final authority rests with the parents.*

Some minors do have the right to self-determination. Examples include those who are considered to be emancipated because they are married and those who are living independently of parents as prescribed by law. In most states, minors can give consent for care related to reproduction, such as birth control, abortion, and treatment for sexually transmitted diseases. The facility where you practice should have specific policies that are based on applicable state law and court decisions to guide you in knowing who can legally give consent for care. One of your responsibilities is to review these policies.

Self-determination means that the patient has the right to accept or refuse any aspect of care and the right to decide whether to use the healthcare system at all, to use any part of the system, to ask for adaptations of the system, or to totally refuse the care available. It is the care provider's responsibility to give sufficient information to enable the patient to make decisions with an adequate understanding of related consequences. For example, if you ask the patient to consent to having a procedure such as an enema, you are responsible for making sure the patient understands the purpose of the enema and the possible consequences of *not* having it at that time. The patient's choice is then truly informed.

Sometimes consent is implied by the patient's previous actions or statements. When a patient consents to have surgery, there is implied consent to procedures and routines that are necessary for successful preparation for and recovery from the surgery. *Although a patient is free at any time to change his or her mind with regard to the original procedure or to refuse any aspect of care, care proceeds on the basis of the implied consent.* Another factor to be considered in such a situation is the patient's current health status. *The individual who has just had surgery and is weakened and in pain is not in a position to make the best decisions about care.* Thus, immediately after surgery, do not ask a patient if he or she is willing to turn. You say, "It is time to turn now." When you believe that pain medication is needed, you say, "It is time for your pain medication. It will help you to rest more comfortably and move as you need to." The patient does have the

---

[1]Note that the rationale for action is emphasized throughout the module by the use of italics.

© 1996 by Lippincott-Raven Publishers

right to refuse the pain medication, but this seldom happens; the patient is interested in recovery and willing to accept the care provider's judgment as to the best action.

Consent is also implied by the patient's behavior in response to your statements. If you say, "It is time for your injection," and the patient rolls over to receive the injection, this is considered implied consent. If you offer a patient an oral medication and he or she reaches for it, implied consent is present.

Decision making is shared between the care provider and the patient in some situations. The nurse instructs a new diabetic in how to give an insulin injection. At some point, the patient will need to perform the procedure independently. The nurse and patient will consider the progress the patient has made in learning, and together they will agree on when the patient is ready to take on this responsibility. The nurse must agree that the patient has the necessary knowledge and skills, and the patient must agree that he or she is ready to undertake the task. For many situations in nursing, joint decision making is the most appropriate course of action.

Nurses and other care providers do make all the decisions for certain patients in certain situations. The patient who is disoriented as to time and place is sometimes not able to make decisions about safety and care. In such cases, the nurse will decide that, for example, raised side rails or other safety devices are necessary to prevent falls. For a newborn, nurses must decide on the amount of covering needed to maintain proper body temperature, the optimum position for safety, and other details of the infant's daily routine. If the patient is unconscious, all aspects of daily life must be controlled by those responsible for care. Decisions such as the amount of a feeding, the length of time to lie in one position, and more technical aspects of care must all be made by caregivers.

Correctly assessing the patient's ability to make decisions is an important responsibility for the nurse. Consult with your instructor and more experienced staff nurses to make sure you are providing maximum self-determination consistent with the patient's health status.

Right to Information on Which to Base Decisions

The patient has the right to information on which to base decisions. This means that the nurse has an obligation to provide information related to the care that he or she is giving. When you take blood pressure, you have an obligation to state what the reading is, if the patient asks. You do not, however, speak for others. Thus, when the patient asks what the medical diag-

nosis is, explain that this question should be directed to the physician who has made the diagnosis. It is then the physician's responsibility to discuss the diagnosis with the patient.

Care providers are often reluctant to give information to patients for fear that it will upset them and increase their anxiety. This fear is usually groundless. *Not knowing what is happening usually produces much more anxiety than knowing the truth. Fear of the unknown can be paralyzing to the patient. Some people prefer not to have information about their health status because it would make them anxious. These people will simply avoid asking for information with which they are not ready to cope.* Therefore, the patient should be your guide in deciding how much information to share.

In some instances, it is essential that patients have information regarding their current health status. A patient who is on a special diet, for example, must have sufficient information to manage self-care. In these instances, the nurse does not wait for the patient to ask questions but initiates discussion and specifically plans for health teaching.

Right to Privacy/Confidentiality

The patient has the right to have confidential information carefully protected. In today's complex society, it is too easy for confidential information to spread to those who have no need for it. Keep in mind that *people can be harmed when information is spread unnecessarily.* The information might cause a change in someone's attitude toward the patient, adversely affect the patient's employment opportunities, or result in financial loss, to name only a few possibilities. *Even when no objective harm is demonstrated, the individual may feel exposed and vulnerable.*

To maintain patient privacy, you should discuss information about a patient only with those who have a need for that information, such as nurses or the healthcare team. Discussions should take place only where you will not be overheard by others. An appropriate place might be a conference room, a patient room, or the nurses' station. Even these places, however, may be inappropriate. For example, a nurses' station with several visitors at the desk might be too public. The cafeteria or elevator are *never* appropriate, and anywhere outside of the facility is inappropriate.

Written communication must also be safeguarded. Watch your notes carefully, and do not leave them in patient rooms or in the cafeteria. When you no longer need informal notes, discard them in the waste basket; do not leave them around on desks. Charts should be read only by those involved in care, those who have the patient's permission, and those involved in healthcare education. This means that you should not read a patient's chart or access a computer record if you do not have a valid need to know about that patient.

The use of patient information for learning experiences is valid but requires you to take special care. Do not identify patients by name when you have chosen them as subjects for a paper. *This would be a breach of confidentiality.* When using a patient as an example in a class discussion, share only information pertinent to the topic. *Some information of a personal or private nature should perhaps not be shared.*

When gathering information from a patient, explain that you will be sharing information you receive with the nurse assigned to the patient's care or with your instructor. Because you are a beginner, you should not accept the responsibility of receiving confidences that cannot be shared in these ways. Doing so might put you in a situation that would be difficult to manage. If the patient asks you to promise to tell no one what is said, explain that you cannot make that promise. State that to plan appropriate care, you need to be free to discuss concerns with your instructor or the staff nurse, and if the patient does not want the information shared in this way, then perhaps he or she should not share it with you. This does not indicate rejection of the patient but clearly outlines your obligations. *The patient is then free to choose what to share, and you are free to consult with others as necessary.*

Right to Safe Care

The patient has the right to expect that those who are providing care are knowledgeable and competent and will provide safe care. This means that the patient will receive safe care no matter who is providing it. Therefore, as a nursing student you are held to the same standard of safety in care as a registered nurse. The patient cannot be expected to accept poor-quality care because you are learning. It is your responsibility to learn skills before you perform them, to know the necessary safety precautions, and to seek supervision. *These actions safeguard the patient and protect you from legal action.* To function safely at all times requires constant self-evaluation and a willingness to accept help and strive toward excellence.

Rights Supported by Ethics

These rights are based on ethical beliefs as to what constitutes high-quality care. *They are concerned with supporting optimum health for the patient, not merely with ensuring the absence of harm.* In most cases, these

rights would not be upheld by a court. If they were violated, recourse would come only from within the healthcare system or from community pressure.

Right to Personal Dignity

The patient has the right to care that respects personal dignity and worth, unrestricted by considerations of nationality, race, creed, color, status, age, or gender. Respecting a person's dignity means that you treat each person as if he or she has intrinsic value at all times. Although this attitude is an internal characteristic, you give it meaning through your behavior.

One behavior that reflects this attitude is addressing the patient by the name he or she chooses. Therefore, the older person who prefers to be addressed as Mr. or Mrs. is so addressed, and the person who asks to be called by his or her first name or a nickname is addressed in that way. *You also can show respect for the patient's dignity by displaying concern for privacy and modesty, for example, by knocking on closed doors, pulling curtains, and providing appropriate garments and draping. You show respect for individual dignity when you help a person have the best possible appearance through careful attention to hygiene and personal care. By doing so you reflect your view of the patient as a human being who is valuable to you and to others.*

The attitude you convey to patients by the manner in which you communicate with them is very important. *Listening to the thoughts and concerns of the patient conveys respect. By his or her attitude, an attentive, concerned listener says, "What you have to say is important." Explaining expectations and new situations so that the individual is more able to cope reflects your belief that the patient is capable of coping when given the opportunity and the necessary information.*

Accepting the individual's feelings without judging them as right or wrong is another way of showing respect. Feelings are personal and arise from internal and external circumstances. Even though you may not understand a patient's feelings, you can accept them.

Right to Individualized Care

The patient has the right to individualized care related to his or her unique needs and lifestyle. Each of us is unique, with a different combination of physical attributes, thoughts, feelings, values, and beliefs. *Care that is precisely uniform will fit no one precisely. Adaptations in care plans are made to provide for each patient's special needs and attributes.* You might adapt a bathing method to respect a patient's attitude about modesty. You might alter visiting hours to help maintain an important family bond. You might request a special dietary consultation to fit the patient's cultural

© 1996 by Lippincott-Raven Publishers

background. The patient has the right to expect this kind of individualized approach to planning care.

Right to Assistance Toward Independence

Being able to care for oneself is important in building one's self-esteem and is critical to being able to function as an independent person. Patients have the right to expect that care will have the goal of returning them to maximum independence. Nurses can support this right in many ways. Put simply, this means that you will allow the patient to perform self-care whenever possible. When bathing a patient, you might encourage the patient to wash his or her own face. When helping the patient move in bed, take the extra time to give directions carefully *so that the patient can move independently without strain. To function independently at home, the person with a health problem may need considerable knowledge and skill.* The nurse is typically the person who must plan and carry out the teaching program.

Right to Evaluate and Obtain Changes in Care

The patient has the right to evaluate care, criticize when care has not been of high quality, and obtain changes to improve the quality of care. To do this, the patient needs some knowledge of what constitutes good care. *Providing healthcare consumers with this knowledge provides them with more power.* In the past, some healthcare providers have been reluctant to share this information with consumers for fear of being harshly evaluated. The reality is that healthcare consumers will always evaluate providers, but if they have no objective standards, they will do so on the basis of attractiveness, demeanor, or other superficial criteria.

Some hospitals now provide patients with a form that lists evaluation criteria and asks the patient to respond. In a less formal way, patients may be given information on admission as to what they can expect with regard to care. Some facilities provide patients with a list of their rights so they can knowledgeably exercise them. *Legal recourse is always available when care has been so poor as to cause harm; however, this is a complex process that is not suited to lesser issues that are nevertheless important to the patient.*

Some facilities now have someone in the position of "patient advocate" or "ombudsman." It is this person's responsibility to discuss problems with the patient and then work with the healthcare system to improve the patient's care. In many facilities, however, no one is officially designated to do this job, and the role of patient advocate falls to the nurse. It is logical for the nurse to fulfill this role, because nurses are the only care providers who are in contact with the patient 24 hours a day, 7 days a week. Nurses also understand the institutional structure and can interface with that structure on behalf of the patient. This role is not an easy one. It demands a great deal of understanding of human behavior, understanding of the institution, and excellent communication skills.

You can support this right by listening carefully to patients' concerns and complaints and then discussing them with your instructor or a knowledgeable nurse on the unit. There may be simple remedies that you can implement, or you may begin the process by which others will resolve the patient's concerns. When you are criticized, do not become defensive, but carefully consider how this information might help you to provide better care to all patients.

RESEARCH BASE FOR NURSING PRACTICE

Although nursing is moving toward a research base for its practice, this does not yet exist for many nursing procedures and skills. References to the research that is available to support certain methods or approaches to a skill are given in the modules. Future research may further refine what nurses do or significantly alter how they proceed. For some nursing skills, there is little or no research base. In these instances, the skills should be based on past practice and sound deductive reasoning from known facts. Future research may support traditional methods or it may not, even though the reasoning behind them may seem logically correct.

Because nursing is an applied science, nurses' knowledge is incomplete. Given this reality, it is the responsibility of all nurses to be aware of the reasoning or rationale underlying what they do, to evaluate this rationale, and to be willing to alter their practice when research brings more specific information.

THE NURSING PROCESS

The nursing process is a thoughtful, deliberate use of a problem-solving approach to nursing. This process forms a structure within which you can function. You will need to consult a nursing theory text for a complete understanding of the nursing process. Each step is defined here, followed by a discussion of how that step is used in the performance of nursing skills.

© 1996 by Lippincott-Raven Publishers

Assessment

Assessment is the process of gathering information, analyzing information, and identifying problems. The basic purpose of some skills is to gather information. These skills are grouped together in Unit II. For every skill that you use, however, you must gather the necessary information to implement it appropriately and safely. In each module, directions for carrying out the skill begin by indicating the assessment data you must gather before you proceed.

In addition to carrying out the specific assessment listed, you should always be observant while carrying out the procedure. It is an excellent time to gain further information about the patient. You may extend your knowledge of existing problems or gain insight that will lead you to identify new ones.

Analysis/Nursing Diagnosis

Analysis may be considered either an entirely separate step in the nursing process or the second phase of assessment. *Analysis includes the intellectual processes of sorting and classifying the data collected, recognizing patterns and discrepancies, comparing these with norms, and identifying patient responses to health problems that are amenable to nursing intervention.* This process is referred to as analysis because you are analyzing the data obtained. In many instances, analysis results in a statement of a patient concern or problem called a nursing diagnosis. The problem-solving processes involved in assessment, planning, implementation, and evaluation are always appropriate, but in the context of specific skills, a nursing diagnosis may not be appropriate. The purpose of the assessment is to enable you to gather data, individualize the procedure to the patient, and ensure safety. Although you may identify concerns, these may not fall into the classifications currently accepted by the North American Nursing Diagnosis Association. During the process, you may uncover data that contribute significantly to the development of nursing diagnoses for the patient. In many instances, a skill is used to help resolve a patient problem or nursing diagnosis that has already been identified.

Two nursing diagnoses that are commonly identified in patients receiving treatment are Knowledge Deficit related to the specific procedure and Anxiety related to the specific procedure.

Planning

Planning is the phase during which you identify specific desired outcomes for the patient and determine what actions will be needed to reach those outcomes. Planning often includes a group of nursing measures needed to combat a particular problem. Some of the actions planned will require specific technical skills. Within each skill there is also a planning phase. The general guidelines given for evaluation must be examined and translated into specific desired outcomes for the patient. Equipment must be identified and obtained. Timing must be determined. Careful planning is the main factor in organization.

Implementation

This is the phase of the nursing process during which you carry out the actions you planned. The specific nursing skills you use are only part of the implementation for a given problem. Nursing implementation includes your task, along with your attitude toward and communication with the patient. Because implementation is the most visible part of nursing, some people make the mistake of thinking that it is the most important. It is important, but it can never be more important than the careful data gathering and planning that goes before it.

For each technical skill presented, step-by-step instructions are given to guide you in your implementation of the skill. The implementation phase is the "hands-on" segment of any procedure.

Evaluation

Evaluation is the process by which you identify the outcomes of your nursing action. The central aspect of evaluation is the evaluation of the patient. However, you also want to evaluate your own nursing ability and whether you functioned well.

For each skill, specific factors that can help you to identify outcomes are listed. You will need to adapt those factors to the specifics of individual situations. For example, if one of the steps of evaluation states that you should recheck the patient's vital signs to determine response, it is essential to identify what the specific desired vital signs are for this particular patient.

Documentation

Documentation is establishing a written record of the assessment, the care provided, and the patient's responses. It usually is not considered an independent step in the nursing process, but rather an extension of each of the other steps. That is, you assess and then you record your assessment; you plan and then you record your plan and so forth. For the beginner, it is often much easier to consider all documentation at the same time. Therefore, we have grouped all

© 1996 by Lippincott-Raven Publishers

information about documentation as a fifth section in each skill. You will find more complete information about documentation in Module 5, Documentation.

TECHNICAL COMPETENCE

Technical competence has four components: the technique, the organization, the dexterity, and the speed with which you implement nursing skills.

Appropriate Technique

Appropriate technique is always the most important component of technical competence because it maintains safety and is most likely to achieve the optimum outcome for the patient. In each module, appropriate technique is outlined and discussed in detail in the implementation phase. Some elements of each procedure may be different, depending on the circumstances and the policy in your facility. These elements are carefully pointed out. When practicing a skill, the most important element is to make sure that you always use appropriate technique, regardless of how slow or awkward it may be at first.

Organization

Having an organized approach to technical skills has many advantages. First, *if you are well organized, you do not waste your time or others' time.* Second, *being well organized makes you appear competent and enhances the patient's trust in your skill.* Third, *you are less likely to make errors in technique when you are well organized; therefore, you will give safe care.*

During the planning of any procedure, you will be organizing your work. One part of this is carefully identifying all the equipment you will need so that you can obtain it all at once. Nothing makes one look more disorganized than repeated trips to get forgotten items. Trips of this kind also take time and energy that can be better spent in other ways. The equipment needed for each skill is listed in the planning phase of the directions. You will often find a list of equipment specific to your facility when you consult the procedure or policy book there.

Another part of organization is determining at what point in your schedule it is most appropriate to carry out a task. For example, an irrigation that is likely to result in a wet bed should be done before the bed linen is changed so that you do not end up changing the bed twice. *The patient's schedule and needs must also be considered when deciding when to perform a procedure.* The patient may wish to have a bath after a procedure to feel fresher. In other instances, the patient should have the bath before the procedure so that after the procedure, the patient can rest without interruptions. Because planning for the timing of any procedure is a highly individual matter, it is not included in the directions for each skill. You will need to keep it in mind, however, in each situation.

Dexterity

Dexterity refers to your skill or adroitness in the use of your hands. When you are dexterous, your movements are deliberate, coordinated, and purposeful. You do not use awkward or inappropriate movements. Dexterity requires practice. *To increase your dexterity, you must work with the equipment enough to develop the neural pathways that coordinate your movements.* You develop your sense of touch to provide accurate feedback about the position of your hands and the equipment. Although some people are naturally more dexterous than others, everyone needs practice to develop dexterity with a new skill. Going slowly and thinking carefully about your movements at first will help you to develop dexterity.

Speed

The speed with which you carry out a nursing skill can be important. *When you perform a procedure quickly, you help yourself in terms of overall time management, and more importantly, you also help the patient.* If a procedure is uncomfortable and you perform it in 5 minutes instead of 15, the patient is only uncomfortable for 5 minutes. If a procedure creates anxiety, the anxiety is lessened if you are quick and dexterous. The value to yourself in terms of time management is a serious consideration. Nurses often find that the many demands on their time can lessen the quality of patient care. *When you perform an individual skill more quickly, you are more free to plan for all patients' needs.* Be cautious, however, in your quest for speed. Never sacrifice appropriate technique or neglect patient rights. Developing your organizational ability and your dexterity are the first steps in gaining speed in performance. After you have mastered the appropriate technique, developed your organizational ability, and achieved some dexterity, you can work on speed alone.

METHODS FOR DEVELOPING TECHNICAL COMPETENCE

Developing technical competence in routine nursing skills is an important part of your education as a nurse. Various techniques will help you in this endeavor.

© 1996 by Lippincott-Raven Publishers

Reading the Module

Before attempting any skill, you should first read through the entire module. This provides you with the background information to understand the procedure and an overview of what you will be doing. Read as though you will be expected to teach the procedure to someone else. This will often be true. You may be required to teach or assist patients, their families, and other caregivers. Look carefully at photos and drawings to help you identify new equipment and relate these to the steps of the procedure. You may also wish to point out the photos and drawings as you teach.

Mental Practice

Mental practice is a technique to help you establish the mental patterns that govern your actions when performing the procedure. In mental practice, you imagine yourself performing the actions in the procedure. You should attempt to "feel" and "see" yourself doing the movements and skills as they are described and illustrated as you go through each step. Bucher (1993) found that students who had used mental and physical practice increased their competence slightly more than those who used all of their time for physical practice. Because mental practice may be done at home or in a study room, it is an efficient use of your time and resources.

Physical Practice

When you go to your practice setting to physically practice skills, the most important aspect is the time you spend doing the task. Focus your attention so that you do not waste this valuable time. Repeat the procedure following the module directions. When you believe you have learned the skill, try doing it with just the checklist to remind you of the steps. When you are able to do this satisfactorily, you are ready to ask a partner to check your performance, using the checklist.

If you are not able to complete the entire procedure and check off in one practice session, use mental practice before you go to the practice setting again. This will maximize your ability to perform the skill.

CRITICAL THINKING EXERCISES

- You have been caring for Mrs. Banks for 3 sequential days. On the third day of care, Mrs. Banks begins to share personal information with you as you are bathing her. You believe this information should be shared with others on the healthcare team, because it has implications for approaches to her care. Mrs. Banks has not said that you must keep the information confidential. Describe how you should proceed.

Reference

Bucher, L. (1993). The effects of imagery abilities and mental rehearsal on learning a nursing skill. *Journal of Nursing Education, 32*(7), 318–324.

© 1996 by Lippincott-Raven Publishers

? **Q U I Z**

Short-Answer Questions

1. List patients' rights in eight major areas that are of special concern to nurses.

a. _____

b. _____

c. _____

d. _____

e. _____

f. _____

g. _____

h. _____

2. Give an example of a behavior that demonstrates respect for the individual.

_____

3. List the steps of the nursing process.

a. _____

b. _____

c. _____

d. _____

e. _____

4. Define assessment. _____

_____

5. List four components of technical competence.

a. _____

b. _____

c. _____

d. _____

6. If research is not available, how is the decision made as to what nursing action is correct?

_____

_____

7. What is the purpose of evaluation in nursing practice?

_____

_____

8. Describe the process of mental practice.

_____

_____

© 1996 by Lippincott-Raven Publishers

MODULE

2

BASIC INFECTION CONTROL

M O D U L E   C O N T E N T S
_____

RATIONALE FOR THE USE OF THIS
  SKILL
NURSING DIAGNOSIS
PRINCIPLES OF BASIC INFECTION
  CONTROL
How Microorganisms Spread
Universal Precautions for Blood and Body
  Fluids
Standard Precautions
Handwashing
PROCEDURE FOR HANDWASHING
Personal Hygiene
CRITICAL THINKING EXERCISES

P R E R E Q U I S I T E
_____

Successful completion of the following module:

VOLUME 1
Module 1 An Approach to Nursing Skills

© 1996 by Lippincott-Raven Publishers

OVERALL OBJECTIVE

To apply principles of basic infection control when practicing all aspects of nursing, with particular emphasis on handwashing.

SPECIFIC LEARNING OBJECTIVES

Know Facts and Principles	Apply Facts and Principles	Demonstrate Ability	Evaluate Performance
1. Movement of microorganisms State five ways in which microorganisms move from one area to another.	Given a situation, state methods to prevent microorganisms from moving from dirty to clean items or areas.		
2. Basic infection control related to general nursing 　a. *Handling linens* 　b. *Disposition of soiled articles* State basic infection control guidelines related to handling linens and disposition of soiled articles.	State rationale for holding linen away from uniform, not shaking or tossing linen, and keeping clean items separate from dirty items.	Hold linen away from uniform. Do not shake or toss linen. Keep clean items separate from dirty items.	Evaluate own performance with instructor using Performance Checklist.
3. Universal Precautions List nine body substances included in Universal Precautions. Identify situations in which gloves, eye protection, masks, gowns or aprons are needed.	Given a situation, state what precautions are necessary to prevent transmission of blood-borne infections.	Wear gloves in appropriate situations. Wear eye protection, masks, gowns, or aprons in appropriate situations for Universal Precautions.	Evaluate use of appropriate precautions with instructor.
4. Standard Precautions List five body substances for which gloves are worn that are not included in Universal Precautions.	Given a situation, state what precautions would be used for Standard Precautions.	Wear gloves in appropriate situations for Standard Precautions. Wear eye protection, masks, gowns, or aprons in appropriate situations for Standard Precuations.	Evaluate use of gloves with instructor.
5. Handwashing State when handwashing is indicated.	State rationale for washing hands before and after each patient contact, before handling food, after using toilet, after blowing nose or sneezing, and after touching hair.	Wash hands at appropriate times.	Evaluate own performance with instructor using Performance Checklist.

(continued)

© 1996 by Lippincott-Raven Publishers

SPECIFIC LEARNING OBJECTIVES (continued)

Know Facts and Principles	Apply Facts and Principles	Demonstrate Ability	Evaluate Performance
6. Handwashing procedure a. *Friction* b. *Running water* c. *Cleansing agents*			
State effect of friction, running water, and cleansing agents on handwashing. Describe correct handwashing telchniques.	State rationale for use of friction, running water, and cleansing agents during handwashing.	Use friction, running water, and cleansing agents when washing hands, using correct handwashing techniques.	Evaluate own performance with instructor using Performance Checklist.
7. Personal hygiene a. *Hair* b. *Fingernails* c. *Jewelry*			
State personal hygiene guidelines related to hair, fingernails, and jewelry.	Describe manner of fixing own hair that conforms to guidelines given.	Wear hair short or restrained. Keep fingernails clean and trimmed. Do not wear jewelry in clinical facility.	Evaluate own performance with instructor using Performance Checklist.

© 1996 by Lippincott-Raven Publishers

LEARNING ACTIVITIES

1. Review the Specific Learning Objectives.
2. Read the section on asepsis (in the chapter on infection), focusing especially on the chain of infection in Ellis and Nowlis, *Nursing: A Human Needs Approach,* or comparable material in another textbook.
3. Look up the module vocabulary terms in the glossary.
4. Read through the module, and mentally practice the skill. Study the material so you will be able to teach it to others.
5. Practice putting on clean gloves and taking them off in a way that protects you from contamination.
6. Practice handwashing techniques.
7. In the practice setting, practice safe handwashing techniques, using the procedure as a guide and the Performance Checklist as an evaluation tool. When you are satisfied with your ability, have your instructor evaluate you.
8. In the clinical setting, demonstrate handwashing to your clinical instructor.
9. In the clinical setting, demonstrate Standard Precautions to your clinical instructor.

VOCABULARY

bacteria	droplet nuclei	interdigital	pathogenic organism
barrier	face shield	invasive	Standard Precautions
blood-borne	friction	medical asepsis	subungual
body substances	goggles	microorganism	Universal Precautions
contaminate	immunosuppression	nosocomial	

© 1996 by Lippincott-Raven Publishers

Basic Infection Control

Rationale for the Use of This Skill

Infection control includes all of the practices used to prevent the spread of microorganisms that could cause disease in a person. Traditionally, infection control procedures have been divided into medical asepsis and surgical asepsis.

Medical asepsis *is the practice of techniques and procedures designed to reduce the number of microorganisms in an area or on an object and to decrease the likelihood of their transfer. Medical asepsis is sometimes referred to as "clean technique." The practice of medical asepsis takes on added importance in the presence of individuals who are more susceptible to infection because of illness, surgery, or immunosuppression.*

Because the nurse may be in contact with a number of patients during any day, he or she must be aware of the principles of medical asepsis to avoid transferring microorganisms from a patient to the nurse, from the nurse to a patient, from the nurse to a coworker, or from one patient to another. Microorganisms can also be transferred by way of equipment.

Intact skin is an effective barrier to microorganisms. Skin that is not intact and areas of the body that are normally sterile (such as the eyes and inside of the bladder) require additional precautions to prevent the entry of infection-causing microorganisms. These additional precautions are called surgical asepsis.

Surgical asepsis includes all the sterile procedures and techniques used to exclude all microorganisms from an area. Surgical asepsis is described in Module 33, Sterile Technique, and Module 34, Surgical Asepsis: Scrubbing, Gowning, and Gloving.[1]

▼ NURSING DIAGNOSIS

> Infection control measures are used for all patients in all settings. However, some patients are more susceptible to infection because of compromised immune systems, breaks in the normal defense barrier of the intact skin, or invasive devices. For these patients, the nursing diagnosis Risk for Infection is used.

PRINCIPLES OF BASIC INFECTION CONTROL

How Microorganisms Spread

Microorganisms move on air currents. Because of this movement, avoid shaking or tossing linens, which can create air currents on which microorganisms can be transported. *To reduce the spread of microorganisms,* most hospitals are built in such a way that the ventilation system does not circulate air from one section to another. Be sure that all doors leading to rooms used for respiratory isolation are kept closed *to stop air currents.*

Rooms designed to be used for patients with airborne infections, such as tuberculosis, have air systems that create negative pressure in the room. *When the door is opened, air from the corridor moves into the room, and potentially contaminated air from the room does not move outward.* In operating rooms, the air systems are designed to provide positive pressure. *When the door is opened, potentially contaminated air does not move into the operating room. Instead, air from the extra clean environment tends to move out into the corridor.*

Microorganisms are transferred from one surface to another whenever objects touch. Both clean and dirty items are present in a hospital. Even among ostensibly clean items, some are more clean than others. *When a clean item touches a less clean item, it becomes "dirty," because microorganisms (which are not visible) are transferred to it.* Therefore, keep your hands away from your own hair and face, keep linens away from your uniform, and always keep clean items separate from dirty ones. If you drop anything on the floor, consider it dirty.

Microorganisms are transferred by gravity when one item is held above another. Avoid passing dirty items over clean items or areas *because it is possible for microorganisms to drop off onto a clean item or area.* When storing items in a bedside stand, place clean items on upper shelves and potentially dirty items, such as bedpans, on lower shelves.

Microorganisms are released into the air on droplet nuclei whenever a person breathes or speaks. Coughing or sneezing dramatically increases the number of microorganisms released from the mouth and nose. Avoid having a patient breathe directly into your face, and avoid breathing directly into a patient's face. If the patient has a cough, wear a mask when giving care.

Whenever you cough or sneeze, cover your nose and mouth with a tissue, and discard it immediately. Whenever you have coughed, sneezed, or blown your nose, wash your hands before you touch anything else. Teach the patient to handle coughing and sneezing in the same way. If you handle tissues that a patient has used when coughing or sneezing, always wash your hands thoroughly.

Microorganisms move slowly on dry surfaces but quickly through moisture. For this reason, use a dry paper towel when you turn off faucets, and dry a bath basin before you return it to a bedside stand for storage.

[1]Note that the rationale for action is emphasized throughout the module by the use of italics.

© 1996 by Lippincott-Raven Publishers

Proper handwashing removes many of the microorganisms that can be transferred by the hands from one item to another. Wash your hands not only when they are obviously soiled, but whenever you move from one patient to another or from patient contact to contact with the general environment or vice versa.

Blood-borne infections may be spread to another person through contact between blood and body substances that contain the blood-borne organism and open wounds, sores, or mucous membranes and through penetrating injuries (such as those caused by needle sticks or cuts) with contaminated items. Healthcare workers can protect themselves from these blood-borne infections by using precautions that prevent contact with blood and body fluids that transmit blood-borne pathogens. These precautions are called **Universal Precautions for Blood and Body Fluids** and are described below.

Some body substances, such as feces, urine, nasal secretions, vomitus, and sputum, do not contain blood-borne organisms, but they may contain such large quantities of bacteria that their removal through handwashing is difficult. Additionally there are drug-resistant organisms present in the health care environment. Therefore, in 1994 the Centers for Disease Control and Prevention released a draft of a new infection control standard termed **Standard Precautions**. This set of precautions is similar to **Body Substance Precautions** that had been instituted by many healthcare agencies, in which the use of gloves was expanded beyond Universal Precautions to include gloves for all contact with feces, urine, nasal secretions, vomitus, and sputum to decrease the potential for transmission of bacteria found in these substances. Standard Precautions are discussed further on in this module.

Universal Precautions for Blood and Body Fluids

The Centers for Disease Control and Prevention (CDC) of the US Department of Health and Human Services provides the basic guidelines for actions used in infection control (CDC, 1988). A major concern is protection from blood-borne and body fluid–borne viruses, especially human immunodeficiency virus (HIV), which causes acquired immunodeficiency syndrome (AIDS), and hepatitis B virus. The CDC recommends that the following **Universal Blood and Body Fluid Precautions** be used in all patient contacts (that is, universally) because you will not know which individual is infected with these viruses. The body fluids included in these precautions have the potential for communicating a blood-borne virus if it is present in the patient. Table 2–1 lists the specific body fluids included in this policy.

The Occupational Health and Safety Administra-

Table 2–1. Substances Included in Universal Precautions for Blood and Body Fluids	
Blood	Pleural fluid
Semen	Peritoneal fluid
Vaginal secretions	Pericardial fluid
Cerebrospinal fluid	Amniotic fluid
Synovial fluid	

Note: Universal Precautions do not apply to nasal secretions, sputum, urine, feces, saliva, sweat, tears, or vomitus unless there is visible blood in them (CDC, 1988).

tion (OSHA) has established regulations mandating that healthcare agencies provide educational sessions regarding Universal Precautions before any employee contacts patients. In addition, OSHA regulations require that agencies provide an annual review of these practices for every employee. Every agency must provide the necessary supplies to enable employees to carry out Universal Precautions. Any agency that does not provide appropriate supplies or in which personnel are violating these standards is subject to a substantial fine. You will be accountable for carrying out these procedures in all healthcare settings.

Although OSHA is now planning its regulatory response to the CDC's establishment of Standard Precautions, Standard Precautions are not required by OSHA regulations at the time this text goes to press.

UNIVERSAL BLOOD AND BODY FLUID PRECAUTIONS

1. Wear clean latex or vinyl gloves whenever there is potential for contact with any of the body fluids listed in Table 2–1. *This protects you by preventing any accidental contact of a substance that could carry a blood-borne pathogen through breaks in your skin.*
   a. Know the specific situations in which gloves are recommended by the CDC *because the potential for contact with blood and body fluids is high.* These include situations in which you are doing the following:
      (1) Performing phlebotomy (if the nurse is learning phlebotomy technique; if the nurse has cuts, scratches, or other breaks in the skin; and when hand contamination with blood may occur)
      (2) Performing finger or heel sticks on infants and children

© 1996 by Lippincott-Raven Publishers

(3) Performing procedures involving contact with mucous membranes and diagnostic procedures that do not require sterile gloves

(4) Changing or manipulating intravenous lines when blood contamination is possible

(5) Handling dressings soiled with body fluids

(6) Handling urine or feces if gross blood is visible

(7) Providing care (such as perineal care) that could result in contact with the previously named body fluids

b. Change gloves between patient contacts. *Gloves can carry pathogens from one patient to another.*

c. Do not wash or clean examination gloves. *They are not designed for this heavy use and develop small holes and weakened areas that diminish their effectiveness.*

2. *Handwashing removes blood-borne pathogens from intact skin. Microorganisms multiply rapidly on the warm, moist skin under gloves.* Wash your hands thoroughly:

a. Immediately after accidental contact with body substances containing blood

b. Between patients

c. Immediately after gloves are removed.

3. Wear masks and protective eyewear or face shields to *protect the mucous membranes of your mouth, nose, and eyes* during procedures that may generate droplets or splashes of blood or other body fluids specified. Goggles, plastic eye glasses, or shields that fit over eyeglass frames may be used as protective eyewear. A face shield may be attached to the top of a mask or to a head band.

4. Wear a disposable, moisture-proof apron or gown during procedures likely to generate splatters of blood or body fluid and soil your clothing. *This protects you from accidental contact with pathogens and prevents you from carrying contaminated substances to others.*

5. Wear general purpose utility gloves (such as rubber household gloves) for housekeeping chores and instrument cleaning. *This type of glove is thicker and stronger and provides better protection against accidental glove breaks when dexterity and touch are not concerns.* These gloves may be decontaminated and reused. They should be discarded if they are peeling, cracked, or discolored or if they have punctures, tears, or other evidence of deterioration *because they will no longer provide an effective barrier.*

6. Wear sterile gloves for procedures involving contact with normally sterile areas of the body (see Module 33, Sterile Technique). *The sterile gloves*

protect the patient from environmental pathogens while protecting you from the patient's pathogens.

7. Dispose of equipment and secretions properly. *Accidental penetrating injuries and contact with contaminated substances are serious occupational hazards for healthcare workers.*

a. Needles, disposable syringes, scalpel blades, and other sharp instruments should be placed in puncture-resistant containers for disposal. These items should not be recapped, broken, or carried from one area to another but disposed of directly in an appropriate container in the area where used. *Any manipulation or uncovered transporting of the object increases the potential for accidental injury.*

b. Carefully pour bulk blood, suctioned fluids, and excretions that contain blood and named body fluids down drains to the sewer. *The sanitary sewer system is designed to prevent pathogens from contacting people in the community.*

8. Put all specimens of blood and listed fluids in moisture-proof containers with secure lids to prevent leakage during transport. Avoid contaminating the outside of the container *to protect those who will handle the container.* In many settings, specimen containers are placed inside a plastic bag to protect further against potential leakage. *These actions protect transporters and laboratory personnel from accidental contamination.*

9. Handle soiled linen correctly. Hold it away from your uniform, and handle it as little as possible and with minimal agitation *to prevent contamination of the air and of people handling the linen.*

a. Hold linen away from your uniform.

b. Do not shake or toss linen.

c. Place and transport linen soiled with blood or body fluids in leakage-resistant bags *to prevent accidental contamination of those who handle linens.*

10. Follow your facility's policies for cleaning contaminated surfaces and materials and for disposing of infective wastes.

a. Clean visible soil from objects and surfaces before disinfection *because pathogens can live inside of or under visible soil despite contact with disinfectants.*

b. Use a commercial germicide solution for cleaning. In the absence of a commercial germicide, household bleach in a 1:10 dilution is an effective disinfectant. *These solutions can destroy all blood-borne pathogens and most other microorganisms.*

11. Use mouthpieces, resuscitation bags, or other ventilation devices for cardiopulmonary resuscitation whenever possible. *Saliva has not been implicated in HIV transmission, but other infections*

© 1996 by Lippincott-Raven Publishers

are transmitted by saliva. Facilities are urged to place these devices in areas where their need is predictable.

12. Healthcare workers with open or draining lesions should refrain from all direct patient care and from handling patient care equipment until the lesions are resolved. *This prevents any possible contact between contaminated substances and the lesions of the healthcare worker who is at high risk if accidental contact occurs. This also protects the patient from a healthcare worker who may have a blood-borne infection.*

Standard Precautions

In November of 1994, the Centers for Disease Control and Prevention published "Draft Guideline for Isolation Precautions in Hospitals: Part I. Evaluation of Isolation Practices" and "Part II. Recommendations for Isolation Precautions in Hospitals." These guidelines were developed by HICPAC (Hospital Infections Control Practices Advisory Committee) in cooperation with the NCID (National Center for Infectious Diseases). All healthcare providers were asked to respond to these suggested changes.

At the time of this publication, the CDC final guideline has not been published but experts expect the standard will be basically those published in the Draft Guideline. The revised guideline contains two tiers of precautions. The first tier, termed Standard Precautions, was designed to provide a greater margin of safety for healthcare providers and consumers than would be provided by the use of Universal Precautions only.

The second tier "Transmission-based Precautions" was designed for patients documented or suspected of being infected or colonized with highly transmissable or important microorganisms. These precautions are discussed in Module 32, Isolation Technique.

For Standard Precautions the actions of Universal Precautions are extended to include contact with (1) blood, (2) all body fluids, secretions, and excretions regardless of whether or not they contain visible blood, (3) nonintact skin, and (4) mucous membranes (CDC, 1994). Standard precautions are included in all modules.

STANDARD PRECAUTIONS

1. Wear clean latext or vinyl gloves whenever there is potential for contact with any of the body fluids listed in Table 2–2 or any moist body surface.

Table 2–2. Substances Included in Standard Precautions

Wear gloves for contact with:

1) Blood
2) All body fluids, secretions, and excretions regardless of whether or not they contain visible blood. Include:
   a. sputum
   b. urine
   c. feces
   d. nasal secretions
   e. vomitus
   f. spinal fluid
   g. semen
   h. cerebrospinal fluid
   i. synovial fluid
   j. pleural fluid
   k. peritoneal fluid
   l. pericardial fluid
   m. amniotic fluid
3) Nonintact skin
4) Mucous membranes

This protects you by preventing any accidental contact of a substance that could carry a microorganism through breaks in your skin.

a. Know the specific situations in which gloves are recommended by the CDC *because the potential for contact with body substances is high.* These include situations in which you are:
   (1) Performing phlebotomy (if the nurse is learning phlebotomy technique; if the nurse has cuts, scratches, or other breaks in the skin; and when hand contamination with blood may occur)
   (2) Performing finger or heel sticks on infants and children
   (3) Performing procedures involving contact with mucous membranes and diagnostic procedures that do not require sterile gloves
   (4) Changing or manipulating intravenous lines when blood contamination is possible
   (5) Handling dressings soiled with body fluids
   (6) Handling urine or feces
   (7) Providing care (such as perineal care) that could result in contact with moist body surfaces or body fluids

b. Change gloves between patient contacts. *Gloves can carry pathogens from one patient to another.*

c. Do not wash or clean examination gloves.

© 1996 by Lippincott-Raven Publishers

They are not designed for this heavy use and develop small holes and weakened areas that diminish their effectiveness.

2. Wash your hands thoroughly:
   a. Immediately after accidental contact with body substances or moist body surfaces
   b. Between patients
   c. Immediately after gloves are removed. *Handwashing removes microorganisms from intact skin. Microorganisms multiply rapidly on the warm, moist skin under gloves.*

3. Wear masks and protective eyewear or face shields to *protect the mucous membranes of your mouth, nose, and eyes* during procedures that may generate droplets or splashes of any body fluids. Goggles, plastic eye glasses, or shields that fit over eyeglass frames may all be used as protective eyewear. A face shield may be attached to the top of a mask or may attach to a head band.

4. Wear a disposable, moisture-proof apron or gown during procedures likely to generate splatters of body fluid and soil your clothing. *This protects you from accidental contact with pathogens and prevents your carrying contaminated substances to others.*

5. Wear general purpose utility gloves (such as rubber household gloves) for housekeeping chores and instrument cleaning. This type of glove is thicker and stronger and provides better protection against accidental glove breaks in situations where dexterity and touch are not concerns. These gloves may be decontaminated and reused. They should be discarded if they are peeling, cracked, or discolored or if they have punctures, tears, or other evidence of deterioration *because they will no longer provide an effective barrier.*

6. Dispose of equipment and secretions properly. *Accidental penetrating injuries and contact with contaminated substances are a serious occupational hazard for health care workers.*
   a. Needles, disposable syringes, scalpel blades, and other sharp instruments should be placed in puncture-resistant containers for disposal. These items should not be recapped, broken, or carried from one area to another, but disposed of directly into an appropriate container in the area where used. *Any manipulation or uncovered transporting of the object increases the potential for accidental injury.*
   b. Carefully pour bulk blood, suctioned fluids, and excretions down drains to the sewer. *The sanitary sewer system is designed to prevent pathogens from contacting people in the community.*

7. Put all specimens in moisture-proof containers with secure lids to prevent leakage during transport. Be sure to avoid contaminating the outside of the container *to protect those who will handle the container.* In many settings, specimen containers are placed inside a plastic bag to further protect against potential leakage. *These actions protect transporters and laboratory personnel from accidental contamination.*

8. Handle soiled linen correctly. Hold it away from your uniform and handle it as little as possible and with minimal agitation *to prevent contamination of the air and of people handling the linen.*
   a. Hold linen away from your uniform
   b. Do not shake or toss linen
   c. Place and transport linen soiled with body fluids in leakage-resistant bags *to prevent accidental contamination of those who handle linen.*

9. Follow your facility's policies for cleaning contaminated surfaces and materials and for disposing of infective wastes.
   a. Clean visible soil from objects and surfaces before disinfection because pathogens can live inside of or under visible soil despite contact with disinfectants.
   b. Use a commercial germicide solution for cleaning. In the absence of a commercial germicide, household bleach in a 1:10 dilution is effective as a disinfectant. These solutions can destroy all blood-borne pathogens and most other microorganisms.

10. Use mouthpieces, resuscitation bags, or other ventilation devices for cardipulmonary resuscitation (CPR) whenever possible. Saliva has not been implicated in HIV transmission, but other infections are transmitted by saliva. Facilities are urged to place these devices in areas where their need is predictable.

11. Healthcare workers with open or draining lesions should refrain from all direct patient care and from handling patient care equipment until the lesions are resolved. This prevents any possible contact between contaminated substances and the lesions of the healthcare worker who is at high risk if accidental contact should occur. This also protects the patient from a healthcare worker who may have an infection.

Handwashing

The most important procedure for preventing the transfer of microorganisms, and therefore nosocomial infection, is correct and frequent handwashing. Proper handwashing protects the patient, your coworkers, you, and your family.

Handwashing should be done in all of the following instances:

- At the beginning of every work shift
- Before and after prolonged contact with a patient
- Before invasive procedures
- Before contact with especially susceptible patients
- Before and after touching wounds
- After contact with body substances, even when gloves are worn
- Any time you are in doubt about the necessity for doing so
- At the end of every shift before leaving the healthcare facility

For medical aseptic purposes, the CDC recommends at least a vigorous 10-second handwashing procedure that includes "a rubbing together of all surfaces of lathered hands followed by rinsing under a stream of water." Further, they comment that in situations in which hands are visibly soiled, "more time" may be required (Garner & Favero, 1985). Some nurses prefer to use a 30-second hand wash all of the time *as an extra safety precaution.*

Friction, running water, and a cleansing agent are necessary to remove microorganisms or other material that may be present on the hands. The cleansing agent may be plain soap in all situations except those involving the care of newborns, between patients in high-risk units, and before the care of immunosuppressed patients. In these situations, antimicrobial products should be used.

A deep sink with controls that can be operated by foot, leg, or elbow is ideal for handwashing. Where faucets are operated by hand, it is recommended that you use a dry paper towel as a barrier when turning the water off *because a dirty hand was used to turn it on.*

Because the handwashing procedure causes microorganisms to accumulate in the sink, you should avoid touching the sink as you wash and avoid splashing dirty water on your uniform.

PROCEDURE FOR HANDWASHING

1. Roll your sleeves above your elbows, and remove all jewelry and your watch. If your watch has an expansion band, move it up above your elbow *to allow you to wash well up your arms.* After the initial handwash of the shift, wash your hands well above the wrists, unless you have been in a situation that you feel necessitates more thorough washing.
2. Do not touch the sink.
3. Turn on the water, and adjust the temperature. *Warm water removes fewer oils from the skin than hot water and removes microorganisms more effectively than cold water.*
4. Dispense liquid or powdered soap, preferably with a foot control. Bar soap is not recommended *because it may harbor microorganisms.* If only bar soap is available, lather and rinse the bar thoroughly *to remove the outside layer of soap before you use it.*
5. Lather your hands and arms well.
6. Clean your fingernails as needed with a nail file or orangewood stick. (If these utensils are not provided, do this before you leave home.) *The subungual area (under the fingernails) is especially important because it is an area where bacteria multiply and is frequently missed in handwashing.* It is not necessary to clean your nails each time you wash your hands.
7. Wash your hands and arms up to your elbows, adding soap as needed *to maintain a lather. Microorganisms are suspended in the lather and later rinsed off.* Keep your hands lower than your elbows at all times.
   a. Rub briskly, using friction and a rotary motion (as opposed to a back-and-forth motion) *to contact all surfaces more effectively.*
   b. Pay particular attention to the areas between your fingers (the interdigital spaces), your knuckles, and the outside surfaces of the fifth or "little" fingers, *because these areas are often missed.*
   c. Leave the water running during the entire procedure.
8. Holding your hands and forearms lower than your elbows, rinse thoroughly, starting at one elbow and moving down the arm (Fig. 2–1). Then repeat this step for the other arm. *This position prevents microorganisms from being rinsed up your arms from your hands, which are frequently the most contaminated.*
9. Dry your hands thoroughly from fingers to forearms. Most facilities provide paper towels for this purpose. Blotting with a paper towel *is easier on the skin* than rubbing.
10. Use a dry paper towel to turn off the faucet if it is hand operated.
11. Use lotion if needed *to maintain your skin condition. Because frequent handwashing can lead to dry, cracked skin in some individuals,* the use of lotion may be encouraged *to help keep skin intact, thus preventing possible invasion by microorganisms.* In some settings, however, you may be asked not to use lotion during the work day *because it can be an excellent medium for bacterial growth in the healthcare environment.*

© 1996 by Lippincott-Raven Publishers

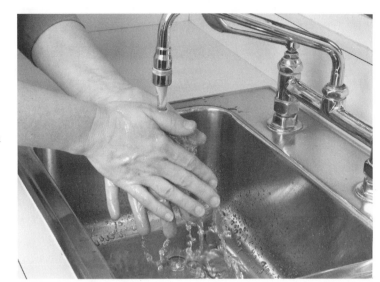

Figure 2–1. Handwashing with hands lower than elbows. (Courtesy Ivan Ellis)

Personal Hygiene

Obviously, *to enhance infection control,* you must practice good personal hygiene. *Also, it is much more pleasant for patients to be near someone who smells fresh and who is wearing a clean uniform.* Use the following important guidelines for personal hygiene:

1. Arrange your hair in a way that does not contribute to contaminating the patient or the environment and that will protect you from contaminating your hair with microbes you may have contacted with your hands. Hair should not fall forward when you lean forward (for example, when you examine a patient). *When hair falls over an area, microorganisms can drop from the hair (by gravity) onto the patient, or the hair itself may fall onto trays or wounds.* Keep your hair short or restrain it in some way *so that it does not fall forward.* Also avoid any style in which you are constantly brushing your hair out of your eyes or back from your face. *If your hands have just been washed, you may transfer microbes from your hair to your hands. If your hands have not just been washed, you may transfer microbes from your hands to your hair.*

2. Keep your fingernails clean and trimmed or filed short, *so you do not endanger patients by scratching them or by harboring bacteria.* If you use polish, it must be intact; *chipped polish also is a place for bacteria to lodge.*

3. Wear only a minimum of jewelry, *because jewelry is a place for microorganisms to lodge.* Plain studs or posts for pierced ears and plain wedding bands or other plain rings are the most jewelry you should wear in a clinical setting. *Necklaces and large hoop or dangling earrings are a hazard not only in terms of infection control, but also because a patient can grab them and hurt you and the jewelry.*

These guidelines often are not enforced by the employing agency; therefore, your knowledge of the rationale for such guidelines and your conscience must guide your actions.

CRITICAL THINKING EXERCISES

• Mr. Smith is a resident in a long-term care facility where you are having clinical experience. You note that he has a cough. Identify the specific infection control measures you should institute with Mr. Smith. Determine which infection control measures you should teach him.

• You are in a hospital room, and the patient cries out, "I just caught my IV tubing in the bed rail, and I've pulled it out. I'm bleeding! Do something!" Identify the infection control principles and directives that apply in this situation. Explain your concerns, and describe the actions you should take to protect yourself.

References

Centers for Disease Control (1994, November 7). Draft Guideline for Isolation Precautions in Hospitals: Part I. "Evolution of Isolation Practices" and Part II. "Recommendations for Isolation Precautions in Hospitals." *Federal Register, 59, (214),* 55552–55570.

Centers for Disease Control (1988, August 21). Recommendations for prevention of HIV transmission in health care settings. *Morbidity and Mortality Weekly Report Supplement, 36,* 25–185.

Garner, J. S., & Favero, M. S. (1985).Guideline for Handwashing and Hospital Environmental Control. Atlanta: Centers for Disease Control and Prevention.

© 1996 by Lippincott-Raven Publishers

✔ PERFORMANCE CHECKLIST

Standard Precautions	Needs More Practice	Satisfactory	Comments
1. Wear gloves (clean or sterile as required by the patient's situation) for contact with (1) blood, (2) all body fluids, secretions, and excretions regardless of whether or not they contain visible blood, (3) nonintact skin, and (4) mucous membranes.			
2. Wash hands: **a.** Between patients			
b. Immediately after gloves are removed			
c. Immediately after accidental contact with blood, any body fluid, secretion or excretion, nonintact skin, or mucous membrane.			
3. Wear masks and protective eyewear whenever there is the possibility of splash of any type of body fluid.			
4. Wear moisture-proof apron or gown whenever there is the potential of a body fluid contacting your clothing.			
5. Wear utility (household) rubber gloves when cleaning equipment or surfaces.			
6. Wear sterile gloves to protect the patient as appropriate.			
7. Dispose of equipment so that no patients or health care providers are endangered by accidental contact.			
8. Dispose of secretions so that no patients or health care providers are endangered by accidental contact.			
9. Handle soiled linens correctly. **a.** Hold linen away from uniform.			
b. Do not shake or toss linen.			
c. Transport linen contaminated with blood or body fluids in leakage-proof bags.			
10. Clean contaminated articles and surfaces. **a.** Clean visible soil first.			
b. Use an appropriate disinfectant.			
11. Use mouthpieces, resuscitation bags, or ventilation devices for cardiopulmonary resuscitation when possible.			
12. Do not care for patients if you have open or draining lesions.			

(continued)

© 1996 by Lippincott-Raven Publishers

Procedure for Handwashing	Needs More Practice	Satisfactory	Comments
1. Roll sleeves above elbows and remove all jewelry and watch.			
2. Do not touch outside or inside of sink.			
3. Turn on water and adjust temperature to warm.			
4. Dispense liquid or powdered soap.			
5. Lather hands and arms well, using rotary motion.			
6. Clean fingernails.			
7. Hold hands and forearms lower than elbows. Wash hands and arms to elbows, with running water, using rotary motion and giving special attention to areas between fingers. Leave water running during entire procedure.			
8. Rinse thoroughly, keeping hands lower than elbows.			
9. Dry hands thoroughly from fingers to forearms.			
10. Turn off water with dry paper towel if faucet is hand operated.			
11. Use lotion if appropriate.			
Personal hygiene			
1. Keep hair restrained.			
2. Keep fingernails clean and short.			
3. Do not wear jewelry, or wear only a minimum.			

© 1996 by Lippincott-Raven Publishers

? Q U I Z

Multiple-Choice Questions

_____ **1.** In which of the following situations should nurses wash their hands?

 a. At the beginning of the shift
 b. Before going to lunch
 c. After removing gloves used while handling body substances
 d. All of these

_____ **2.** Which of the following are essential components of the handwashing procedure? (1) friction, (2) running water, (3) foot-operated water controls, (4) cleansing agent

 a. 1 only
 b. 1 and 4
 c. 2, 3, and 4
 d. 1, 2, and 4

_____ **3.** Which of the following areas should the nurse _not_ touch during the handwashing procedure? (1) the inside of the sink, (2) the outside of the sink, (3) a hand-controlled faucet, (4) own hair

 a. 1 only
 b. 2 only
 c. 1, 2, and 3
 d. All of these

_____ **4.** Which of the following should receive attention during the handwashing procedures? (1) palms, (2) elbows, (3) spaces between the fingers, (4) fingernails

 a. 1 and 4
 b. 1, 3, and 4
 c. 2, 3, and 4
 d. All of these

_____ **5.** Which body substance transmits blood-borne pathogens, such as human immunodeficiency virus and hepatitis B virus?

 a. Feces
 b. Sputum
 c. Urine
 d. Vaginal secretions

_____ **6.** How may blood-borne pathogens enter the body?

 a. Through breathing contaminated droplet nuclei
 b. By skin-to-skin contact with the infected person
 c. Through open wounds and mucous membranes that have been contacted by blood and certain body substances
 d. By contact with objects that have been handled by the infected person

Short-Answer Questions

7. State the rationale for the following actions.

 a. Avoid shaking or tossing linens. _____

 _____

 b. Keep your hands away from your hair and face. _____

 _____

© 1996 by Lippincott-Raven Publishers

    c. Avoid passing dirty items over clean items or areas. _____

_____

    d. Use a dry paper towel when you turn off faucets. _____

_____

    e. Wear goggles and mask or face shield when there is a potential for splashing of blood.

_____

_____

    f. Do not recap or break contaminated needles. _____

_____

    g. Wear gloves when handling feces. _____

_____

    h. Wear goggles or face shield when irrigating a wound. _____

_____

MODULE

3

SAFETY

MODULE CONTENTS

RATIONALE FOR THE USE OF THIS
  INFORMATION
ENVIRONMENTAL SAFETY AGENCIES
SAFETY IN INSTITUTIONS
Safe Staff Behavior
  Use Good Body Mechanics
  Walk; Avoid Running
  Keep to the Right in Hallways
  Turn Corners Carefully
  Open Doors Slowly
  Use Stretchers Properly
  *Use Brakes on Beds, Wheelchairs, and
    Stretchers*
  *Place Elevators on "Hold" when Loading or
    Unloading*
Safety in Working Spaces, Halls, and
  Corridors
  Lighting
  Floor Surfaces
  Needles and Other Sharp Objects
  Dangerous or Caustic Substances or Materials
  Uncluttered Hallways
Safety in the Patient's Room
  Lighting
  Floor Surfaces
  Oxygen
  Furniture
  Medications and Dangerous Substances
  Doors
PROTECTING THE DEPENDENT PATIENT
The Dependent Adult
  Position of the Bed
  Side Rails
  Positioning
  Protection from Sharp Objects
  Eyes
  Air Passages

The Dependent Child
OTHER SAFETY CONSIDERATIONS
SAFETY DEVICES AND RESTRAINTS
Nursing Diagnoses
Hazards of Using Safety Devices and
  Restraints
Use of Restraints and the Law
Types of Restraints
  Belt Restraints
  Vest Restraints
  Jacket Restraints
  Elbow or Knee Restraints
  Wrist or Ankle Restraints
  Mitt Restraints
Knots Used with Safety Devices
Nonrestraint Safety Devices
  Types of Nonrestraint Safety Devices
GENERAL PROCEDURE FOR APPLYING
  SAFETY DEVICES AND RESTRAINTS
  Assessment
  Planning
  Implementation
  Evaluation
  Documentation
SMOKING AS A HAZARD IN THE
  HEALTHCARE FACILITY
FIRE PLANS
FIRE CODE PROCEDURE
DISASTER PLANS
Internal Disaster Codes
External Disaster Codes
Fire and Disaster Drills
INCIDENT REPORTS
LONG-TERM CARE
HOME CARE
CRITICAL THINKING EXERCISES

© 1996 by Lippincott-Raven Publishers

P R E R E Q U I S I T E S [1]

Successful completion of the following modules:

VOLUME 1
Module 1   An Approach to Nursing Skills
Module 2   Basic Infection Control
Module 4   Basic Body Mechanics
Module 5   Documentation
Module 6   Introduction to Assessment Skills
Module 15 Moving the Patient in Bed and Positioning
Module 19 Basic Infant Care
Module 22 Range-of-Motion Exercises

[1]The need for safety is implicit in the skills outlined in all
the modules. Keep safety in mind at every step.

© 1996 by Lippincott-Raven Publishers

OVERALL OBJECTIVE

To provide a safe environment for staff, visitors, and all people receiving care in hospitals, long-term care facilities, and the home by being constantly vigilant for unsafe conditions; to apply a variety of safety devices or physical restraints, taking into account the comfort and safety of the patient.

SPECIFIC LEARNING OBJECTIVES

Know Facts and Principles	Apply Facts and Principles	Demonstrate Ability	Evaluate Performance
1. Safe behavior			
State seven behaviors that are important to safety.	State rationale for each behavior, and explain the consequences if safety measures are not carried out.	In the clinical setting, document own behavior and that of others.	Discuss documentation with instructor.
2. Safety in working spaces, halls, and corridors			
List five physical aspects of safety in working spaces, halls, and corridors.	State rationale for each aspect.	In the clinical setting, document safety by describing: a. A working space b. A hallway c. A corridor	Discuss documentation with instructor.
3. Safety in the patient's room			
Name seven safety precautions specific to patients' rooms.	State rationale for each precaution as it relates to the patient.	In the clinical setting, identify and document safe and unsafe conditions in a patient's room.	Discuss documentation with instructor.
4. Protecting the dependent patient			
Discuss additional safety precautions to protect dependent patients.	Identify reason for each precaution or action.	If the opportunity to care for a dependent patient is available, add any appropriate safety measures to the care plan.	Evaluate with instructor.
5. Reasons for safety devices or physical restraints			
List two reasons for applying safety devices or restraints.	State reason in a given situation.	In the clinical situation, understand reason for application.	
6. Hazards of restraints			
List six hazards related to the use of restraints.	Given a situation, state potential hazards of restraints.	In the clinical setting, identify potential hazards of restraining a specific patient.	
7. Alternatives to restraints			
List three alternatives to the use of restraints.	Given a situation, state possible alternative(s) to the use of restraints.	In the clinical setting attempt alternative interventions.	Evaluate with instructor.

(continued)

© 1996 by Lippincott-Raven Publishers

SPECIFIC LEARNING OBJECTIVES (continued)

Know Facts and Principles	Apply Facts and Principles	Demonstrate Ability	Evaluate Performance
8. *Legal implications*			
State reason for obtaining order.		Check order before applying, or take steps to obtain order.	
9. *Choice of safety device or restraint*			
Know various safety devices and restraints used. State factors to consider in use of particular device.	Adapt choice to patient's needs.	With an individual patient, choose appropriate device.	Evaluate own performance with instructor.
10. *Application of safety devices or restraints*			
Explain how to use particular safety devices or restraints.		Apply device chosen, taking into account comfort and safety factors.	Evaluate own performance using Performance Checklist.
11. *Documentation*			
List data to be recorded.		Make complete record of entire procedure, including assessment demonstrating need for safety device or restraint, time applied or removed, and condition of skin and circulation.	
12. *Smoking policy in the healthcare facility*			
State policies that healthcare facilities use to contain or monitor smoking behavior.	Give rationale underlying policies regarding smoking behavior.	In the clinical setting, observe which policies regarding smoking are in effect.	Identify whether changes in policies regarding smoking in your facility are needed. Share with instructor.
13. *Fire plans*			
List the 12 steps of most fire plans.	Read the plan in use in your facility, and compare steps with module list.	In the clinical setting, identify specific fire procedures for assigned unit.	Evaluate with instructor using Performance Checklist.
14. *Disaster plans*			
Briefly discuss disaster plans, both internal and external.	Explain how each type of disaster plan applies to the staff nurse.	In the clinical setting, identify specific disaster plan for your department.	Evaluate with instructor.

(continued)

© 1996 by Lippincott-Raven Publishers

S P E C I F I C   L E A R N I N G   O B J E C T I V E S   (c o n t i n u e d)

Know Facts and Principles	Apply Facts and Principles	Demonstrate Ability	Evaluate Performance
15. *Fire and disaster drills*			
State two reasons for holding drills.	Give examples of how drills make codes more effective.	Attend a debriefing session if possible.	Evaluate with instructor.
16. *Incident reports*			
Give the three main purposes of incident reports.	State rationale regarding legal importance of reporting.	In the clinical setting, fill out an incident report, using the facility's form and a hypothetical situation.	Discuss the completed report with the instructor.

© 1996 by Lippincott-Raven Publishers

LEARNING ACTIVITIES

1. Review the Specific Learning Objectives.
2. Read the sections on safety in Ellis and Nowlis, *Nursing: A Human Needs Approach,* or comparable material in another textbook.
3. Read through the module as though you were preparing to teach the content to another person.
4. In the practice setting, form groups of three to five students. Taking turns, discuss which steps in the following modules could lead to unsafe conditions for patients, visitors, or staff. You may refer to the modules.
     14: Bedmaking
     15: Moving the Patient in Bed and Positioning
     16: Feeding Adult Patients
     18: Hygiene
     20: Transfer
     27: Applying Heat and Cold
5. In the practice setting:
   a. Inspect the various safety devices and restraints.
   b. Have a partner apply various safety devices and restraints to you. Answer the following questions:
       Which are the most comfortable?
       Which are the least comfortable?
       Why?
       Describe some of your feelings regarding the experience.
   c. Apply the various safety devices and restraints to your partner. Check them for comfort and safety.

6. In the clinical setting:
   a. Read the sections of the policy or procedure manual dealing with general safety.
   b. Familiarize yourself with the types of safety devices (restraints and restraint alternatives) used in the facility.
   c. Observe any safety devices or restraints being used. Have they been applied correctly and safely?
   d. When the opportunity arises, apply an appropriate safety device or restraint with your instructor's supervision.
   e. Using the Performance Checklist, evaluate your performance with your instructor's help.
   f. Document pertinent data regarding the application of the safety device or restraint. Check your documentation with your instructor.
   g. Read the fire plan, and locate exits and extinguishers.
   h. Examine the incident report forms used by the facility.
   i. Find out whether your facility has a printed disaster plan, internal or external; if it does, read it.
   j. Visit a patient in a room. Observe potential safety hazards. After the visit, share these with a classmate in a conference.
   k. Note on paper any risks to safety you see in the hallways, work spaces, or nursing station. Share these observations with your instructor.

VOCABULARY

AIDS
antineoplastic
caustic
critical care

external disaster
fetal
internal disaster

isotope
neurosensory
pavilion

scalpel
triage
vesicant

[handwritten annotations:]

a community disaster that may threaten the med. facility

fetal — pertaining to fetus

triage — prioritization of patience according to their injuries

fetal

Caustic — ability to burn, corrode by chem. action

Critical care = healthcare provider for acute life threatening illness

internal disaster w/in the medical facility

isotope same # of protons but diff. # of neutrons.

pavilion grp. of bldgs composing a hospital, annex also

Vesicant — agent that can cause blistering or necrosis, the sloughing of tissue

scalpel — a sharp surgical knife.

© 1996 by Lippincott-Raven Publishers

Safety

Rationale for the Use of This Information

Because of its complexity, the healthcare setting is potentially dangerous. The structure is usually spacious, with heavily traveled hallways, steps, and elevators. For reasons of economy, most hospitals are constructed on a high-rise or pavilion plan. Monitoring areas for unsafe conditions and needed maintenance constantly poses problems and requires the vigilance and assistance of staff.

Patient rooms, on the other hand, usually are not spacious. They are often confining—even more so if special equipment is needed for care. The space provided for nurses' stations has also been increasingly taken up by the records, monitoring equipment, and computer terminals that have been added as nursing and medical practice have grown more sophisticated.

The variety of equipment used within the modern healthcare environment adds to the difficulty of maintaining safety. Equipment as diverse as a simple thermometer and a complicated ventilator are included in the repertoire of practicing nurses today. The nurse must be skilled not only in operating equipment but also in detecting and correcting any problems that arise.

The unfamiliarity of the healthcare facility for most individuals adds to the potential for accident or injury. Members of the nursing staff should have the knowledge to protect themselves and act as advocates for others regarding safety. Nurses should be cognizant of the ethical and legal issues as well as the skills relative to the application of safety devices and restraints.

Fire and natural disasters pose an especially serious threat in any facility containing a large number of people, especially when many of these people are ill or dependent. An important goal for every practicing nurse is to be knowledgeable and prepared in all aspects of safety.

Providing a safe environment is important for the nurse practicing in a long-term care facility because of the advanced age and fragility of most of the residents. In addition, the increasing number of nurses involved in home care have the added responsibility of monitoring the home environment for safety hazards.[2]

ENVIRONMENTAL SAFETY AGENCIES

A number of agencies are concerned with maintaining safety for staff and patients in healthcare facilities. Some have a regulatory function, whereas others are advisory. These agencies also conduct or support research *to understand better what hazards exist and how to diminish them.*

The National Institute for Occupational Safety and Health gathers and interprets data regarding safety collected by other organizations *so that changes in practice can be made to ensure safety.*

The Occupational Safety and Health Administration (OSHA) is an official body with regulatory powers allowing fines to be imposed on institutions that violate safety regulations. Each state has its own occupational safety agency that randomly inspects facilities with 11 or more workers for violations that may endanger the safety of workers. Safety regulations stemming from these organizations are written into the state codes.

The Centers for Disease Control and Prevention (CDC) is an advisory organization, largely concerned with preventing the spread of infection. Violations of physical safety, such as cluttered hallways and storage areas, are monitored by each state's Department of Health and Human Services or comparable agency.

SAFETY IN INSTITUTIONS

A patient has the right to a safe environment in the healthcare facility (Fig. 3–1).

Whether you are in a patient's room, the hallway, in utility rooms, or at the nurses' station, similar safety precautions apply. These precautions include safe behavior at all times, constant vigilance for unsafe conditions, and the protection of dependent patients. When a breach in safety occurs and an incident results, it is important to know how to report it properly *to protect the patient, the staff, and the healthcare facility.*

Safe Staff Behavior

Many of the habits of safe behavior may seem to be nothing more than common sense, but they are of great importance to safety.

Use Good Body Mechanics

Although you will learn good body mechanics in connection with moving patients, using proper body mechanics in daily activities is just as important. As you carry out your duties, which require much standing and walking, an erect posture in good body alignment *protects you from strain.* Stretching, reaching, and carrying or moving heavy objects can take their toll on poorly aligned muscles. Using good body mechanics and reminding others of their importance is a basic part of safe behavior.

---

[2]Note that rationale for action is emphasized throughout the module by the use of italics.

© 1996 by Lippincott-Raven Publishers

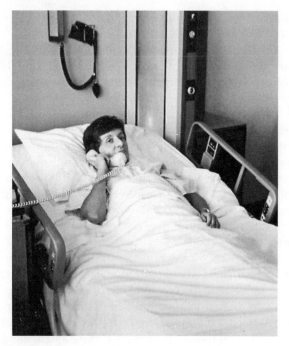

Figure 3–1. Patient in a safe environment. (Courtesy Ivan Ellis)

Walk; Avoid Running

It is sometimes imperative that you run, in a patient emergency, for example. Even at these times, however, remember that *running is risky and leads to falls.* Often the same task can be accomplished just as rapidly by brisk walking, which is much safer. *For safe movement,* well-fitting shoes are essential. Some facilities have policies that prohibit clogs and other shoes with open toes or heels. Such shoes can prove hazardous, particularly if running becomes necessary, *because they may slip off and trip the wearer.*

Keep to the Right in Hallways

It is easy to run into someone else whose attention is diverted. Therefore, as a general practice, always walk to the right. This provides for a smoother flow of traffic.

Turn Corners Carefully

Most collisions take place when two people are rounding a corner. Always keep to the right, slow your pace, and turn corners carefully. This is of particular importance when you are pushing a stretcher or cart. Safety organizations have mandated the placement near the ceiling of mirrors on intersecting walls *to allow you to see around the corner and avoid such collisions.*

Open Doors Slowly

An opening door may easily strike someone on the other side. If it is opened slowly, it is less likely to cause injury.

© 1996 by Lippincott-Raven Publishers

With swinging doors that have a glass insert, it is possible to see whether anyone is on the other side of the door. Even with this safety precaution, however, *distractions can interfere with full vision,* and a door can strike another person.

Use Stretchers Properly

When *pushing a patient on a stretcher, keep the patient's head toward your body.* This is done *so that the head, which is highly vulnerable to impact injury, is protected, and the feet, which are less vulnerable, are outward.*

When pushing a stretcher, occupied or unoccupied, or a cart or conveyance of any kind, keep your eyes to the front at all times. *Looking away for even a second can result in a collision and possible injury to another.*

Use Brakes on Beds, Wheelchairs, and Stretchers

When beds, wheelchairs, and stretchers are stationary, apply the brake or brakes. On beds and stretchers, the brake is usually a flat metal "rocking" bar near the wheels. Pushing down on one side of the bar with your foot applies the brake, and pushing on the opposite side releases it. On wheelchairs, the brake is usually a small handle near the wheel. Moving the handle toward the occupant causes a bar to compress the rubber wheel and prevent it from moving. When a patient is being transferred to one of these pieces of equipment or when it is standing still, *the braking action prevents accidental movement that may lead to injury.*

Place Elevators on "Hold" When Loading or Unloading

When you are pushing a patient in a wheelchair or stretcher, place elevator operating buttons on "hold." *This will keep the doors open until you and the patient are safely in or out of the elevator.* Back into the elevator with an occupied wheelchair *so that if the door does not hold with the hold request button and suddenly closes, you, rather than the patient, will receive the impact* (Fig. 3–2).

Safety in Working Spaces, Halls, and Corridors

Lighting

Ensure that working spaces are lighted well enough *to allow objects and people to be seen clearly.* During the late evening hours, hallways are sometimes dimmed *so that patients can rest more comfortably,* but lighting should always be at a level *that will ensure clear visibility.*

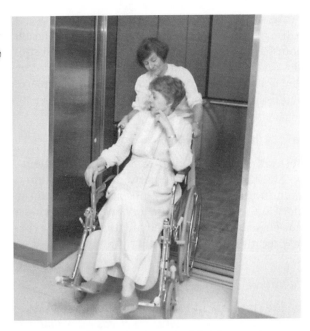

Figure 3–2. Back the patient in a wheelchair into an elevator, so that if the door closes prematurely, the patient will not be injured.

Floor Surfaces

Whether the flooring is of tile, linoleum, or carpeting, surfaces should be smooth. Cracked tiles, raised linoleum, or torn carpeting *can easily lead to falls.* Highly polished floors *also can cause skidding, falls, and injury.* Dropped materials, such as tissues or food substances, should be retrieved immediately, *because they can cause a staff member, a visitor, or a patient to skid.* Wipe up liquid spills immediately. Calling a custodian or maintenance person *could cause a delay long enough to expose someone to the danger of a fall.* If mopping is in progress, "Danger, Wet Floor" signs should always be posted.

Electrical Appliances

Ensure that all electrical appliances being used are in good working order and have a cord weight that is adequate for the appliance. A frayed or damaged cord or plug should never be used *because it may cause sparks or fire, injuring the operator or endangering the surrounding area.* All plugs should be the three-pronged ground type (Fig. 3–3) *so that the third prong carries any unexpected, potentially dangerous bursts of electricity to the ground.*

When an appliance, such as an electric floor polishing machine, is being used in a hallway or work area, the cord should not lay where people can trip over it. Cords that have to remain in place should be taped to the floor away from walking areas. The policy of most healthcare facilities is to prohibit any electrical appliance that is brought into the facility

from home or to require that such appliances be inspected by an electrician. Unused electrical outlets in settings where young children are present should have a safety cover in place *to protect children from electrical shocks.*

Needles and Other Sharp Objects

Most needle sticks are sustained when the nurse is attempting to recap a needle. Based on the recommendation of the CDC, OSHA has established a regulation that hospital personnel should never manually recap contaminated needles. A nurse doing so is considered in violation of the regulation and the employing agency could be cited and fined if this action were documented by an inspector. This regulation is enforced *to reduce the chance of needle sticks and the risk of exposure to diseases transmitted by blood and body fluids,* such as hepatitis and acquired immunodeficiency syndrome (AIDS). Specifically, the needle should be either instantly deposited into a bedside "sharps" receptacle (Fig. 3–4) after use, or if such a receptacle is not close by, the cap can be placed on a flat surface and "scooped up" with the needle.

The capped needle can then be safely carried to the nearest receptacle. You should develop the habit of never recapping any used needle. Recapping sterile needles does not violate the regulation, although carrying an uncapped needle down a hallway is in violation. Razor blades, scalpels (surgical knife blades), and other small, sharp instruments may also be put in these sharps receptacles. Hospitals and long-term care facilities are required to provide such receptacles in patients' rooms and medication areas. Directions for safely handling contaminated needles are provided in Module 50, Giving Injections.

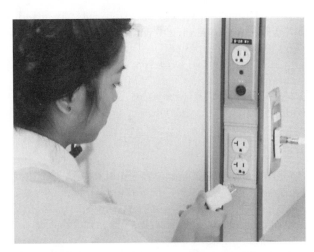

Figure 3–3. A three-pronged plug provides grounding for electrical current.

© 1996 by Lippincott-Raven Publishers

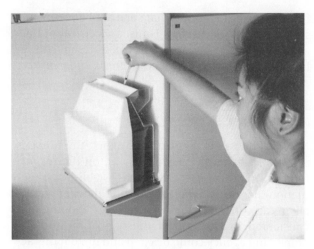

Figure 3–4. A receptacle used for needles and sharp objects to avoid needle sticks.

Dangerous or Caustic Substances or Materials

OSHA's Hazard Communication Standard of August 1988 directed all industries, including healthcare facilities, to provide workers who handle hazardous substances with guidelines for minimizing risks. Those requiring gloves or masks for protection must be clearly designated.

Evidence indicates that nurses are increasingly exposed to potentially hazardous procedures and substances. For example, the administration of even low-level antineoplastic drugs has been suspected of causing miscarriages in pregnant nurses (Jacobson, 1990). Inhaling the particles in the air surrounding laser surgery or having unprotected eyes exposed to the laser beam can be dangerous. Also, a number of transmittable viruses in hospital patients were previously not identified as hazardous. The Infection Control staff person within the hospital can provide you with more specific data.

All products, regardless of where they are used, should be clearly labeled to warn of any risks or dangers. They should never be left within easy reach of others in hallways or work spaces, including nurses' stations. *They could be ingested by children or by people who are confused or incompetent.* A liquid substance could be spilled, *causing burns or injury.*

Uncluttered Hallways

Government codes usually prohibit the presence of equipment in hallways. *In a fire or emergency, such equipment could block the access of emergency personnel and equipment and interfere with the evacuation of patients and staff* (Fig. 3–5).

Some facilities, however, have hallways with "nurse servers" attached to the corridor walls for each patient or for several patients in adjacent rooms. These contain charts, medications, and supplies and provide a charting area. *Making such items more accessible greatly saves staff time,* and this placement is in compliance with fire codes.

Safety in the Patient's Room

Most falls and other injuries occur in the patient's room (Cutchins, 1991). Many of the precautions taken in other areas of the hospital also pertain to safety in the patient's room. Review those previously discussed, and pay particular attention to the special precautions that follow.

Lighting

Be sure that patient rooms have enough light *to allow the ambulatory patient to see objects easily that may be in the way and to allow staff to work without difficulty.* At night most patients who have slept in complete darkness at home are not disturbed by the use of a wall nightlight. *This light helps to orient both the bedridden patient and the patient who is able to get out of bed to use the bathroom.*

Floor Surfaces

Ensure that floors are smooth and in good repair. *An unsteady patient is more likely to slip than an able-bodied visitor or staff member.*

Provide nonslip mats or a bath towel for use on the floor of a shower or on the bottom of a bathtub *to prevent slipping.* It also is a good idea to have hand rails and a call cord within reach *to ensure the safety of the patient.*

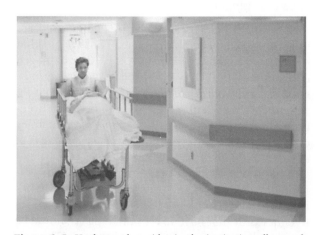

Figure 3–5. Uncluttered corridor in the institution allows safe movement for patients and staff.

© 1996 by Lippincott-Raven Publishers

Oxygen

If oxygen is in use, take special precautions *to ensure that sparks and flames never occur in the vicinity.* Oxygen, as a gas, does not itself explode, *but it supports rapid combustion, and materials will burn at an explosive rate in its presence*

Post a "No Smoking" sign on the door of the room to remind the patient and visitors not to smoke. Keep in mind that electrical appliances, including electric razors, are not to be used when oxygen therapy is in use. These precautions are of utmost importance for safety.

Furniture

Be sure that all furniture in the patient's room is arranged to allow easy access to the wash basin, bathroom, closet area, and door. *This protects ambulatory patients and staff members from bumps or falls.* Some beds may have a bedside stand that contains a console used for summoning the nurse and operating the television. This stand is attached in such a way that it swings out away from the bed. Although *consoles are more convenient for the patient,* remember that stretching toward a stand that is just out of reach has caused serious falls for many patients.

Medications and Dangerous Substances

Remove medications and dangerous substances from the bedside *to prevent a visitor or someone for whom they were not intended from ingesting them.* A physician may authorize medications to be kept at the bedside for the patient to self-administer. Check the policy of your facility regarding where these are to be stored. If a liquid used in treatment, such as a saline or hydrogen peroxide solution, is to be kept at the bedside, the container should be clearly marked.

Doors

Fully open or fully close entrance doors and bathroom, closet, and cabinet doors at all times *to eliminate the possibility of people colliding with them.* If door latches are not functioning properly, have them fixed or replaced.

PROTECTING THE DEPENDENT PATIENT

The Dependent Adult

It is part of the nursing role to protect patients who are partially or completely unable to protect themselves. Patients at special risk for falls and injury include children; those who are elderly or confused; those who have sensory deficits, impaired mobility, a history of falls, or a history of substance abuse; and those who are receiving medications that interfere with normal functioning. Rader (1991) found that certain modifications in space, lighting, furniture, and equipment decrease the possibility of falls. A few important environmental considerations follow.

Position of the Bed

Ensure that all occupied beds remain in the low position unless bed height is needed for care procedures. In this way, *if the patient should fall, the distance is lessened.*

Side Rails

Side rails are reminders to the patient of the narrow boundaries of the bed and may prevent falls and injury. Use them thoughtfully. If there is any doubt about the patient's safety, however, a nursing judgment can be made to use them. Some falls occur when patients attempt to climb over raised rails. *To prevent this,* a device can be used that will alert the nurse when a patient attempts to climb over a rail or get abruptly out of bed. The device consists of a slim, plastic-covered rod placed widthwise under the mattress. An electric alarm box fits underneath the bed. If the patient suddenly rises up and reduces pressure on the mattress, the alarm sounds. Casual movements, such as position changes and turning, will not activate the alarm. These devices are usually obtained from the housekeeping or central supply department.

Positioning

Position the unconscious or immobile patient in good body alignment, making sure that extremities are not caught beneath the heavier portions of the body or on the side rails. *Failure to do this could lead to nerve impingement and permanent damage.* The patient's position should be changed every 2 hours *to prevent pressure ulcers and maintain comfort.*

Protection from Sharp Objects

Dropped instruments, utensils, pieces of debris, fingernail clippings, and even minute loose hairs between the patient's body and the bed *can cause irritation and eventual skin breakdown.* Ensure that such items are not dropped into the bed, and inspect and

© 1996 by Lippincott-Raven Publishers

rearrange linens frequently *to safeguard the dependent patient.*

Nurses should be discouraged from wearing nail polish, but if they do, it must be kept in good repair *so that it does not chip and fall into the bed.*

Eyes

Routinely examine the eyes of the comatose patient not only for irritation, but for the *presence of foreign bodies that may cause harm.* Keep all sharp objects away from eyes. If the eyes of the patient in a coma are open and do not blink enough *to lubricate the cornea,* it is sometimes necessary to pad and tape the lids closed *to protect the eyes from ulceration.*

When caring for contact lenses, follow the guidelines for the specific lens worn. Removal and care of contacts for patients who are unable to care for their own lenses is discussed in Module 18, Hygiene. *Failure to remove and clean contact lenses properly can lead to damage or infection of the eyes.*

Air Passages

Protect the patient's airway at all costs. *To eliminate the risk of aspiration,* never use linty cloth, loose cotton balls, or caustic substances around the air passages of the dependent patient. When patients are unable to swallow saliva, they should be positioned on their side *so that the saliva will drain from the mouth rather than occlude the airway and be aspirated.*

The Dependent Child

Because children are in the early stages of development, they may be at a higher risk for injury than adults. It is essential that staff acknowledge the responsibility to provide the same kind of safety precautions that are taught to parents. All the precautions just discussed for the dependent adult patient are applicable to the dependent child. There also are some additional responsibilities. Each situation requires careful assessment and discretion.

To prevent falls, never leave infants and small children unattended when they are lying on a high surface, such as an examination table. Never leave them unattended in tubs, *where they might slip and drown.* Lock up or make inaccessible all medications and products used on the unit *so that nothing can be taken unintentionally* and cause harm. Use glass thermometers with a pediatric patient only when the child can safely hold one in the mouth without biting it. Protect the airway at all costs *to maintain adequate ventilation.* Ensure that foods are of a consistency that allows them to be chewed and swallowed

without choking. Mints, nuts, and popcorn are not appropriate for a small child *because of the high risk of choking.* Inspect toys for evidence of loose small parts *that could be detached and swallowed.* Place protectors over electrical outlets *to prevent a child from inserting fingers or small objects, which could lead to electric shock.* Nurses caring for infants or children must intensify their vigilance for possible safety hazards.

OTHER SAFETY CONSIDERATIONS

Other environmental considerations are important for those working and being cared for in healthcare settings. Unstable temperature control, inadequate ventilation, and improper food preparation or waste disposal are just a few examples of conditions *that could endanger patients, staff, and visitors.* Report any of these conditions immediately to the supervisor of that area, such as the engineer or custodian responsible for temperature control, ventilation, or waste disposal. Notify the nutritionist or kitchen manager of any concerns you may have about food preparation.

Many therapeutic agents used to treat disease have specific safety hazards. Chemotherapeutic agents and radio isotopes used for treating cancer are just two of these potentially dangerous therapeutic agents.

Discussion of the specific hazards of these agents is beyond the scope this text. However, it is your nursing responsibility to investigate therapeutic agents in use as to their safe administration and the possible hazards they pose for patients and healthcare providers.

Protection against harmful microorganisms is a constant concern and responsibility for the nurse. See Module 2, Basic Infection Control; Module 32, Isolation Technique; and Module 33, Sterile Technique for specific information related to providing safety from infection.

Nurses can do many things to become more resistant to the many disease-causing organisms that are always present to some extent in the hospital environment. General good health habits, such as proper nutrition, adequate rest, and lessened stress, *enhance the body's immune system and decrease the chances of infection.*

SAFETY DEVICES AND RESTRAINTS

Safety devices include a wide variety of devices that can keep individuals with specific problems safer. These devices include both physical and chemical restraints and nonrestraint devices.

© 1996 by Lippincott-Raven Publishers

▼ NURSING DIAGNOSES

A nursing diagnosis to keep in mind when considering the use of any safety device is Risk for Injury. Patients can be injured by falls, manipulating or removing equipment necessary to therapy, or scratching irritated areas.

Another nursing diagnosis that can be related to the use of physical restraints is Risk for Violence: Self-directed or directed at others. This nursing diagnosis might be appropriate for patients who exhibit suicidal behavior or who are overtly hostile or aggressive toward staff members.

Hazards of Using Safety Devices and Restraints

Although these devices are almost always used with safety for the patient or staff as a goal, the restrained patient may feel punished rather than safe and may react by becoming more distressed and angry, at least for a while. This increased agitation can lead to falls or other injuries (bruises, lacerations) that occur when the patient attempts to "escape."

Later, resignation and withdrawal may set in. In addition, all safety devices or restraints impose some degree of immobility, which can be hazardous. Contractures, pressure ulcers, dehydration, chronic constipation, functional incontinence, loss of bone mass, muscle tone, and the ability to move about independently have all been known to occur at least partially as the result of safety devices or restraints being applied *to provide safety*(Blakeslee, Goldman, Papougenis, & Torell, 1991).

Use of Restraints and the Law

The federal Omnibus Budget Reconciliation Act (OBRA) of 1987 included a provision that patients in healthcare settings have the right to be free from unnecessary physical and chemical restraints. Restraints were defined as "any manual method or mechanical device, material or equipment . . . that the individual cannot remove easily which restricts freedom of movement or normal access to one's body" (Federal Register, 1989). The word "restraint" can be offensive because it suggests denying a person's dignity and self-determination by restricting the ability to move. To ensure that right, all healthcare facilities are mandated to meet strict guidelines regarding the use of any type of restraint in order to qualify for Medicare and Medicaid reimbursement. Since this Act was im-

plemented in 1991, some healthcare facilities have adopted a "restraint-free environment" policy. To support these actions, many nonrestraint safety devices have been developed. Although acute care facilities were not initially included in these regulations, they are now required to meet these standards.

A wide variety of medications can be used to restrict an individual's behavior or activity. These medications are sometimes referred to as *chemical restraints.* Although valuable in some situations, there is a great potential for abuse of these drugs by caregivers who use chemical restraints as a substitute for personal attention and care for the patient.

Information specific to the use of safety devices and restraints with infants and toddlers can be found in Module 19, Basic Infant Care.

Types of Restraints

Many restraints are available to provide safety for the patient. Each restraint has a specific purpose; using the least restrictive device that maintains adequate protection is a legal and professional standard for the nurse. The manufacturer's directions for use must be followed. All restraints are considered medical devices and therefore must receive FDA approval. Facility-produced devices do not have FDA approval and therefore do not meet this standard.

Belt Restraints

Belt restraints are threaded at the back and are used to prevent the patient from falling out of the bed or chair (Fig. 3–6). The belt is fastened around the pa-

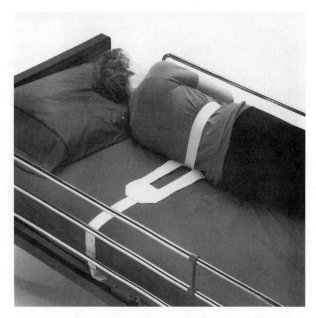

Figure 3–6. Belt restraints prevent the patient from falling out of bed or chair.

© 1996 by Lippincott-Raven Publishers

tient's waist, and the ties are fastened to the bed or wheelchair frame. Disposable belt restraints also are available.

Vest Restraints

These canvas or mesh vests have long ties that are secured to the bed frame (Fig. 3–7). The ties may cross at the front or back, depending on the design of the vest. Vest restraints are used when the patient needs more support or a stronger reminder than a simple belt provides. Attach the ties to the nonmovable part of the bed.

Some vest restraints have shoulder loops. If the patient is unable to maintain an erect posture, short straps can be passed through the loops and slipped over the wheelchair handles *to prevent leaning forward.*

Jacket Restraints

Jacket restraints fit over the patient's head. The neck opening is secured with a zipper or Velcro closure. There are secure ties fixed to the waist of the jacket. These ties may then be tied to the bed or wheelchair frame.

Elbow or Knee Restraints

These are canvas or mesh wraparound ties that have lengthwise rigid stays *to prevent joint flexion* (Fig. 3–8). They are used most often to prevent the pediatric or confused patient from disturbing a tube or dressing or from scratching a rash.

Wrist or Ankle Restraints

Commercial wrist or ankle restraints are cloth straps with a thread-through buckle device or Velcro cuff. They are usually used to restrict motion of a limb for therapeutic reasons, such as to maintain an IV or prevent the patient from pulling out a tube (Fig. 3–9).

Slip the device on the patient's wrist or ankle, thread it, and tie it to the bed frame; never tie it to a side rail because *if the rails were suddenly lowered, the patient could be injured.* Attach wrist and ankle ties to the movable portion of the bed frame *so that if the head or foot of the bed is raised, the ties will not be pulled.* Disposable wrist and ankle restraints, made of fabric or soft but strong paper, also are available.

Mitt Restraints

Mitt restraints (Fig. 3–10) are used for patients who absentmindedly pull at tubes or appliances or who may injure themselves by scratching a rash or picking at a wound. They restrict only the hand and fingers and *allow the arm to move freely.*

Mitts are available commercially, or they can be made by wrapping the hands loosely with strips of soft fabric or rolls of dressing material. Secure the wrapping with paper tape *to prevent skin irritation and allow easy removal.* Remove the mitts periodically, as

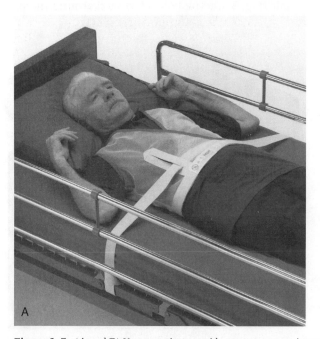
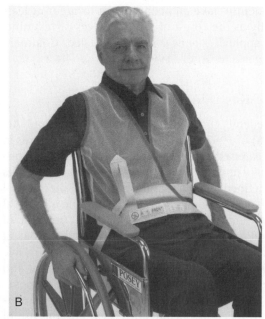

Figure 3–7. (**A** and **B**) Vest restraints provide support to a patient who is confined to bed and can aid the patient in a chair to maintain a more erect posture.

© 1996 by Lippincott-Raven Publishers

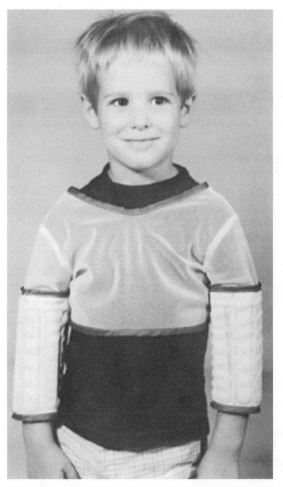

Figure 3–8. Elbow restraints are often used to prevent a pediatric patient from disturbing a tube or dressing. (Courtesy J. T. Posey Company, Arcadia, California)

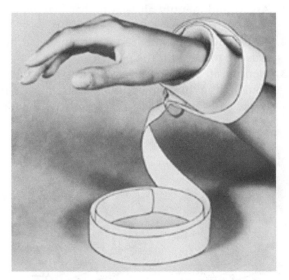

Figure 3–9. Wrist or ankle restraints are always tied to the bed frame, never to a side rail. (Courtesy J. T. Posey Company, Arcadia, California)

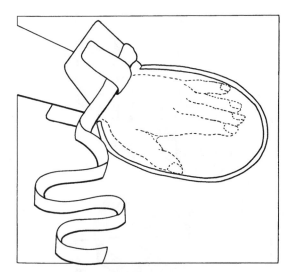

Figure 3–10. The mitt restraint restricts only the hand and fingers and allows the arm to move freely.

you would other devices, *to clean and exercise the hands and fingers.*

Knots Used With Safety Devices

Traditionally the clove hitch and the square knot were used to secure safety devices. The *clove hitch* allows the patient some movement. *Because this knot is relatively loose* and does not tighten with movement of an extremity, circulation to the part is not restricted (Fig. 3–11). The *square knot* is used more often to secure a tie to the bed frame or back of a wheelchair *because it will not slip.*

Concerns about patient safety in case of an emergency have led all long-term care facilities and hospitals to adopt quick release knots for restraints. Ties are looped around the outside frame twice and then tied with a knot that can be released quickly. Although these may be more easily released by the patient, the added safety in case of fire or disaster is mandated by the OBRA regulations (Fig. 3-12). Placing them out of reach of the patient is essential.

Some facilities are adopting restraints that fasten with Velcro closures and attach to the bed or wheelchair with clips. These are easy and quick to use and do not rely on every individual remembering how to tie appropriate quick-release knots. Many existing restraints can be modified by the addition of clips. "D" rings may be fixed to bed and wheelchair frames by a variety of techniques. These further facilitate the use of either appropriate knots or clips for fastening.

Nonrestraint Safety Devices

Nonrestraint safety devices are those that the patient can release independently for desired movement.

© 1996 by Lippincott-Raven Publishers

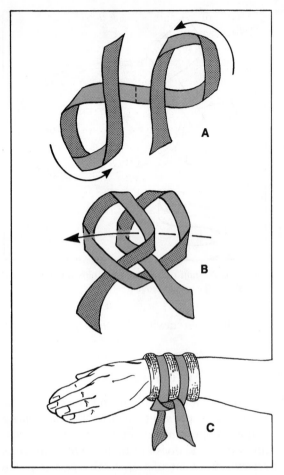

Figure 3–11. Clove hitch: Pad wrist or ankle with gauze or cloth. (**A**) Using a 54-inch strip of gauze, make two loops. (**B**) Place loops together, and put wrist or ankle through loops. (**C**) Allowing 1/2 inch for comfort, tie a half hitch to secure. Tie free ends to bed frame.

Types of Nonrestraint Safety Devices

A *wedge cushion* may be placed in a wheelchair with the thicker end toward the front of the seat so that the main weight of the patient's body rests more securely in the chair. With the weight at the back of the seat, it is more difficult for the patient to slide out

or to arise unaided. There is no restriction for the patient, and this may be all that is needed to keep a patient safely in a chair (Fig. 3–13).

A *safety belt* may be placed around a chair and a patient's lap. This may have either an airline style quick-release or a Velcro fastener. The safety belt slows the patient's progress in standing unaided, allowing staff to come to assist. A safety belt also prevents falls from a wheelchair caused by the patient's weakness or instability. Because the patient is able to release the belt, it is not considered a restraint. People are accustomed to safety belts in cars and airplanes and therefore do not have adverse feelings about using them.

A *lap-board* over the front of a chair may prevent a patient from falling forward out of a chair and provide support for the very weak patient. Patients often respond very differently and favorably to a lap-board than to a restraint that prevents their falling.

A *torso support* with a front Velcro closure may be used to support the individual who does not have enough body strength to remain upright in a chair. Because the device can be released by the patient, it is not considered a restraint.

Large foam bolsters that fit on the arms or sides of a wheelchair also may be used for the individual who lacks the ability to maintain stability of the trunk. These help the patient to comfortably maintain an upright position.

GENERAL PROCEDURE FOR APPLYING SAFETY DEVICES AND RESTRAINTS

Assessment

1. Assess and identify all factors that may be contributing to the patient's risk for injury.
2. Assess the environment to determine what hazards are present for the patient.
3. Identify all types of safety devices available in your setting. In some facilities, restraints are referred to as *protective devices*. In others, they are

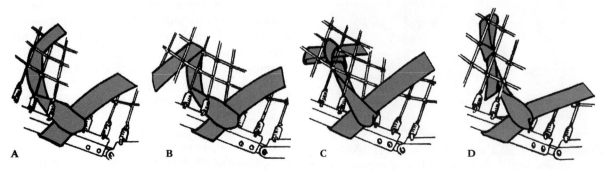

Figure 3–12. (**A–D**) The "quick release" knot provides safety for the patient in the event of an emergency.

© 1996 by Lippincott-Raven Publishers

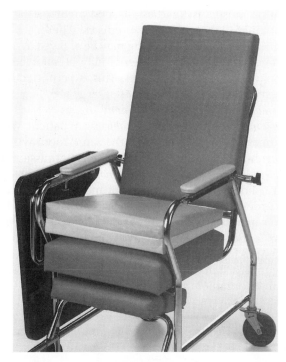

Figure 3–13. Using a wedge cushion in a chair prevents the patient from sliding downward and assists the patient to rise.

commonly called *Poseys*, after a leading manufacturer of safety devices and restraints.

4. If the patient already has a safety device or restraint in place, assess the need for the device. *The situation that made the device necessary may have changed, or the patient may need a different type of restraint.* The decision to apply a safety device or to restrain a patient physically must always be made after careful assessment. Restrict the patient's movements as little as possible to accomplish your purpose.

Planning

5. If a restrictive restraint is applied, a physician's order must be secured unless the safety consideration is an emergency. In such a situation, it is permissible to seek the order *after* the safety device has been applied. *If the immediate safety of a patient or of the staff is in question,* apply restraints at once, and secure an order at the earliest possible moment. A new standard of the Joint Commission for the Accreditation of Healthcare Organizations is that of a "time-limited" physician's order for any type of restraint used. This means that a physician's order for this action must be obtained by the nurse within a reasonable period of time. If this procedure is not followed, *the patient could take legal action against you.* You should be aware of state law in your locale and agency policy regarding the use of restraints.

Restraints should be used, however, only when absolutely necessary, and then only until an alternative intervention can be devised. Sometimes the presence of a family member or friend makes restraining the patient unnecessary, at least for a time. Nonrestraint safety devices do not need a physician's order.

6. When a restraint is required, choose the least restrictive device necessary to protect the patient or staff effectively. For example, if a patient is attempting to remove a nasogastric tube with the left hand, and the right upper extremity is paralyzed, you can use a wrist restraint only on the left wrist. You might leave the tie loose enough *to allow some flexion of the elbow,* though not enough to let the patient reach the nasogastric tube. You can always modify what you have chosen to use later if necessary.

7. Wash your hands *for infection control.*

8. Plan for any assistance that may be needed. You may need help with positioning or perhaps to calm the confused or irrational patient.

9. Obtain the chosen device.

Implementation

10. Identify the patient *to be sure you are carrying out the procedure for the correct patient.*

11. When possible, provide for the patient's elimination needs before applying any device. *This adds to the patient's comfort and lessens the chance that you will have to remove the safety device or restraint to provide for elimination immediately after it is in place.*

12. Regardless of how irrational a patient might be, always explain what you plan to do and why. Never convey the impression that a restraint is used as punishment. For example, you might say that the device is to "remind" the patient not to lean too far forward in the chair. *This often makes the procedure more acceptable.*

13. Apply the device, using an appropriate knot if needed. If the patient is in bed, never knot the ties to the side rails *because if the rails were suddenly lowered, the patient could be injured.* Knot the ties to the bed frame instead. Be careful not to secure any restraint too tightly *so that you do not cause the patient discomfort, impair circulation, or restrict function. For example, a vest restraint that is too tight could restrict breathing.*

14. If the patient is extremely restless or has fragile skin, add extra padding to the restraint *to protect the tissues.* You can use clean cloths, stockinette or gauze padding.

15. Reassure the patient.

16. Remove any safety device or restraints every 2

© 1996 by Lippincott-Raven Publishers

hours or less, *so that the patient's position can be changed and the body part under restraint can be inspected and exercised.* Never leave a restraint on for longer than 2 hours without checking and moving it.

17. Reapply the safety device or restraint if necessary.

18. Wash your hands *for infection control.*

Evaluation
19. Evaluate using the following criteria:
  a. Patient comfort
  b. Effectiveness of the safety device or restraint
  c. Continued need for the safety device or restraint

Documentation
20. Record on the nurses' notes or flow sheets:
  a. The type and location of the safety device or restraint
  b. The time and the reason for application. If you do not yet have a physician's order, note that the physician has been notified of your action.
  c. The condition of skin under the restraints, distal circulation, and removal of restraints for skin care and range-of-motion as appropriate. There may be a flow sheet for this purpose.

SMOKING AS A HAZARD IN THE HEALTHCARE FACILITY

Smoking has become a major health hazard in our society, and it can pose unique problems in a healthcare facility. Not only can fires be started accidentally, but smoking is known to have harmful effects on both those who smoke and those around them. Many health organizations have clearly documented harmful physical effects on nonsmokers who inhale smoke produced by others. For some time, cigarettes have not been sold in healthcare facilities *to discourage what is recognized as a major health risk.*

Most hospitals have established a complete "no smoking" policy on their premises. There are, of course, exceptions. Smoking may be allowed in designated areas. Certain patients may be allowed to smoke with a doctor's order. This is permitted because *the stress to a long-term smoker of not being able to smoke, when added to the many stresses of being ill, can compound the patient's problems.* A patient who smokes cannot be placed in the same room with a nonsmoker without the nonsmoker's permission, *to protect the nonsmoker's right to a smoke-free environment.* Any patient who is confused or medicated and has an order to permit smoking should do so only under the supervision of a staff person *to prevent accidental fires.* If the staff does not have time to closely monitor smoking, ask the patient to refrain from smoking until a staff member is available. Only nonflammable containers should be used as ashtrays.

FIRE PLANS

Healthcare facilities must adhere to fire code standards. Nurses must know what to do in the event of a fire of any size. Fire plans vary somewhat in different facilities, but all have similar basic principles. The plan is written into the procedure or policy manual of the facility. Basically, most plans follow the fire code guidelines given below.

FIRE CODE PROCEDURE
1. Know the fire code and initiating procedure in your facility. *To avoid alarming patients and visitors,* a code is used both to report the fire and to notify others in the building. There may be a special number on the telephone that signals the telephone operator in the building to call the fire department and notify those in the facility. The overhead paging system is commonly used to voice-page a code, frequently in the form of

DATE/TIME		
6/14/99 1020	S	*"I'm sorry I keep slipping down in the chair, I feel like I'm going to fall."*
	O	*Patient's buttocks slipping forward when in wheelchair even though wearing vest restraint.*
	A	*Unable to move self upright in chair.*
	P	*Use wedge cushion in wheelchair. Explain its use to patient.* — W. Dickinson, RN

Example of Nursing Progress Notes Using SOAP Format

© 1996 by Lippincott-Raven Publishers

a number or code name. Some facilities have a fire bell that sounds softly but insistently. Whatever the system, become familiar with it.

2. If you are actually at the location of the fire, first and foremost remove any patient to a safe distance before taking the time to "call" the fire code. This prevents harm to the patient.

3. Initiate the fire code according to the policy at your facility.

4. If you do not "call" the fire code yourself but hear the code paged or the fire bell, return immediately to your nursing unit. The rationale for this procedure *is to mobilize all personnel who might be useful in the emergency.*

5. Never use elevators to return to your unit or for any other purpose. They must remain free so that firefighters and emergency equipment can be transported. Also, elevators may cease to work if the fire involves electrical wiring, causing them to resemble chimneys in a fire, rapidly filling with smoke.

6. On the unit, return patients who are in the hallways to their rooms. Close all doors to rooms. This is done to contain the fire and keep smoke from spreading through the environment.

7. Be available to calm patients and visitors.

8. Follow any additional directions of the person in charge. If the danger is immediate, take action. This may include the use of fire extinguishers. Although all fire extinguishers now are red rather than color-coded, each has its classification clearly designated on the container along with words and pictures of the items against which it is effective. Class A is a water or solution type, designed to be used on paper and linens; Class B is a foam extinguisher, designed to be used on grease and other chemicals; and Class C is a carbon dioxide or a dry chemical type, designed to be used on electrical fires. On patient units, most facilities have a variation of the Class C extinguisher that is multipurpose and can be used for paper or linens or on electrical fires. Some facilities hold in-service classes on using fire extinguishers. If your facility does not, this equipment is usually described for you in the unit manual. Read this section closely, and locate and examine any fire extinguishers that are on your unit so that you are prepared if the need arises.

9. If there are no specific directions, stand quietly in the hallway, where you will be visible in case an evacuation of patients is ordered.

10. *Because smoke and fire are real dangers to the health of patients,* those in charge may order an evacuation. If this occurs, move patients according to procedure. *The goal is to move the most patients in the shortest time.* To accomplish this, direct those who are ambulatory to exits first *because they can move more rapidly.* Then help out those in wheelchairs or using assistive devices. Finally, move those who are bedridden and who need transfer. Remaining calm is essential. Lifting patients is sometimes more hazardous to the patient and the nurse than simply lowering patients to blankets on the floor and pulling them to safety. Remember to assure people who are restrained or in a confining device, such as a cast, that they will be promptly evacuated. Your actions during this time will depend on those in charge and on your own decision-making ability. Being prepared can be comforting and useful should the need arise.

11. Remain calm.

12. Wait for further directions or the sound of the all-clear signal.

DISASTER PLANS

Disaster plans usually cover hazardous occurrences other than fire. Disaster plans are of two types: internal and external. Internal disasters include explosions, collapse of a part of the building, or damage to the building as a result of earthquakes, flooding, or toxic fumes. External disasters may affect the facility but have more to do with disaster in the community. In this category are such happenings as aircraft, train, and transit crashes; earthquakes; collapses of buildings; uncontained fires involving sections of a city; extensive flooding; landslides; and widespread toxic fumes.

To differentiate between external and internal disaster codes, facilities use one of several methods. Some call them by color (eg, a red or green disaster code); others may call the internal code "A" and the external one "B." Be familiar with the system used in your facility before the need arises.

Internal Disaster Codes

Just like fire plans, disaster plans assign a specific role to each staff person in the event of a disaster. Usually, this involves a return to the unit, where further assignments may be given. A special part of the facility is designated as a "triage" area. Triage means prioritization of patients according to their injuries *so that the most expedient and appropriate treatment can be given to a large number of people.*

Personnel with special skills, such as starting intravenous therapy or suturing wounds, for example,

© 1996 by Lippincott-Raven Publishers

may have specific assignments. Others may transport or maintain patients who are injured or emotionally upset. *Because internal disaster plans vary,* you should carefully read and become knowledgeable about the plans of the facility in which you practice.

External Disaster Codes

These plans are regional so that several facilities within the community can respond. In large urban areas, one hospital takes responsibility for continually monitoring the availability of critical care beds for those who need immediate life-saving medical intervention and acute care beds for those who need close monitoring and more intensive nursing care. The hospital supervisor or coordinator, after notifying the administrator, usually has the responsibility of activating the plan within the facility. All personnel are categorized according to their skills, and travel times from home are catalogued so that additional personnel can be summoned quickly. Different facilities may take on responsibility for different types of care; a hospital with a burn unit, for example, may receive patients with burns, while other facilities receive patients with other types of injuries. Again, become acquainted with the policy in your facility and community.

Fire and Disaster Drills

To evaluate the effectiveness of the staff's response to a fire or disaster code, drills are held occasionally. All participants respond as if a real code had been called. Some think a drill response is most effective if the institution's staff does not know whether or not a real emergency exists. All workers have the responsibility to review the emergency policies of a facility and determine their specific role in the event a code is called.

After a drill, it is useful to hold a debriefing session with all who participated *so that the process can be evaluated and suggestions given for more effectiveness in the future.* The more drills and debriefings held, the more calm and purposeful is the behavior on the part of those involved.

INCIDENT REPORTS

The incident report is used to document any unusual occurrence, accident, or error, not just errors in administering care or medications. Some facilities use different forms for different kinds of events (for example, medication errors and falls), whereas others use one standard form for all incidents. Figure 3–14 is an example of a patient or visitor accident report.

Incident reports serve several purposes. First, they *objectively document the event.* Second, because of this, *they are a record for insurance and legal reference.* Last, *they help identify the need to modify or correct procedures, policies, or situations within the healthcare facility.*

The incident report is completed by the staff person who discovers or is involved in the incident. *Because it may become a legal document,* it should contain good usage of language, pertinent facts, and the exact times and proper sequence of events. Only facts—not opinions or conclusions—are documented. If a report concerns a patient, the report is not incorporated into the patient's chart but is sent to the immediate supervisor and finally to administration. A notation about the incident is made in the chart. The report does not constitute an admission of liability, and the fact that one was filed is not documented in the chart. Complete and file an incident report in timely fashion, *because recall is more difficult if time has elapsed.*

An important issue in healthcare today is that of quality assurance (QA), which means measurement and ongoing monitoring of the quality of patient care. Most healthcare facilities have an active QA committee composed of a variety of staff members, including nurses. The incident report is useful for determining quality of the care provided and can facilitate improvements. The incident report may be called a quality assurance report.

LONG-TERM CARE

It is particularly important that precautions be taken for the protection of residents in long-term care facilities. *Many of these people are elderly, have impaired mobility, and have problems with neurosensory function.* As you review the various precautions for patients in hospitals, remember the many limitations of those in long-term care. For example, elderly people may fall because of disturbances in balance and gait. These people also may have difficulty feeling temperatures and sharp objects. The use of safety devices may not always prevent falls of elderly residents (Magee, et al., 1993). Because the needs of each resident are different, thorough assessment is essential. Assessment will be discussed in Module 6, Introduction to Assessment Skills.

© 1996 by Lippincott-Raven Publishers

INCIDENT REPORT

IDENTIFICATION	SEX	AGE	REPORT DATE	INCIDENT DATE	INCIDENT SHIFT	INCIDENT TIME	LOCATION OF INCIDENT
☒ Patient ☐ Visitor ☐ Employee (Non-injury) Dept.:	☐ MALE ☒ FEMALE	71	2/23/99	2/23/99	☒ 1ST ☐ 2ND ☐ 3RD	0700— 1500 (24 HR. CLOCK)	DEPT.: _Medical Unit - 7N_ ROOM NO: _781_

PATIENT CONDITION BEFORE INCIDENT:

☒ Oriented
☐ Disoriented
☐ Sedated
☐ Unconscious
☐ Other: _____

If **EMPLOYEE** injury, report to Health Nurse or Emergency Dept. in her absence.

INCIDENT INVOLVES: Describe incident below:

☐ Falls
☐ Blood
☐ Narcotic count incorrect
☒ Medication incident
☐ IV incident
☐ Equipment, supplies, waste
☐ Order on wrong patient

☐ Broken or lost article
☐ Loss of hospital requisition
☐ Equipment malfunction
　* (see below)
☐ Patient permit incorrect
☐ Other: _____

OTHER INFORMATION
☐ Bed rest
☒ Up with assistance
☐ Ambulatory

BED RAILS
☐ Up ☒ Down

HILO BED
☐ Up ☐ Down

POSEY IN USE
☐ Yes ☒ No

IF PATIENT - Diagnosis

Berta Simmons - angina pectoris

IF VISITOR - Reason for presence

ROOM NO: 781	ATTENDING PHYSICIAN: _Dr. Peter Adams_	HOME PHONE: (　　)

STATE INJURY:

none apparent

GIVE A BRIEF DESCRIPTION OF INCIDENT (Continue on reverse)

Prepared patient's medications; overlooked 9 a.m. Persantine 50 mg.

Did not discover ommission until 1 p.m. when next dose was due.

SIGNATURE: _Pam Bennett, N.S._　　TITLE: _nursing student_　　DEPARTMENT: _Eastern College_

NAMES/ADDRESSES OF WITNESSES (indicate if employee): _____
Sue Haggart, Instructor

✻EQUIPMENT INVOLVED:　　　　MANUFACTURER:　　　　SERIAL NO:

STATE ACTION TAKEN, INDICATE IF FURTHER INVESTIGATION REQUIRED (continue on reverse).

Observed patient for possible effect of omitted dose.

SUPERVISOR'S SIGNATURE

Was person seen by physician?	☒ YES ☐ NO ☐ REFUSED	If yes, record time (24 Hr.): _1330_ _2/23/94_	PHYSICIAN NAME/TIME NOTIFIED _Dr. Peter Adams_

RESIDENT FINDINGS:

RESIDENT'S SIGNATURE
Peter Adams, M.D.

ADDRESSOGRAPH OR NAME AND ADDRESS

SIMMONS, Berta　　F
_276-72-7134　　71_

SWEDISH HOSPITAL MEDICAL CENTER
Seattle, WA 98104

Figure 3–14. Incident report.

© 1996 by Lippincott-Raven Publishers

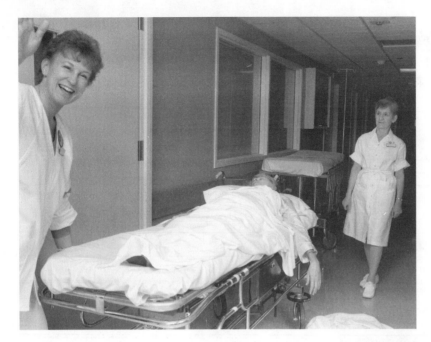

Critical thinking exercise: Identify the unsafe practices depicted in this photograph.

HOME CARE

Because many elderly and incapacitated people reside in private homes, safety becomes an issue. Nurses practicing in hospitals or long-term care facilities can review with the family a list of precautions to be taken when the patient is discharged. Attention should be given to proper lighting, eliminating physical obstacles, and providing smooth floors. Many other precautions can be taken. One example is the simple but important elimination of small floor rugs, *which can cause falls.* Homes should be evaluated for electrical safety before medical equipment is put into use. If the application of any safety device becomes necessary, the nurse should carefully instruct the care providers in its use.

The nurse who provides care in the home can also be effective in assessing the home environment for safety and acting as a valuable resource to the family. Suggestions can be made concerning specific changes *to minimize hazards.* Public funds are available in some states to alter the environment of those who are disabled to provide the maximum in safety. *Because the home is increasingly being used as a care setting,* more emphasis must be placed on providing safety. In the home setting, where family or other care providers are involved in client care, teaching the proper and safe use of equipment and maintaining a safe environment are major nursing responsibilities.

CRITICAL THINKING EXERCISES

• Your patient is an elderly woman who suffered a stroke a few days ago. She is semiconscious and slumped in a wheelchair. Her right side is flaccid with her right hand hanging over the arm of the chair and her right foot positioned between the footrests. Identify the safety hazards that are present. Describe the nursing actions you might take to protect the patient. For each nursing action, explain the rationale.

• Examine the photograph above and identify the unsafe practices that you observe.

References

Blakeslee, J. A., Goldman, B. D., Papougenis, D., & Torell, C. (1991). Making the transition to restraint free care. *Journal of Gerontological Nursing, 17*(2), 4–8.

Cutchins, C. H. (1991). Blueprint for restraint-free care. *American Journal of Nursing, 91*(7), 36–42.

US Department of Health and Human Services (1989). *Guidelines for prevention of transmission of human immunodeficiency virus and hepatitis B virus to health-care and public safety workers.* Atlanta: Centers for Disease Control.

Jacobson, E. (1990). New hospital hazards: How to protect yourself. *American Journal of Nursing, 90*(2), 36–41.

Magee, M., Hyatt, E. C., Hardin, S. B., Stratmann, D., Vonson, M. H., & Owen, M. (1993). Institutional policy: Use of restraints in extended care and nursing homes. *Journal of Gerontological Nursing, 19*(4), 31–39.

Rader, J. (1991). Modifying the environment to decrease use of restraints. *Journal of Gerontological Nursing, 17*(2), 8–13.

© 1996 by Lippincott-Raven Publishers

✔ PERFORMANCE CHECKLIST

Safe Staff Behavior	Needs More Practice	Satisfactory	Comments
1. Use good body mechanics.			
2. Walk; avoid running.			
3. Keep to the right in hallways.			
4. Turn corners carefully.			
5. Open doors slowly.			
6. Use stretchers properly.			
7. Use brakes on beds, wheelchairs, and stretchers.			
8. Place elevators on "hold" when loading or unloading.			
Safety in Working Spaces, Halls, and Corridors			
1. Obtain adequate lighting.			
2. Ensure that floor surfaces are in good repair, smooth, and free of spills and foreign material.			
3. Inspect electrical cords, and do not use those that are frayed or damaged.			
4. Never recap needles. Dispose of needles and other sharp objects in designated receptacles.			
5. Never leave dangerous or caustic substances unattended.			
6. Ensure that equipment never blocks hallways.			
Safety in the Patient's Room			
1. Obtain adequate lighting. Encourage the use of a nightlight.			
2. Ensure that floor surfaces are in good repair, smooth, and free of spills and foreign material.			
3. Keep oxygen away from sparks or flames. Check electrical equipment. Make sure that no one is smoking.			
4. Be sure furniture allows free access to wash basin, bathroom, and closet area.			
5. Never leave medications and dangerous substances in full view at the patient's bedside.			
6. Fully open or close entrance, bathroom, closet, and cabinet doors to prevent collisions with them.			
Protecting the Dependent Patient			
1. Ensure that beds remain in low position unless height is needed for a care procedure.			
2. Use side rails only to protect the patient from possible fall and injury.			

(continued)

© 1996 by Lippincott-Raven Publishers

Protecting the Dependent Patient *(Continued)*	Needs More Practice	Satisfactory	Comments
3. Position the patient so that extremities are not caught beneath body or on side rails.			
4. Prevent sharp objects and foreign materials from falling into the bed.			
5. Protect the eyes from foreign materials and possible ulceration.			
6. Protect air passages from aspirating foreign substances, materials, and fumes at all costs.			
General Procedure for Applying Safety Devices and Restraints			
Assessment			
1. Identify factors that may place the patient at risk for injury.			
2. Assess environment for hazards.			
3. Identify safety devices and restraints available in facility.			
4. If device is in place, assess current need.			
Planning			
5. If the safety consideration is emergent, apply device and obtain a physician's order in a timely manner. Otherwise, obtain an order.			
6. Choose least restrictive safety device or restraint.			
7. Wash your hands.			
8. Plan for any assistance needed.			
9. Obtain appropriate device for individual situation.			
Implementation			
10. Identify patient.			
11. Provide for elimination needs.			
12. Explain what you plan to do and why.			
13. Apply safety device or restraint.			
14. If needed, protect body tissues with padding.			
15. Reassure patient.			
16. Remove safety device or restraint every 2 hours for inspection and exercise.			
17. Reapply safety device or restraint if necessary.			
18. Wash your hands.			

(continued)

© 1996 by Lippincott-Raven Publishers

General Procedure for Applying Safety Devices and Restraints *(Continued)*	Needs More Practice	Satisfactory	Comments
Evaluation			
19. Evaluate using the following criteria: **a.** Patient comfort			
b. Effectiveness of the safety device or restraint			
c. Continued need for the safety device or restraint			
Documentation			
20. Document: **a.** Type and location of safety device or restraint			
b. Time and reason for application			
c. Condition of skin, circulation, skin care			
Fire Plans			
1. Know the fire code and initiating procedure in your facility.			
2. If you are at location of fire, remove any patient in the vicinity.			
3. Call the fire code.			
4. If you are not near the fire or if you do not call, return immediately to your unit.			
5. Do not use elevators.			
6. Return patients to their rooms, closing doors.			
7. Be available to calm patients.			
8. Follow directions of persons in charge.			
9. Stand quietly in hallway, available for any duties.			
10. If there is an evacuation, move patients according to procedure.			
11. Remain calm.			
12. Wait for further directions or sound of all clear.			

© 1996 by Lippincott-Raven Publishers

? **Q U I Z**

Short-Answer Questions

1. Give three reasons why providing a safe environment in the healthcare facility is important.

   a. _____

   b. _____

   c. _____

2. List five of the seven behaviors that demonstrate a concern for safety on the part of the nurse.

   a. _____

   b. _____

   c. _____

   d. _____

   e. _____

3. Describe a safe floor surface. _____

   _____

4. Discuss electrical safety precautions. _____

   _____

5. State why attempting to recap the needle of a syringe is unsafe and how needles and syringes are disposed of properly. _____

   _____

6. Describe a safe environment for the patient who is bedfast. _____

   _____

7. What is the most important safety precaution for the dependent patient in your care?

   _____

   _____

8. What rules or policies do healthcare facilities have about smoking? _____

   _____

   _____

9. Briefly, give the steps of responding to a fire code. _____

   _____

10. What might be the role of the staff nurse in a disaster plan? _____

    _____

11. What are the two main purposes for holding debriefing sessions after a fire or disaster drill?

    _____

    _____

© 1996 by Lippincott-Raven Publishers

12. In addition to reasons for safety in the hospital, name three additional reasons safety becomes even more important when working in a long-term care setting. _____

_____

_____

13. What could you do to help the family ensure safety for the person residing in a private home?

_____

_____

14. What are the three purposes of incident reports?

a. _____

b. _____

c. _____

MODULE

4

BASIC BODY MECHANICS

MODULE CONTENTS

RATIONALE FOR THE USE OF THIS
   SKILL
NURSING DIAGNOSIS
PRINCIPLES OF BASIC BODY
   MECHANICS
LONG-TERM CARE
HOME CARE
CRITICAL THINKING EXERCISES

PREREQUISITES

Successful completion of the following modules:

VOLUME 1

Module 1 An Approach to Nursing Skills
Module 3 Safety
Module 15 Moving the Patient in Bed and Positioning
Module 21 Ambulation: Simple Assisted and Using Cane, Crutches, or Walker

© 1996 by Lippincott-Raven Publishers

OVERALL OBJECTIVE

To apply the principles of body mechanics to conserve energy; to decrease the potential for strain, injury, and fatigue; and to promote safety.

SPECIFIC LEARNING OBJECTIVES

Know Facts and Principles	Apply Facts and Principles	Demonstrate Ability	Evaluate Performance
1. Principles of body mechanics			
State principles of body mechanics.	Given a situation, correctly identify which principles could apply, and state why.	In the clinical setting, use body mechanics correctly.	Evaluate own performance with instructor using Performance Checklist.
2. Using body mechanics			
Identify tasks of the nurse and patient that may require facts and principles of body mechanics.	Given a situation, select the principle needed to guide correct body movement.	Correct own body movement, or instruct patient in proper use of principles of body mechanics.	Evaluate own application of principles of body mechanics with instructor.

© 1996 by Lippincott-Raven Publishers

LEARNING ACTIVITIES

1. Review the Specific Learning Objectives.
2. Read the section on posture and body mechanics (in the chapter on activity and rest) in Ellis and Nowlis, *Nursing: A Human Needs Approach,* or comparable material in another textbook.
3. Look up the module vocabulary terms in the glossary.
4. Read through the module as though you were preparing to teach the contents to another person. Mentally practice the techniques.
5. Do the following in the practice setting, with a partner observing:
   a. Stand with your weight balanced over your base of support.
   b. Stand 3 ft from a table or counter. Try to place a book on the table without enlarging your base of support. Begin again, and place the book on the table using an enlarged base of support. Compare your stability in the two situations.
   c. Stand in a normal position. Have your partner take your arms and pull until you begin to tip forward. Using the same base of support, squat low and have your partner pull again. Compare the force needed to disrupt your stability in the two positions.
   d. Stand with your feet 8 in apart, but side by side, and try to push a bed. Now enlarge your base of support in the direction in which you are pushing, and note the difference.
   e. Practice tightening your abdominal muscles upward and your gluteal muscles downward. Relax. Tighten the muscles again. Do this before you attempt any task.
   f. Face the bed. While keeping your feet in the same position, turn your upper body 90 degrees to the right as if reaching for something; note the feeling of strain and pull on your back muscles. Try bending from this position; note the lack of stability.
   g. Face the bed. Turn 90 degrees to the right by moving your right foot and turning your whole body; note that your back is straight. Now try bending and reaching; note the increased stability in this position.
   h. Pick up an object from the floor or other low surface, bending your knees and keeping your back straight. Use this posture whenever you need to reach something on the floor.
   i. With your partner assisting, try to move another person up in bed with the head of the bed at a 30-degree angle. Now place the bed in a flat position and repeat the activity. Compare the amount of energy required. Have your "patient" evaluate the experience.
   j. Again, with your partner assisting and with the bed in a flat position, move your "patient" up in bed without a turn sheet and against a wrinkled bottom sheet. Now tighten the bottom sheet and use a turn sheet for the same activity. Compare the experiences. Ask your "patient" to comment.
   k. Hold a 10-lb object (brick, book) with both hands directly in front of and close to your body for 3 minutes. Now do the same thing holding the object at arm's length from your body. Compare the amount of energy required for each task.
   l. With a turn sheet, turn your "patient" from a supine position to a lateral position, using your weight as a counterbalance. Note the ease with which you can do this.
   m. Have one person lie in the bed. Try to move the "patient's" shoulders closer to the far edge of the bed by pushing. Then push the hips and feet toward the far side of the bed. Next, move the patient's shoulders toward you by slipping your arms under the shoulders and pulling. Do the same for the hips and feet. Note the difference in ease of movement when pushing and pulling.
   n. Trade places with the person in the bed, and repeat the exercise of pushing and pulling. Compare how it felt to be pulled and how it felt to be pushed.
   o. When you feel you have practiced enough, perform all the above tasks *correctly* for your instructor, using your partner as a "patient" when necessary.
6. In the clinical setting, apply basic body mechanics whenever possible. If you are unsure or need help, consult your instructor.
7. Identify a patient who would gain by using body mechanics principles. This may be a patient with limitation of one or both lower extremities. Instruct the patient in the correct use of body mechanics with the help of your instructor.

© 1996 by Lippincott-Raven Publishers

base of support   counterbalance
body mechanics   supporting muscles
center of gravity   torsion

Basic Body Mechanics

Rationale for the Use of This Skill

A nurse engaged in clinical practice daily performs a variety of physical tasks, including reaching, stooping, lifting, carrying, pushing, and pulling. Practiced incorrectly, any of these has the potential to cause strain, fatigue, or injury to the nurse or patient. With practice, using the principles of body mechanics, the nurse will move smoothly and surely, minimizing personal strain, conserving energy, and enhancing the safety, comfort, and confidence of patients.[1]

▼ NURSING DIAGNOSIS

Patients may experience Knowledge Deficit related to principles of body mechanics specific to their illness or injury. For example, the practice of correct body mechanics can prevent injury or reinjury related to ambulation, changing position, or lifting or moving heavy objects.

PRINCIPLES OF BASIC BODY MECHANICS

Learning the principles of body mechanics is an essential task for the nurse and is often taught to patients. The promotion of proper body mechanics is, in itself, a valid nursing intervention (Glick, 1992).

Assess each physical task encountered to determine the most appropriate way to accomplish it for both your own and the patient's safety. You may need to obtain supplies, such as a lift sheet or a gait (transfer) belt, before you undertake the necessary task. You may also need another staff person or a mechanical lift to ensure safety for all involved.

The following principles of body mechanics have been selected because of their applicability to commonly encountered nursing situations. Examples of how they can be applied are included as illustrations.

[1]Note that rationale for action is emphasized throughout the module by the use of italics.

1. *Weight is balanced best when the center of gravity is directly above the base provided by the feet. In this position, an individual can maintain balance and stability with the least amount of effort.* When this posture is *not* maintained, the potential for strain, fatigue, and poor stability is increased.

2. *Enlarging the base of support increases the stability of the body.* Changes in position should not cause the center of gravity to fall beyond the edge of the base. Therefore, when you assist a patient to move or the patient moves in a standing position, each will be more stable if the feet are apart than if they are close together.

3. *A person or an object is more stable if the center of gravity is close to the base of support.* Apply this principle when an object is picked up from the floor by bending the knees and keeping the back straight (thus keeping the center of gravity directly above and close to the base of support), rather than by bending forward at the waist.

4. *Enlarging the base of support in the direction of the force to be applied increases the amount of force that can be applied.* Place one foot forward when you push a heavy object (such as a bed with a patient in it), or place one foot back when you move a patient toward the side of the bed.

5. *Tighten or contract your supporting muscles before beginning a lifting task to prevent injury.* Supporting muscles are the muscles of the abdomen and lower back that provide stability and support to the lower spine. If you practice tightening the supporting muscles continually, you will eventually do it automatically when you prepare for any activity. This technique can also be taught to patients.

6. *Facing in the direction of the task to be performed and turning the entire body in one plane (rather than twisting) lessens the susceptibility of the back to injury.* When the back is twisted, one group of muscles is stretched while the other is contracted. Muscles that are stretched are weaker and more susceptible to injury. Also, the spine functions less effectively when it is twisted. Teach this principle to patients who are standing and reaching for objects or clothing (Fig. 4–1).

7. *Lifting should be undertaken by bending the legs and using the leg muscles rather than by using the back*

© 1996 by Lippincott-Raven Publishers

dividual, the employer, and society. Back problems are the major reason people seek medical care (Gonet & Kryzwon, 1991).

8. *It takes less energy to move an object on a level surface than to move it up a slanted surface against the force of gravity.* Therefore, you will need less effort to move a patient up toward the head of the bed if you first lower the head of the bed. Be sure to check to see whether the patient can tolerate the flat position before lowering the head of the bed. Patients can use this principle to move themselves up in the bed.

9. *Less energy is required to move an object when friction between the object and the surface on which it rests is minimized. Because friction opposes motion,* you can make the task of moving a patient in bed easier by working on a smooth surface such as a taut sheet. A smooth sheet also allows patients to move more effectively.

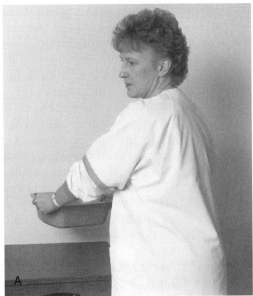
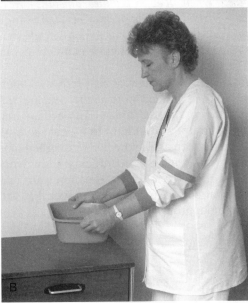

Figure 4–1. A: Avoid torsion of the spine. **B:** Facing in the direction of the task to be performed lessens the susceptibility of the back to injury.

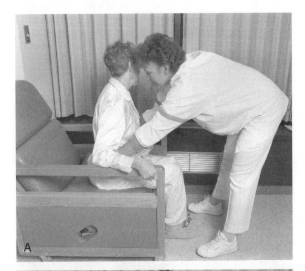
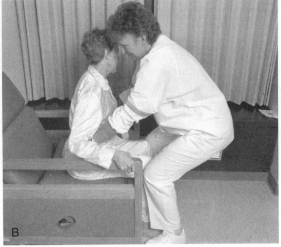

Figure 4–2. A: When lifting, avoid using the smaller muscles of the back, which tire more easily. **B:** Lifting is better undertaken by bending the legs and using the large muscles of the legs.

muscles. Because large muscles tire less quickly than small muscles, you should use the large gluteal and femoral muscles rather than the smaller muscles of the back. The large, compact muscles of the legs are stronger and less prone to injury than the broad, flat muscles of the back (Fig. 4–2). In addition, if the back muscles are strained they may be injured. Ligaments, tendons, and even the intervertebral disks may be injured as well. Back injuries are one of the major health problems in adult workers, resulting in pain, disability, and economic loss to the in-

© 1996 by Lippincott-Raven Publishers

10. *It takes less energy to hold an object close to the body than at a distance from the body; it also is easier to move an object that is close. Muscles are strongest when contracted and weakest when stretched.* Therefore, hold heavy objects close to your body, and move the patient near to your side of the bed (for bathing, for example) to conserve energy. Patients walking with equipment, such as an intravenous pole or walker, should be instructed to keep the equipment close to the body (Fig. 4–3).

11. *The weight of the body can be used as a force to assist in lifting or moving.* When you help a patient stand, you can use the weight of your body by rocking back, counterbalancing the patient's weight, as illustrated in Figure 4–2. You can use the patient's weight by placing his or her legs in a knees-up position before moving him or her from side to side or up in bed. It is essential to explain this maneuver to the patient to elicit cooperation. Patients will also be able to move themselves more easily if they use their body weight to facilitate turning.

12. *Smooth, rhythmic movements at moderate speed require less energy than rapid, jerky ones. Smooth, continuous motions also are more accurate, safer, and better controlled than sudden, jerky movements.* You will work more effectively if not hurried. Also caution patients not to feel hurried when moving.

13. *When an object is pushed, it absorbs part of the force being exerted, leaving less force available to move the object. When an object is pulled, all of the force exerted is available for the task of moving.* Using this principle, when moving patients, pull steadily rather than pushing, which is much less effective.

14. *It takes less energy to work on a surface at an appropriate height (usually waist level) than it does to stoop or stretch to reach the surface.* The back is susceptible to injury and fatigue from excessive bending. Therefore, raise the bed or overbed table to an appropriate height for maximum working comfort *to prevent fatigue.* If patients are using a working surface of any type, be sure that surface is at an appropriate height.

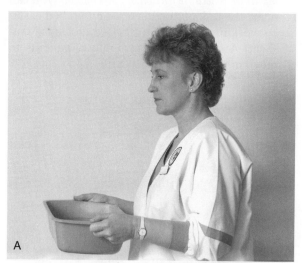

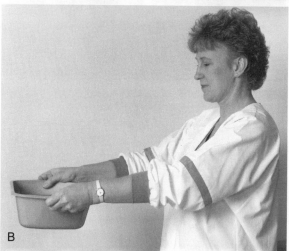

Figure 4–3. It takes less energy to hold an object close to the body (**A**) than at a distance from the body (**B**).

LONG-TERM CARE

The same principles of basic body mechanics apply in the long-term care setting as in the acute care setting. However, the residents in this setting may need more assistance from you, and you may need to secure more help before attempting a task. In addition, because many caregivers in long-term settings are nursing assistants, you may need to teach these principles to them. The example you set by the body mechanics you use is important to those with whom you work.

© 1996 by Lippincott-Raven Publishers

HOME CARE

The client receiving care at home and the family and other caregivers will need to be taught appropriate principles of body mechanics to ensure safety for all concerned. You may need to assess family members and caregivers for adequacy of knowledge, skill, and equipment to handle a client in a particular situation. The height of the chair or bed, the distance to the bathroom or kitchen, the size of the client and the caregiver, and the availability of mechanical assistive devices should be considered during this assessment.

CRITICAL THINKING EXERCISES

• You are to transfer a surgical patient from a chair to a standing position. Review the principles presented in the module, then determine which ones are essential for this task. Identify the rationale for each principle you will follow. After planning for the task, state which directions you will give the patient so that he or she can assist you.

References

Glick, O. J. (1992). Interventions related to activity and movement. *Nursing Clinics of North America, 27*(2), 541–568.

Gonet, L., & Kryzwon, A. (1991). Preventing back pain through education. *Nursing Standard, 5*(24), 25–27.

© 1996 by Lippincott-Raven Publishers

Basic Body Mechanics	Needs More Practice	Satisfactory	Comments
1. Keep weight balanced above base of support.			
2. Enlarge base of support as necessary to increase body's stability.			
3. Lower center of gravity toward base of support as necessary to increase body's stability.			
4. Enlarge base of support in direction in which force is to be applied.			
5. Tighten abdominal and gluteal muscles in preparation for all activities.			
6. Face in direction of task, and turn body in one plane.			
7. Bend hips and knees (rather than back) when lifting.			
8. Move objects on level surface when possible.			
9. Slide (rather than lift) objects on smooth surface when possible.			
10. Hold objects close to body, and stand close to objects to be moved.			
11. Use body's weight to assist in lifting or moving when possible.			
12. Use smooth motions and reasonable speed when carrying out tasks.			
13. When moving patients, use a pulling motion whenever possible.			
14. Raise the working surface to your waist level when possible.			

© 1996 by Lippincott-Raven Publishers

? Q U I Z

True-False Questions

_____ **1.** The body is less stable when the center of gravity falls beyond the edge of the base of support.

_____ **2.** Stability is increased when the center of gravity is close to the base of support.

_____ **3.** Facing in the direction of the task to be performed is not recommended.

_____ **4.** Friction enhances movement.

_____ **5.** It takes less energy to hold an object close to the body than at a distance from the body.

_____ **6.** When carrying out a task, the faster one moves, the better.

Short-Answer Questions

7. Why is lifting or pulling using the back muscles contraindicated?

_____

_____

8. Which principle of body mechanics is the basis for a decision to put the head of the bed down before moving the patient?

_____

_____

9. Which principle of body mechanics is the basis for a decision to spread your feet farther apart before trying to lift a patient?

_____

_____

10. Which principle of body mechanics is the basis for a decision to move closer to the patient's bed before attempting to move the patient?

_____

_____

© 1996 by Lippincott-Raven Publishers

DOCUMENTATION

MODULE CONTENTS

RATIONALE FOR THE USE OF THIS
  SKILL
TYPES OF RECORDS
Temporary Records
The Permanent Record
  The "Chart"
  The Computerized Record
RECORD CONTENT
SYSTEMS FOR ORGANIZING CONTENT
CONTENT OF THE NURSING RECORD
MECHANICS OF CHARTING
Meeting Legal Standards
  Errors
  Spaces
  Signature
  Time
  Right to Privacy

Using Special Terminology and
  Abbreviations
Using Chart Forms Correctly
WRITING PROGRESS NOTES
Narrative Notes
Problem-Oriented Medical Records
  Special Notes
  Choosing Which Problems to SOAP
Charting by Exception
Focus Charting
CHARTING PROCEDURE
LONG-TERM CARE
HOME CARE
CRITICAL THINKING EXERCISES
PRACTICE SITUATIONS

PREREQUISITES

Successful completion of the following modules:

VOLUME 1
Module 1 An Approach to Nursing Skills
Module 6 Introduction to Assessment Skills

© 1996 by Lippincott-Raven Publishers

OVERALL OBJECTIVE

To provide effectively written records of nursing care to facilitate care by the entire healthcare team and maintain a legal record.

SPECIFIC LEARNING OBJECTIVES

Know Facts and Principles	Apply Facts and Principles	Demonstrate Ability	Evaluate Performance
1. Purposes Explain rationale for use of chart as a legal record, for determining quality of care, and for communication.	Given a situation in which someone wants information from a record, determine whether that should be permitted.	Maintain privacy of patient's record. Use record to gain information regarding patient, and maintain legal standards in documentation.	Evaluate own performance.
2. Content List types of information to be recorded. Give rationale for use of objective terminology. State situations in which subjective terminology is appropriate.	Given a situation, do sample charting containing all appropriate information. Given a situation, describe it in objective terminology.	Record all needed information as outlined on Performance Checklist. Use objective terminology for all observations. Identify subjective material clearly. State problems correctly. Describe nursing actions taken. Record evaluation of patient response.	Evaluate own performance using Performance Checklist.
3. Systems for organizing List two systems for organizing contents of record.	Given a sample chart, identify system of organization in use.	Document appropriately given system of organization.	Evaluate with instructor.
4. Styles of progress notes List three styles of writing progress notes.	Given a situation, write progress notes using each style.	Document in style appropriate to facility.	Evaluate documentation with instructor.

© 1996 by Lippincott-Raven Publishers

LEARNING ACTIVITIES

1. Review the Specific Learning Objectives.
2. Review the abbreviations in Ellis and Nowlis, *Nursing: A Human Needs Approach*, or those in the procedure manual of your facility and those in Tables 5–1 through 5–4 in this module.
3. Read the section on written communication in Ellis and Nowlis, *Nursing: A Human Needs Approach*, or comparable material in another textbook.
4. Look up the module vocabulary terms in the glossary.
5. Read through the module.
6. If charting samples are available in your practice setting, review them.
7. Practice charting using the situations provided in the module. Make a sample form for practice charting that is similar to the one used in your facility.
8. Exchange your practice charting with another student and check each other's work. Review and rewrite your own charting based on this critique.
9. Have your instructor review your practice charting.
10. Review your instructor's comments and rewrite your practice charting if necessary.
11. Chart data regarding a patient to whom you are assigned. Make a first draft on a piece of paper and have your clinical instructor review it before you write in the patient's record.
12. Continue to chart on patients assigned in the clinical area. Have your first draft reviewed before writing in patients' records until your instructor directs you to do otherwise.

VOCABULARY

assessment
computerized record
data
exception
excretion
flow sheet
focus charting

graphic
infused
ingested
legibility
military (24-hour)
    clock
minimum data set

narrative charting
objective
password
problem-oriented
    medical record
problem-oriented
    record

SOAP
subjective

© 1996 by Lippincott-Raven Publishers

Documentation

Rationale for the Use of This Skill

The patient's official record is used by all members of the healthcare team to communicate the patient's progress and the current treatment. Therefore, entries in the record must be clear. The chart also serves as a legal record of care and the patient's progress. It is used to determine the appropriateness and quality of care being given; therefore, accuracy, legibility, clarity, and completeness are very important. Finally, each healthcare facility establishes its own format for patients' records. This format must be used for all documentation in the facility. [1]

TYPES OF RECORDS

All healthcare agencies keep many different records. All recording systems, however, share characteristics that will make it easier for you to adapt to any system you encounter.

Temporary Records

A nursing unit will almost always have a variety of temporary records that are used to facilitate communication or to maintain information for easy accessibility. These are valuable, but they must be recognized as temporary and should not be the only record of important information about the patient. Although they are temporary, these records do need to be accurate.

A "vital signs list" is typically maintained. This form may include the temperature, pulse, respiration, and blood pressure of every patient on the unit. If one person is assigned to take all these measurements, a one-page form is a convenient way to record the data as they are obtained. This list also is a quick reference for a nurse in charge of the unit. It may be used for immediate access; the information is later transferred to the patient's permanent record by the nurse responsible for care or by a unit secretary.

There may be a page in the front of the chart on which the nurses make brief notations to remind physicians of pertinent timelines, such as "The narcotic order is due for renewal within the next 24 hours." These are to facilitate communication, but the official record of these matters is elsewhere in the chart.

Many nursing units maintain a white board or

other display for noting patients' special needs. This board might, for example, indicate patients who are not allowed to take oral food and fluids, are to be weighed daily, have intravenous infusions, or are going for special tests or surgery. This allows staff members to obtain information quickly and conveniently. These must be updated whenever a change in the patient's plan of care occurs *so that care can be appropriately adjusted.*

Temporary records may also be placed at the bedside to facilitate carrying out specific measures. An example would be a "turning record" that specifies when the patient is to be turned and which position is to be used. Having the information at the bedside makes it easier for the staff person to check what needs to be done and when.

Another common temporary record is a fluid intake and output worksheet. This is used to document all fluids taken and lost by a patient. This might be kept on the bathroom door for easy accessibility. The information may be transcribed onto the permanent record once each shift (see Module 10, Intake and Output, for further instructions).

Temporary bedside records that are designed to be discarded must be differentiated from actual chart forms that are kept at the bedside in some facilities. For example, a neurologic assessment flow sheet might be placed at the patient's bedside to facilitate documentation. When the flow sheet has been filled out, it is then transferred to the permanent chart.

In some facilities, the nursing care plan is kept on a card file (such as a Kardex) and changed as the patient's needs change. This record may be written in pencil and considered temporary. In most settings, however, the nursing care plan is now considered a permanent part of the record and is written in ink and retained along with the other permanent parts of the chart.

The Permanent Record

The permanent patient record may be a paper chart or a computerized record. In either situation, the information in the permanent record constitutes a legal and confidential document.

The "Chart"

A permanent paper record of the patient's healthcare is called the "chart." This record is the *legal-record* of care; it is the proof of the patient's condition and care in legal proceedings. It also is proof of care rendered for reimbursement purposes. During the patient's stay in a healthcare facility, the chart is a means of communication among members of the

---

[1]Note that the rationale for action is emphasized throughout the module by the use of italics.

© 1996 by Lippincott-Raven Publishers

healthcare team in regard to the patient's condition and care. It also is used to evaluate the quality of care given. In addition, data from the chart are used for teaching and research.

The Computerized Record

Computerized information systems are used in many healthcare facilities, and the trend is toward increasing use. Some systems may be limited to only one or two functions, such as patient location and laboratory or diagnostic test results. This information may be printed and then placed in a permanent paper record. In other facilities or agencies, comprehensive patient care information systems provide a complete "paperless" record and include all aspects of nursing assessment, care planning, charting, scheduling, and patient information input and retrieval. Some acute care hospitals now have computer terminals at each patient's bedside *to facilitate immediate entry and retrieval of data.*

The components of these computerized systems vary, but they generally include a keyboard and a screen, or monitor, and possibly a light pen and a printer. Information is input using the keyboard, although some systems use hospital-defined menus to reduce typing to a minimum. The screen displays information and, in many cases, questions (Fig. 5–1).

Responses are generated by typing in words, phrases, or actual narrative, or the system may include a light pen, which, when touched to the screen, inputs information. A printer may be available to provide written documents as needed by staff members.

In most healthcare facilities, staff members must use a special password to gain access to patient information. Access to system functions may be limited by job category, level of authorization, and loca-

tion of the terminal being used. For example, some data may be available only on the unit where the patient is located. Limiting by occupation may permit only registered nurses to change the nursing care plan but other nursing personnel (such as nursing assistants or students) to read it. Level of authorization may limit access to certain information to only a limited number of people.

Computerized patient information systems are typically unique to the setting in which they are found.

RECORD CONTENT

All patient records provide personal data. This includes home address and telephone number, next of kin, insurance coverage, and attending physician. The admitting diagnosis and the date of admission to the agency or facility also are included.

Every type of care given is documented in the record. The physician documents the history and physical examination and then continues with medical progress notes and medical orders for care. All diagnostic and laboratory data are permanently documented in the record. Other healthcare groups, such as physical therapy, occupational therapy, or respiratory therapy, are responsible for documenting their contributions to the patient's healthcare.

Nursing personnel are responsible for documenting all nursing care. Medication administration may be documented on a medication administration record that is kept separately; however, it will be placed with the chart for permanent storage. This same process is often used with the nursing care plan. It may be kept separately for ease of use, but then it is added to the patient record at discharge when the record is permanently stored. As more facilities use computerized systems, the need to keep parts of the record in separate locations is decreased. Each location may have access to all parts of the record through a computer terminal.

SYSTEMS FOR ORGANIZING CONTENT

The two major systems for organizing the information in a patient's record are the source-oriented system and the problem-oriented record (POR) or problem-oriented medical record (POMR) system. A facility may use one system or a combination of these two systems to meet its needs and staff preferences.

In the *source-oriented method*, the majority of the

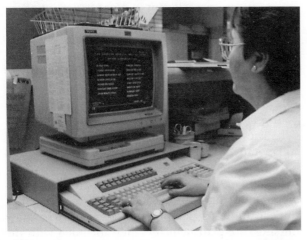

Figure 5–1. The nurse responds to a computer-generated screen.

© 1996 by Lippincott-Raven Publishers

information is organized according to the source of that information. Progress notes written by the physician are found in the medical progress notes. Nursing progress notes are on another page of the chart. Notes written by other disciplines, for example by the respiratory therapist or the dietitian, are found on other forms in the patient's record. Some facilities combine certain of these records *to facilitate effective use.*

The POR in its purest form is organized according to the identified problems of the patient. All members of the healthcare team write progress notes about the same problem on the same form in the chart.

Both systems contain the following elements:

1. *Data base.* This includes the initial physician's history and physical examination, original laboratory and diagnostic test results, social and financial data, and the nursing admission interview. The term *data base* may not be used, but this type of information is part of every record.
2. *Flow sheets.* These forms are arranged in columns or graphs that allow information to be recorded quickly and progress to be monitored with ease. Some facilities use many different flow sheets; others use only a few. Usually you will use flow sheets to record vital signs, intake and output, medications given, and routine nursing care, although a more complex parameter, such as patient teaching, may also be recorded on a flow sheet. Again, the term *flow sheet* may not be used, but the charts and graphs that compose this element are easily recognized.

    Flow sheets facilitate review of information to determine patterns and trends. Because they do this so effectively and require less time for data entry, many facilities are developing flow sheets to replace other types of documentation. Computer records lend themselves particularly well to the use of flow sheets.
3. *Progress notes.* The most obvious difference between the systems of charting is the structure of the progress notes. In source-oriented records, progress notes are separated by discipline: There is one form for the physician's progress notes, another for the nurses' notes, and still others for the notes of other healthcare groups (physical therapists, respiratory therapists, occupational therapists). Source-oriented records may use fewer flow sheets; therefore, you may find most information in the progress notes. With problem-oriented records, all progress notes (from all sources) use the same form. The notes have a formal, specific structure (page 85), which makes them easier to use.

4. *Problem list.* A fourth feature, the problem list, was once seen as unique to POR, but is now found in other documentation systems as well. This list is a combination table of contents and index to the patient's condition and progress. Each problem is numbered and titled for easy reference. Titles may refer to medical diagnoses, patient problems, or nursing diagnoses, depending on the setting. The date when the problem was initially identified is included, and when the problem is resolved, that fact and the date of resolution are added.

CONTENT OF THE NURSING RECORD

To provide a complete nursing record, you must determine what information to include in your charting. This is a complex responsibility, and one in which you will become more skilled with experience. The Joint Commission on the Accreditation of Healthcare Organizations (JCAHO), the accrediting body for hospitals and many other healthcare agencies, requires a system for documenting nursing care that is pertinent and concise and reflects patient status. The standards further expect nursing documentation to address the patient's needs, problems, capabilities, and limitations and to include information on nursing interventions and evaluation (JCAHO, 1993). You must try to provide a clear and concise record of the nursing process in relation to the individual patient. This includes aspects of assessment, nursing diagnosis or analysis, planning, intervention, and evaluation.

Assessment data include both subjective and objective information (see Module 6, Introduction to Assessment Skills, for a discussion of subjective versus objective data). You will have to decide which assessment data are relevant in a particular situation. As a general guideline, record assessment data when they reflect findings that relate to the patient's reason for being hospitalized, any abnormal findings, and normal findings that relate to previously noted problems.

In addition to these data, you must also record your analysis to indicate any new problems identified. These may be recorded as nursing diagnoses, collaborative problems, or general problems that have not yet been categorized.

Depending on the policies of your facility, *planning* may or may not be included in the chart. In some institutions, planning is recorded on a separate nursing care plan, which is then included with the rest of a patient's record at the time of discharge.

© 1996 by Lippincott-Raven Publishers

Planning information may also include referrals made to other healthcare providers, such as the patient's physician or the respiratory therapist. Some facilities have developed protocols or standards for care for specific problems or situations. These may then be individualized as needed for the patient. When a problem or nursing diagnosis is identified, the appropriate standard or protocol is then activated. When records are computerized, this is particularly easy.

Intervention data include nursing actions that are taken in response to an existing nursing diagnosis and measures taken to prevent problems. Even actions that are part of routine care, such as those related to hygiene, usually are noted in some manner. Also important are actions taken to maintain patient safety and those that were ordered by the physician to support the medical plan of care.

Evaluation data document the effectiveness of nursing and all other actions and therapies. These data identify the patient's progress toward the desired outcomes of care. They are vital for determining whether care has been effective and for planning future care.

MECHANICS OF CHARTING

Meeting Legal Standards

As a legal record, a chart must conform to certain legal standards of legibility, clarity, and accuracy. All entries in a paper chart must be in ink *so that changes are noticeable and the record is permanent.* Your facility may specify a particular color of ink to be used. If it has no policy, remember that black or dark blue ink reproduces especially well on microfilm. Legibility is critical; obviously *statements that are not legible are not usable either for care or in court.*

Computerized patient records maintain this legal standard by not permitting changes once the information has been entered into the record. The healthcare worker can usually edit the note being composed, but after permanently entering the information in the record, the computer program blocks any changes. Errors in documentation, blank spaces, legal signatures, time frames, and privacy are all major legal concerns in documentation.

Errors

If you make an error, draw a single line through the incorrect entry so that it remains legible. Traditionally the word "error" followed by initials (or first initial, last name, and title) was written above the lined-out entry. Recently, some attorneys have suggested that entering the word "error" may give an uninformed lay person the idea that this means an error was made in care. To avoid this, include a note as to the nature of the error. This is helpful if the chart is needed in a legal proceeding. Such a note might read "charted on wrong chart" or "mistaken entry" and your initials. This notation and the traditional "error" are both legally correct, so follow the policy of your facility. If it has no policy, the more descriptive notation is preferable.

Documentation errors should never be corrected by erasing, using correction fluid, or obliterating the first entry. This may create the impression that the information recorded was damaging to the care provider or is being hidden for other reasons. When the mistake can be clearly read, the situation can be evaluated more readily.

If you have omitted information that should have been included in earlier charting, it may be essential to record that information. For example, you may have noted a series of assessments on a pocket note pad and failed to record them on the patient's chart in a timely manner. This information may help to identify an ongoing pattern in the patient. It is legally acceptable to add a notation as long as it is clear when the notation was made. Your facility may have a policy on how to note this. If there is none, a heading that indicates "delayed entry" with a date and time will clearly indicate that these data were collected in a timely manner but not recorded at the appropriate time.

A delayed entry for the purpose of protecting oneself or the agency from legal liability is more problematic. This may arouse suspicion as to whether the entry is accurate. If this situation arises, consult with an instructor or supervisor before making an entry.

Computer systems have individualized approaches to correcting errors. When the error has been entered, a subsequent note is written to correct or clarify the error.

Spaces

If you are using the narrative form of charting, chart on consecutive lines and do not leave any blank spaces. Draw a single line through any empty spaces to prevent subsequent entries from being made above your signature (Fig. 5–2). Some facilities specify that you place your signature at the end of the note and follow it with a line to the margin.

In some PORs, the standard is to start each segment of the note on a separate line. You would then draw a straight line through any unused space on a line before starting the next segment. Computerized

© 1996 by Lippincott-Raven Publishers

DATE / TIME	
12-26-99	*Ambulated to bathroom c̄ one person assist. Urinated 250 ml clear urine. Up in chair until after dinner.*
1815	*Completed all activities c̄ no complaint of breathing difficulty or fatigue. Stated "I'm so glad I can get*
	around some now. I was so short of breath when I cam in." Returned to bed after dinner. Resting quietly.
	———————————————————————————————————— S. Chin, NS
1900	*Husband in to visit. —————————————————————————————— S. Chin, NS.*

Mansch, Paulina F-83
516-30-2250
Dr. Salisbury

SWEDISH HOSPITAL MEDICAL CENTER
Seattle, WA 98104

Figure 5–2. Draw a single line through any empty spaces.

charting omits this problem. Each entry is recorded independently and the computer maintains separation.

Signature

When you sign a notation on a patient's record, use your first initial and full last name followed by the abbreviation of your position. If you were a nursing student named Jane Smith, you would sign the record "J. Smith NS." In large facilities where there is more chance of two individuals having the same initials, the facility may require that you sign your full name.

Traditionally, nursing students used the abbreviation *SN* (student nurse) to designate their position; however, most now use the abbreviation *NS* (nursing student). If more than one nursing program uses the facility or agency, you may also need to add initials designating your educational institution, for example, "Jane Smith NS, SCC." Your instructor will indicate the notation your facility prefers. In some cases, the facility may require your instructor to cosign your progress notes, flow sheets, or medication records.

You must use the designation appropriate to your position. For instance, a licensed practical nurse who is enrolled in a program preparing registered nurses would use the SN or NS designation while working as a student. The nurse would use the LPN designation only when employed by and working for the facility as an LPN.

Flow sheets are often signed once per shift in a designated signature section where the signature and the initials are documented together. All data entries are then identified by the initials of the person collecting the data. You may be asked to use two initials or, in some facilities, three initials. This often depends on the size of the facility and the likelihood that there is more than one person with the same initials.

Signatures in computerized records rely on each individual having a password to identify who is making the entry. Keeping your password secret is important to your own integrity of nursing practice. Some facilities require that passwords be changed at regular intervals to safeguard the system from illegal entry.

Time

Notations of time and date are important *for healthcare reasons and legal reasons. Time sequences can be crucial in certain problems.*

You can note time in conventional notation or according to the 24-hour, or military, clock. The 24-hour clock works as follows: when the time reaches 12:00 noon (or 1200), instead of returning to 1:00 PM, the time goes on to 1300, continuing until 2400 is reached at midnight. The hours before noon are

© 1996 by Lippincott-Raven Publishers

Table 5–1. Time may be indicated by using conventional 12-hour notation or by using the 24-hour clock.			
Conventional Time	**24-hour Clock**	**Conventional Time**	**24-hour Clock**
1 AM	0100	1 PM	1300
2 AM	0200	2 PM	1400
3 AM	0300	3 PM	1500
4 AM	0400	4 PM	1600
5 AM	0500	5 PM	1700
6 AM	0600	6 PM	1800
7 AM	0700	7 PM	1900
8 AM	0800	8 PM	2000
9 AM	0900	9 PM	2100
10 AM	1000	10 PM	2200
11 AM	1100	11 PM	2300
12 noon	1200	12 midnight	2400

recorded as 0100, 0200, 0300, and so on (Table 5–1). The 24-hour clock eliminates confusion as to whether something took place before noon (AM) or after noon (PM). In some facilities, this confusion is lessened by using different ink colors for different shifts or different times of day. This method is quite effective in the original, but when records are photocopied or microfilmed, the color distinction is lost, and certain colors do not reproduce as well as others. Therefore, most facilities use black ink.

On flow sheets, the times that events occurred or actions were taken are noted with initials in the "Time" column. This is clear on most records.

Policies differ regarding time notations on narrative or SOAP progress notes. The policy in most facilities is to note in the "Time" column the time you write on the nursing progress notes, rather than the time the event occurred. The time of the event can be reflected in the body of the note, if that is appropriate to the charting. Often the charting reflects a process or series of events rather than one event. For particularly important events, such as a sudden change in a patient's condition, your documentation may be done immediately.

Some facilities, however, have a policy of noting the time of the events in the "Time" column on the narrative or SOAP progress notes even if they are documented later. It is critical that you understand the policy of the facility in regard to this time notation.

Computers have internal clocks and calendars that allow times and dates to be automatically appended to any entry. You will have to specify the time of the event if you are charting after the fact.

Right to Privacy

A chart or computerized record is a legally protected, private record of a patient's care. Access to a chart is restricted to those in the facility using it for care and, in some instances, for research or teaching. A chart may not be photocopied except following careful procedures designed to protect the patient's privacy. If you, as a student, are using a chart as a learning tool, it is your responsibility to protect the patient's privacy by not using the patient's name or any identifying statements in any notations you make for your own use. Papers or case studies based on a patient's care should likewise protect the anonymity of the patient.

The medical record is the *property* of the hospital, but a patient *has* a right to the *information* contained in that record (state laws differ as to whether or not a patient has the legal right to review the chart). Usually, however, the patient must follow a procedure to obtain this information, and you must know what that procedure is. This should be found in the facility's policy and procedure manual. If there is no such procedure, you should notify the nursing supervisor for assistance. Clear and timely explanations and progress reports to patients and families may result in fewer requests to see the chart.

The same policies cover computerized charting. Privacy is maintained by limiting access to those with an appropriate password. Even those with a password, however, do not have a right to access the computerized record unless they are participating in care in some way. Many computer systems have a program that traces all computer access to any record. Therefore, it is possible to identify any breaks in computer security.

Using Special Terminology and Abbreviations

Traditionally, a great deal of specialized medical terminology and word patterns have been used in charting. As a beginner, concentrate on describing what you see. Even if you do not know the medical terminology, you will be understood if you clearly describe what you observe.

As you progress in your nursing and related studies, you will pick up a large medical vocabulary. You must use this vocabulary effectively and correctly. For example, a false belief is called a delusion. Rather than charting that a patient has a delusion, chart the exact nature of the belief. *This is certainly more informative to others using the chart. (It can also save you from jumping to conclusions; sometimes what appears to be a false belief is true.)*

© 1996 by Lippincott-Raven Publishers

Table 5–2. Descriptive Charting Terms

1. Body Location	Use specific anatomic terms. For example:
	    Right upper quadrant
	    Left upper quadrant
	    Right lower quadrant
	    Left lower quadrant
	    Distal/proximal

2. Body functions	Urinate—void
	Have a bowel movement—defecate
	Profuse sweating—diaphoresis
	Walk—ambulate
3. Skin description	Intact—not open, broken, or blemished
	Moist/dry
	Smooth, roughed, cracked
	Warm, brown (light, medium, dark): describes healthy color of the black- or brown-skinned person
	Warm, pink: describes healthy color of what is usually termed white skin
	Warm, tan: healthy color of most Asians and those termed dark-complected
	Dull, ash brown: African-American person's skin without adequate blood supply
	Dull, gray-brown: African-American or dark-complected person's skin with unoxygenated blood apparent
	Pale, pallor: white person's skin without adequate blood supply
	Cyanotic: blue-gray color in skin of white person and in conjunctiva, mucous membranes, and nail beds of all people with unoxygenated blood apparent

4. Nutrition	List portion of meal eaten:
	    ¼, ½, ¾; all (*not* poor or good)
	    Specify types of foods eaten when more specific information needed

5. Urine description	Color: pale, yellow, amber, dark amber
	Clarity: clear, cloudy, smoky
	Contents: mucus, clots, sediment
6. Stool description	Color: black, brown, clay-colored (gray)
	Consistency: liquid, watery, semiformed, soft, formed, hard
	Tarry: indicates black, sticky
	Mucoid: indicates contains mucus

7. Drainage or secretions	Quantity:
	    Exact measurement preferred
	    Estimate milliliters if you have a standard to compare
	    Specify number of dressings saturated
	    Other terms: slight, scanty, small, moderate, large, copious, profuse

	Character:
	    Watery, thin
	    Thick, tenacious
	    Stringy
	    Mucoid (like mucus)
	    Serous (like serum)
	    Sanguineous (with blood)
	    Serosanguineous (serum and blood mixed)
	    Purulent—containing pus

© 1996 by Lippincott-Raven Publishers

Table 5–2. Descriptive Charting Terms (*Continued*)

8. *Mental attitude or mood*	When you observe behavior, ask patients for an appraisal of their own feelings. Chart both your description of a patient's behavior and the patient's statement of feelings.

Patient's statement of feelings	*Behaviors observed*
a. "I feel depressed." "I feel sad."	Does not smile Avoids eye contact Drooping posture Cries when alone
b. "I am glad to go home." "I am happy."	Speaks with animation Smiles and jokes Moves about room briskly
c. "I am worried." "I feel anxious."	Asks many questions Paces the floor In constant movement Short attention span Worried look on face
d. "I am mad." "I feel angry."	Loud and belligerent Frown on face Vigorous movements

Abbreviations are used in charting *to save time and space*. Most nursing texts include a list of common abbreviations, and healthcare facilities often have their own lists of approved abbreviations. Use the approved abbreviations for the facility in which you are working. Although certain abbreviations are in general usage, others are used only in one geographic area. When in doubt, use the full term, which will be understood regardless of local custom. This is particularly true for initials used as abbreviations. (See Tables 5–2 through 5–5 for special terminology and abbreviations.)

In charting, sentences are typically reduced to their essential components *to lessen work and decrease the space used*. Thus, articles (*a, an, the*) and even verbs may be omitted. *Because the entire chart is about an individual patient,* the subject of a sentence is omitted when it represents the patient (Table 5–6).

Do not omit the subject if it represents someone other than the patient. Also, when you omit words, be careful that your meaning remains clear. Begin each statement with a capital letter and end it with a period, even if the statement is not a complete sentence. *This helps to clarify meaning.*

Correct spelling of terminology is essential to a legally correct record. A misspelled term may indicate an entirely different concept and therefore give incorrect information to anyone reading the record. An entry that contains many misspelled words may be given less attention because the reader may assume that the individual who cannot spell the terms used may not understand their meaning or use them appropriately.

Using Chart Forms Correctly

Many different chart forms are in use. You must become familiar with all the forms used in your facility *so that you know where to look for information and where to record your own data.* Initially, concentrate on forms that nurses are responsible to maintain. These usually include a graphic chart for vital signs (see Module 7, Temperature, Pulse, and Respiration), an intake and output record (see Module 10, Intake and Output), a checklist or flow sheet for routine care (Fig. 5–3), a medication record (see Module 47, Administering Medications Overview), and the nursing progress notes (Fig. 5–4). Other forms that may be your responsibility are the parenteral fluid record (see Module 52, Preparing and Maintaining Intravenous Infusions), the subcutaneous injection flow sheet (for recording urine testing, blood sugar results, and insulin given; see Module 50, Giving Injections), the blood pressure graph (see Module 8, Blood Pressure), the patient teaching flow sheet (see Module 45, Postoperative Care), and the admission and transfer forms (see Module 13, Admission, Transfer, and Discharge).

© 1996 by Lippincott-Raven Publishers

Table 5–3. Common Abbreviations

Abbreviation	Latin Meaning	English Meaning	Abbreviation	Latin Meaning	English Meaning
@		at	OS	oculus sinister	left eye
abd.		abdomen	OT		occupational therapy
ac	ante cibum	before meals	OU	oculus uterque	each eye
ADL		activities of daily living	pc	post cibum	after meals
ad lib	ad libitum	at will	po	per ora	by mouth
ax		axillary	prn	pro re nata	when needed
bid	bis in die	twice a day	PT		physical therapy
BM		bowel movement	qad or qod	quaque altera die	every other day
BP		blood pressure	q2h		every 2 hours
BRP		bathroom privileges	q3h, etc.		every 3 hours, etc.
c̄	cum	with	qd	quaque die	each day
cap		capsule	qh	quaque hora	every hour
c/o		complains of	qid	quarter in die	four times a day
DOA		dead on arrival	qs	quantum sufficiat	sufficient quantity
et	et	and	RLQ		right lower quadrant (of abdomen)
Frax, Fx		fractional, fracture			
gtt	gutta	drop	ROM		range of motion
h	hora	hour	RUQ		right upper quadrant (of abdomen)
H/P		history and physical	s̄	sine	without
hs	hora somni	hour of sleep (bedtime)	sob		short of breath
IM		intramuscular	sos	si opus sit	if necessary
IV		intravenous	spec		specimen
KVO		keep vein open (with intravenous infusion)	stat	statim	immediately
			sub q		subcutaneous
			tab		tablet
LLQ		left lower quadrant (of abdomen)	tid	ter in die	three times a day
LUQ		left upper quadrant (of abdomen)	TKO		to keep open (intravenous infusion)
NPO	non per os	nothing by mouth	TLC		tender loving care
nr	non repetatur	not to be repeated	TPR		temperature, pulse, and respiration
"o"		orally			
od	omni die	every day	UA		urinalysis
OD	oculus dexter	right eye	ung	unguentum	ointment

Flow sheets allow information to be recorded in tables or graphs. This facilitates charting in that *it takes less time to record information on a table than to write it in a paragraph.* In most instances, *it also is easier to review data or to recognize relationships among data when they appear in a table or graph.*

All systems of charting use some standard flow sheets, such as a graph for temperature, pulse, and respirations and a table for intake and output. Some facilities have more flow sheets than others. In the source-oriented system of charting, anything that does not fit onto one of the existing forms is written into the appropriate disciplinary progress notes (see below).

© 1996 by Lippincott-Raven Publishers

Table 5–4. Abbreviations of Medical Conditions

Abbreviation	Condition	Abbreviation	Condition
AIDS	acquired immunodeficiency syndrome	DTs	delirium tremens
AK Amp	above-knee amputation	FUO	fever of undetermined origin
ALL	acute lymphocytic leukemia	FX	fracture
AML	acute myeloid leukemia	GB	gallbladder
ARDS	adult respiratory distress syndrome	GC	gonococcal infection
ASCVD	arteriosclerotic cardiovascular disease	HCVD	hypertensive cardiovascular disease
ASH	acute subdural hematoma	LTB	laryngotracheobronchitis
ASHD	arteriosclerotic cardiovascular disease	MI	myocardial infarction, mitral insufficiency
ASH	acute subdural hematoma		
ASHD	arteriosclerotic heart disease	MRSA	methicillin-resistant *Staphylococcus aureus*
BE	bacterial endocarditis		
BK Amp	below-knee amputation	MS	multiple sclerosis
BMT	bone marrow transplant	PAP	primary atypical pneumonia
BPH	benign prostatic hypertrophy	PID	pelvic inflammatory disease
Ca	cancer (carcinoma)	PVD	peripheral vascular disease
CF	cystic fibrosis	RDS	respiratory distress syndrome
CHD	coronary heart disease	RF	rheumatic fever
CHF	congestive heart failure	RHD	rheumatic heart disease
CLL	chronic lymphocytic leukemia	SBE	subacute bacterial endocarditis
CML	chronic myeloid leukemia	SIDS	sudden infant death syndrome
COPD	chronic obstructive pulmonary disease	T&A	tonsillectomy and adenoidectomy
		TB or TBC	tuberculosis
CSH	chronic subdural hematoma	TIA	transient ischemic attack
CVA	cerebrovascular accident	TURB	transurethral resection of the bladder
D&C	dilation and curettage (of uterus)	TURP	transurethral resection of the prostate
DIC	disseminated intravascular coagulation	URI	upper respiratory infection
DM	diabetes mellitus	UTI	urinary tract infection

In the POR system, you are encouraged to initiate flow sheets whenever you will be collecting data or performing actions on a regular basis. Blank forms are usually available for this purpose. Thus, it will be your responsibility to figure out how best to represent the information in a table. Be sure you provide a place to note the date and time of each item in your table. Some computer programs do this for you.

WRITING PROGRESS NOTES

Narrative Notes

Narrative notes are a narration, or telling, of information. Most narrative charting is done in chronological order. You begin your statement with the data that were observed or that occurred first and move forward in time (Example 5–1).

This type of narration is easy to follow, and most people find that it traces thought patterns well. Finding relevant data regarding a single problem can be difficult, however, because a great deal of material must be read to gather specific data. Thus, many healthcare agencies have made some modifications to narrative charting. The narration itself may be organized according to functional assessment categories, body systems, or a focus of concern. In this case, you would chart in chronological order all the information appropriate to one category before going on to another category (Examples 5–2 and 5–3).

Problem-Oriented Medical Records

In this style of patient record, progress notes are written for significant data regarding any problem, and detailed data may be entered by any member of the

© 1996 by Lippincott-Raven Publishers

Table 5–5. Combining Forms

The combining form may appear at the beginning of, within, or at the end of a term. By identifying the meaning of each combining form contained in a word, it is possible to discern the meaning of the word. A dash preceding the form indicates that it is most commonly a suffix (appearing at the end of a term); a dash following the form indicates that it is most commonly a prefix (appearing at the beginning of a term).

Form	Meaning	Form	Meaning
a-, an-	without	hepato-	liver
ab-	away from	histo-	tissue
ad-	to, toward	hyper-	excessive
adeno-	gland	hypo-	low, lesser
-algia	pain	hystero-	uterus
ambi-	on two sides	-iasis	condition, formation of, presence of
angio-	vessel		
ano-	anus	ileo-	ileum (part of small intestine)
ante-	before, forward	ilio-	ilium (part of pelvic bones)
arterio-	artery	intra-	within
arthro-	joint	-itis	inflammation of
bis-	two	laparo-	loin, flank, abdomen
broncho-	bronchus	laryngo-	larynx
cardi-, cardio-	heart	latero-	side
-cele	hernia, tumor, protrusion	-lith	stone
-centesis	puncture	lympho-	lymph
cepha-, cephalo-	head	-lysis	dissolution, breaking down
cerebro-	cerebrum of brain	macro-	large
cervico-	neck	mal-	bad, poor
chole-	bile	-malacia	softening
cholecysto-	gall bladder	masto-	breast
chondro-	cartilage	medio-	middle
circum-	around	-megaly	enlargement
cranio-	head	meningo-	meninges
cysto-	sac, cyst, bladder (most often urinary bladder)	micro-	small, microscopic
		mono-	single
-cyte	cell	myelo-	bone marrow, spinal cord
derm-	skin	myo-	muscle
dys-	abnormal, painful	naso-	nose
-ectasis	expansion, dilation	neo-	new
-ectomy	excision	nephro-	kidney
-emia	blood	neuro-	nerve
encephalo-	brain	non-	not
endo-	within, inner layer	oculo-	eye
entero-	intestines	odonto-	tooth
ex-	out, out of, away from	-oma	tumor
exo-	outside, outer layer	oophoro-	ovary
gastro-	stomach	ophthalmo-	eye
hem-, hema-,	blood	oro-	mouth
hemo-,		-orrhaphy	suture/repair of
hemato-		os-	bone, mouth
hemi-	half	-osis	condition, disease, increase

© 1996 by Lippincott-Raven Publishers

Table 5–5. Combining Forms (Continued)

Form	Meaning	Form	Meaning
osteo-	bone	-ptosis	falling, drooping
-ostomy	artificially created opening into an organ	pyo-	pus
		retro-	behind
oto-	ear	rhino-	nose
-otomy	incision into	salpingo-	Fallopian tube
ovario-	ovary	sclero-	hard
para-	beside, along with	-spasm	involuntary contraction
-pathy	disease	spleno-	spleen
-penia	deficiency, decrease	sterno-	sternum
peri-	around	super-, supra-	above, more than
-pexy	suspension, fixation	teno-	tendon
pharyngo-	pharynx	thoraco-	thorax, chest
phlebo-	vein	thyro-	thyroid
-plasty	surgical correction, plastic repair of	tracheo-	trachea
		trans-	across, throughout
-plegia	paralysis	urethro-	urethra
pneumo-	lungs, breath	uro-	urine, urinary
post-	after	utero-	uterus
pro-	in front of, before	vaso-	blood vessel
procto-	rectum	veno-	vein
pseudo-	false		

healthcare team. The following format is frequently used (sometimes not all components are included).

Problem—identified by number and title.

Subjective data—the patient's perception or statements regarding the problem.

Objective data—your observations regarding the problem. Sometimes it is appropriate to summarize or refer to specific information found on flow sheets, for example, the pattern of an elevated temperature or the progression of a falling blood pressure.

Assessment/analysis—the conclusions you reach based on the data gathered. (This use of the term assessment is slightly different from the common meaning of assessment within the nursing process, which is why the term analysis also is used for this section.) The analysis may consist of a newly identified nursing diagnosis, a general problem area, or a summary of the evaluation of the patient's progress.

Plan—your plan of action to deal with the problem. This format is commonly called *SOAP notation,* and the process has been called *SOAPing* (Examples 5–4 through 5–6), from the terms subjective, objective, assessment, and plan. Although the SOAP format was developed for use with POR, it may be used for progress notes even when the record is not entirely problem oriented.

The actual implementation of the plan is documented on flow sheets. When a one-time action has been taken, some facilities suggest adding an "I" to the format of the note for the purpose of recording "intervention."

On occasion, facilities modify the POMR and use a more traditional style for progress notes. It also is common for facilities to make individual modifications in charting style. You should consult the procedure book in your clinical setting for specific policies and procedures related to documentation.

Special Notes

At times, information must be recorded that does not seem to fit within the scope of a single problem, and therefore SOAPing may not be appropriate. In-

Table 5–6. Using the Minimum Number of Words

Thought	Charted
The patient ate all of the soft diet.	Ate all of soft diet.
Bedbath was given to the patient by the nurse.	Bedbath given.

© 1996 by Lippincott-Raven Publishers

SHIFT	23–07	07–15	15–23	23–07	07–15	15–23	23–07	07–15	15–23	23–07	07–15	15–23
PERSONAL HYGIENE:	bedbath c̄ assist	back rub	Ø									
ACTIVITY: (Bedrest, Amb c̄ help, Dangle, Chair c̄ / s̄ help, Up Ad Lib.)	up in chair 15"	amb c̄ help 50 ft.	up to bath room									
ELIMINATION: BM (Number & Description)	Ø	ī med soft brown	Ø									
SLEEP PATTERNS: (Naps, 1 hour intervals, etc.)	nap 90"	slept 2130 – 23	slept 23 – 03 04 – 07									

DIET 2 gm. Na	Breakfast	Lunch	Dinner	Breakfast	Lunch	Dinner	Breakfast	Lunch	Dinner	Breakfast	Lunch	Dinner
Type	soft	soft	reg.									
Amount taken (All, none, fraction)	All	3/4	3/4									

ADDITIONAL NURSING ACTIONS & TREATMENTS: I.E. (Restraints, Decubitus Care, T.C.D.B., Wound Care, Dressing Changes, Traction Anti-Embolic Stockings, ROM, Suctioning, Positioning, Cath. Care, O₂, etc.)

O₂ @ 2 liters per nasal prong prn		11 – 13	18 – 21	Ø								

ONE TIME ONLY NURSING ACTIONS & TREATMENTS:

SIGNATURES:	23–07			A. Carlson R.N.								
	07–15	R. Gomez NS										
	15–23	K. Jones R.N.										

DATE:	3–17–99			3–18–99								

ADDRESSOGRAPH:

WATERS, VERNON M-57
539-74-0629
DR. SALINAS

SWEDISH HOSPITAL MEDICAL CENTER
Seattle, Washington 98104

Figure 5–3. A flow sheet facilitates documentation of routine care, including activities of daily living and treatments. The time that each activity occurred is documented when pertinent.

formation of this kind is placed in the progress notes and identified as a special note. Some types of special notes used are temporary problems, discharge planning, family involvement, and interim notes.

Temporary problems are concerns that could be SOAPed but that are so quickly resolved it is inappropriate to place them on the problem list. An example might be a misplaced valuable that is found or urinary retention that is resolved through nursing action (Example 5–7).

© 1996 by Lippincott-Raven Publishers

DATE / TIME	NURSES PROGRESS NOTES
3-17-99 1400	Reluctant to get up and take bath. Agreed to partial bedbath c̄ assist. Ate only 3 bites of cereal for breakfast. Refused toast, banana and coffee, c/o being S.O.B. after going to bathroom. Voided 150 ml dark amber urine @ 1100. Ate 1/2 of soup and 2 crackers for lunch. Napped from 1230–1300. ———————— R. Gomez SN
3-17-99	Lasix 40 mg given @ 1800. Voided 550 ml clear straw urine @ 1930 (1½ hrs. after Lasix given.) O₂ at 2 liters per nasal prongs 1800–2100.
2300	States "I feel some better now." Resting quietly @ 2300 ———————— J Paulson, R.N.

DATE	INTERDISCIPLINARY NOTE CONTINUED
3-17-99 1300	Given list of foods high in sodium and booklet of recipes low in sodium. Encouraged to write questions down. ———————— S. Kelly RD
3-17-99 1400	Reluctant to get up and take bath. Agreed to partial bedbath c̄ assist. Ate only 3 bites of cereal for breakfast. Refused toast, banana and coffee, c/o being S.O.B. after going to bathroom. Voided 150 ml dark amber urine @ 1100. Ate 1/2 of soup and 2 crackers for lunch. Napped from 1230–1300. ———— R. James NS
3-17-99 1700	c/o "a little short of breath" & "not much appetite." Crackles heard in lower 1/3 of both lungs. Ankles slightly puffy. (Less than 1+ edema) Will order prn O₂ @ 2 liters and Lasix 40 mg bid. ———— J. Abernathy M.D.
3-17-99 2300	Lasix 40 mg given @ 1800. Voided 550 ml clear straw urine @ 1930. O₂ at 2 liters per nasal prongs 1800–2100. States "I feel some better now." Resting quietly @ 2300 ———————— J Paulson, R.N.

Munsch, Paulina F-83
516-30-2250
Dr. Salisbury

SWEDISH HOSPITAL MEDICAL CENTER
Seattle, WA 98104

Figure 5–4. (**A**) Nurses' progress notes. The nurse may document on progress notes specific to nurses. (**B**) Interdisciplinary progress notes. The nurse may document on interdisciplinary progress notes.

DATE/TIME	
1/1/99 7:00 AM	AM care. Up in chair c̄ assistance for 30 minutes. No c/o weakness or fatigue. IV running @ 22 gtt/min into R forearm. Abd dressing dry and intact. ———————— J. Jones, RN
7:30 AM	Assisted back to bed. Voided 250 ml clear straw-colored urine. Moderate-sized, soft, dark brown BM. Demerol 75 mg IM given for moderate abd incisional pain. Stated relief in 20 min. ———————— J. Jones, RN
8:30 AM	Complete bedbath given. ROM done. ——— J. Jones, RN
10:30 AM	Rested quietly in bed. No further c/o pain. ——— J. Jones, RN

Example 5–1. Simple Narrative Progress Note.

© 1996 by Lippincott-Raven Publishers

DATE/TIME	
1/1/99 10:30 AM	Hygiene: AM care ā bkft. Complete bedbath. Activity: Up in chair c̄ assistance for bkft. No c/o fatigue or weakness. ROM p̄ bath. Nutrition: Ate all of soft diet. Elimination: Voided 250 ml clear amber urine @ 8:00. Moderate amt soft, dark brown BM @ 8:00. Pain: c/o abd incisional pain, 3 on scale of 1–5, @ 8:00. Demerol 75 mg IM given. Stated relief in 20 min. No further pain in AM. Fluids and Elec: IV running at 22 gtt/min into R forearm. Site s̄ redness, pain, swelling. J. Jones, RN

Example 5–2. Assessment Category Modified Narrative Progress Note.

DATE/TIME	
1/1/99 10:30 AM	Circ: IV running at 22 gtt/min into R forearm. Abd drg dry and intact. GI: Ate all of soft diet. Mod amt soft, dark brown BM @ 8:00. GU: Voided 250 ml clear amber urine @ 8:00. Musc-Skel: Up in chair c̄ assistance for 30 minutes. No c/o weakness or fatigue. ROM to lower extremities p̄ bath. Rested p̄ ROM. Neur: c/o abd incisional pain, 3 on scale of 1–5, @ 8:00. Demerol 75 mg IM given. Stated relief in 20 min. No further pain in AM. J. Jones, RN

Example 5–3. Body Systems Modified Narrative Progress Note.

DATE/TIME	
1/22/99 3:30 PM	3. Abd discomfort related to retained gas. S States pain relieved by passing flatus but has not been able to pass flatus. O Abd feels tense and hard. Guards when moving. A Has retained gas. P Increase ambulation. Encourage movement in bed. J. Jones, RN

Example 5–4. POMR Progress Note in SOAP Format Using Patient Problem as a Title.

DATE/TIME	
12/21/99 3:30 PM	4. Congestive Heart Failure S States cannot walk farther than doorway without shortness of breath. Feels as if cannot get enough air. O Resp 24, shallow, rales over both lung bases. Became cyanotic when moving to chair. A Fluid in lungs causing decreased aerating surface. Not enough O_2 exchange for activity. P Minimize activity. Provide supportive care to lessen O_2 need. Encourage coughing and deep breathing and turning to remove secretions. J. Jones, RN

Example 5–5. POMR Progress Note in SOAP Format Using Medical Diagnosis as a Title.

© 1996 by Lippincott-Raven Publishers

DATE/TIME	
12/28/99	3. Pain related to developing wound infection.
11:30 PM	S Has c/o of "increased pain" in incisional area changed from 3 to 4.
	O Had pain med q4h yesterday and q3h today (see Med Record). Temp increasing steadily to 101.6 (see graphic). Wound drainage has increased from scant serosanguineous to moderate and odorous (see Drsg Flow Sheet).
	A Wound infection developing.
	P Notify Dr. Jones immediately. Culture wound drainage. Increase fluid intake to a minimum of 3000 ml/24 h. Change drsg q 2 h. Establish dressing isolation.
	———— John Stuart, RN

Example 5–6. POMR Progress Note in SOAP Format Using Nursing Diagnosis as a Title.

DATE/TIME	
3/10/99	Temporary problem: Missing hearing aid
1600	S Wife thought it was with patient when he entered through Emergency Room.
	O Hearing aid not listed in initial personal effects list and not found in belongings.
	A
	P 1. Emergency Room to be contacted.
	2. Wife to search at home for hearing aid.
	3. Recheck tomorrow evening when wife visits.
	J. Jones, RN
3/11/99	Temporary problem: missing hearing aid, resolved:
1700	Wife brought in hearing aid this evening. ——— J. Jones, RN
3/11/99	3. Urinary incontinence
2000	S States: "I think I'm doing better, I was only wet once today."
	O Voiding when offered urinal on q2h schedule. See flow sheet.
	A Current program successful.
	P Continue bladder rehab. program without change.
	———— J. Jones, RN

Example 5–7. Temporary Problem in SOAP Format.

DATE/TIME	
12/30/99	Discharge Planning
3:30 PM	S Mrs. E. wishes to go to her own home for convalescence.
	O Resources for home care equipment and assistance with care discussed. Expected activity limitations reviewed.
	A Pt will be able to manage home care only with some outside assistance.
	P Contact social services.
	———— M. Rosen, RN

Example 5–8. Discharge Planning in SOAP Format.

DATE/TIME	
1/15/99 2100	Family Involvement ⸻ Rules regarding visiting hours discussed with relatives (two brothers, mother, aunt, and cousin). Family asked to arrange for not more than two people at the patient's bedside at any one time, to allow adequate rest for both patients in room. Special arrangements will be made for a larger number to be with the patient when the grandfather arrives to visit. Other family members may wait in lounge area. Family agreed to make these arrangements. Nurses will give the family notice when procedures are to be done so that an appropriate family member can be present to offer support for the patient. ⸻ M. Sanchez, RN

Example 5–9. Family Involvement in Narrative Style.

Discharge planning is important for a patient, but it often encompasses many problems and cannot be SOAPed in the conventional manner. A section of the progress notes is titled *Discharge Planning*, and the relevant information is recorded (Example 5–8).

Recognition of the family's role in the patient's life has led to an increased emphasis on including the family in care. This may be done by teaching family members and discussing the patient's care needs with them. When family involvement occurs, it is appropriate to make a legal record of it. This is done by writing a note titled *Family Involvement* in the progress notes (Examples 5–9 and 5–10).

Another type of special note is the *interim note*. This note is most often used to provide a legal record of nursing action that is not directly related to observations of the patient. For example, if a patient's condition is becoming worse and you are unable to locate the physician, your interim note might be a series of entries recording your attempts to contact the physician, your conferences with the nursing supervisor, and your contact with another physician. This provides the necessary legal record that appropriate nursing action was taken. Your obser-

vations of the patient would be recorded in a conventional SOAP note. An interim note might also be used to record the time of departure and return of a patient leaving a facility on a temporary pass (Examples 5–11 and 5–12).

Choosing Which Problems to SOAP

Most facilities have a policy that states the minimum intervals for SOAPing the active problems on the problem list. A common policy is that a SOAP note should be written if there are any significant changes, new data, or new insights or if there is a new plan of care. Additionally, the facility may require that each problem on the problem list be SOAPed at least once every 24 hours, even if there are no significant changes. In some facilities the nursing care plan indicates how often a problem must be SOAPed if it is not necessary every 24 hours (for example, "document on Mondays and Thursdays" or "document every Wednesday").

As a student, you should review the problems listed for the patient as you review your assessment data. Identify problems for which there are changes

DATE/TIME	
1/15/99 2200	Family Involvement ⸻ Growth and development information regarding common 2-yr-old behavior discussed with mother. Mother encouraged to let nurse know when she must leave and to be direct with Robbie and not sneak out. Reassured mother that nurses understand why he cries when she leaves and this is OK. ⸻ R. Filipi, SN

Example 5–10. Family Involvement in Narrative Style.

© 1996 by Lippincott-Raven Publishers

DATE/TIME	
1/23/99	*Interim Note*
11:30 PM	*Phone call to Dr. Johnson regarding patient's condition. His answering service was notified that immediate contact is needed.*
	C. Chang, RN
11:45 PM	*Call to Dr. Johnson has not been returned. Nursing Supervisor notified of pt's condition and of call placed to physician.*
	C. Chang, RN
12:00 midnight	*Supervisor here. Dr. Johnson's answering service contacted again. Unable to reach him. ER doctor contacted and arrived at 12:10 PM.*
	C. Chang, RN

Example 5–11. Using Interim Notes to Document Needed Medical Care.

to report. If you have not identified any changes, identify the problems that were the most significant for the patient while you were there and that have not been noted within the previous 24 hours. Plan to do a SOAP note on these problems if the facility policy requires it.

Your SOAP note should not just duplicate information on the flow sheets. It will summarize data and may even refer to a flow sheet for specific data.

Charting by Exception

In an effort to increase the efficiency and effectiveness of documentation, nursing departments have recently increased their use of flow sheets and decreased their use of narrative and SOAP notes, especially those that duplicate what has already been noted elsewhere or merely indicate "normal" or expected assessments or progress. As with other documentation methods, adaptations are made by individual healthcare agencies, but essentially the emphasis is on variations from the norm.

An example of one flow sheet developed by hospital nurses using charting by exception is shown on pages 92–93 (Figures 5–5 and 5–6). Side 1 is completed using functional independence measures (FIM). The FIM key is printed at the top of the form. Normal assessment parameters are printed on side 2. A normal assessment is indicated by a check (√)

in the box on the flow sheet. An asterisk (*) indicates a variation from the norm as specified in the assessment parameters. A narrative entry is then written on the flow sheet in the area corresponding with that shift and assessment area. An arrow (→) indicates that the variation continues but is unchanged since the previous assessment. Hence, variations from the norm stand out because they are the only narrative entries on the flow sheet.

Flow sheets may be kept at the bedside to allow for immediate documentation of data, thereby eliminating transcription of data (eg, from any temporary record to the permanent record). Trends in patient status are easily seen, and routine care and "normal" assessments are documented concisely.

There is usually a section in which a more traditional narrative note or SOAP note (depending on the policy of the facility) may be entered. This section is used for identifying new problems in a SOAP format or recording data that do not fit into the flow sheet format.

Focus Charting

Focus charting is another method of making narrative notes more clear and organized. The focus note has three parts to each entry: "D," the data; "A," the nursing action; and "R," the patient response. The data section contains both subjective and objective

DATE/TIME	
1/27/99	*Interim Note*
	Pt left on pass at 1:00 PM. Plans to return at 7:00 PM.
	P. Jensen, NS

Example 5–12. Using an Interim Note to Document a Specific Event.

© 1996 by Lippincott-Raven Publishers

KEY FIM

1. TOTAL ASSIST.	4. MINIMUM
2. MAXIMUM	5. SUPERVISION č CUES
3. MODERATE	6. INDEP. č EQUIP.

7. INDEPENDENT
NE (NOT EVALUATED)

DATE

HYGIENE

2300 - 0700	FIM	0700 - 1500	FIM	1500 - 2300	FIM
BATH AT___		BATH AT _08_	7	BATH AT___	
ORAL CARE X___		ORAL CARE X___		ORAL CARE X _1_	7
PERI CARE X___		PERI CARE X___		PERI CARE X _1_	5
OTHER___		OTHER___		OTHER___	

MEALS

COMMENT:	BREAKFAST	LUNCH	DINNER
	TYPE _2 gm Na_ FIM _7_	TYPE _2 gm Na_ FIM _7_	TYPE _2 gm Na_ FIM _7_
	% EATEN _20_	% EATEN _40_	% EATEN _70_
	COMMENTS _nausea_	COMMENTS___	COMMENTS___

TUBE FEEDING TYPE___	TUBE FEEDING TYPE___	TUBE FEEDING TYPE___
STRENGTH___ RATE___	STRENGTH___ RATE___	STRENGTH___ RATE___
RESIDUAL q̄ 8°___	RESIDUAL q̄ 8°___	RESIDUAL q̄ 8°___

ACTIVITY

BED MOBILITY	FIM	BED MOBILITY	FIM	BED MOBILITY	FIM
TURNED X___	7	TURNED X___	7	TURNED X___	7
AMBULATION X___		AMBULATION X___		AMBULATION X___	
DISTANCE___		DISTANCE___		DISTANCE___	
CHAIR TRANSFER X___		CHAIR TRANSFER X___		CHAIR TRANSFER X___	
TIME IN CHAIR___		TIME IN CHAIR___		TIME IN CHAIR___	

EQUIPMENT REQUIRED ▶ ☐ BELT ☐ WALKER ☐ CANE ☐ OTHER___
EQUIPMENT REQUIRED ▶ ☐ BELT ☐ WALKER ☐ CANE ☐ OTHER___
EQUIPMENT REQUIRED ▶ ☐ BELT ☐ WALKER ☐ CANE ☐ OTHER___

SAFETY

☑ 2 SIDE RAILS UP ☐ OTHER___	☑ 2 SIDE RAILS UP ☐ OTHER___	☑ 2 SIDE RAILS UP ☐ OTHER___
☐ 4 SIDE RAILS UP ___	☐ 4 SIDE RAILS UP ___	☐ 4 SIDE RAILS UP ___
☐ RAILS PADDED ___	☐ RAILS PADDED ___	☐ RAILS PADDED ___
☐ RESTRAINTS, TYPE___	☐ RESTRAINTS, TYPE___	☐ RESTRAINTS, TYPE___

INVASIVE LINES
(√) If site has NO Swelling, Redness. WRITE IN COMPLICATIONS.

	LOCATION	SITE		LOCATION	SITE		LOCATION	SITE
PERIPHERAL	RA	√	PERIPHERAL	RA	infiltration	PERIPHERAL	LA	√
PERIPHERAL			PERIPHERAL	LA	√	PERIPHERAL		
CENTRAL			CENTRAL			CENTRAL		
CENTRAL			CENTRAL			CENTRAL		
HICKMAN/GROSHONG			HICKMAN/GROSHONG			HICKMAN/GROSHONG		
IVAD			IVAD			IVAD		
OTHER			OTHER			OTHER		

SLEEP / REST

PT REPORTS DIFFICULTY SLEEPING ☐ YES ☑ NO
REASON___
___
___
EFFECT OF SLEEPING MEDICATION: ___

COMMENT:

COMMENT:

MEDICATION — PRN

EFFECT

ANALGESIC		Tylenol 650 mg po - 09 Pain 3 relieved to 1	

OTHER		Senokot 0.5 tsp po 08 mod. loose stool @ 1330	

PAIN SCALE ▶ 0-NONE, 1-MILD, 2-DISCOMFORT, 3-DISTRESSING, 4-HORRIBLE, 5-NO RELIEF
PAIN SCALE ▶ 0-NONE, 1-MILD, 2-DISCOMFORT, 3-DISTRESSING, 4-HORRIBLE, 5-NO RELIEF
PAIN SCALE ▶ 0-NONE, 1-MILD, 2-DISCOMFORT, 3-DISTRESSING, 4-HORRIBLE, 5-NO RELIEF

SIGS.

P Jones RN	R. Gomez, RN	J Paulson, RN

ADDRESSOGRAPH

ANDERSON, MILDRED F-62
542-37-1407
DR. KINDER

NORTHWEST HOSPITAL
SEATTLE, WA
ACUTE CARE FLOW SHEET
© NORTHWEST HOSPITAL

SIDE 1

M-439
(7/90)

Figure 5–5. An acute care flow sheet to accompany a charting by exception form. The functional independence measures key is printed at the top of the form.

© 1996 by Lippincott-Raven Publishers

☑ ASSESSMENT DONE FINDINGS WITHIN ESTABLISHED CRITERIA	☐ NO ASSESSMENT DONE	⊡ ASSESSMENT DONE – FINDINGS OUTSIDE OF ESTABLISHED CRITERIA	⇥ ASSESSMENT DONE VARIATION CONTINUES

INDICATE TIMES IN NARRATIVE

	24	01	02	03	04	05	06	07	08	09	10	11	12	13	14	15	16	17	18	19	20	21	22	23
CARDIO-VASCULAR	✓								✓								✓							
RESPIRATORY	✓								✓				*				⇥		*				*	

RESPIRATORY narrative:
1200 - c/o being S.O.B. p̄ going to bathroom at 1100. Resp. 26 twenty min. p̄ return to bed. Rules in lower lobes bilat.

1800 - c/o S.O.B. p̄ being O.O.B. to eat dinner. Resp. 30 twenty min. p̄ return to bed. O₂ at 2 liters per nasal prongs. 2100 - O₂ removed.

	24	01	02	03	04	05	06	07	08	09	10	11	12	13	14	15	16	17	18	19	20	21	22	23
GASTRO-INTESTINAL	✓								*				✓				✓							

GASTRO-INTESTINAL:
- BM: _____   *0800 - c/o "a little nauseated." Ate only 3 bites of cereal.*   BM: ꝑ lg
- HEMOCCULT _____   HEMOCCULT ⊖
- GASTROCCULT _____   GASTROCCULT _____
- BM: _____
- HEMOCCULT _____
- GASTROCCULT _____

	24	01	02	03	04	05	06	07	08	09	10	11	12	13	14	15	16	17	18	19	20	21	22	23
GENITO-URINARY	✓								⇥								⇥							

GENITO-URINARY (CIRCLE):
- PAD COUNT _____ — (FOLEY) — SUPRAPUBIC — CONDOM — ADULT BRIEFS
- PAD COUNT _____ — (FOLEY) — SUPRAPUBIC — CONDOM — ADULT BRIEFS
- PAD COUNT _____ — (FOLEY) — SUPRAPUBIC — CONDOM — ADULT BRIEFS

	24	01	02	03	04	05	06	07	08	09	10	11	12	13	14	15	16	17	18	19	20	21	22	23
NEUROLOGICAL	✓								✓								✓							

NEURO FLOW SHEET IN USE ☐ (YES)   NEURO FLOW SHEET IN USE ☐ (YES)   NEURO FLOW SHEET IN USE ☐ (YES)

	24	01	02	03	04	05	06	07	08	09	10	11	12	13	14	15	16	17	18	19	20	21	22	23
MUSCULO-SKELETAL	✓								✓								✓							

NEURO VASCULAR FLOW SHEET IN USE ☐ (YES)   NEURO VASCULAR FLOW SHEET IN USE ☐ (YES)   NEURO VASCULAR FLOW SHEET IN USE ☐ (YES)

	24	01	02	03	04	05	06	07	08	09	10	11	12	13	14	15	16	17	18	19	20	21	22	23
SKIN	✓								✓								✓							

	24	01	02	03	04	05	06	07	08	09	10	11	12	13	14	15	16	17	18	19	20	21	22	23
BEHAVIOR	✓								✓								✓		*			✓		

BEHAVIOR narrative:
1800 c/o "scared" when S.O.B. required O₂. 2100 "I feel some better now."

SIGNATURE: *P. Jones RN*   SIGNATURE: *R. Gomez RN*   SIGNATURE: *J. Paulson RN*

ASSESSMENT PARAMETERS

CV – REGULAR PULSE RATE; NO PEDAL EDEMA; NO DIAPHORESIS	**NEURO** – ALERT; ORIENTED TO PERSON, PLACE, TIME WHILE AWAKE
RESP – LUNGS CLEAR BILATERALLY; RESPIRATIONS QUIET, REGULAR RHYTHM, 10-20/MIN. AT REST; NON-PRODUCTIVE COUGH; ON ROOM AIR	**MUSCULOSKELETAL** – MOVES EXTREMITIES WITH EQUAL STRENGTH & SYMMETRY
GI – BOWEL TONES PRESENT; ABDOMEN NON-DISTENDED; NO NAUSEA OR VOMITING	**SKIN** – NO RASHES OR REDNESS; DRY, INTACT; ANY INCISIONS CLEAN & DRY; ORAL MUCOSA MOIST, INTACT
GU – CONTINENT OF URINE WITHOUT DEVICES; NO DYSURIA OR FREQUENCY	**BEHAVIOR** – APPROPRIATE TO SITUATION

DATE *March 17, 1998*	PATIENT NAME *ANDERSON, MILDRED F-62*	ACUTE CARE FLOW SHEET	SIDE 2 M-439 REV. 7/90

Figure 5–6. Charting by exception assessment flow sheet. The normal assessment is described at the bottom of the page and is indicated by a "√" in the box on the flow sheet.

© 1996 by Lippincott-Raven Publishers

DATE/TIME	
1/28/99	*Shortness of breath: Data: Able to walk to bathroom with O² @ 2L, without shortness of breath, Became S.O.B. with R 32 and labored after shower without O₂. Action: O₂ restarted at 2L. Response: Respirations became less labored and rate @ 22 in 10 min.*
	— J. Jones R.N.

Example 5–13. Focus Note Based on Patient Problem.

information and an identified problem if one exists. The nursing action section documents any intervention that was taken in relation to the information presented. The patient response section provides for an evaluation of the effectiveness of the action taken (Examples 5–13 and 5–14).

CHARTING PROCEDURE

The following is a general approach to assist you in organizing your documentation.

Identify Relevant Information to Record

Use the nursing process as a framework to guide your review and help you identify the relevant information.

Assessment

Consider all of the assessment data you have obtained throughout your time of care. Use a systematic plan to help you identify all *abnormal findings*, *changes in status*, and *information significant to the patient's nursing diagnoses, specific problems, or medical diagnoses*. Include all substances draining from the patient or the condition of dressings, tubes, or other devices. Use objective and descriptive terminology for these data, not judgments or conclusions. Do not forget the subjective data that the patient has shared or the indicators of psychosocial adjustment. Sub-

jective data should be clearly identified as originating with the patient. If your facility uses no organizing framework, the basic needs framework presented in this text may be helpful *to promote inclusion of all significant information.*

Nursing Diagnosis/Analysis

Note if you have identified a new *nursing diagnosis* for the patient or if there is a *collaborative problem*. Make a professional judgment regarding the meaning of the data, but be sure to differentiate between your subjective impressions or beliefs and a *professional* judgment regarding the nature of the patient's problem.

Planning

Note care plans that have been developed. Have *new plans* been made for addressing any of the patient's problems? Was a standardized plan of care, a protocol, or a nursing standard initiated for this patient?

Implementation

Note the nursing actions you have taken during the time you cared for this patient. Review the *routine care activities* that should be recorded and any *special procedures and interventions* (eg, prn medications, treatments, dressing changes, fluids instilled or infused), *patient or family teaching*, or *psychosocial interventions*.

Evaluation

Note your evaluation of the *patient's progress or response* to any nursing actions or medical therapies.

DATE/TIME	
1/28/99	*Heart failure: Data: Edema of ankles has decreased from a 3+ to 2+. Able to ambulate around unit without shortness of breath. Pulse strong this a.m. Action: Instructed in activity and rest management and low sodium diet. Response: Able to repeat instructions correctly. States she is looking forward to discharge.*
	— J. Jones R.N.

Example 5–14. Focus Note Based on Medical Diagnosis.

© 1996 by Lippincott-Raven Publishers

Identify Where to Document Data

1. *Flow sheets*: Start with the flow sheets, the specialized checklists and graphs in the chart. Fill in each one appropriately, including assessment data and actions taken. The forms will also help to remind you what data need to be recorded. Review each form thoroughly to make sure you have not forgotten anything, and then sign each form as required by your facility.
2. *Progress notes*: Turn to the form on which you will record your nursing progress notes (the nurses' notes or progress notes). Do not repeat information that you have placed on flow sheets unless the facility specifically requests that some information be documented in more than one place. Not only does duplicating records waste time, it also makes the record larger and more cumbersome.
   a. Using the format required by the facility, plan a nursing progress note. If this is a POR system, you will first identify which problems should be addressed at this time. Follow the directions given previously for a SOAP note. If the system requires a different orientation, such as a focus note, systems organization, or functional health patterns organization, determine the subject of your note. A progress note is most commonly used to *evaluate* the patient's progress.
   b. Date, time, and sign your charting as required.

Do a Final Self-Check

1. Reread your progress notes to make sure that they are legible and understandable.
2. Make sure that your charting is complete. Although it may make the record less neat in appearance, correcting errors or adding information that was omitted may be essential to the accuracy and clarity of the record.
3. Check that you have used the correct format required by the facility.
4. After you have finished, recheck everything to make sure that dates, times, and signatures are present and correct.

Although as a beginning student you will be expected to write out your charting on a separate piece of paper for approval before putting it in the actual record, you should develop the habit of double-checking yourself. It is easy to forget a time or a signature. Notify your instructor that you have completed your documentation if your facility requires the instructor to cosign any aspect of student documentation. Display 5–1 shows the charting procedure in outline form.

DISPLAY 5–1. CHARTING PROCEDURE

1. Identify relevant information to record.
   a. Assessment data obtained
      (1) Abnormal findings
      (2) Changes in status
      (3) Information significant to the patient's diagnosis and problems, such as drainage and excretions; condition of devices, tubes, and dressings; feelings and concerns expressed
   b. New nursing diagnosis or problem identified
   c. Plans developed for care
   d. Nursing interventions completed
      (1) Routine care activities and safety measures
      (2) Special procedures and interventions, such as prn medications, treatments, dressing changes, fluids instilled or infused
      (3) Patient or family teaching
      (4) Psychosocial interventions
   e. Evaluation of patient's status and progress
2. Identify where to document data.
   a. Complete each flow sheet with information, date, times, signatures.
   b. Complete progress note on information not on flow sheets.
      (1) Use correct format for facility.
      (2) Include date, time, and signature.
3. Do a final self-check.
   a. Legibility
   b. Completeness
   c. Correct format
   d. Date, time, and signature

© 1996 by Lippincott-Raven Publishers

LONG-TERM CARE

The regulations for documenting nursing care in long-term care facilities are federally mandated and interpreted at both federal and state levels. Specifically, these regulations state that the director of nursing services "ensures that all nurses' notes are informative and descriptive of the nursing care provided and of the patient's response to care" (The Federal Register, p. 49). With regard to the patient care plan, the surveyor is charged to verify that "the record indicates that the plan of care is followed and the goal of care is being met" (The Federal Register, p. 53).

All of the information in this module generally applies to documentation in the long-term care facility. Check the policies and procedures in the individual facility for further guidelines.

In long-term care facilities, admitting assessments and monthly assessments must be recorded on a form known as the minimum data set (MDS). This form is required by the federal regulations regarding reimbursement by Medicare and Medicaid. The MDS standardizes the collection of data on long-term care residents and thus facilitates policy making and research. Based on the MDS data, ongoing assessment is specified by resident assessment protocols (RAPs). These protocols help to standardize follow-up on actual or potential problems frequently seen in long-term care residents. Most facilities have a specific form on which to record the data required by the RAP.

In long-term care facilities, summary narrative notes are often written monthly. These notes may address each problem that appears on a resident's nursing care plan, providing an evaluation of that problem.

Many nursing homes use computerized systems that integrate all of the required data. For example, the nurse may enter the assessment data on a computerized MDS. If these data include "triggers" for the resident assessment protocols, they may be automatically included in the nursing care plan. As the nursing care plan is developed, the nurse indicates who is to perform each specified aspect of care. From this information, the computer will compile work lists for nursing assistants. The computer program facilitates accurate and complete documentation that meets all relevant regulations.

HOME CARE

The federal government and third-party payers require specific types of documentation to justify paying for home care. In home healthcare, documentation is directed toward nursing activities that are reimbursable. Reimbursement for home care is usually available only when a person is homebound and continues to need acute or skilled (not chronic) care. Because specific terminology is used in reimbursement policies, the documentation of visits must use correct terminology. To facilitate this type of documentation, many home care agencies have special forms with headings that guide documentation.

Some home care agencies have developed computerized systems that allow home care nurses to document care using a laptop computer and then communicate that information to the main agency computer through a modem or by transferring files at the office location. Whatever the system used, each visit must be correctly documented for the agency to receive reimbursement.

CRITICAL THINKING EXERCISES

• You are working in a facility that uses a POR system for charting. Jed Watson, 78 years old, was admitted for a radical prostatectomy. Since his admission 4 hours ago, he has been lying in bed. You have noted that Mr. Watson is very thin and has developed a bright reddened area over his coccyx. Design a flow sheet to monitor his skin condition and to record actions taken to prevent skin breakdown.

• You will be assessing pulse, respiratory rate, and blood pressure every 15 minutes after a patient returns from a procedure. In addition, your instructor has stated that every 5 minutes you should assess popliteal and pedal pulses on the right leg and make sure that a sandbag stays in place over the right groin to prevent bleeding where an arterial catheter was removed. To ensure that you do all of this correctly, design a working form for the bedside to help you remember all details and keep records as you care for the patient.

© 1996 by Lippincott-Raven Publishers

PRACTICE SITUATIONS

The following are clinical situations to be used for practicing documentation. Each focuses on a situation in which you are providing bedside care and assistance. You can use these situations on your own to practice writing various styles of progress notes, filling in forms used in your facility, or designing flow sheets. Alternatively, your instructor may direct you to other activities based on these situations. Evaluate your own documentation based on the instructions given in the module.

Situation 1

You worked as a student nurse from 7:00 AM until 10:30 AM. During that time you cared for Mr. Oscar Johanson. He is 66 years old and is in the hospital for bronchial pneumonia. This is his third hospital day. You assisted him with a bed bath; you washed his back and legs and he did the rest. He sat in a chair while you made his bed. At the end of 15 minutes, he felt tired and asked to return to bed. For breakfast he was served and ate hot cereal with cream, toast with margarine and jelly, orange juice, and coffee. His blood pressure was 146/84, his pulse was 78, and his respirations were 22. He coughed intermittently, but the cough was nonproductive.

Situation 2

You worked as a nursing student from 7:00 AM until 11:00 AM at Cascade Vista Nursing Home, caring for Paulina Munsch. She is 84 years old and has mild congestive heart failure. She is somewhat unsteady on her feet but can usually ambulate from her room to the dining room, the chapel, and the activities room. She is normally cheerful, cooperative, and interested in the scheduled activities at Cascade Vista. Today you noticed that she was slow to wake up and reluctant to participate in her care. Although she normally eats all of her breakfast, today she ate only a few bites of cereal and refused the rest of the meal. On the way back to her room she asked to stop and rest twice. At 10:30 AM, when it was time to bake cookies, she stated she wished to stay in her room and rest. She had an occasional nonproductive cough, and vital signs were as follows: T, 97.8°F; P, 88; R, 22; BP, 148/86.

Situation 3

You worked as a student nurse from 4:30 PM to 8:30 PM, caring for Mrs. Effie Sturdevan. She is 45 years old and had a hysterectomy 2 days ago. Her postoperative course has proceeded smoothly. She had a soft diet for dinner and had a large, soft bowel movement after dinner. She complained of abdominal pain, noted as 7 on a scale of 0 to 10 and was given a pain pill by the medication nurse at 7:00 PM. At 7:30 PM she stated that the pain was now reduced to a 3 on the same scale. During visiting hours, her husband and daughter were present. After they left, you observed that she was quiet, did not speak, and had tear-stained cheeks.

You helped her to ambulate at 4:30 PM and again at 8:00 PM. Then you helped her get ready for bed and gave her a back rub. While you were giving her the back rub, she said that she knew the surgery had been necessary, but she somehow felt like a different person. After you listened to her for 10 minutes, she seemed more relaxed and said she felt she would be able to sleep.

Situation 4

You worked as a student nurse from 0700 to 1200, caring for Mr. John Steiner, 36 years old. He is recovering from abdominal surgery to remove his gall bladder, which had been filled with large gallstones. This is his second postoperative day, and you helped him bathe himself and gave him back care. For breakfast, he ate a small serving of cooked cereal with milk and drank a small glass of apple juice and a cup of tea. You assisted him in ambulating the length of the hall and back, after which he asked for and was given his pain medication. His vital signs were as follows: T, 98.8°F; P, 78; R 14; BP, 134/86. His pulse and respiration were unchanged after ambulation.

Situation 5

During clinical laboratory practice, from 1300 to 1600, you cared for Mrs. Jennie Johnson, 77 years old. She had a mild stroke 2 weeks ago and is now on the transitional care unit. She has some difficulty speaking and cannot use her right arm. You washed her hair and set it, read a newspaper article to her, and helped her select her menu for the next day. She understood what you asked her about the menu and nodded yes or no about food selection. She could not comb her hair with her left hand; she held the comb awkwardly and kept dropping it. Her speech was not clear, but with enough time, she made some appropriate verbal responses. She said, "toilet" and urinated when taken to the bathroom. Her right arm was in a supportive sling. When you took her arm out to exercise it, her elbow flexed easily but her shoulder was stiff.

© 1996 by Lippincott-Raven Publishers

Situation 6

Your clinical time was from 0700 to 1100. You were assigned to care for Mrs. Dorothy Wu, 88 years old. Mrs. Wu was transferred from a nursing home for diagnostic studies related to decreasing functional ability. She is totally dependent and on complete bed rest. You did complete morning hygiene, including a bed bath and oral, nail, and hair care. You turned her every 2 hours and gave her a back massage each time you turned her. At 0800 you fed her breakfast. She ate a bowl of oatmeal, a dish of applesauce, and a glass of milk (240 mL); she would not take coffee and could not chew toast because she had no dentures. She was incontinent of urine twice and had an incontinent stool after breakfast.

Situation 7

Between the hours of 3:00 PM and 7:00 PM, you cared for Mr. Joseph Gonzales, 38 years old. He had surgery to repair a right inguinal hernia at 8:00 AM today. He returned to the surgical nursing unit from the postanesthesia room at 12:00 noon.

You took his blood pressure, pulse, and respiration every 2 hours, and they were as follows: 4:00 PM, 130/82, 68, 14; 6:00 PM, 128/82, 66, 16. He took 200 mL of liquid during the 4 hours you were present and had no nausea. You helped him walk to the bathroom and stand to void. He voided 150 mL. When you examined his dressing, you noted that there was no drainage and the dressing was clean. He had pain in the incisional area that he indicated was a 4 on a scale of 0 to 5. You gave him 50 mg of meperidine (Demerol) IM at 6:00 PM. He stated that this reduced his pain to about a 1 . He moved around in bed with ease and deep-breathed well when directed to do so.

Situation 8

From 7:00 AM to 3:30 PM, you were on a general medical unit as a nursing student. You cared for Mr. Thomas Brown, 32 years old. Mr. Brown has been diagnosed as having hypertension and is hospitalized to establish control of his blood pressure through an appropriate medication regimen. He is on a 500-mg sodium diet and allowed up ad lib. He had routine morning care. He ate all of his breakfast and borrowed salt from his roommate, which he used liberally on his eggs. He complained that the food was tasteless. He was dizzy when he got up to go to the shower. His blood pressure at 9:00 AM was 180/100 while lying, 130/80 while sitting, and 118/70 when standing. His pulse was 72, respirations 20, and temperature 98.4°F. At noon, he ate all of his lunch plus some potato chips brought in by a friend. He rested in the afternoon. At 1:00 PM, his blood pressure was 176/98 lying, 128/76 sitting, and 122/70 standing.

Situation 9

You cared for Mr. Wayne Jefferson this morning. He is 60 years old and had a right inguinal hernia repair. He ate all of a general diet for breakfast. He has been constipated, and you gave him a Fleet's enema at 8:30 AM. He then had a large, formed, brown stool. He bathed himself at the bedside. You washed his back and gave him a back rub. Vital signs checked at 7:30 AM were as follows: T, 97.8°F; P, 62; R, 18; BP, 144/90. He has had no incisional pain. He walked around the room and down the hall twice. He napped for an hour from 11:00 AM until noon, when you left.

Situation 10

From 3:00 PM to 7:00 PM, you cared for Mrs. Bessie McDonald, who was admitted 4 days ago with mild heart failure. At 4:00 PM, you assisted her to walk to the bathroom, where she urinated 250 mL clear urine. She then sat in a chair until after she had eaten all of her dinner. She said, "I'm so glad I can get around some now. I was so short of breath when I came in." You noted that there was no shortness of breath and that she did not seem fatigued from her activity. She returned to bed after dinner and rested quietly. As you were leaving at 7:00 PM, her husband arrived to visit.

References

Long term care facility interpretive guidelines. (1989). *The Federal Register.*

Joint Commission on Accreditation of Healthcare Organizations (1993). *Accreditation manual for hospitals.* Chicago: Author.

© 1996 by Lippincott-Raven Publishers

✔ PERFORMANCE CHECKLIST

Charting Procedure	Needs More Practice	Satisfactory	Comments
1. Identify relevant information to record. a. Assessment data obtained (1) Abnormal findings			
(2) Changes in status			
(3) Information significant to the patient's diagnosis and problems, such as drainage and excretions; condition of devices, tubes, and dressings; feelings and concerns expressed			
b. New nursing diagnosis or problem identified			
c. Plans developed for care			
d. Nursing interventions completed			
(1) Routine care activities and safety measures			
(2) Special procedures and interventions, such as prn medications, treatments, dressing changes, fluids instilled or infused			
(3) Patient or family teaching			
(4) Psychosocial interventions			
e. Evaluation of patient's status and progress			
2. Identify where to document data. a. Complete each flow sheet with information, date, times, signatures.			
b. Complete progress note on information not on flow sheets.			
(1) Use correct format for facility.			
(2) Include date, time, and signature.			
3. Do a final self-check. a. Legibility			
b. Completeness			
c. Correct format			
d. Date, time, and signature			

© 1996 by Lippincott-Raven Publishers

❓ Q U I Z

Multiple-Choice Questions

_____ 1. Ink is used for all charting because (1) it looks neater; (2) it is more permanent; (3) changes or erasures can be seen; (4) it is a custom.

       a. 1 and 2   **c.** 3 and 4
       b. 2 and 3   **d.** 1 and 4

_____ 2. If a 24-hour clock is in use, the correct term for 4:00 PM would be

       a. 0400   **c.** 1600
       b. 0800   **d.** 2000

_____ 3. In problem-oriented medical records, the progress notes are often written in a standard form. This form is abbreviated

       a. SOAP   **c.** COAP
       b. SOLD   **d.** PROP

Short-Answer Questions

4. List two systems for organizing the contents of the chart.

    a. _____

    b. _____

5. What are two methods of writing progress notes?

    a. _____

    b. _____

6. Why should objective terminology be used in charting?

    _____

7. In the following sample, underline the subjective terms:

    Crying. States upset over upcoming surgery.
    Paced the room for an hour before bedtime.

8. On the following charting sample, an error was made in the quantity of urine. The correct amount was 175 mL. Correct the sample as if it were a real chart.

    Up in chair for 30 min. No sign of fatigue.
    Assisted to BR to urinate. 225 mL clear
    yellow urine.

9. To whom does the physical chart or medical record belong?

    _____

10. Discuss the patient's right to the information contained in his or her own chart.

    _____

    _____

© 1996 by Lippincott-Raven Publishers

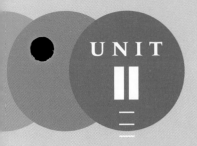

Assessment Skills

MODULE 6
Introduction to Assessment Skills

MODULE 7
Temperature, Pulse, and Respiration

MODULE 8
Blood Pressure

MODULE 9
The Nursing Physical Assessment

MODULE 10
Intake and Output

MODULE 11
Collecting Specimens and Performing Common Laboratory Tests

MODULE 12
Assisting With Diagnostic and Therapeutic Procedures

MODULE 13
Admission, Transfer, and Discharge

MODULE

6

INTRODUCTION TO ASSESSMENT SKILLS

MODULE CONTENTS

RATIONALE FOR THE USE OF THIS
    SKILL
METHODS OF GATHERING DATA
Consultation With Other Members of the
    Healthcare Team
Review of the Literature
Interview
General Observation
Basic Techniques for Physical Assessment
    Inspection
    Palpation
    Auscultation
    Percussion
Additional Skills to Enhance Physical
    Assessment
PUTTING ASSESSMENT SKILLS
    TOGETHER
BASIC DATA GATHERING
HUMAN NEEDS APPROACH
Physical Needs
    Activity
    Circulation

Elimination
Fluid and Electrolyte Balance/Hydration
Nutrition
Oxygenation
Protection from Infection/Safety
Regulation and Sensation/Comfort
Rest and Sleep
Skin Integrity/Hygiene
Psychosocial Needs
    Development
    Mental Health (Self-Esteem, Love, and
        Belongingness)
    Sexuality
    Social, Cultural, and Ethnic Identity
    Values and Beliefs
IDENTIFYING THE PATIENT'S
    PROBLEMS: THE DIAGNOSTIC
    PROCESS
LONG-TERM CARE
HOME CARE
CRITICAL THINKING EXERCISES

PREREQUISITES

Successful completion of the following modules:

VOLUME 1
Module 1 An Approach to Nursing Skills
Module 2 Basic Infection Control
Module 3 Safety
Module 4 Basic Body Mechanics
Module 5 Documentation

© 1996 by Lippincott-Raven Publishers

OVERALL OBJECTIVES

To gain an appreciation for the components of a complete nursing assessment; to achieve beginning skills in organizing assessment data and performing basic physical assessment skills; and to accurately state nursing diagnoses from the data collected.

SPECIFIC LEARNING OBJECTIVES

Know Facts and Principles	Apply Facts and Principles	Demonstrate Ability	Evaluate Performance
1. Methods of gathering data			
State five methods of gathering assessment data.	Given a list of information needed, identify appropriate assessment method for that information.	Gather assessment data using all five methods.	
2. Physical assessment methods			
a. Inspection			
Define *inspection*. List six areas to be included in inspection.		Include color, odor, size, shape, symmetry, and movement appropriately when performing inspection.	Evaluate own performance with instructor
b. Palpation			
Define *palpation*. List four areas or conditions that can be identified using palpation.	Given patient situations, choose parameters to be measured by palpation.	Using palpation, identify softness, rigidity, temperature, position, and size appropriately.	Evaluate own performance with instructor.
State two items of information to be included in explanation to patient prior to palpation.	Given a patient situation, state what should appropriately be included in explanation to patient.	In the clinical setting, give appropriate explanation to patient before palpating.	Evaluate with instructor using Performance Checklist.
c. Auscultation			
Define auscultation. State two ways in which nurse can help control environmental noise level.	Given a patient situation, state what might be done to control noise level.	Take steps to control noise level before attempting auscultation.	Evaluate with instructor using Performance Checklist.
d. Percussion			
Define *percussion*. Describe percussion procedure. Define *resonance, tympany, dullness,* and *flatness.* State where and in what situation(s) each sound might be heard.	Given a patient situation, state what sound might be heard on percussion.	In the clinical setting, demonstrate percussion of chest and abdomen.	Evaluate with instructor using Performance Checklist.

(*continued*)

© 1996 by Lippincott-Raven Publishers

SPECIFIC LEARNING OBJECTIVES (continued)

Know Facts and Principles	Apply Facts and Principles	Demonstrate Ability	Evaluate Performance
3. Areas of assessment			
Using the human needs approach, list and define 11 areas to be assessed.	Given patient data, determine to what areas data are pertinent.	Gather assessment data in all areas.	Evaluate own performance using Assessment Guide.

4. Analysis of data
    a. Objective data (signs or objective symptoms)
    b. Subjective data (symptoms or subjective symptoms)			

Differentiate between objective and subjective data.	Given data and their source, identify them as subjective or objective.	Include and appropriately identify subjective and objective information.	Evaluate differentiation of data with instructor.
5. Statement of nursing diagnoses			
State components of nursing diagnosis.	Given a list of assessment data, identify problem area, and state nursing diagnosis correctly.	In clinical setting, correctly identify nursing diagnosis, and state on patient's record.	Verify accuracy of nursing diagnosis with instructor.

© 1996 by Lippincott-Raven Publishers

LEARNING ACTIVITIES

1. Review the Specific Learning Objectives.
2. Read the chapter on assessment in Ellis and Nowlis, *Nursing: A Human Needs Approach,* or comparable material in another textbook.
3. Look up the module vocabulary terms in the glossary.
4. Read through the module as though you are preparing to teach the information and skills to another person.
5. Practice the following activities with a partner:
   a. Select an assessment approach (the one suggested by your program, the one used at your facility, or the one included in this module), and write its assessment categories on one side of a blank piece of paper.
   b. Observe each other without speaking or touching. Write all the data you can gather for each area. You may use the module as a reference while observing each other.
   c. Compare your lists. Discuss the differences and similarities in the data collected. Review your lists together, and put a star next to each item that is truly objective.
   d. Show your lists to your instructor for suggestions or corrections.
   e. Gather additional data without speaking but using touch and contact. Compare your lists again, discuss the data collected, and put a star next to objective data. Show your lists to your instructor again for suggestions or corrections.
   f. Interview each other to gather additional data in each area. Note the kinds of questions that elicit helpful answers and those that do not.
   g. Discuss these data. What data gathered by interview would cue you to make further observations? Also, what data gathered by observation over a longer period might be needed? What data are unique and obtainable only by interview? Underline the subjective data.
   h. Show these lists of data to your instructor.
6. In the clinical setting:
   a. Select an assessment approach, and write its assessment categories on one side of a blank piece of paper.
   b. Consult with your clinical instructor before choosing a patient to observe. Choose a patient who will not be upset or disturbed by your visit.
   c. When you are with the patient, explain your task in a way that will make the person feel comfortable. You can simply say that you are trying to improve your observational skills. Observe the patient for 5 to 10 minutes. Write all data gathered by observation. You may socialize with the patient during this time, but do not do an interview. At the end of the time, excuse yourself and look over your list. If it will not upset the patient, two students may work together. In that instance, you can compare lists.
   d. Consult with your instructor regarding the data collected. If you or your instructor feel it would be beneficial to you, repeat the activity with another patient.
7. Again, in the clinical setting:
   a. Look at an available patient record. Locate the healthcare practitioner's history and physical examination records, records related to laboratory and diagnostic studies, and the records of other specialists working with the patient.
   b. Note the documentation format (or blend of formats) used by nurses and other healthcare professionals in the facility. Is the format easy to understand? Share your observations with your classmates.
8. Look at an available clinical record. From the record, gather only what you think is pertinent assessment data. List the data under appropriate assessment areas. Mark each item *O* for objective or *S* for subjective. From these assessment data, identify and write what you consider the patient's problems to be, and formulate nursing diagnoses. Consult with your instructor regarding your determinations.

© 1996 by Lippincott-Raven Publishers

VOCABULARY

auscultation	flatness	protuberance	tremor
bell	inspection	resonance	tympany
consolidation	lesion	stethoscope	vibration
diaphragm	objective data	subjective data	
distention	palpation	symmetry	
dullness	percussion	symptom	

Introduction to Assessment Skills

Rationale for the Use of This Skill

Assessing patients is a major responsibility of the registered nurse. In every care setting, the nurse is expected to gather data that will be analyzed to determine patients' problems and strengths, formulate nursing diagnoses, establish treatment priorities, and plan care.

An important aspect of the information collected involves performing a nursing physical assessment to identify physical or physiologic problems. Many skills are part of nursing assessment. This module introduces the basic skills that underlie more complex tasks. Subsequent modules in this unit introduce you to additional skills that will assist you in gathering data.

Consultation with other members of the healthcare team, review of the literature, general observation, interview, and physical assessment will all be included in your total nursing assessment, although they may not all be a part of each assessment encounter.

Observations, augmented by skills in inspection, palpation, auscultation, and percussion, give the nurse a better data base for nursing care and give the physician valuable input into the medical diagnosis and treatment of patients.

Development of the skills presented in this module requires frequent practice. Acquiring these skills will provide a part of the foundation to enable you to do a more complete nursing assessment.[1]

METHODS OF GATHERING DATA

Assessment involves gathering all possible patient data *to identify problems and strengths*. Methods of gathering data include consultation with other members of the healthcare team through records

and reports related to the patient and through verbal interaction; review of the literature; interview; general observation; and physical assessment. Inspection, palpation, auscultation, and percussion are the only aspects of the physical assessment that are included in this module. They introduce the remainder of the skills related to nursing physical assessment found in Modules 7, 8, and 9.

Data are gathered from five sources: records of the patient's present and past health status, other members of the healthcare team, written information regarding the problem or problems and treatment facing the patient and family members, friends, and associates.

Consultation With Other Members of the Healthcare Team

The most basic method of acquiring information from other members of the healthcare team is through the change-of-shift report. You may or may not have an opportunity to look at the patient's chart before you hear the report.

A patient's chart or record contains essential information regarding identified problems. Consult the healthcare practitioner's history and physical examination records, the results of laboratory and diagnostic studies, the various nursing records, and the records of other specialists working with the patient. It is not always possible to review a record completely before your initial patient contact, but a thorough nursing assessment cannot be made without reference to the data contained in the record. Records of previous hospitalizations also may be useful. Module 5, Documentation, provides more information on using the patient's record.

In addition to reviewing the record, you may wish to consult verbally with other individuals who are or have been involved in the patient's care. Depending on the situation, the nurses, healthcare practitioner, dietitian, chaplain, or physical therapist may be able to share useful information regarding the patient.

---

[1]Note that rationale for action is emphasized throughout the module by the use of italics.

© 1996 by Lippincott-Raven Publishers

DISPLAY 6–1. EXAMPLES OF QUESTIONS
YOU MIGHT ASK THE PATIENT
DURING THE INTERVIEW*

Tell me in your own words what is "going on."

Is this what caused you to seek help regarding your medical problems?

Have you ever had this problem before?

What do you think makes it worse?

Is there anything you have tried that seems to help?

How do your problems affect your family and your life?

Is your family concerned about your health?

How can those of us in healthcare be of help to you?

By changing the wording, the same questions could be asked of the family.

Review of the Literature

Consulting textbooks and journals to gain more information about the patient's medical diagnosis, common problems related to that diagnosis, usual diagnostic tests, medications, and other forms of treatment can be an invaluable part of the data-gathering process. Although your patient will probably not fit the "textbook picture" in every way, you will be better able to plan care if you have updated or expanded your knowledge in this way.

Interview

The interview is a conversation with the patient through which you can gain information related to the patient's health problem(s), feelings, and perceptions, which can assist you as you provide care. Because it may be the first time you meet the patient, it can be the beginning of a trusting nurse-patient relationship. You must have a manner that reflects genuine interest, attentive listening, and a nonjudgmental attitude. The information provided by the patient is *subjective data*. If the patient is not able to participate fully in the interview because of physical or psychological impairments, include the family or those significant to the patient.

The first questions establish the patient's or family's perception of the patient's level of wellness before the present health problems. This part also contains other aspects of the health history, such as allergies and chronic conditions. The next set of questions focuses on the patient's present health sta-

tus and responses to illness. Display 6–1 gives examples of interview questions.

Note that a nursing history is a formalized tool for interviewing patients. Module 13, Admission, Transfer, and Discharge, provides an example of an initial patient interview. Whatever format is used, when a patient expresses a problem or describes a symptom, you need to elicit specific information related to the problem or symptom. For example, you can ask the patient the following questions (see Display 6–2 for a condensed version):

1. To determine the location: "Where does it hurt?"
2. To determine the onset and duration: "When did it start?" and "How long has it persisted?"
3. To determine the quality (eg, sharp or dull): "What word would you use to describe the pain?"
4. To determine the intensity or severity: "Using a scale from 0 (no pain at all) to 5 (worst possible pain), can you describe its intensity?"
5. To determine other affecting factors: "What makes it worse?" and "What makes it better?"
6. To determine functional effects: "Does it affect your ability to carry out routine activities of daily living or to perform other important tasks?"
7. To determine how the patient perceives the problem or symptom, which may range from insignificant to requiring a career change to life-threatening: "How do you perceive the problem or symptom?"

You may not need to ask each question specifically to elicit this information. Sometimes several areas are included in the answer to one question.

The interview will sometimes be abbreviated based on the situation and the reason for the assess-

DISPLAY 6–2. SYMPTOM ASSESSMENT

1. Location (*Where* is the problem?)
2. Onset and duration (*When* did the problem start, and *how long* has it been happening?)
3. Quality (How does the person describe the problem?)
4. Intensity or severity (What is the *magnitude* of the problem?)
5. Affecting factors (What makes the problem *increase* or *decrease*?)
6. Functional effects (How does the problem affect the person's *ability to perform activities of daily living*?)
7. Meaning of the problem *to the person* (Is the problem perceived as *significant* or *insignificant*?)

© 1996 by Lippincott-Raven Publishers

ment. For example, factors affecting the length of the interview may include the patient's current condition or symptoms (extreme fatigue, shortness of breath, or pain), the patient's schedule (appointment for physical therapy or a procedure in another part of the facility), or your need for only one or two specific pieces of information.

General Observation

While you interview the patient, you can, with practice, make many observations. General observation refers to what is seen, heard, and smelled while standing or sitting at the bedside. Whenever you contact a patient, observe carefully, paying close attention to detail. Your observational skills will improve with practice and experience. The information you gather through observation and performing a physical assessment is called *objective data.*

Look at the patient and the environment. *(Maintaining an environment that is therapeutic for the patient is a nursing responsibility.)*

When observing, no detail is unimportant. Are there any apparent lesions, depressions, or protuberances? Observe the patient's facial expressions and gestures, noting whether they are appropriate to what is spoken and to the situation. Note whether the general color of the skin is that expected for the patient's ethnic origin. Note also if the body is generally symmetrical. Do you see any problems with posture or with movement of the extremities? You may detect abnormal tremors of the face or extremities. Observe the patient's breathing, watching for abnormal movements and listening carefully to the sound of the breathing. Is it quiet and easy or labored and noisy?

Listen carefully to speech, and determine whether it is clear and understandable. Investigate thoroughly any differences from normal, distinct speech.

Note odors that are present. Smells are often difficult to describe, but comparing them to something familiar can help. For example, odors are associated with wounds and drainage, with the breath, and sometimes with the body itself. Be familiar with these smells; they all are important.

Basic Techniques for Physical Assessment

Physical assessment is the process of gathering data related to a patient's physical status. Combined with the data already acquired by reviewing the chart, consulting with other members of the healthcare team, reviewing the related literature, interviewing the patient or family and friends, and making general observations, these data assist you to reach conclusions regarding the patient's problems and strengths and to plan individualized nursing care.

Techniques basic to physical assessment include inspection, palpation, auscultation, and percussion. Terminology and a general overview are included here. You will find a detailed discussion of the application of these skills in Module 9, The Nursing Physical Assessment.

Inspection

Inspection is closely related to general observation, but it involves more specific, precise, and close examination of the body. Inspection may require that clothing or dressings be removed, the patient be turned, or a body part moved to permit examination. Although it is primarily visual, inspection also includes the sense of smell.

Work out your own system for the inspection process *to avoid missing any area.* You can use the body systems approach, a head-to-toe approach, or a combination of the two, but the emphasis should be on a *systematic* approach.

Whichever system you use, inspection should include observations of color, odor, size, shape, symmetry, and movement (or lack of it). In each instance, you will be comparing what you see with what is "normal" for someone of the patient's age group (Display 6–3).

When you observe something significant, you must elicit information about the finding. Use the questions presented in the section on interviewing to elicit further information.

You will use inspection when making specific assessments, for example as you assess pupils, breasts, and capillary refill (see Module 9).

Palpation

Palpation involves the sense of touch and in most cases is used simultaneously with inspection. Using the palms, fingers, and tips of the fingers, the nurse

---

DISPLAY 6–3. ESSENTIAL ELEMENTS OF INSPECTION

1. Color
2. Odor
3. Size
4. Shape
5. Symmetry
6. Movement

© 1996 by Lippincott-Raven Publishers

can identify softness, rigidity, masses, and temperature and determine position and size (Display 6–4). You also will use palpation to measure the rate and quality of the peripheral pulses. To carry out palpation *and* percussion safely and effectively, your fingernails should be kept short, extending only to the tips of your fingers.

Explanation is extremely important in gaining the patient's cooperation as you palpate. Explain what is being done, why it is being done (if appropriate), and what the patient can do to make it easier for both of you.

Auscultation

Auscultation refers to listening (usually with a stethoscope) to sounds produced by the body *to differentiate normal from abnormal sounds*. To perform auscultation, you must first be able to recognize the normal variation in sounds. Gradually, through constant practice, you will begin to recognize deviations from normal. Only a sophisticated practitioner can evaluate the significance of the abnormal sounds.

Stethoscopes come equipped with a bell, a diaphragm, or preferably both. With this last type, you can switch from one to the other by turning the chestpiece or by flipping a lever. Low-pitched sounds are better heard with the bell placed lightly against the skin; high-pitched sounds are better heard with the diaphragm pressed firmly against the skin. Many nurses purchase their own stethoscopes *to ensure quality and consistency.*

A critical aspect of auscultation is the control of the noise level in the environment. This is extremely important *to detect all sounds*. In addition, instruct the patient not to talk during this aspect of the examination. You will learn to auscultate, for example, blood pressure, lung, heart, and bowel sounds (see Module 9, The Nursing Physical Assessment).

Percussion

Percussion involves striking a body surface *to produce sounds that enable an experienced examiner to determine whether the underlying tissues are air filled, fluid filled, or* solid. The examiner hears (sounds change with the density of the tissue beneath) and feels the effects of percussion.

Because percussion penetrates only about 5 to 7 cm into the body, it will not detect deep lesions.

Types of Sounds. *Resonance* is the normal sound heard when the lung is percussed. You can elicit this sound by percussing the lung at the right anterior portion of the third interspace. The sound is low in pitch and not loud.

Tympany results from air trapped in an enclosed chamber. It is loud and high in pitch, somewhat like a drum. You can hear this sound if you percuss over the stomach. It is especially marked after a carbonated beverage has been consumed.

Dullness is a short, high-pitched sound heard over solid organs, such as the liver, spleen, or diaphragm. It also occurs with consolidation or increased density of lung tissue, as with pneumonia.

Flatness is a short, high-pitched sound completely without resonance or vibration. Fluid in the chest or abdomen can produce this sound. You can hear the sound by percussing over solid tissue—your thigh, for example.

Percussion Process. In this module, the percussion process is presented along with examples of the kinds of sounds that can be elicited (for the actual procedure, see Module 9). To be able to detect abnormal sounds, you will first have to practice on healthy individuals *to become familiar with normal sounds.*

1. Prepare the patient for the percussion process.
2. Place the middle finger of your nondominant hand firmly against the body surface to be percussed. Keep the palm and other fingers off the skin.
3. With the tip of the middle finger of your dominant hand, strike the base of the distal phalanx of the stationary finger twice, just behind the nail bed (Figure 6–1). Use a wrist action, and make the blows brief and even. Remove the striking finger immediately *to avoid diminishing the vibrations.*
4. Listen carefully to the sound produced *to identify its character*.

Additional Skills to Enhance Physical Assessment

Module 7 (Temperature, Pulse, and Respiration) and Module 8 (Blood Pressure) introduce knowledge and skills that make your nursing assessment more comprehensive. Measurement of *body temper-*

DISPLAY 6–4. ESSENTIAL ELEMENTS OF PALPATION

1. Softness/rigidity
2. Masses
3. Temperature
4. Position
5. Size

© 1996 by Lippincott-Raven Publishers

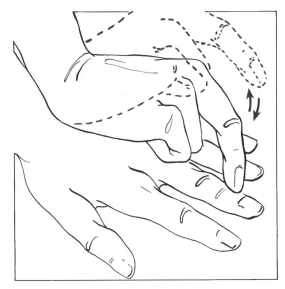

Figure 6–1. Percussion. With the tip of the middle finger of your dominant hand, strike the base of the distal phalanx of the stationary finger twice, just behind the nail bed.

ature along with knowledge of normal values for various age groups will assist in detecting signs of infection, inflammation, or both. Measurement of *cardiac pulse* (heart rate, rhythm, and quality) and peripheral pulses will elicit information related to cardiac and vascular status. Measurement of *respiratory rate*, along with observations related to depth and character of respirations, will assist you in assessing acute and chronic respiratory problems. Finally, measurement of *blood pressure*, along with knowledge of normal values for various age groups, will give you an overall indication of circulatory status.

PUTTING ASSESSMENT SKILLS TOGETHER

Although you will learn each skill independently, the goal is to combine your skills in a systematic way as you perform increasingly more thorough nursing assessments. The section that follows, Basic Data Gathering, assists you to visualize nursing assessment in its most comprehensive form. If you learn best from being able to see the entire process before you learn the parts, you may wish to read it now. If you learn better by viewing the parts before seeing the total picture, you may wish to study Modules 7 and 8 before reading this section. Module 9 presents details of various aspects of the nursing physical assessment and a comprehensive head-to-toe assessment. Module 10, Intake and Output; Module 11, Collecting Specimens and Performing Common Laboratory Tests; and Module 12, Assisting

With Diagnostic Examinations and Therapeutic Procedures, provide additional knowledge and skills to augment those you already have. With each new fact, concept, and skill you learn, you will move closer to being able to provide a complete nursing assessment.

BASIC DATA GATHERING

This module presents an approach to assessment data organized around human needs. An overview of each area is presented. If your program uses another approach to assessment, the human needs approach can be integrated into that one easily.

As you study the physiology and pathophysiology related to each of the categories listed, you will recognize the complexity of assessment. This discussion does not cover all the data relating to specific areas. Rather, it is an outline of major components to give you a beginning framework. Some components relate to skills and knowledge you have now. Others require skills you will learn in the future. As you learn, you will add more detail to your patient assessments.

Because a person is a whole entity, not simply a collection of parts, you may find it difficult to determine whether certain data are more applicable to one area or to another. In such cases, note the data under two or more categories. At other times, the problem may be clear, in which case list the data in the area that pertains to the known problem. The location of data is not as critical as your ability to identify related data and to recognize problems.

You must appreciate that no one system is perfect, but many have been used successfully. For example, Orem (1990) developed the "self-care" model; Neuman (1989) presented a system that focuses on the stressors and strengths of the patient; Roy (1984) developed the adaptation system of assessment; and Gordon (1993) used a functional health pattern model. (For details on one or all of these systems, consult the appropriate reference given within this module or a nursing text.)

Whichever system you use, assess the total person. The same data are required, but the organization will differ. The differences in the data-gathering systems stem from differing approaches to the organization of concepts relating to people and nursing. If you choose your own system, become familiar with the various systems, comparing and contrasting the terminology and the data organization. Consider the system you choose in light of your own approach to nursing and to people, and identify the one that will work most comfortably for you.

© 1996 by Lippincott-Raven Publishers

HUMAN NEEDS APPROACH

This system is based on organizing data around human needs. It is used most often by those who approach nursing with the objective of meeting human needs or preventing interference with the meeting of needs. The physical needs are identified separately, and the psychosocial needs are grouped together (see "Basic Data Gathering Guide," pages 119–120).

Physical Needs

Activity

This component pertains to the patient's ability to move and exercise for optimal functioning. You may see the term "functional assessment" used to describe this aspect of assessment. Functional assessment is usually an evaluation of the patient's ability to carry out activities of daily living. Consider the patient's usual exercise at home, diversional choices, and the effects of exercise. Note any recent variation from the norm, such as joint or muscle pain or disability. The individual's posture and positioning and the level of activity ordered by the physician are other items of concern. Note the pathophysiology of bones, joints, and muscles and the use of traction, bedboards, or assistive devices. Note also any medications prescribed for the patient that relate to this area.

Circulation

Under this category, collect all data that relate to the delivery of nutrients and oxygen to the cells and the removal of wastes from the cells. Objective data include pulses and blood pressure; color and warmth of the skin; medications taken for heart, blood pressure, or other cardiovascular problems; and any symptoms specific to cardiovascular problems. Include laboratory data that relate to hematology and blood chemistry in this category.

During your interview, try to elicit the patient's or family's perception of any current cardiovascular problems and the medications and treatment prescribed. You also must identify any cardiovascular risk factors that may exist, including whether the patient is a smoker or has diabetes. Other risk factors include high blood pressure, inadequate exercise, and a family history of cardiovascular disease or stroke.

Elimination

This category covers the excretion of wastes from the large intestine and the urinary system. Assess the patient's bowel habits and the type and frequency of stools. Listen for bowel tones. Ask about the patient's normal pattern of bowel movements and characteristics of the stool, noting those that are unusual. Elicit any history of constipation or diarrhea, along with pertinent information about medication. Be aware of the pathophysiology of the gastrointestinal system and of any relevant medications or laboratory tests ordered by the physician.

The urinary system handles the excretion of waste products by the kidneys through the urethra and bladder. Note usual patterns of urination and the appearance and odor of the urine. Note whether a catheter of any kind is present. Measure urinary output and compare it with fluid intake. Note any problems with incontinence, urinary pathophysiology, and medications taken for urinary problems.

Fluid and Electrolyte Balance/Hydration

This category deals with keeping the proper fluid and electrolyte composition within the body. Observe fluid intake and output, including the type and amount of intravenous fluids being given. Note changes in alertness or mental capacity and changes in muscle tone. Observe for changes in respiration that are not related to exertion and changes in cardiac rate and rhythm that are not due to heart disease. Alteration in the amount of fluid present in the tissues may be demonstrated by poor skin turgor or edema and by changes in daily weight. An increase in body weight may be the first indication of excess body fluid. Note serum electrolyte levels and any medications being received that might affect fluid and electrolyte balance.

Nutrition

This category deals with getting nutrients into the body. Observe the patient's eating habits (the amount of food taken and the kinds of foods preferred), noting particularly variations related to the patient's culture. Ask the patient about food likes and dislikes, the amount of fiber consumed, and any dietary modifications. Consider the patient's knowledge of proper nutrition and understanding of any special dietary restrictions. What is the patient's perception of ideal body weight? Both weight gain and weight loss (especially when the person is not trying to lose weight) are significant to nutritional data. These data should be considered in light of whether the patient has changed dietary intake or was seeking to change weight and whether the weight loss was intended.

© 1996 by Lippincott-Raven Publishers

Oxygenation

This category includes all data concerned with getting oxygen into the lungs and carbon dioxide out of the lungs. Note breathing patterns and changes in these patterns. Include observations of chest symmetry and the rate, depth, and rhythm of respirations. Auscultate all lung lobes. Listen for indications of impaired airways and for signs or symptoms of breathing difficulty. If the patient is receiving oxygen, note the rate and mode of administration. Note whether the patient coughs and whether sputum is produced. Describe color, consistency, and odor of sputum. Note whether suction is being used to help clear secretions. Ask what medications the patient is using at home as well as those being given in the healthcare setting. Note any chronic or acute pathophysiology present (eg, asthma, chronic obstructive pulmonary disease, bronchitis, or pneumonia).

Note respiratory risk factors, such as smoking and exposure to air pollutants. Some work settings predispose a person to an increased risk for respiratory problems. A history of frequent colds or upper respiratory infections should be listed as a risk factor.

Protection from Infection/Safety

These data are concerned with the effect of the total environment on the patient. Consider the environment in light of the patient's ability to respond to it and in terms of safety from microorganisms for the patient and others. Include data concerning the care of equipment, the position of side rails, handwashing procedures, and isolation provisions. Consider such factors as room temperature, cleanliness, drafts, lighting, and noise. Note whether the patient is able to reach the call light. Also note the accommodations (private or nonprivate room), the impact of other patients on your patient, and the location of the patient's room in relation to the nurses' station. Depending on the situation, the patient's immunization status may be important, especially in cases of acute trauma or infection.

The ability to communicate with others is essential to maintaining safety and must be investigated. Can the person speak? If speech is not possible, is another method of communication being used? For a young child, find out what words are used for communicating body functions, such as urination and defecation. Try to determine the extent of the child's vocabulary and the general pattern of speech.

Regulation and Sensation/Comfort

This category includes all characteristics associated with the central and autonomic nervous systems, including special senses and pain. It also includes levels or states of consciousness. Special senses include visual and auditory acuity or lack of it and sensitivity to touch or lack of it. The pain component includes the nature of pain, its location and duration, the patient's perception of its intensity, the pathophysiology involved, the length of time it has been present, medications used to control it, and the patient's perception of what is most effective. Sometimes it is more appropriate to list pain under another area, for example, when the pain is known to relate to a specific problem. Include any pathophysiology of the nervous system (eg, unconsciousness, tremor) and any related observations you have made.

You can check vision by asking the patient to read a name tag or a menu. Ask whether the patient regularly wears glasses or contact lenses. Assess hearing by noting the patient's response to your questions and comments. If you stand behind or to one side of the patient, you can be sure that the patient can actually hear you and is not reading your lips. If you suspect a problem, always validate your assumptions by asking if the patient feels there is a vision or hearing problem.

Rest and Sleep

Included in this category are data related to the patient's normal sleep and rest patterns; any bedtime rituals, such as bathing or reading before sleep; and data that reflect how illness or hospitalization may have affected those patterns and rituals. Observe the patient's appearance. Does the patient appear tired or rested? What amount of sleep does the patient normally need, and what is the usual bedtime? Are any sleep aids required (warm milk, medications) or any special equipment (special mattress, extra pillows)? The patient's physical and psychological status are important. Identify factors, such as pain, equipment (interference with comfort or normal position), and distracting noises that might interfere with the amount or quality of sleep the patient is getting. Consider the patient's diagnosis and what that means in terms of the need for extra sleep and rest periods.

Skin Integrity/Hygiene

Note the condition of the skin (turgor, hydration, color, lesions, wounds, rashes, scars, tattoos, and needle injection scars). List any skin sensitivity to soaps or lotions. Include hygienic needs, such as the care of mouth, hair, and nails.

Psychosocial Needs

Psychosocial assessment is complex and involves many different components. You will need to explore the patient's development; mental health; sexuality; social, cultural, and ethnic identity; and values and beliefs.

Development

A person's life stage reflects that person's stage of development. To understand life stage clearly , you must know the person's age, gender, occupation, and role in the family. For example, one client may be a 28-year-old woman who has a full-time job, a husband, and two children. This woman's response to hospitalization will most likely be different from that of a 68-year-old retired man who lives alone. The problems surrounding adaptation to illness will be different. Try to learn people's perceptions of how well they meet their own and society's expectations related to their stage in life.

Mental Health (Self-Esteem, Love, and Belongingness)

Observe for behaviors, and document any statements that indicate how patients feel about themselves and their own life situations. What kind of immediate family or close support does each patient have? Is assistance available at home? Will the patient have visitors? How do the patient and significant others interact? What statements does the patient make regarding feelings about others and their support and about the patient's relationship with them? Note eye contact, tone of voice, affect, and level of anxiety.

Sexuality

Gather information about sexual difficulties, menstruation, and menopause. Note medications taken or pathophysiology relating to the reproductive system.

It is especially important to gather information about sexuality when the person has had an illness or surgery that affects the reproductive system or gynecologic, breast, or urologic surgery. The patient may share with you that there are problems with sexual performance. Sexuality is a sensitive area for most people, so word your inquiries carefully, and avoid offending the patient or making him or her

feel you are prying into matters that do not concern you.

Social, Cultural, and Ethnic Identity

You will need to assess patients within the context of their cultural or ethnic environment and determine how this affects the reaction to illness or hospitalization. Is the patient able to speak and understand English? Will general care customs, dietary restrictions or preferences, or religious practices make a difference in the way you approach the care of this patient? What are the family's expectations regarding their participation in care? They may be accustomed to visiting in large groups, providing much of the care (especially any intimate aspects), and providing food for the patient. Does the patient have insurance or the ability to pay for care? How will this illness affect the patient's job status or ability to return to work?

Values and Beliefs

These may be based on an organized religion or on a general philosophical system. Note any religious preference listed on the hospital admission form. Ask the patient whether a religious advisor, pastor, or church should be notified. Observe religious or philosophical reading materials in the patient's room and conversation related to such matters. Consult your hospital chaplain or written materials about any religious group with which you are not familiar, or ask the patient if there is any way you can help.

IDENTIFYING THE PATIENT'S PROBLEMS: THE DIAGNOSTIC PROCESS

After you have gathered data related to your patient, analyze the data to determine the nature of the problems that are present. You may identify medical problems that need to be referred to a physician, social problems that must be referred to a social worker, or nutritional problems that will require the intervention of a nutritionist. The focus here is on identifying nursing diagnoses that are the responsibility of the nurse.

Nursing diagnoses are conclusions you reach based on the data you have collected. A nursing diagnosis includes a statement of an actual or potential problem for which the nurse is accountable and responsible to treat. In addition, a complete nursing

© 1996 by Lippincott-Raven Publishers

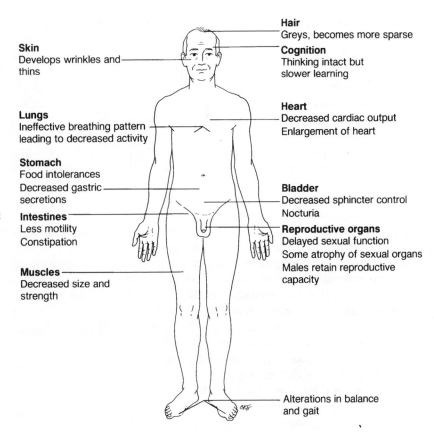

Figure 6–2. Changes in aging that affect assessment of the elderly.

Skin
Develops wrinkles and thins

Lungs
Ineffective breathing pattern leading to decreased activity

Stomach
Food intolerances
Decreased gastric secretions

Intestines
Less motility
Constipation

Muscles
Decreased size and strength

Hair
Greys, becomes more sparse

Cognition
Thinking intact but slower learning

Heart
Decreased cardiac output
Enlargement of heart

Bladder
Decreased sphincter control
Nocturia

Reproductive organs
Delayed sexual function
Some atrophy of sexual organs
Males retain reproductive capacity

Alterations in balance and gait

diagnosis usually includes a statement indicating the etiology or etiologies of that problem.

The North American Nursing Diagnosis Association (NANDA) approved the following definition of a nursing diagnosis at its ninth conference: "A nursing diagnosis is a clinical judgment about individual, family or community responses to actual or potential health problems/life processes." The Association further states, "Nursing diagnoses provide the basis for selection of nursing interventions to achieve outcomes for which the nurse is accountable." A list of approved nursing diagnosis terms has been compiled by NANDA. New terms are added at a conference of the group every other year.

The possible etiologies and defining characteristics of each identified nursing diagnosis also are established. The etiology of the problem is especially important because your nursing intervention could vary depending on the cause or causes of the problem. For example, your nursing diagnosis might be Constipation related to lack of privacy. Change the etiology to "medications," however, and the appropriate intervention would be different.

Nursing diagnosis provides a common language for nurses to use when identifying patient problems. With frequent use, you will begin to feel comfortable with this "new language." The use of nursing diagnoses helps to ensure continuity of care for the patient who moves from one area of a healthcare setting to another or who must change facilities. You can find a current listing of NANDA terms in any fundamentals text or in one of the many books available on nursing diagnosis.

LONG-TERM CARE

Accurate assessment of a resident in a long-term care setting is just as important as it is in the acute care facility. Unless a thorough assessment is carried out, the resident's problems may either be misinterpreted or go undetected. Although the majority of residents in long-term care are elderly, each is a unique individual, and problems cannot be identified without sufficient assessment data. People who have lived for many years have been affected by the various influences of a lifetime.

Some areas should be particularly closely assessed in elderly people (Fig. 6–2). The heart

(continued)

© 1996 by Lippincott-Raven Publishers

LONG-TERM CARE (Continued)

and lungs do not work as efficiently, resulting in problems with circulation and oxygenation. Mobility may be reduced, and coordination and balance may be impaired. Gastrointestinal disturbances of aging may lead to degrees of food intolerance, urinary incontinence, or constipation. The five senses may not be as acute as they were previously. Cognition and memory function vary with the individual. Certainly, assessment of the environment should not be omitted *because safety with this age group is a major concern.*

The person entering a long-term care setting is initially assessed for problems and needs using the federally required Minimum Data Set (MDS) form. This data set does not contain all the possible assessments needed, but it is designed to provide a common baseline. Individualized assessment should be added as needed. A standard procedure has been established for analyzing the MDS. Certain patterns of information on the MDS are used to identify the need for specific ongoing assessment, such as monitoring for possible skin breakdown. The protocols for these specific assessments are called Resident Assessment Protocols (RAPs). The MDS and resulting RAPs must be updated on a regular basis because the resident's condition may change. By doing this, *risk factors can be recognized and interventions taken to avoid serious or dangerous situations.*

To add to the assessment and gain more complete data, document the perceptions of both the physician and the family. By including the perceptions of the family, you gain insight into problems that may not have been evident on examination. The family also gains a sense of participation in the welfare of the older relative.

HOME CARE

The nurse in home care must perform a careful and detailed assessment. This represents a baseline on which newer data can be measured as the status of the client changes. Identifying whether the client is home bound is important, because funding for home care often requires that the person be home bound. In this setting, the family becomes central in giving information regarding the changing problems and needs of the ill person. It is helpful to use a consistent system for data gathering, which clearly outlines areas where problems exist. These can be updated and deleted, if resolved. Home care does not mean less assessment but a different view toward planning care appropriate to the home.

CRITICAL THINKING EXERCISES

You have been assigned to care for an 82-year-old female nursing home resident. You have 1 hour this afternoon to collect data about this resident to prepare for caring for her tomorrow morning. Identify your sources of information. Write out the approach to data collection that you believe will be the most effective, including the specific questions you will ask. Share your work with another student in your group, and critique each other's work.

References

Gordon, M. (1993). *Manual of nursing diagnosis, 1993–1994.* St Louis: C.V. Mosby.

Neuman, B. (1989). *The Neuman systems model* (2nd ed.). Norwalk, CT: Appleton-Lange.

Orem, D. (1990). *Nursing: Concepts of practice* (4th ed.). St. Louis: C.V. Mosby.

Roy, C. (1984). *Introduction to nursing: An adaptation model.* (2nd ed.). Englewood Cliffs, NJ: Prentice-Hall.

© 1996 by Lippincott-Raven Publishers

BASIC DATA GATHERING GUIDE

Human Needs Approach

Patient Initials _____ Room _____ Major Health Problem _____

Physical Needs

I. Activity
  A. Posture
  B. Ability to move
  C. Gait
  D. Activity ordered
  E. Abnormalities
  F. Assistive devices
  G. Medications
II. Circulation
  A. Blood pressure
  B. Pulse
    1. Radial
    2. Apical
    3. Pedal
    4. Rhythm
  C. Skin and mucous membrane color
  D. Nailbed color
  E. Skin temperature
  F. Diagnostic/laboratory
  G. Medications
  H. Risk factors
III. Elimination
  A. Bowel
    1. Date of last BM
      a. Description
      b. Stool specimen?
    2. Control?
    3. Bowel sounds
    4. Medications
  B. Bladder
    1. Urination patterns
    2. Appearance/odor of urine
    3. Urinary control?
    4. Urinalysis results
    5. Medications
IV. Fluid and Electrolyte Balance/Hydration
  A. Intake and output
  B. Intravenous fluids
    1. Type
    2. Amount
  C. Abnormalities
  D. Daily weight?
  E. Skin turgor

  F. Serum electrolytes
  G. Medications
V. Nutrition
  A. Diet ordered
  B. Likes and dislikes
  C. Height and weight
  D. Amount eaten
  E. Abnormalities
  F. Medications
VI. Oxygenation
  A. Respiration
    1. Rate
    2. Rhythm
    3. Depth
    4. Chest movement
  B. Breath sounds
  C. Secretions
    1. Amount
    2. Appearance
  D. Cough?
  E. Diagnostic/laboratory
  F. Medications
  G. Respiratory risk factors
VII. Protection from Infection/Safety
  A. Temperature
  B. Speech/Communication
  C. Environment
    1. Side rails
    2. Call light
    3. Accommodations
    4. Room temperature
  D. Gait
  E. Medications
VIII. Regulation and Sensation/Comfort
  A. Level of consciousness
  B. Special senses
    1. Vision
    2. Hearing
    3. Tactile sense
  C. Pain
    1. Description
    2. Location
    3. Duration
    4. Medications

(*continued*)

© 1996 by Lippincott-Raven Publishers

BASIC DATA GATHERING GUIDE

Human Needs Approach (*Continued*)

IX. Rest and Sleep
   A. Normal sleep patterns
   B. Sleep aids?
   C. Appearance
   D. Factors interfering with rest/sleep
X. Skin Integrity/Hygiene
   A. Skin temperature
   B. Color
   C. Integrity
   D. Lesions/wounds/scars?
   E. Rash?
   F. Hydration
   G. Sensitivity to soap/lotion?
   H. Hygiene
   I. Medications

Psychosocial Needs

XI. Development
   A. Age
   B. Life stage
   C. Occupation
   D. Role in family unit
XII. Mental Health
   A. Self-esteem
      1. Feelings about self
      2. Behaviors exhibited
   B. Love and belongingness
      1. Immediate family
      2. Help at home
      3. Feelings about relationships
      4. Behaviors exhibited
XIII. Sexuality
   A. Gender
   B. Last menstrual period (LMP)—menstrual history
   C. Gravida; para?
   D. Significant other
   E. Concerns expressed
   F. Diagnostic/laboratory
   G. Medications
XIV. Social, Cultural, and Ethnic Identity
   A. Country of origin
   B. Language?
   C. Special needs?
   D. Insurance/financial support?
XV. Values and Beliefs
   A. Religious preference
   B. Notification desired?
   C. Special needs?

© 1996 by Lippincott-Raven Publishers

? **Q U I Z**

Multiple-Choice Questions

For questions 1–4, indicate which data gathering method would be most useful in acquiring the information indicated: (a) interview, (b) general observation, (c) physical assessment, (d) consultation with other members of the healthcare team, or (e) review of the literature.

_____ **1.** The best way to learn whether a patient has had a bowel movement during your shift

_____ **2.** The best way to learn whether a patient is developing edema (tissue swelling from retained fluid)

_____ **3.** For a night nurse, the best way to learn the sleeping patterns of a patient

_____ **4.** The best way to learn the potential side effects of a medication the patient is taking

For questions 5–9, mark *O* if the data are objective and *S* if they are subjective.

_____ **5.** The patient says he or she has severe nausea.

_____ **6.** After ambulation, the patient is pale and has a pulse rate of 100.

_____ **7.** The patient feels depressed.

_____ **8.** The patient is breathing shallowly at a rate of 30 respirations per minute.

_____ **9.** The laboratory report indicates that the patient has a hemoglobin level of 8.

Short-Answer Questions

10. List five elements that should be included in inspection.

　　a. _____

　　b. _____

　　c. _____

　　d. _____

　　e. _____

11. List three elements that the nurse should include in the explanation to the patient prior to palpation.

　　a. _____

　　b. _____

　　c. _____

© 1996 by Lippincott-Raven Publishers

MODULE

7

TEMPERATURE, PULSE, AND RESPIRATION

MODULE CONTENTS

RATIONALE FOR THE USE OF THIS SKILL
NURSING DIAGNOSES
VITAL SIGNS
Temperature
 Types of Thermometers
 Sites for Measuring Temperature
Pulse
 Peripheral Pulses
 Apical Pulse
Respiration
PROCEDURE FOR MEASURING TEMPERATURE, PULSE, AND RESPIRATION
 Assessment
 Planning
 Implementation
 Evaluation
 Documentation
LONG-TERM CARE
HOME CARE
CRITICAL THINKING EXERCISES

PREREQUISITES

Successful completion of the following modules:

VOLUME 1
Module 1 An Approach to Nursing Skills
Module 2 Basic Infection Control
Module 3 Safety
Module 5 Documentation
Module 6 Introduction to Assessment Skills

© 1996 by Lippincott-Raven Publishers

OVERALL OBJECTIVE

To measure and document patients' temperature, pulse, and respiration (TPR) accurately and safely, recognizing deviations from the norm.

SPECIFIC LEARNING OBJECTIVES

Know Facts and Principles	Apply Facts and Principles	Demonstrate Ability	Evaluate Performance

1. Body temperature
  a. Normal body temperature
  b. Methods of measurement
  c. Measurement procedures
  d. Documentation			

State normal oral, rectal, and axillary temperature range in Celsius and Fahrenheit measurements.	Give examples of factors that can cause variations in body temperature.	Demonstrate taking patient's temperature, using Fahrenheit and Celsius thermometers, observing proper technique and safety precautions. On graphic and nurses' notes, record data clearly and accurately.	Evaluate own performance using Performance Checklist.

2. Pulse
  a. Normal pulse rate
  b. Pulse rate procedure
  c. Documentation			

Define normal pulse rates for different age groups.	Identify factors that influence pulse rate.	Count patient's radial and apical pulse accurately. On graphic, record pulse in proper location; on nurses' notes, record pulse in numeric and descriptive terms.	Evaluate own performance using Performance Checklist.

3. Respiration
  a. Normal respiratory rate
  b. Respiratory rate procedure
  c. Documentation			

Identify normal respiratory rates for different age groups.	Relate factors that influence respiratory rates.	Determine patient's respiratory rate using correct technique. Record rate and character of respiration on graphic and nurses' notes.	Evaluate own performance using Performance Checklist.

© 1996 by Lippincott-Raven Publishers

LEARNING ACTIVITIES

1. Review the Specific Learning Objectives.
2. Read the chapter on oxygenation, circulation, and neurologic function in Ellis and Nowlis, *Nursing: A Human Needs Approach,* or a comparable chapter in another textbook.
3. Look up the module vocabulary terms in the glossary.
4. Read through the module, noting the graphic chart used to record vital signs (see Fig. 7–1). Read as though you were preparing to teach the content to another person.
5. Review the steps of the procedure in the Performance Checklist.
6. Do the following in the practice setting:
   a. Inspect and become familiar with the TPR equipment.
   b. Select a partner. Take your partner's oral and axillary temperatures using a standard mercury thermometer. Compare the two findings.
   c. Record the oral temperature reading on the vital signs graphic chart (see Fig. 7–1).
   d. Have your partner drink a glass of cold water and retake the oral temperatures in 15 minutes. How does this reading compare with the one taken previously?
   e. If an electronic or tympanic thermometer is available, retake your partner's temperature using these thermometers, and compare this reading with the reading from the glass or mercury thermometer.
   f. With your partner in a supine position, count the radial pulse, and record it. Record the quality of the pulse felt on a progress sheet or a piece of paper.
   g. After your partner has exercised briskly (running in place) for 3 minutes, retake the pulse and compare the rate and quality with that of the radial pulse taken previously.
   h. Choose another student in the practice setting. With your partner, take an apical-radial pulse on the student. What would you consider normal? Why?
   i. Repeat steps f and g, this time measuring respiration.
   j. Complete the vital signs graphic, and turn it in to your instructor.
7. Do the following in the clinical setting:
   a. Check the form used by your facility, the type of equipment being used, and the cleaning method for thermometers and stethoscopes.
   b. Take a TPR on a patient. Follow the procedure with supervision, and record your results.
   c. If possible, repeat the TPR procedure 4 hours later on the same patient, and compare the two readings. Which of the measurements has changed? To what factors might you attribute this change?

VOCABULARY *Know*

Temperature

afebrile	centigrade	fever	remittent
antipyretic	circadian rhythm	intermittent	Sims' position
axilla	Fahrenheit	metabolism	tympanic
Celsius	febrile	reflectance	

Pulse

apical pulse	dorsalis pedis artery	pulse deficit	temporal artery
bounding pulse	femoral artery	pulse pressure	thready pulse
bradycardia *slow*	midclavicular line	radial artery	
carotid artery	pedal pulse	tachycardia	

Respiration

apnea	dyspnea	orthopnea	symmetry
bradypnea	eupnea	rhythm	tachypnea
Cheyne-Stokes respirations	Kussmaul's respirations	stertorous	thermistor

© 1996 by Lippincott-Raven Publishers

Temperature, Pulse, and Respiration

Rationale for the Use of This Skill

Because temperature, pulse, and respiration (TPR) are basic measurements that are helpful when assessing patients' conditions, it is essential that the practicing nurse be able to take and record them accurately. TPRs are taken by professional and nonprofessional staff in healthcare settings. Both can perform the mechanics of the procedure equally well. The professional nurse, however, has the responsibility for understanding the deviations from normal on which assessments and interpretations are based.

After completing this module, you should be able to define these signs accurately, measure them, and record them. You should also be able to adapt this procedure to both well and ill individuals of any age and appropriately interpret your findings. You will then be able to move on to Module 8, Blood Pressure, which will complete the material on vital signs.[1]

▼ NURSING DIAGNOSES

A major nursing diagnosis that is frequently used is Hyperthermia. The patient could have a fever that is related to a variety of factors, including infection, dehydration, vigorous exercise, or an unusually warm environment. Another nursing diagnosis is Hypothermia or reduction in body temperature. Factors for this nursing diagnosis are often related to the environment or to inadequate clothing. Other factors include malnutrition and dehydration. When risk factors are present, the diagnosis is written Risk for Hyperthermia or Hypothermia.

The nursing diagnosis Ineffective Thermoregulation refers to persons who may have an inadequately controlled or unstable body temperature. In the infant, the risk factor may be an immature regulatory system; in the elderly, the regulatory response may not be as vigorous.

Decreased Cardiac Output is a collaborative diagnosis that could be related to the presence of an excessively slow or excessively rapid pulse rate. The nursing diagnosis would relate to the patient's problems. A very rapid pulse and respiratory rate may be associated with Activity Intolerance.

Sleep Pattern Disturbance and Ineffective Breathing Pattern could both be related to an abnormality in the respiratory rate or pattern.

[1]Note that rationale for action is emphasized throughout the module by the use of italics.

© 1996 by Lippincott-Raven Publishers

VITAL SIGNS

Taking vital signs (including TPR) is important *because it indicates a patient's health status.* Most institutions have routine times for taking TPR, often twice a day (b.i.d.), *but a patient's illness or certain other conditions may dictate more or less frequent measurement.* For example, you would make an independent nursing decision to take the temperature of a flushed patient who complains of feeling warm. Routine TPR is usually taken on a number of patients at one time, and the readings recorded at the bedside on paper or directly into a bedside computer terminal. Readings recorded on paper are then transcribed to a central clipboard at the nurses' station or directly on the graphic record in the patient's chart (Fig. 7–1).

Temperature

Body temperature is the balance between heat produced and heat lost by the body. It is surprisingly consistent in healthy individuals; that is, a normal oral reading is 98.6° Fahrenheit or 37° Celsius (sometimes called *centigrade*). Actually, body temperature can register 97° to 99°F or 36.1° to 37.2°C and still be considered normal in healthy individuals. Researchers have long studied the mean or average body temperature of adults, and the measurement 98.2°F or 36.8°C appears to be more accurate than the long-held measurement of 98.6°F or 37°C. However, whichever value is used, the variation within individuals is the most important factor to consider (Winslow, 1994). You will need to ascertain the standard your facility uses regarding "normal" temperature.

A normal daily temperature variation results from the body's circadian rhythm. The lowest temperature occurs between about 2 AM and 6 AM, and the highest between about 4 PM and 8 PM.

Studies of oral temperatures in healthy older adults indicate that the normal body temperature decreases as age increases. In addition, infectious processes are not always accompanied by an elevated temperature in older adults. Because of these factors, those who care for older adults need to know what "normal" is for each resident, so they will be aware of any change and take steps to initiate any necessary treatment.

Many factors—age, infection, temperature of the environment, amount of exercise, metabolism, and emotional status—can affect a patient's temperature and should be considered when evaluating a temperature reading. If the temperature is elevated, the patient is *febrile,* that is, has a fever. If the temperature is normal, the patient is *afebrile,* that is, without fever. Depending on the pattern of fluctuations of the elevation, the temperature can be described as *remittent* or *intermittent* (see glossary).

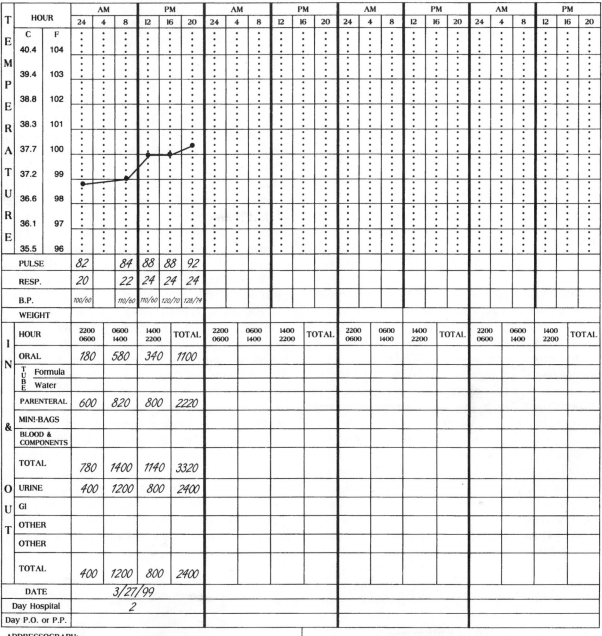

Figure 7–1. Vital signs graphic form. You can easily identify relationships between serial vital signs when a graphic flow sheet is used.

Types of Thermometers

With a *standard glass thermometer* containing mercury, temperature can be measured orally, rectally, or by placing the thermometer in the axilla. The mercury in the thermometer expands as it is heated. Therefore, when the thermometer comes into contact with warm body tissues, the mercury warms, expands, and rises inside the glass tubing. The top of the column of mercury can be identified and the temperature is read from number markings on the glass.

The oral glass thermometer has a slender bulb designed *to provide a large surface for exposure when it is placed under the tongue.* The rectal glass thermometer has a pear-shaped bulb, and the multiuse glass ther-

© 1996 by Lippincott-Raven Publishers

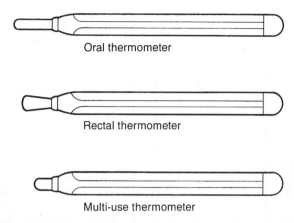

Oral thermometer

Rectal thermometer

Multi-use thermometer

Figure 7–2. The oral thermometer has a slender bulb. The rectal thermometer has a pear-shaped bulb. The multiuse thermometer has a blunt tip.

mometer has a blunt, stubby tip. This latter type of thermometer may be used at the oral, rectal, or axillary site and is commonly used for children, *because it is considered the safest* (Fig. 7–2).

A thermometer sheath can be used *to keep the thermometer from direct contact with the patient*. The sheath is a tube of very thin plastic that comes wrapped in a paper strip. To use it, strip back the paper to expose the open end of the sheath. Insert the glass thermometer into the sheath, and push down until it is completely protected except for the end that you will hold in your hand. Discard the paper covering. Insert the sheath-covered thermometer into the patient's mouth or rectum. Wait the appropriate time, and then remove the thermometer. Pull the sheath down over itself and discard. Read the thermometer. Although most microorganisms are enclosed in the sheath, the thermometer should be washed with soap and cool water *to ensure infection control.*

The obvious disadvantage of the glass thermometer is that it is breakable and could cause injury at any site if not used with care. Although mercury from a broken glass thermometer can give off harmful vapors when exposed to air, the amount of mercury in an individual thermometer is so small that it is of little consequence. If ingested, it is not toxic because it oxidizes too slowly to be absorbed.

Electronic thermometers (Fig. 7–3) are available for oral and rectal use. These thermometers use a component called a thermistor at the end of a plastic and stainless steel probe to sense the temperature. While the thermometer is being used, the probe is covered with a disposable probe cover, which is discarded after each use.

The temperature is read on a digital display that resets itself when the probe is replaced in the body of the battery-powered device. Some electronic thermometers include a timer that may be used to measure pulse, respiration, intravenous drip rate, or any other time measurement. It functions like a stopwatch and may be restarted at any time. The electronic thermometer is carried from one patient to another, along with a sufficient supply of disposable probe covers. It therefore is not useful for patients with infectious disease, unless it can stay in the room and be used by one patient only. Most facilities do not own enough electronic thermometers to use them in this way, so glass or disposable thermometers are commonly used in such situations.

Another type of electronic thermometer, a *tympanic thermometer*, is increasing in use. This type of thermometer uses infrared technology (reflectance) to measure temperature on the tympanic membrane.

A covered probe is placed at the external opening of the ear canal, where it senses the infrared energy produced by the tympanic membrane (Fig. 7–4).

It is essential that the probe be placed at the proper angle, sealing the ear canal. (Directions from the manufacturer will delineate the correct angle.) The tympanic temperature is registered on a digital display in about 1 second. *Because the ear canal has no mucous membranes*, it is not easily influenced by evaporation or other ambient changes and has demonstrated reliable correlation with the body's core temperature. A study conducted by Davis (1993) concluded that the use of the tympanic thermometer is accurate when compared with oral, rectal, or axillary temperature measurement in adults and children, but it is not accurate in temperature measurement of newborns. To ensure accuracy, Davis recommends that tympanic thermometers be used only in children older than 3 years.

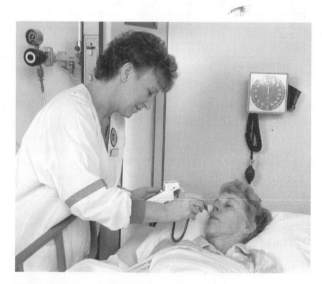

Figure 7–3. The display panel on an electronic thermometer will register the temperature reading in 30–50 seconds.

© 1996 by Lippincott-Raven Publishers

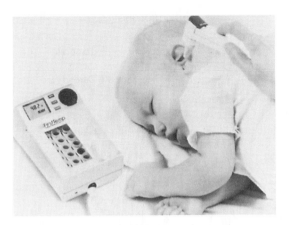

Figure 7–4. The tympanic thermometer. The same nonintrusive probe covers may be used for infants and adults.

Cerumen does not affect the integrity of the readings, and if one ear shows evidence of otitis, the other can be used. The same nonintrusive probe covers may be used for children and adults.

Chemical dot thermometers are disposable and consist of a flat plastic device holding many temperature-sensing chemical "dots" that change color when they reach a certain temperature (Fig. 7–5). These thermometers have two advantages: They are inexpensive and unbreakable. One disadvantage is that they are considered somewhat less precise than glass, electronic, or tympanic thermometers. Also, the sharp plastic can cause a minor cut in the mouth if the patient is not alerted to the danger.

Temperatures may also be measured centrally by means of a pulmonary artery catheter equipped with a thermistor. This is usually used in intensive care settings or during surgery.

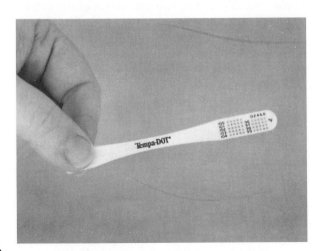

Figure 7–5. Chemical dot thermometer. The chemical "dots" change color as the temperature rises.

Sites for Measuring Temperature

The oral site is most common for measuring the patient's temperature in the clinical setting, with the thermometer placed in the left or right posterior sublingual pocket (Fig. 7–6). *The sublingual area has an abundant blood supply from the nearby carotid arteries and the central circulation at the heart.*

Contraindications to use of the oral site include pain, injury, or inflammation of the mouth or the inability of a small child or confused or unconscious patient to cooperate. Also, if a patient has recently ingested hot or cold food or beverages or has smoked, you should wait 15 minutes before taking an oral temperature *to ensure accuracy* (Eady, 1994). Research indicates that oral temperatures may be taken in patients who are receiving oxygen by nasal cannula without concern about inaccuracy.

The rectal site may be used when the oral site is contraindicated. Although measurement taken by a rectal thermometer is normally about 1 degree higher than the reading taken orally (0.7°F or 0.4°C higher), the rectal site is generally more accurate *because fewer factors can alter measurement*. The rectal site also is more accurate *because it measures the core temperature of the body* (Porth, 1994).

Disadvantages are that the rectal site is commonly frightening to infants and small children, and

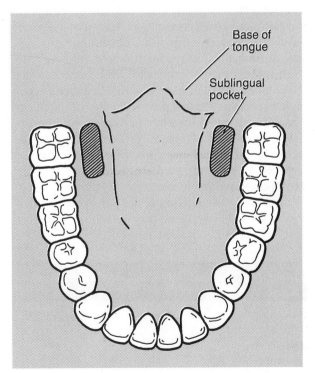

Figure 7–6. The most common site for measuring the patient's temperature in the clinical setting is the oral site, with the thermometer placed in the left or right posterior sublingual pocket.

© 1996 by Lippincott-Raven Publishers

there is the remote danger of rectal ulceration or perforation because of the very small anal cavity. Research indicates that, contrary to popular belief, the rectal site is safe as an alternative site for cardiac patients; *there is little evidence to support the belief that reflex slowing of the heart occurs as a result of vagal stimulation.*

The axilla is generally considered the least desirable site in the adult patient *because it is not close to major blood vessels, and it is more likely to be affected by the environmental temperature.* (An axillary temperature is normally lower than an oral one by 1°F or 0.6°C.) It is, however, recommended for infants and small children *because it is less frightening and safer.* Your facility may have policies concerning specific age groups or situations.

The ear canal is increasingly being used as a site for measuring body temperature for adult and pediatric patients. Temperatures can be measured accurately in as little as 10 seconds.

Pulse

When the left ventricle contracts, blood is pushed out into the arterial circulation. This can be felt in various places as the arterial pulse. Veins do not register blood flow in synchrony with the heartbeat, so pulses cannot be felt nor heard over veins.

Pulse rates vary greatly among adults. A heart rate of around 80 is often considered "normal," although the American Heart Association states that a normal pulse rate may be 50 to 100 beats/min. Table 7–1 lists normal pulse rates for infants, children, and adults.

The pulse rate can increase or decrease *as a result of changes in body temperature.* Exercise, the application of heat or cold, medications, emotions, hemorrhage, and heart disease can affect pulse rates as well. The term *bradycardia* describes an adult pulse rate below 60 beats/min; *tachycardia* refers to an adult pulse rate above 100.

The quality and rhythm of the pulse must also be observed and described. Terms such as "full" or

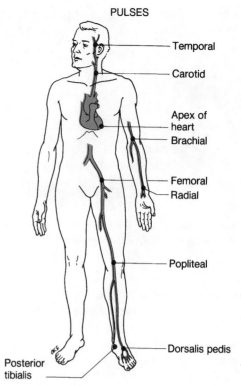

Figure 7–7. The location of the various pulse points.

"bounding" are often used to describe a strong pulse, and "thready" or "weak" might be used to describe a pulse of diminished strength. In some facilities, "grading" of pulses is indicated with a 0 to 4+ scale: 0, absent; 1+, greatly diminished; 2+, slightly diminished; 3+, normal; and 4+, bounding.

A pulse is taken to evaluate the circulation distal to that point and to measure the rate, rhythm, and quality of the heartbeat. Figure 7–7 shows the location of various pulse points.

The nurse must use a variety of special techniques to assess accurately the vascular status of the elderly patient. Among these are interview, inspection, palpation, and auscultation. Also, instead of palpating for a pulse, it may be helpful to use the "bell" portion of the stethoscope rather than the "diaphragm" *to hear more definitive sounds* (Kuhn & McGovern, 1992).

Peripheral Pulses

Some of the peripheral pulses commonly assessed include the following:

- *Radial pulse.* Feel for the radial artery with the patient's arm positioned alongside the body, palm downward. Curl two or three of your fingers around the wrist on the thumb side, and palpate gently. This site is used routinely to measure the

Table 7–1. Approximate Pulse and Respiration Rates by Age		
	Pulse	**Respiration**
Newborn	120	35
4-year-old	100	23
8-year-old	90	20
14-year-old	85	20
Adult	70	18

© 1996 by Lippincott-Raven Publishers

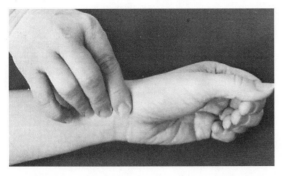

Figure 7–8. The radial pulse site is used routinely to measure the pulse rate because of its convenience and accessibility.

pulse rate because of its convenience and accessibility (Fig. 7–8).

- *Temporal pulse.* Feel for the superficial temporal artery, which passes upward just in front of the ear. Palpate gently, using the tips of two or three fingers. This pulse is often used in infants or when the radial pulse is not accessible (Fig. 7–9).
- *Carotid pulse.* Feel for the carotid pulse by locating the larynx (voice box) and sliding two or three fingers off into the groove beside it. You should feel for the pulse on your side of the patient *to avoid compressing the other carotid artery with your thumb.* If used, the carotid artery should only be compressed for a short time *to avoid impeding blood flow to the brain* (Fig. 7–10). The carotid pulse is used during adult CPR and to assess cardiac function and circulation to the head (see Module 30, Emergency Resuscitation Procedures, and Fig. 30–5).
- *Brachial pulse.* Feel for the brachial artery, which is located near the center of the antecubital space, toward the little finger. Have the patient rest the arm palm upward, and use two or three fingers to locate the pulse. This pulse is commonly used to

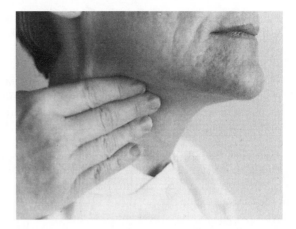

Figure 7–10. The carotid pulse is used during adult cardiopulmonary resuscitation and to assess circulation to the head.

measure blood pressure. (See Module 30 for use of the brachial pulse during infant CPR.)

- *Femoral pulse.* You may need to press harder to locate the femoral pulse, found about halfway between the anterior superior iliac spine and the symphysis pubis, below the inguinal ligament. Respect the patient's privacy when attempting to locate this pulse. It is commonly used to assess circulation to the leg and may be used to evaluate chest compressions during CPR.
- *Popliteal pulse.* With the patient's leg in a flexed position, feel behind the knee in the popliteal fossa. Again, you may need to press more deeply to locate this pulse. This is useful when assessing the circulation to the lower leg and when measuring the blood pressure using the leg (Fig. 7–11).
- *Pedal pulses.* Feel for the *dorsalis pedis pulse* on the dorsum (top) of the foot with the foot plantar flexed if possible. This pulse is easily obliterated, so feel gently. You will find the pulse about

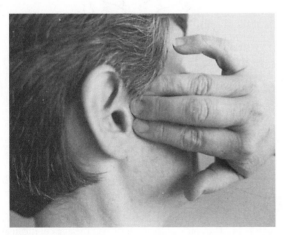

Figure 7–9. The temporal pulse is often used in infants and when the radial pulse is not discernible.

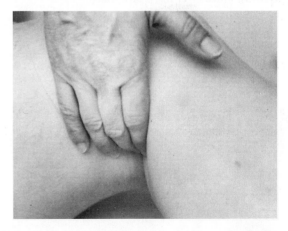

Figure 7–11. The popliteal pulse is useful in assessing the circulation to the lower leg and when measuring the blood pressure using the leg.

© 1996 by Lippincott-Raven Publishers

halfway between the middle of the patient's ankle and the space between the great toe and the second toe (Fig. 7–12).

- *Posterior tibial pulse.* Feel for this pulse by curving your fingers behind and a little below the medial malleolus of the ankle. This pulse is often difficult to feel in obese patients or in those with considerable edema (Fig. 7–13).

These last two pulses are used to assess circulation to the foot. If a patient has had surgery on blood vessels leading to the foot, you may be asked to mark the dorsalis pedis or the posterior tibial pulse with a marking pen so that these pulses can be located more easily by all care providers.

Apical Pulse

The apical pulse is measured by listening over the apex of the heart on the left side of the chest, using a stethoscope. The apex is usually found at the fifth intercostal space just inside the midclavicular line (Fig. 7–14).

You may need to move your stethoscope around in this general area to find where the patient's apical pulse is heard most clearly. The elderly individual with some degree of heart failure typically has an enlarged heart; therefore, you may need to listen laterally to the midclavicular line in such an individual. This pulse should be measured for 1 full minute before administering certain heart medications that might be withheld if the pulse is too fast or too slow. The apical pulse is also used in infants or the elderly, whose pulse rates are often difficult to determine using peripheral sites.

The *apical-radial pulse* is sometimes used when a patient has a cardiovascular disorder. Two people are needed to take this pulse. The first nurse measures the pulse apically using a stethoscope, while at the

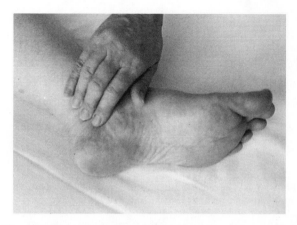

Figure 7–13. Locate the posterior tibial pulse by curving your fingers behind and a little below the medial malleolus of the ankle.

same time the second nurse takes the pulse by palpating the radial artery. The pulse is measured for 1 full minute, using a single watch placed where both nurses can see it. If the radial pulse is lower than the apical, the difference is called the *pulse deficit.* This means that some of the contractions of the heart are not strong enough to push a wave of blood that can be felt at the radial site.

Respiration

The act of breathing is involuntary but can be affected by voluntary control. Respirations are normally regular, even, and quiet, but they can be af-

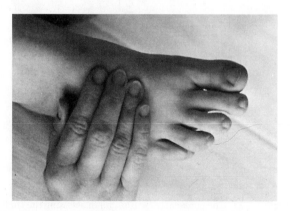

Figure 7–12. Locate the dorsalis pedis pulse about halfway between the great toe and the second toe.

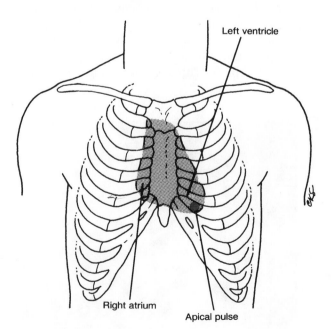

Figure 7–14. The apical pulse is heard over the apex of the heart, usually found at the fifth intercostal space just inside the midclavicular line.

© 1996 by Lippincott-Raven Publishers

fected by all of the same factors that cause the pulse rate to vary. A rate of 16 to 20 is considered "normal" for the adult. The term *eupnea* is used to describe respirations that have normal rate and depth. (See Table 7–1 for the normal respiratory rates for infants, children, and adults.)

The depth and character of respirations must also be observed and described. Respiratory and metabolic disorders can cause variations, as can other acute and chronic problems. The sides of the chest may not rise and fall symmetrically. The term *dyspnea* can be used to describe any breathing difficulty, but a more specific description that includes depth and any pattern that varies from normal should be included as well. The term *Cheyne-Stokes respirations* is used to describe a gradual increase and decrease in the rate and depth of respirations, usually including a period of apnea at the end of each cycle. Any periods of apnea should be timed. (Check the vocabulary list, and refer to the glossary for more terminology related to respiration.)

In this module, the procedure lists the steps for taking the TPR of one patient. Blood pressure measurement is described in Module 8, Blood Pressure. If you are taking routine TPRs on several patients at once, adapt the steps below to accommodate more than one individual.

PROCEDURE FOR MEASURING TEMPERATURE, PULSE, AND RESPIRATION

Assessment

1. A doctor's order is not needed for taking vital signs. Nurses can check TPR at their own discretion to assess the patient's health status. Find out the times at which routine vital signs are taken in your facility.

   When a patient's condition is serious, however, the physician may order vital signs to be taken more often than usual. After surgery, when the patient is in the recovery phase, check the patient's pulse, respirations, and blood pressure every 15 minutes until the patient is alert or the signs are stable. Check the temperature of a patient with a fever hourly. If antipyretic medications are administered to a patient with a fever, check the temperature in 30 minutes *to determine if the medication has been effective.*

2. Assess the patient's readiness for the procedure. If the patient is smoking, eating, or drinking a hot or cold beverage, the reading will be altered, so wait at least 15 minutes before proceeding. Sometimes, because of a change in the patient's condition, you will have to change the route for taking the temperature. If you are taking TPRs on a number of patients at the same time, you may be carrying out this assessment as part of the procedure at the bedside of each.

Planning

3. Wash your hands for infection control.
4. Choose the equipment you will need.
   a. Temperature: glass, electronic, or tympanic thermometer from central storage area or from patient's bedside; if using a rectal thermometer, lubricant
   b. Pulse and respirations: a watch, digital or with a sweep second hand
   c. Vital signs board or paper and pencil
   d. Tissues

Implementation

5. Identify the patient to be sure you are performing the procedure on the correct patient.
6. Explain what you are going to do.
7. Be sure lighting is adequate for you to read the thermometer accurately.
8. Assist the patient to a comfortable position.
9. Proceed with the following:
   a. Temperature
      (1) *Oral.* Shake down the mercury thermometer with a quick snap of the wrist. It should register below 95°F or 36°C before you begin. Place the thermometer carefully in either the left or right posterior sublingual pocket at the base of the tongue. Ask the patient to hold the mouth open until you see that the thermometer is correctly placed, then instruct the patient to close the lips gently and breathe through the nose. Leave the thermometer in place for 8 minutes *to ensure accurate measurement.* Some argue that although the difference between the temperature after 3 minutes and after 8 minutes is *statistically* significant, it is not *clinically* significant. Consider the factors in each situation (such as the patient's clinical status, time of day, and environmental temperature) when you decide how long to leave the thermometer in place, especially because temperature is often measured in the morning, when it is the lowest in its normal daily cycle.

      Remove the thermometer, and wipe it with a tissue using a twisting motion from your fingers to the bulb, *from clean to soiled.* Discard the tissue. Holding the thermometer at eye level—without touching

© 1996 by Lippincott-Raven Publishers

the bulb end—read it, and write your finding on paper. Then shake down the thermometer.

(2) *Rectal*. Shake down the mercury as you would an oral thermometer. Lubricate the clean rectal thermometer *to prevent damage to the rectal mucosa*. Have the patient turn on the side in a Sims' position. Insert the bulb end at least 1.5 in or 3.8 cm into the rectum. Always hold the thermometer with your hand *to prevent displacement or breakage if the patient moves suddenly*. Leave the thermometer in place for 3 minutes. Remove, clean, and read the thermometer as before. When you transfer the patient's temperature to the graphic form, mark (*R*) next to it to indicate that it was taken rectally.

(3) *Axillary*. Take axillary temperatures using the same general procedure as for oral and rectal temperatures. Place the tip of the thermometer in the center of the axilla, and keep the patient's arm held tightly against the side of the chest for 9 minutes in the adult. Remove and read the thermometer. Research has shown that 3 minutes may be adequate for infants weighing less than 6.5 lb, 5 minutes for children weighing between 6.5 and 13 lb, and 7 minutes for children between 14 and 66 lb. Again, when you transfer the patient's temperature to the graphic form, mark (*A*) next to it to indicate axillary measurement.

(4) *Electronic thermometer*. Follow the manufacturer's instructions that come with the device. A clean rigid plastic probe cover is used each time a temperature is measured. Insert the probe into a cover (see Fig. 7–3), and place the probe in the patient's mouth as described for glass thermometers. The display panel will register the temperature reading in 30 to 50 seconds. Next, push the button on the probe to discard the cover, and replace the probe. This will automatically reset the thermometer, and it will be ready for the next use.

With an electronic thermometer *there is a minimal effect on the result of the temperature measurement if the patient is unable to keep his or her mouth closed during the procedure*. Therefore, you can obtain a valid reading with the patient's mouth closed or open.

When the electronic thermometer is used rectally, the oral probe is replaced by a rectal probe, which is covered with a probe cover, lubricated before use, and discarded after use.

(5) *Tympanic thermometer*. Follow the manufacturer's instructions that come with the device. Remove the thermometer from its power base. Use a clean, plastic probe cover. Gently "seal" the opening of the ear canal with the tip of the probe. Hold for approximately 5 seconds. The reading will be visible on the display panel.

(6) Clean all thermometers according to your facility's policy. If mercury thermometers are used in the clinical setting, each patient often has an individual thermometer. After removing saliva or mucus, using a twisting motion toward the bulb end, wash the thermometer with soap and cool water. Then replace it in the holder by the bedside. When using an oral or rectal electronic thermometer or a tympanic thermometer, discard the probe, and return the main unit to its power base.

b. *Pulse*. You will use the radial artery for routine measurement of the pulse rate in most patients. In some patients, the radial pulse will not be discernible, so you will have to choose another site, such as the temporal or carotid artery (see Figs. 7–9, 7–10, and 30–5). Exert only light pressure *so that the artery is never completely occluded*. *Because a patient's position can modify the pulse*, a resting pulse is usually taken with the patient in a supine position *for consistency*. If the pulse is regular, count for 15 seconds, then multiply by 4 for a full minute count. Any pulse that is irregular should be taken for 1 full minute. Also determine pulse rhythm and quality at this time.

(1) *Radial pulse*. Position the patient's arm alongside the body. Lightly place your first two or three fingers over the radial artery; count for 15 seconds, multiply by 4, and record.

(2) *Pedal pulse*. Place your first three fingers over the dorsalis pedis artery, and count as you would for a radial pulse.

(3) *Apical-radial pulse*. Two nurses are required for this procedure. The first nurse takes the pulse radially; at the same time, the second nurse listens and counts the heart rate with a stethoscope over the apex of the heart. The pulse is measured for 1 full minute, using a single watch.

© 1996 by Lippincott-Raven Publishers

DATE/TIME	
5/29/99	Interim Note
2015	S "I feel like my heart is racing."
	O Radial pulse 96 and strong. Respirations 22 and deep. Has been walking in corridor for 10 min.
	P Return to bed. Recheck pulse and respirations in 15 min. Monitor closely when ambulates next.
	C. Church, RN

Example of Nursing Progress Notes Using SOAP Format.

(4) Pulse rate using the ultrasound (Doppler) *stethoscope*. This device is a battery-powered ultrasound instrument that detects blood flow through vessels by bounding sound waves off the moving blood cells. It is commonly used to determine blood pressure in unstable patients, but it also registers pulse rate accurately and in a manner that is easy to hear.

You will need a Doppler instrument with stethoscope head or receiver probe; earpieces, headphones, or a speaker; and an electrode gel. Place the gel on the end of the sound-sensitive probe. Place the probe or stethoscope head over the artery while you listen with the stethoscope, headphones, or speaker. Adjust the device to increase sensitivity. The pulse becomes audible and can be counted or simply reported as present or absent (see Module 8, Blood Pressure, and Fig. 8–4).

(5) *Newborns and infants*. To take the pulse rate, listen over the apex of the heart with a stethoscope. *Because the pulse rate often is quite labile in infants and children*, it is necessary to do a full 1-minute count.

c. *Respirations*. It is best to count respirations after taking the pulse. If you use this sequence, you can keep your fingers on the patient's wrist and place the patient's arm across his or her chest. The patient should be unaware that you are doing another procedure and thus will continue to breathe naturally. Feeling the rise and fall of the patient's chest, count for the required 30 seconds. Multiply the result by two to determine the rate for 1 full minute. If a patient's respirations are irregular, you may choose to count for 1 full minute *for accuracy*.

Note that less than a full 1-minute count in an infant might be misleading *because an infant tends to breathe with a cyclical pattern*.

Document breathing characteristics, rate, and rhythm.

10. Wash your hands *for infection control*.

Evaluation

11. If the patient has any abnormal vital signs, consider retaking them if you think there is any possibility of inaccuracy.

Documentation

12. When you are assigned to several patients, you will find that readings are sometimes difficult to remember. Keep a piece of paper in your pocket so that after you have washed your hands, you can jot down the figures. Then transfer these numbers to a vital signs clipboard or paper and later to a graphic form in each patient's chart. Check with your facility for the routine to be used. If any of your readings are unusual or abnormal, make a note in the nurses' notes section of the chart.

DATE/TIME	
2/11/99	D: Temperature remains elevated, 102.8 at 8:00 AM. Patient states he has head pain.
1:45 PM	
	A: Physician notified; hypothermia blanket ordered and placed on patient at 9:45 AM.
	R: Temperature 99.4 after 4 hours on blanket. Patient states relief from head pain.

Example of Nursing Progress Notes Using Focus Format.

© 1996 by Lippincott-Raven Publishers

13. Report any abnormal findings to the appropriate person, such as your instructor, the registered nurse, or the physician, in a timely manner.

LONG-TERM CARE

Under ordinary circumstances, TPRs are taken much less frequently in long-term care facilities than they are in acute care hospitals. However, there will be a routine policy, such as once or twice weekly, perhaps on bath day. When a change in TPR or other indicators (often a decline in functional abilities) occurs, caregivers are alerted to the necessity of initiating more frequent monitoring of TPR and perhaps blood pressure.

HOME CARE

The individual giving care in the home setting may need to be taught how to measure TPRs accurately. What you teach will depend on the situation, the equipment available, and your assessment of the caregiver's ability. In some cases, heat-sensitive patches may be adequate to measure body temperature. These are reusable and react to heat by changing color. They are often used in home settings *if less precise temperature readings are acceptable*. At times, people are taught to monitor their own vital signs. Clients who have pacemakers are usually asked to monitor the pulse *to ensure that the cardiac device is performing properly*. A family member or friend may be taught to perform this for the client.

CRITICAL THINKING EXERCISES

• You are caring for three young patients, Megan, Melissa, and Hanna. All share the same room and are between 5 and 7 years old. You take their 4 PM TPR, noting your readings as follows:

Megan—36.2°C, 88, 29

Melissa—37°C, 92, 22

Hanna—37.8°C, 108, 28

Interpret these readings. Are all of the patients within the normal range for children in their age group? If not, which of these patients has an abnormal TPR? Determine whether you should report these findings and if so, to whom.

References

Davis, K. (1993) The accuracy of tympanic temperature measurement in children. *Pediatric Nursing*, *19*(3), 267–272.

Eady, B. (1994). How long do iced drinks affect temperature? *American Journal of Nursing*, *94*(5), 58–59.

Kuhn, J. K., & McGovern, M. (1992). Peripheral vascular assessment of the elderly client. *Journal of Gerontological Nursing*, *18*(12), 35–38.

Porth, C. M. (1994) *Pathophysiology: Concepts of altered health states.* Philadelphia: J.B. Lippincott.

Winslow, E. H. (1994). What's so normal about 98.6°F? *American Journal of Nursing*, *94*(6), 57.

1996 by Lippincott-Raven Publishers

PERFORMANCE CHECKLIST

Temperature, Pulse, and Respiration	Needs More Practice	Satisfactory	Comments
Assessment			
1. Although a doctor's order is not needed for routine TPRs, check the policy of the facility.			
2. Assess patient's readiness.			
Planning			
3. Wash your hands.			
4. Choose type of equipment you will need. **a.** Temperature: type of thermometer			
b. Pulse and Respirations: digital watch or one with a sweep second hand			
c. Vital signs board or paper and pencil			
d. Tissues			
Implementation			
5. Identify patient.			
6. Explain what you are going to do.			
7. Be sure lighting is adequate.			
8. Assist patient to a comfortable position.			
9. Proceed with the following: **a.** Temperature (1) *Oral.* Shake down thermometer and place in left or right posterior sublingual pocket at base of tongue. Time for 8 minutes. Remove. Wipe with tissue using a twisting motion from your fingers to the bulb, and read.			
(2) *Rectal.* Shake down thermometer, and lubricate bulb end. Insert at least 1.5 in (3.8 cm) into rectum. Hold in place for 3 full minutes. Remove, clean, and read thermometer.			
(3) *Axillary.* Place tip of thermometer in center of armpit, and keep arm tight against side of chest for 9 minutes in adult patient. Remove and read.			
(4) *Electronic thermometer.* Using the appropriate probe with a cover, insert the probe orally or rectally. Read the display for measurement.			
(5) *Tympanic.* Remove from power base; insert into cover. Seal ear canal with tip of probe. Read measurement on display panel.			

(continued)

© 1996 by Lippincott-Raven Publishers

Temperature, Pulse, and Respiration *(Continued)*	Needs More Practice	Satisfactory	Comments
(6) Clean mercury thermometer thoroughly according to facility's policy. If washing, use cool water. Replace in holder.			
b. Pulse			
(1) *Radial pulse.* Position patient's arm along side of body. Lightly place first two or three fingers over radial artery, and count for 15 seconds; multiply by 4, and record.			
(2) *Pedal pulse.* Place first three fingers over the dorsalis pedis artery, and count as you would a radial pulse.			
(3) *Apical-radial pulse.* Two nurses are required for this procedure. The first nurse takes the pulse radially at the same time that the second nurse is listening and counting the heart rate with a stethoscope over the apex of the heart. A single watch is used, and the count is for 1 full minute.			
(4) *Doppler pulse.* Place electrode gel on end of sound-sensitive probe of Doppler device. Listen for pulse with stethoscope, earpieces, or headphones. Record rate and quality if audible.			
(5) *Newborns and infants.* Take the pulse rate by listening over the apex of the heart with a stethoscope and counting the heart rate for 1 full minute.			
c. Respiration: With your fingers remaining on the patient's wrist and the arm across the chest, count the respirations for 30 seconds; multiply by 2, and record.			
10. Wash your hands.			
Evaluation			
11. Retake any abnormal signs as necessary.			
Documentation			
12. Record from your piece of paper to either the graphic form or the vital signs board, depending on the practice in your facility. You may have recorded directly on the board and need not record further unless there are any unusual findings to enter in the nurses' notes.			
13. Report any abnormal findings to the appropriate person.			

© 1996 by Lippincott-Raven Publishers

? Q U I Z

Short-Answer Questions

1. The normal oral temperature for the average adult is ＿＿＿＿ °C or ＿＿＿＿°F.

2. Four factors that may significantly change body temperature are

   a. ＿＿

   b. ＿＿

   c. ＿＿

   d. ＿＿

3. The bulb of the rectal thermometer should be lubricated to

   ＿＿

4. The oral mercury thermometer should be held in place ＿＿＿＿ minutes; the rectal thermometer, ＿＿＿＿ minutes; the axillary thermometer, ＿＿＿＿ minutes; the electronic thermometer, ＿＿＿＿ minutes; and the tympanic thermometer, ＿＿＿＿ minutes.

5. Place a *1* beside the most accurate method of obtaining a temperature reading, a *2* beside the next most accurate method, and a *3* beside the least accurate method.

   ＿＿＿＿＿ Axillary

   ＿＿＿＿＿ Rectal

   ＿＿＿＿＿ Oral

6. Normal pulse range for the adult at rest is ＿＿＿＿ to ＿＿＿＿ .

7. Four common factors that can alter pulse rate are

   a. ＿＿

   b. ＿＿

   c. ＿＿

   d. ＿＿

8. Three arteries that can be conveniently used for counting the pulse rate are

   a. ＿＿

   b. ＿＿

   c. ＿＿

9. The normal rate of respiration for the adult at rest is ＿＿＿＿ to ＿＿＿＿ .

10. Four factors that cause changes in respiration are

   a. ＿＿

   b. ＿＿

   c. ＿＿

   d. ＿＿

© 1996 by Lippincott-Raven Publishers

MODULE

8

BLOOD PRESSURE

MODULE CONTENTS

RATIONALE FOR THE USE OF THIS
  SKILL
NURSING DIAGNOSES
NORMS AND VARIABLES
EQUIPMENT
PROCEDURE FOR MEASURING BLOOD
  PRESSURE
  Assessment
  Planning
  Implementation
  Evaluation
  Documentation
MEASUREMENT AT THE THIGH
ALTERNATIVE TECHNIQUES FOR
  MEASUREMENT
LONG-TERM CARE
HOME CARE
CRITICAL THINKING EXERCISES

PREREQUISITES

Successful completion of the following modules:

VOLUME 1

Module 1 An Approach to Nursing Skills
Module 2 Basic Infection Control
Module 3 Safety
Module 5 Documentation
Module 7 Temperature, Pulse, and Respiration

© 1996 by Lippincott-Raven Publishers

OVERALL OBJECTIVE
To accurately measure and document blood pressure using a cuff, sphygmomanometer, and stethoscope.

SPECIFIC LEARNING OBJECTIVES

Know Facts and Principles	Apply Facts and Principles	Demonstrate Ability	Evaluate Performance

1. Definition
  a. Systolic BP
  b. Diastolic BP
  c. Norms
  d. Variables			

Define systolic and diastolic blood pressures. State norms for adults and children. List variables that affect blood pressure.	Given a patient situation, identify variables that might affect blood pressure. Given a patient situation, identify potential relationships between blood pressure and pulse. State rationale for taking blood pressure.	Promptly report blood pressures not within textbook norms and significant variations from baseline for particular patient.	Evaluate with instructor.

2. Equipment
  a. Cuff
  b. Bladder
  c. Hand bulb and valve
  d. Sphygmomanometer (mercury gauge and aneroid gauge)
  e. Stethoscope			

Identify equipment involved in taking blood pressure. State use of equipment involved in taking blood pressure.	Identify missing or malfunctioning equipment.		Evaluate own performance with instructor using Performance Checklist.

3. Procedure
  a. Placement of cuff
  b. Estimation of systolic pressure
  c. Korotkoff's sounds
  d. Systolic pressure
  e. Diastolic pressure			

State how blood pressure is correctly measured.	Given a patient situation, identify correct and incorrect aspects of procedure.	In the clinical setting, accurately measure patient's blood pressure.	Blood pressure measurement by student is within 4 mm Hg of that taken by instructor.
4. Documentation			
Know how to record pressure on graphic and narrative records.	Given a patient situation, identify correct recording of blood pressure.	Accurately document blood pressure on appropriate records.	Evaluate own performance with instructor.

© 1996 by Lippincott-Raven Publishers

LEARNING ACTIVITIES

1. Review the Specific Learning Objectives.
2. Read the section on circulation (in the chapter on basic vital functions) in Ellis and Nowlis, *Nursing: A Human Needs Approach,* or comparable material in another textbook.
3. Look up the module vocabulary terms in the glossary.
4. Read through the module as if you were planning to teach the material to another person, and mentally practice the skill.
5. Do the following in the practice setting:
   a. Look over and identify the parts of the blood pressure equipment in the practice setting and the clinical facility. How are they alike? Are there ways in which they differ?
   b. After reading over the procedure carefully, practice it, using another student as a patient, until you feel you can perform it adequately.
   c. Using a double, or "teaching," stethoscope (if one is available), measure your partner's blood pressure with your instructor. If no teaching stethoscope is available, have your instructor check your blood pressure measurement on the same arm 1 to 2 minutes later. Repeat, using palpation. Repeat again, measuring thigh pressure if suitable equipment is available.
   d. Record the arm blood pressure measurement on a graphic and a narrative record, including some mock observations of your "patient." Have your instructor evaluate and make suggestions.
6. In the clinical setting, under your instructor's supervision, measure a patient's blood pressure and document it appropriately.

VOCABULARY

aneroid manometer	diaphragm	popliteal artery	stethoscope
antecubital space	diastolic blood pressure	postural hypotension	supine
auscultatory gap	intravenous infusion	radial artery	systole
brachial artery	Korotkoff's sounds	shock	systolic blood pressure
dialysis cannula	palpation	sphygmomanometer	

© 1996 by Lippincott-Raven Publishers

Blood Pressure

Rationale for the Use of This Skill

Blood pressure is the force exerted by the blood against the walls of the arteries of the body. In combination with other observations, it indicates the circulatory status of patients. Many complications related to prescribed medications and medical procedures are identified partly through the changes in blood pressure that may occur.

The nurse must be able to measure and record blood pressure accurately and to interpret that measurement as it relates to particular patients. To do this effectively, the nurse must be aware of the norms and variables that affect blood pressure.[1]

▼ NURSING DIAGNOSES

Blood pressure measurements are used to assess all patients. Ongoing monitoring of blood pressure is part of the nursing and medical plans of care for many clients. In particular, those with the nursing diagnoses of Decreased Cardiac Output, Fluid Volume Deficit, and Altered Peripheral Tissue Perfusion will need frequent blood pressure monitoring.

NORMS AND VARIABLES

Generally, blood pressure is lowest in the newborn (approximately 40/20) and gradually increases during childhood and adolescence to the adult level (approximately 120/80). Blood pressure, however, varies considerably among people. Hence, a normal reading is usually identified as being within a certain range. For example, the normal range for adults is 110 to 140/60 to 90. A systolic blood pressure of over 160 or a diastolic blood pressure over 100 is termed *hypertensive;* a systolic blood pressure below 100 is termed *hypotensive.*

Blood pressure also varies for the same individual from time to time. Several blood pressure measurements taken one after the other may vary slightly. Therefore, a single blood pressure reading is never considered an absolute indicator of a problem. Several measurements taken at different times are used to determine an individual's usual blood pressure. The trend of a changing blood pressure, whether rising or falling, and the rate of change also are significant.

[1]Note that rationales for action are emphasized throughout the module by the use of italics.

Blood pressure may also differ between the right and left arm. This may be caused by anatomic differences in the blood vessels or by vessel disease. A baseline physical examination often includes taking the blood pressure in both arms *to identify whether such a situation exists for the individual being examined.* Blood pressure, however, is only one indication among many and must be evaluated in the context of an entire situation, not as an isolated event.

Many factors can affect blood pressure. Activity, anxiety, strong emotion, recent intake of food, disease, pain, and drugs can all cause a rise in blood pressure. A fall in blood pressure is caused by blood loss or anything that causes blood vessels to dilate. Postural, or orthostatic, hypotension is a sudden drop in blood pressure caused by a change in position, for example, from lying to sitting or standing. It may cause dizziness, fainting, or falling. When postural blood pressures are ordered, they should be recorded in the same order as they are taken: first lying, then sitting, then standing. The position of the patient during the measurement is often recorded by drawing simple "stick" figures beside the recording.

EQUIPMENT

What is commonly referred to as the *blood pressure cuff* consists of an oblong rubber bag, or *bladder,* covered with a nonexpandable fabric called the *cuff* (Fig. 8–1).

Correct width of the blood pressure cuff is essential to ensure accurate measurement. According to the American Heart Association (AHA), the cuff should be 40% of the circumference of the midpoint of the limb on which it is being used. *If the cuff is too narrow, the reading may be higher than the correct one; if it is too wide, the reading may be lower than the correct one.* Although the AHA recommends the availability of a wide range of sizes, including newborn, infant, child, small adult, adult, large adult, and thigh, these are not available in all settings (AHA, 1994). Most facilities have at least three sizes: child (which can be used for a very thin adult), adult, and thigh (which also is used for arm pressures in obese people). *The circumference of the arm, not the age of the patient, determines cuff size.*

The *hand bulb* is a device attached to the bladder by a rubber tube through which air is pumped (see Fig. 8–1). The hand bulb has a valve, regulated by a thumbscrew, that allows air to escape from the bladder at the desired rate. In automated blood pressure devices, the hand bulb is not needed.

Mercury manometers are manufactured in a variety

© 1996 by Lippincott-Raven Publishers

cuff is inflated with air, then falls as the air is released. Rubber tubing connects the mercury reservoir with the cuff (Fig. 8–2).

The *aneroid manometer* is an air pressure gauge that registers the blood pressure by a pointer on a dial (see Fig. 8–1). The dial generally attaches to the cuff by hooks that fit into a small pocket. The aneroid manometer should be recalibrated approximately every 6 months to ensure accuracy (AHA, 1994).

The *stethoscope* is an instrument used for listening to body sounds. The bell head of the stethoscope is usually used for listening when blood pressure is measured (see Fig. 8–1). (*The low-pitched sounds associated with blood pressure are heard more easily with the bell head of the stethoscope than with the diaphragm.*)

PROCEDURE FOR MEASURING BLOOD PRESSURE

Assessment

1. Check the medical orders and the nursing care plan to determine how frequently blood pressure is to be measured and to see whether any special procedures—for example, postural blood pressure measurements—are to be carried out. Blood pressure also may be measured when the nurse determines that this information is needed.

2. Assess the patient to determine whether any factors are present that might affect how the blood pressure is taken. For example, the presence of

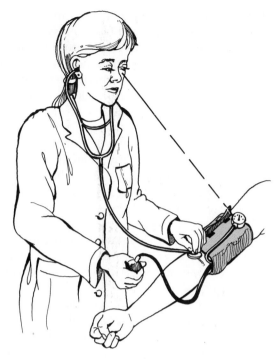

Figure 8–1. Equipment for measuring blood pressure with an aneroid sphygmomanometer.

of models, including a floor model (which can be moved from one place to another), a portable model (which comes in a box), and a wall model (which is probably the most common). The mercury rises in a calibrated glass tube registering the pressure as the

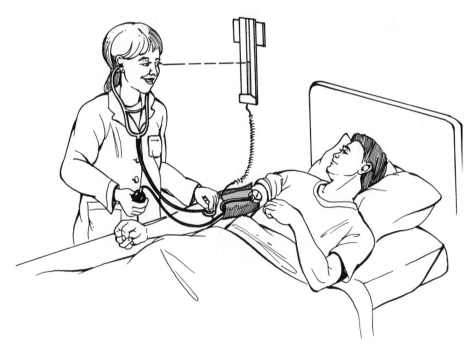

Figure 8–2. When using a mercury manometer, the manometer must be on a level surface, and you must read the meniscus of the mercury in the tube from eye level.

© 1996 by Lippincott-Raven Publishers

an intravenous infusion or a cannula for dialysis in one arm would indicate that the blood pressure should be taken in the other arm. In some patients, there are anatomic or physiologic reasons why the blood pressure should not be taken on one arm or the other. This information may be found on the patient care plan, or it may even be a part of the physician's orders.

Planning

3. Wash your hands for *infection control.*

4. Take the necessary equipment to the patient's bedside. Some facilities have a wall-mounted mercury gauge and a cuff, and sometimes even a stethoscope, at the bedside. In other places, you will have to bring all the necessary equipment with you.

Implementation

5. Identify the patient *to be sure you are performing the procedure on the correct patient.*

6. Introduce yourself to the patient, and explain what you plan to do. Allow the patient to ask questions. Many variables can affect blood pressure. Be aware of such things as medications, recent activity, position, emotional state, recent meals, and pain.

7. Diminish room noise (radio, television, visitors' conversation). Also remind the patient not to talk while you are measuring the blood pressure.

8. Position the patient. Blood pressure is usually measured with the patient in the sitting or supine position, but it can be measured with the patient in a standing position if so ordered. The patient's arm should be fully supported on a flat surface at heart level. *Blood pressure increases as the arm is lowered from heart level and decreases as the arm is raised above this position.* Usually either arm can be used, although the presence of a cast, bandage, or intravenous infusion are some reasons why you might choose one arm over the other. Serial measurements are more reliable if the same arm is used. In the rare cases when it is not possible to take an arm pressure, you can use the patient's leg. In any case, you should either remove any clothing in the way or roll up the patient's sleeves or pant legs. Do not attempt to apply the cuff over any bulky materials.

9. Wrap the blood pressure cuff around the arm above the elbow, making sure the rubber bladder is centered over the brachial artery. The lower edge of the cuff should be about 1 in above the antecubital space (fossa). The bladder should extend 80% of the way around the arm for an adult and 100% of the arm for a child (AHA, 1994). When the blood pressure equipment you are using is attached to the wall, the cuff may be inverted so that the tubing extends out of the top of the cuff. This is often necessary if the tubing is too short to allow you to wrap the cuff with ease. Wrap the cuff smoothly and snugly, and attach it securely. There are many ways to secure the cuff; the most common method is a Velcro closure. If an aneroid gauge is attached to the cuff, place it where you can easily read it. The mercury manometer should be at eye level.

10. Place the stethoscope earpieces in your ears. If you are not using your own stethoscope, wipe off the earpieces with alcohol before using them *to prevent cross-contamination with other users of the same stethoscope.*

11. Palpate for the brachial artery, which is located near the center of the antecubital space, toward the little finger. (The radial artery at the wrist can also be used.)

12. Keeping your fingers over the brachial artery, turn the valve on the hand bulb clockwise until it is tight.

13. Palpate the brachial artery while you pump the hand bulb to fill the rubber bladder in the blood pressure cuff with air. As you pump, the gauge will register the pressure in the cuff. Pump until you no longer feel a pulse and continue for 30 mm Hg beyond that point. *This will prevent you from missing the top sound as a result of the auscultatory gap.* An auscultatory gap refers to a period in which no sounds are heard after they initially started. The sound is initially heard and then fades out completely. The pressure drops 10 to 40 mm Hg before the sound is heard again. An auscultatory gap is most common in those with hypertension. Failure to hear the sounds above the auscultatory gap will result in an erroneously low blood pressure measurement.

14. Place the bell head of the stethoscope over the previously palpated brachial artery.

In screening situations, the AHA (1994) recommends that the blood pressure be measured using palpation first and then measured a second time while auscultating. This allows for identification of the auscultatory gap, if present, and alerts the examiner to the area where sounds may be heard. In the inpatient setting, referring to the record for preliminary data makes this less essential. It also lessens the stress on the patient of multiple measurements.

15. Open the valve on the hand bulb (turning it counterclockwise) gradually, releasing the air

© 1996 by Lippincott-Raven Publishers

from the rubber bladder (no faster than 2–3 mm Hg/sec), and watch the pressure registered on the gauge decrease.

16. Listen for the following sounds (called Korotkoff's sounds):

Phase I: The first faint, clear, repetitive tapping sounds are heard.

Phase II: A swishing or murmur is heard.

Phase III: Sounds are crisper and increase in intensity.

Phase IV: A distinct, abrupt muffling or change of sound is heard.

Phase V: The last sound is heard.

17. Note the pressure at which you hear phase I, the first *regular* tapping sounds (see Fig. 7–3). These sounds gradually get louder. Sometimes you

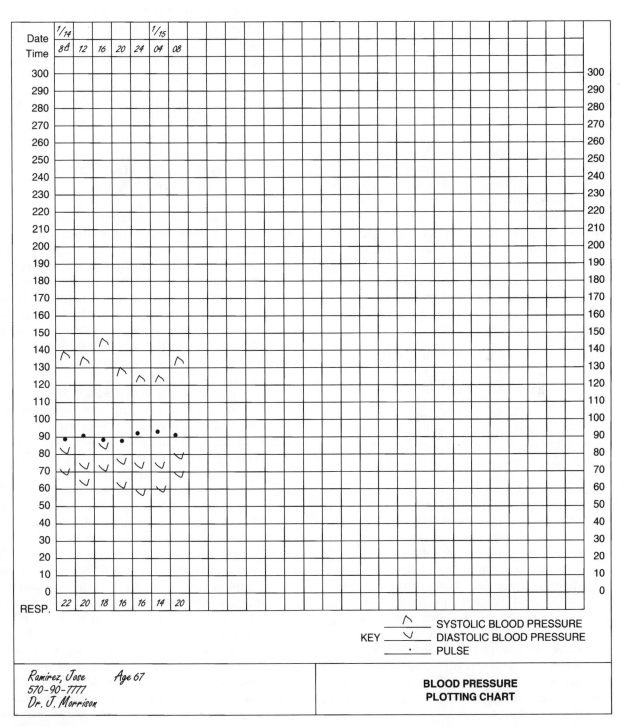

Figure 8–3. Blood pressure graph used to record frequent blood pressure measurements.

© 1996 by Lippincott-Raven Publishers

will hear sounds that you think are first sounds but that are not regular and do not get louder; they are considered extraneous. The pressure at which you hear the first sound is called the *systolic blood pressure*. This occurs when the heart is beating (*systole*) and exerting its greatest force.

18. Note the muffling sound (phase IV) and then the point at which the sound disappears (phase V). True *diastolic pressure* is the point at which the heart is relaxing and filling with blood. The AHA recommends that the onset of muffling (phase IV) be regarded as the best index of diastolic pressure in children and that phase V (when sounds become inaudible) be regarded as the best index of diastolic blood pressure in adults unless this is zero. In those cases the fourth phase, muffling, is a better indicator of true diastolic pressure.

19. If you want to double-check the blood pressure measurement, wait 1 to 2 minutes *to allow the release of blood trapped in the veins,* then repeat on the same arm.

20. Remove your stethoscope earpieces and the cuff from the patient's arm. Wipe the earpieces with an alcohol swab unless it is your personal stethoscope. Wipe the bell head with an alcohol swab between patients to *maintain infection control.* Store the equipment properly.

21. Wash your hands *for infection control.*

Evaluation

22. Evaluate using the following criteria:
    a. Blood pressure is within normal limits for the patient's age and usual blood pressure.
    b. Factors present that might affect the blood pressure have been identified.
    c. If there is reason to believe that the blood pressure recording is inaccurate, it has been repeated after waiting 1 to 2 minutes.

Documentation

23. Document your findings for the adult as follows: 140/80. The first number represents systolic pressure (phase I), and the second number represents diastolic pressure (phase V).

    If you are measuring blood pressure in a child, or if you hear beats all the way to zero (AHA, 1994), record your findings as follows: 140/80/0. The first number represents systolic pressure (phase I), the second number represents muffling (phase IV), and the third number represents cessation of sound (phase V.) The graph shown in Figure 8–3 demonstrates one method of displaying blood pressures for clarity in assessment.

24. Report any abnormality to the appropriate person (instructor, registered nurse, or physician).

MEASUREMENT AT THE THIGH

There will be times when it is necessary to measure blood pressure using the thigh. In such instances, use an appropriately larger cuff (usually 18–20 cm, which is 6 cm wider than the arm cuff), and position the patient on the abdomen. A patient who cannot lie on the abdomen may be placed on the side or in the supine position, with the knee slightly flexed.

Apply the cuff over the midthigh above the knee. Place your stethoscope over the popliteal artery, and measure the patient's blood pressure as before. "Comparison of intra-arterial blood pressures in the arms and legs in humans has shown that the femoral systolic pressure is only a few millimeters of mercury higher, and the diastolic a few millimeters lower than comparable arm pressures" (AHA, p. 18).

ALTERNATIVE TECHNIQUES FOR MEASUREMENT

Electronic blood pressure recording devices have been developed for healthcare settings. The blood pressure cuff is placed on the patient and then the machine is set automatically to take the blood pressure. This may be set to take the pressure at regular intervals, such as every 5 minutes. Warning alarms can be set to signal if the blood pressure goes above or below certain prescribed limits. These are most often used when frequent monitoring is needed and the blood pressure is a critical parameter in determining care and treatment needs.

When you cannot hear Korotkoff's sounds, you can measure systolic blood pressure by palpation. (The diastolic pressure cannot be measured in this manner.) The procedure is the same except that no stethoscope is used, and the pressure shown when the first pulsation is felt is considered the systolic pressure. A palpated blood pressure may be recorded as, for example, 80/P. If you find you can measure blood pressure only by palpation, this should be reported to a registered nurse immediately because it may represent a serious problem.

When Korotkoff's sounds are difficult to hear (as, for example, in cases of shock or with obese patients or infants), a Doppler ultrasound stethoscope can be used. The Doppler, which is used to detect blood flow, consists of a stethoscope or headset attached to a battery-operated ultrasound unit (Fig. 8–4).

To measure systolic blood pressure, use the previous procedure, modifying as follows. Locate the brachial or other pulse desired, apply electrode or contact gel over the pulse site, and gently place the instrument over the pulse point. The systolic blood pressure is recorded as the first point at which the

© 1996 by Lippincott-Raven Publishers

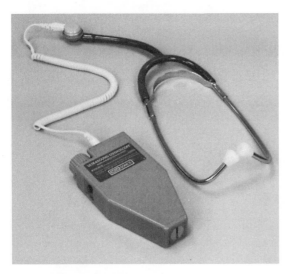

Figure 8–4. Doppler blood-flow detector ultrasound stethoscope is used to detect blood flow when a pulse is not palpable (Courtesy Meda Sonics, Inc.).

pulse is audible. (Volume is adjustable on the machine.) A Doppler blood pressure may be recorded with a "D" to indicate it was obtained by using a Doppler.

Direct arterial blood pressure monitoring also is appropriate when blood pressure measurement is critical. This type of blood pressure monitoring requires sophisticated equipment that includes an intra-arterial catheter, which is usually available only in intensive care settings.

LONG-TERM CARE

In the long-term care setting, blood pressure is not measured daily as a routine. Instead, blood pressure is monitored as it would be for a person living at home. If a resident is on medications that affect blood pressure, monitoring is more frequent than for a resident who is not on such medication. When medications are altered in dose or changed, monitoring may become more frequent until you determine that the resident is stable. The nurse is responsible for determining that additional monitoring is needed when the situation changes.

HOME CARE

Blood pressure may be monitored at home by a home healthcare nurse, or the nurse may teach the client and family how to monitor blood pressure. The directions in this module would be of assistance when teaching this skill to others.

Electronic blood pressure recording devices are available in small units for home use. These enable an individual to monitor personal blood pressure regularly, but they are not usually considered reliable enough for professional use. Equipment for home blood pressure monitoring may include a stethoscope built into the cuff and a digital electronic readout that provides the blood pressure reading after the cuff is pumped up and then released. This enables the individual to manage the equipment while measuring his or her own blood pressure. The calibration of these instruments must be checked periodically to ensure that they remain accurate.

CRITICAL THINKING EXERCISES

• You are caring for an 84-year-old resident of a nursing home. You try to take her blood pressure but are unable to hear the Korotkoff's sounds. Consider the various factors that might contribute to this situation. Recommend actions you can take to modify the situation, the environment, or your technique to increase your ability to obtain an accurate blood pressure reading.

• You note on a patient's record that he weighs 290 lb. You also note that his blood pressure has been varying widely. Describe the factors that might be contributing to a wide variation in blood pressure. Identify which factors in your technique you should modify to ensure that you obtain an accurate reading.

References

American Heart Association (1994). *Human blood pressure determination by sphygmomanometry*. Dallas: Author

© 1996 by Lippincott-Raven Publishers

PERFORMANCE CHECKLIST

Procedure for Measuring Blood Pressure	Needs More Practice	Satisfactory	Comments
Assessment			
1. Check orders.			
2. Assess patient.			
Planning			
3. Wash your hands.			
4. Gather equipment.			
Implementation			
5. Identify patient.			
6. Explain procedure to patient.			
7. Diminish room noise.			
8. Position patient.			
9. Apply blood pressure cuff.			
10. Place stethoscope earpieces in your ears.			
11. Locate patient's brachial artery.			
12. Tighten valve on hand bulb.			
13. Pump hand bulb to 30 mm Hg above last pulse felt.			
14. Place bell head of stethoscope over brachial artery.			
15. Release valve.			
16. Listen for Korotkoff's sounds.			
17. Note pressure at point where you first hear regular sound.			
18. Note pressure at point of muffling and point at which sound disappears.			
19. Wait 2 minutes to double-check, if necessary.			
20. Remove earpieces from your ears and cuff from patient's arm. Clean bell head between patients. Clean earpieces, if appropriate.			
21. Wash your hands.			
Evaluation			
22. Evaluate using the following criteria: **a.** Blood pressure is within normal limits for patient's age and usual blood pressure.			

© 1996 by Lippincott-Raven Publishers

(continued)

Measuring Blood Pressure (*Continued*)	Needs More Practice	Satisfactory	Comments
b. Factors present that might affect blood pressure have been taken into consideration.			
c. If there was reason to believe that blood pressure recording was inaccurate, it was repeated after 1–2 minutes.			
Documentation			
23. Document appropriately, including narrative as necessary.			
24. Report any abnormality to the appropriate person.			

© 1996 by Lippincott-Raven Publishers

❓ Q U I Z

Multiple-Choice Questions

_____ 1. Factors that can affect blood pressure include (1) age, (2) height, (3) recent activity, (4) position, (5) recent meals, (6) pain.

    a. 1 and 3
    b. 1, 2, 3, and 5
    c. 1, 3, 4, 5, and 6
    d. 3, 4, 5, and 6

_____ 2. The usual position for a hospitalized patient to assume during blood pressure measurement is

    a. sitting.
    b. prone.
    c. supine.
    d. lateral.

_____ 3. The bell head of the stethoscope should be placed over which artery to measure blood pressure in the arm?

    a. Radial
    b. Brachial
    c. Femoral
    d. Carotid

_____ 4. The first sound you hear on release of the hand bulb valve indicates

    a. systolic pressure.
    b. diastolic pressure.
    c. pulse pressure.
    d. You cannot tell by one sound.

_____ 5. The point at which the heart is beating and exerting its greatest force is called

    a. systolic pressure.
    b. diastolic pressure.
    c. pulse pressure.
    d. basal pressure.

_____ 6. If you want to double-check a blood pressure measurement, how long should you wait before you remeasure on the same arm?

    a. 30 seconds
    b. 1–2 minutes
    c. 3 minutes
    d. It makes no difference.

Short-Answer Questions

7. The systolic pressure is heard at 140, the point of muffling is heard at 80, and the last sound heard is at 70. Document appropriately. _____

8. Why is the bell head of the stethoscope preferred to the diaphragm for measuring blood pressure?

_____

9. **a.** What is the auscultatory gap? _____

_____

    b. How can you prevent underestimation of the systolic pressure as a result of this phenomenon?

_____

© 1996 by Lippincott-Raven Publishers

MODULE

9

THE NURSING PHYSICAL ASSESSMENT

MODULE CONTENTS

RATIONALE FOR THE USE OF THIS
  SKILL
APPLICATION OF ASSESSMENT
  METHODS
SPECIFIC ASSESSMENT METHODS
Pupils
Procedure for Assessment of the Pupils
The Thorax: Heart, Lungs, and Breasts
  Assessment of the Heart
Procedure for Assessment of the Heart
  Assessment of the Lungs
Procedure for Assessment of the Lungs
  Examination of the Breasts
Procedure for Examining the Breasts
Abdomen/Rectum
  Bowel Sounds
  Vascular Sounds
  Percussion of the Abdomen
  Palpation of the Abdomen and Liver
  Ascites
  Digital Examination of the Rectum

Procedure for Assessment of the
  Abdomen/Rectum
Circulatory Status
  Capillary Refill Time
  Edema
  Neck Veins
Procedure for Assessment of Neck Veins
  Hand Vein Emptying Time
THE COMPLETE NURSING PHYSICAL
  ASSESSMENT
General Procedure for a Comprehensive
  Nursing Physical Assessment
THE "15-MINUTE HEAD-TO-TOE"
  ASSESSMENT
Procedure for A "15-Minute Head-to-Toe"
  Assessment
THE "3-MINUTE HEAD-TO-TOE"
  ASSESSMENT
Procedure for A "3-Minute Head-to-Toe"
  Assessment
CRITICAL THINKING EXERCISES

PREREQUISITES [1]

Successful completion of the following modules:

VOLUME 1

Module 1 An Approach to Nursing Skills
Module 2 Basic Infection Control
Module 3 Safety
Module 4 Basic Body Mechanics
Module 5 Documentation
Module 6 Introduction to Assessment Skills
Module 7 Temperature, Pulse, and Respiration
Module 8 Blood Pressure

[1]The other modules in Unit I should be consulted for specific skills relating to assessment.

© 1996 by Lippincott-Raven Publishers

OVERALL OBJECTIVE

To perform a beginning-level assessment of individual patients, systematically collecting data for all pertinent areas and using all senses.

SPECIFIC LEARNING OBJECTIVES

Know Facts and Principles	Apply Facts and Principles	Demonstrate Ability	Evaluate Performance
Application of assessment methods			
1. Pupils			
List three aspects of pupils to include in inspection. Explain pupillary reaction to light. Explain accommodation. Explain convergence.	Describe patient situations in which inspection of pupils is needed.	Inspect pupils of patient for size, shape, and equality. Check pupillary reaction to light and accommodation. Check pupillary convergence.	Evaluate with instructor using Performance Checklist.
2. Heart, lungs, and breasts			
a. Heart			
List three areas commonly auscultated. List three aspects of heartbeat to be evaluated with use of auscultation. Describe where first and second heart sounds are usually heard most easily.	Describe patient situations in which auscultation of heart is needed.	Accurately discern rate, rhythm, and intensity of heartbeat of assigned patient. Listen for first and second heart sounds in correct locations.	Evaluate with instructor using Performance Checklist.
b. Lungs			
List situations in which breath sounds may be absent or decreased. List conditions that might cause breath sounds to be increased. Define *adventitious sounds*.	Given a patient situation, predict whether breath sounds will be decreased or increased.	In the clinical setting, identify adventitious sounds on auscultation of lungs.	Evaluate with instructor using Performance Checklist.
c. Breasts			
List five parameters to be observed in inspecting breasts of male or female patients. Describe characteristics of breast tissue in younger female, older female, and menstruating female. Describe how to palpate breast.	Given a patient situation, describe what characteristics of breast tissue might be present.	Include size, symmetry, skin color, vascularity, and skin retraction when inspecting breasts of male or female patient. In the clinical setting, palpate breasts of male or female patient.	Evaluate own performance with instructor. Evaluate with instructor using Performance Checklist.

(*continued*)

© 1996 by Lippincott-Raven Publishers

SPECIFIC LEARNING OBJECTIVES (Continued)

Know Facts and Principles	Apply Facts and Principles	Demonstrate Ability	Evaluate Performance
3. Abdomen/rectum			
a. Bowel sounds			
List situations in which bowel sounds may be diminished. List situations in which bowel sounds may be increased. State why auscultation of abdomen should be carried out before palpation and percussion.	Given a patient situation, predict whether bowel sounds will be diminished or increased.	In the clinical setting, listen for bowel sounds in a systematic fashion.	Evaluate with instructor using Performance Checklist.
b. Abdomen and liver			
List four observations to be made when inspecting abdomen. List three parameters that may be demonstrated when palpating abdomen. Describe procedure for palpation of liver.	Describe patient situations in which palpation of abdomen is needed.	Include bulges, bruises, scars, and symmetry when inspecting abdomen of patient. Palpate abdomen, moving systematically and gently. In the clinical setting, palpate for liver of patient.	Evaluate own performance with instructor. Evaluate with instructor using Performance Checklist.
c. Ascites			
Define *ascites*. State how to differentiate between obesity and ascites.	State one problem patient might have as a result of ascites.	In the clinical setting, test for presence of fluid wave.	Evaluate own performance with instructor.
d. Digital exam of rectum			
List signs and symptoms of fecal impaction. Describe procedure for digital exam of rectum.	Describe patient situations in which digital exam of rectum is needed.	In the clinical setting, perform digital examination.	Evaluate with instructor using Performance Checklist.
4. Circulatory status			
a. Capillary refill time			
State how capillary refill time is estimated.	Given a patient situation, state whether peripheral flow is normal or sluggish.	Estimate the rate of peripheral flow using capillary refill time.	Evaluate own performance with instructor.

(continued)

© 1996 by Lippincott-Raven Publishers

Know Facts and Principles	Apply Facts and Principles	Demonstrate Ability	Evaluate Performance
b. Edema			
State four areas of body where dependent edema might be found. Define *periorbital edema* and *pretibial edema*.	Given a patient situation, state where dependent edema might be found.	In the clinical setting, evaluate patient for presence of dependent edema. In the clinical setting, evaluate patient for presence of periobital edema.	Evaluate with instructor using Performance Checklist.
c. Neck veins			
State position in which neck veins are normally collapsed. Describe how to estimate venous pressure without special equipment. State normal venous pressure values in centimeters.	Place patient in position in which neck veins are normally collapsed. Given specific values, state whether venous pressure is within normal limits.	Identify jugular veins of neck and assess. Estimate venous pressure of patient with distended neck veins.	Evaluate with instructor using Performance Checklist.
d. Hand vein emptying time			
State position in which hand veins are normally collapsed.	Place hands in position in which veins are normally collapsed.	Assess hand veins in dependent and above heart level positions. State whether venous pressure is normal or greater than normal.	Evaluate own performance with instructor.
5. Documentation			
State observations that should be included in record with regard to inspection, palpation, auscultation, and percussion.	Given a patient situation, document appropriate items accurately.	In the clinical setting, chart findings of inspection, palpation, auscultation, and percussion completely and accurately.	Evaluate with instructor using Performance Checklist.

© 1996 by Lippincott-Raven Publishers

LEARNING ACTIVITIES

1. Review the Specific Learning Objectives.
2. Read the chapter on assessment and the section on interviewing in Ellis and Nowlis, *Nursing: A Human Needs Approach,* or comparable material in another textbook.
3. Read through the module as though you are preparing to teach these skills to another person.
4. Review the format of Basic Data Gathering in Module 6, Introduction to Assessment Skills, pages 119–120.
5. In the practice setting, with a partner and under supervision:
   a. Test the reaction of your partner's pupils to light and accommodation, and for convergence, using the Performance Checklist as a guide. Document your observations.
   b. Using the diaphragm of the stethoscope:
      (1) Practice listening to your own cardiac rate and rhythm.
      (2) Identify first and second heart sounds, using the carotid pulse as a guide.
      (3) Repeat steps (1) and (2) using your partner as a patient.
   c. Systematically listen to your partner's lungs, both anteriorly and posteriorly. Then listen to your partner's lungs in the supine and side-lying positions. If you hear crackles, ask your partner to cough, and listen again to see whether they have cleared.
   d. Inspect and palpate your partner's breasts. Practice communicating as you would with a patient.
   e. Listen to all four quadrants of your partner's abdomen for bowel sounds.
   f. Observe and palpate the four quadrants of the abdomen.
   g. Palpate for the liver.
   h. Practice the digital examination for fecal impaction on a manikin. Have your partner evaluate your performance, including communication, using the Performance Checklist.
   i. Practice percussion technique on a hard surface, such as a desk or table. Then practice on your thigh to get used to percussing on a body surface. Using the procedure as a guide, practice percussing your partner for resonance, tympany, dullness, and flatness. Do systematic percussion of the chest and abdomen.
   j. Assess your partner's capillary refill time. Explain what you are doing as you would to a patient.
   k. Identify the jugular veins of your partner bilaterally while he or she is lying supine. Gradually elevate the head of the bed to a 45° angle. Note when the jugular veins collapse.
   l. Is your partner's venous pressure within normal limits? Assess your partner for edema of the ankles. If any is present, rate it on a scale of 1+ to 4+. Is periorbital edema present?
   m. Assess your partner's hand vein emptying time. Is it normal or greater than normal?
   n. Have your partner evaluate your technique using the various checklists. Your partner should also evaluate your explanations and your regard for the "patient's" comfort and modesty.
   o. Change roles, and repeat steps a. through n.
   p. When you are both satisfied with your performances, have your instructor evaluate you.
6. For a patient assigned in the clinical area, use the Basic Data Gathering Guide and inspection, palpation, auscultation, and percussion skills to assess the patient, gathering data from all five sources included in Module 6. Have your instructor review this assessment.
7. Continue to use the guide to assess all patients assigned in the clinical area.

© 1996 by Lippincott-Raven Publishers

VOCABULARY

accommodation	crackles	objective	retraction
adventitious sounds	cranium	ophthalmoscope	Snellen chart
alveoli	dependent edema	otoscope	subjective
apex	diastole	para	suprasternal notch
apical pulse	digital	patellar tendon	symphysis pubis
asymmetry	dorsiflexion	pectoralis muscles	systole
base	edema	periorbital edema	trachea
bronchi	gravida	periphery	tuning fork
bruit	gurgles	pinwheel	turgor
caries	Homans' sign	pretibial edema	umbilicus
carotid pulse	impaction	ptosis	uvula
cerumen	intercostal space	rebound tenderness	vaginal speculum
consensual	nares	reflex hammer	venous pressure
constriction	nasal speculum	(percussion	wheezes
convergence	nystagmus	hammer)	xiphoid process

The Nursing Physical Assessment

Rationale for the Use of This Skill
The nurse is expected to perform various aspects of physical assessment on a daily basis when caring for patients. A systematic method of assessment provides a framework for doing an assessment in an orderly, comprehensive way. Without some kind of system, significant areas may be omitted accidentally. This module provides only an initial framework; experience and further education will allow you to expand or change it according to your focus or preference. The module is not meant to provide you with the detail and depth necessary to do a complete physical examination; it is meant to give you a comprehensive overview and the beginning skills to enable you to make a more complete nursing assessment. [2]

APPLICATION OF ASSESSMENT METHODS

In Module 6, Introduction to Assessment Skills, you learned basic information related to inspection, palpation, auscultation, and percussion. Applying these skills proficiently will enable you to do a nursing physical assessment appropriate to the situation in which you find yourself. In some situations, you will need to carry out a comprehensive nursing assessment, and in others you will focus on only one or

two aspects important to the care of the patient at that specific time.

SPECIFIC ASSESSMENT METHODS

Essential individual physical assessments included here are observation of the pupils; examination of the heart, lungs, and breasts; assessment of the abdomen; and evaluation of various aspects of circulatory status. Each can be done alone or incorporated into a comprehensive or focused physical assessment.

Pupils

Frequently it is necessary for the nurse to observe the pupils and their reaction to light. Usually performed as a part of "neuro signs," *this assessment is typically done when neurologic disease is present or suspected.* You will be using inspection when performing this examination.

PROCEDURE FOR ASSESSMENT OF THE PUPILS

1. Determine the need for examination of the pupils. It may be part of an overall general assessment or part of an examination focused on neurologic assessment.
2. Obtain a flashlight or penlight. You may wish to purchase your own penlight *to avoid having to search each time one is needed.*

---

[2]You will note that rationale for action is emphasized throughout this module by the use of italics.

© 1996 by Lippincott-Raven Publishers

ber of centimeters the edema extends up the tibia beyond the malleoli.

Neck Veins

You will often be asked to inspect the distention of the jugular veins for an estimation of venous pressure. When a person is standing, or sitting at an angle greater than 45° to the horizontal, the jugular veins of the neck are normally collapsed. Distention of these veins in a position above 45° indicates an abnormally high venous pressure.

PROCEDURE FOR ASSESSMENT OF NECK VEINS

1. Obtain a centimeter ruler *to measure any venous distention noted.*
2. Have the patient lie flat on the back. Watch for dyspnea. (Patients with distended neck veins are often unable to lie flat without experiencing dyspnea.)
3. Assess the neck veins.
   a. Identify the jugular veins bilaterally.
   b. Gradually elevate the head of the bed to a 45° angle, watching to see when the jugular veins collapse.
   c. If the jugular veins remain distended at 45°, estimate venous pressure by measuring the vertical distance (in centimeters) from the right atrium level to the upper level of distention. *Because the level of the right atrium may be difficult to determine with accuracy,* use the sternal angle, which is approximately 5 cm above the right atrium, as an alternate reference point. Locate the sternal angle by placing two

of your fingers at the suprasternal notch and sliding them down the sternum until they reach a bony protuberance (Fig. 9–10).

Add 5 cm to the distance measured for a rough estimate of venous pressure. Venous pressure of 4 to 10 cm is considered normal.
4. Document the estimated venous pressure on the patient's record and report appropriately.

Hand Vein Emptying Time

Venous pressure is also reflected by distention of the hand veins in nondependent positions. When the hands are allowed to hang freely at the sides, the hand veins will fill and become distended. When the hands are raised to a level above the heart or higher, the veins should be flat. If the hand veins remain distended, the venous pressure is greater than normal.

THE COMPLETE NURSING PHYSICAL ASSESSMENT

After you have made a general survey, as described in Module 6, Introduction to Assessment Skills, perform a complete physical assessment. Take temperature and blood pressure; measure height and weight; palpate, count, and describe the pulse.

You will need a stethoscope for *auscultation* of the lungs, the bowel, and other organs. Although at first you may not recognize what you hear, you will quickly learn to identify normal sounds. Consult with someone else when you hear an unfamiliar sound. Palpate soft areas of the body to check for solid masses or abnormal rigidity.

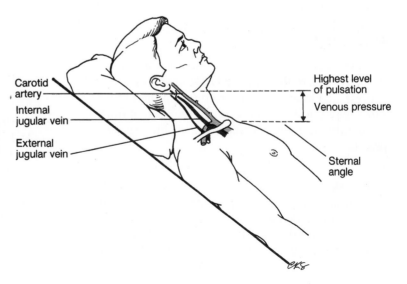

Figure 9–10. To estimate venous pressure, measure the vertical distance from the sternal angle to the upper level of distention in the jugular vein.

© 1996 by Lippincott-Raven Publishers

You can do some parts of a nursing physical assessment while bathing a patient or during other contact. You can examine the skin closely as you assess any area, especially noting hydration, turgor, color, lesions, rashes, and scars, including needle injection scars. Also assess any dressings for degree and nature of drainage and observe the patient's response to activities. All information gathered by observation and examination is *objective data*.

A physical examination is a complex task involving many components, and experience will improve your skill. Still, even at the beginning you can identify normal and abnormal characteristics in general ways. Later, as you study each system of the body in physiology and learn disease entities and nursing care, you will develop new skills to use in physical examinations. Below is a summary of items by body areas included in a complete nursing physical assessment. Although it is beyond the scope of the beginning student, it exposes you to a *comprehensive* nursing physical assessment. You and your instructor can identify which aspects of the assessment are appropriate for you at this point. This format may be the easiest for beginning nursing students. Some nurses prefer a head-to-toe technique somewhat similar to that presented below. Later in the module we will discuss physical assessment using a needs approach. Most facilities provide a form outlining the format they prefer for performing the physical assessment. When completed, it may become a part of or an addition to the patient's care plan. A discussion of all the specific skills needed for a complete physical assessment is beyond the scope of these modules. Many excellent texts on physical examination are available.

GENERAL PROCEDURE FOR A COMPREHENSIVE NURSING PHYSICAL ASSESSMENT

The assessment described here may be more comprehensive than that required in your setting, but it is presented to give you an overview of the kind of nursing physical assessment often required of nurses in nursing homes, clinics, and in independent practice.

1. *Arms, hands, and fingers*
   a. Ask the patient to extend both arms out in front of the body. Inspect the musculature for asymmetry and palpate for turgor. Range the arms, hands, and fingers to assess agility.
   b. Inspect the skin for lesions, spotting, and general color.
   c. Inspect the hands and fingers for color and palpate for temperature.
   d. Inspect and palpate the joints for nodules and enlargements. Observe the hands for any tremors. Note any deviation of alignment in the fingers.
   e. Inspect the nails for hardness and general condition and assess for capillary refill.
   f. Test the grip of each hand.
2. *Head and neck*
   a. *Head*
      (1) Palpate the cranium with the fingers for lumps, abrasions, and asymmetry.
      (2) Inspect the condition of the hair. It should be shiny, with distribution appropriate to the age and sex of the person.
   b. *Neck*
      (1) Palpate the neck for asymmetry, abnormal lymph nodes, and enlarged thyroid.
      (2) Perform range of motion of the neck to detect any limitations.
      (3) Inspect neck veins for distention.
      (4) Auscultate over the carotid artery to listen for bruits (abnormal sounds resulting from circulatory turbulence).
   c. *Face*
      (1) Inspect facial skin for moisture, lesions, and ecchymosis.
      (2) Inspect the face for asymmetry.
      (3) Ask the patient to smile and then to stick out the tongue. The smile should be generally equal on each side, and the tongue should not deviate to one side.
      (4) Note the presence of ptosis (drooping of the eyelids) along with any conditions such as inflammation of the lids.
   d. *Eyes*
      (1) If inspecting the eyes, do so at this time. Use a flashlight or ophthalmoscope (Fig. 9–11) to observe for pupillary response.
      (2) With the ophthalmoscope, inspect each eye for corneal, lens, or vitreous abnormalities while the patient gazes straight ahead. Assess the optic disc for shape and color. The disc should be mushroom shaped and a lemon yellow color.
      (3) Retract each eyelid to observe the color and condition of the conjunctiva. The conjunctivae should be pink without lesions or drainage.
      (4) Check visual acuity using a Snellen chart. This chart has lines of block letters that decrease in size as the reader moves downward. An adaptation of this chart using three-pronged symbols randomly facing

© 1996 by Lippincott-Raven Publishers

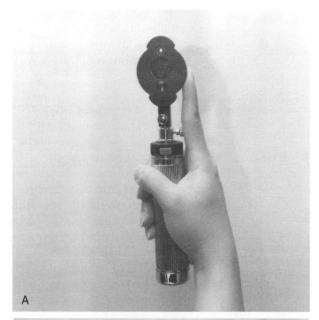

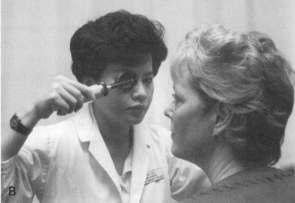

Figure 9–11. Inspecting the eyes. **A.** The nurse holds the ophthalmoscope with the finger on the lens selector dial. **B.** The interior of the eye is examined with the ophthalmoscope. (Courtesy Ivan Ellis)

in different directions can be used for children and illiterate adults. The Blackbird chart uses a modified E to resemble a flying bird and children are asked to identify which way the bird is flying. If corrective lenses (glasses or contact lenses) are worn, check vision with and without the corrective lenses in place. Ask the patient if there have been any recent vision changes.

e. *Nose:* With the patient's head tilted slightly back, inspect each inner nostril using a nasal speculum (Fig. 9–12). Some examiners use the light from the ophthalmoscope instead of room light or a flashlight. Inspect the nares for color and condition of the mucosa, bleeding, and the presence of foreign bodies or masses.

f. *Ears*

   (1) With the patient's head turned, examine each ear with the otoscope for evidence of excess cerumen (ear wax), growths, or redness (Fig. 9–13). Assess the eardrum (tympanic membrane) for signs of swelling or color change and for perforations. Palpate the area around the outer ear for tenderness.

   (2) Test hearing by striking a tuning fork and holding it an equal distance from each ear to test for air conduction (Fig. 9–14). Then place the struck tuning fork on each mastoid process, just below and behind the ears, and on the center top of the cranium to test for bone conduction of sound. A more definitive hearing test may be performed using electronic equipment.

   (3) If the patient uses a hearing aid or aids, check to see that they have working batteries, are free from wax buildup, and are properly placed in the ears. Ask the patient if there have been any recent changes in hearing ability.

g. *Mouth*

   (1) Ask the patient to open the mouth, and inspect it with a flashlight and tongue depressor. The tongue should be medium red, and appear smooth at the margins

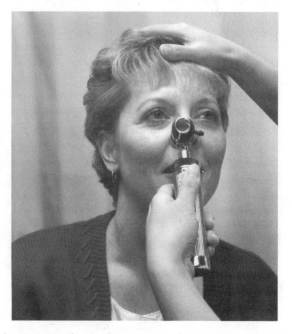

Figure 9–12. The nasal passages can be inspected or treated when dilated with a nasal speculum. (Courtesy Ivan Ellis)

© 1996 by Lippincott-Raven Publishers

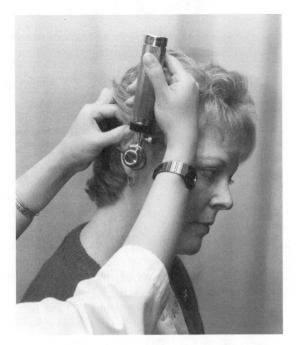

Figure 9–13. The otoscope head is used to inspect the ears. (Courtesy Ivan Ellis)

and rough in the center. When the tongue is lifted, inspect carefully *because this area is often the site of cancerous lesions*. Examine the back of the throat for swelling, redness, bacterial or viral patches, and the position and size of the uvula. Have the patient say "Ah," and inspect the tonsils for redness and swelling.

(2) Inspect the teeth for looseness and the presence of caries. Observe the mucosa of the inner mouth for color and the pres-

ence of lesions. Ask the patient to clench the teeth and smile, which helps in assessing bite and facial musculature. Note the color and smoothness of the lips.

3. *Thorax*

   a. *Back*

     (1) Place the patient in either the prone position or in a sitting position in bed with the back facing you. Expose the back and examine the skin for spots or lesions.

     (2) Note the curvature of the spine and palpate the vertebral column. Check school-age children for scoliosis (lateral curvature of the spine) by 1) looking for asymmetry of shoulders and hips while observing the standing child from behind, and 2) observing for asymmetry or prominence of the rib cage while watching the child bend over so the back is parallel to the floor (Fig. 9–15).

     (3) With the stethoscope, auscultate all lobes of the lungs, anteriorly and posteriorly. (See the section on application of assessment skills that appeared earlier in this module, pp. 164–166, for specific information on examination of the lungs.) Ask the patient about and observe for the presence of cough, sputum, and dyspnea on exertion (DOE).

   b. *Chest:* Remove the gown or pajama top from the male patient. Because a female patient may feel modest about exposing her breasts, untie and part her gown for the chest examination. If more exposure is needed, drop the gown to the waist.

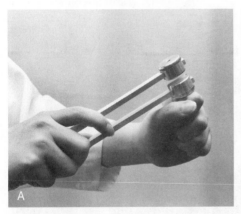
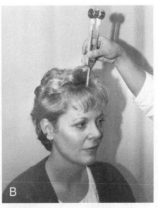
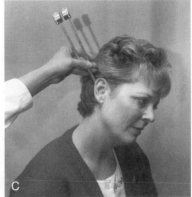

Figure 9–14. Testing hearing. (**A**) The nurse activates the tuning fork by striking the tines gently on the back of the hand. (**B**) Bone conduction can be tested by placing the vibrating tuning fork in the midline of the patient's skull. This test is called the *Weber test*. A normal result is equal sound in both ears. (**C**) Bone and air conduction are tested using the *Rinne test*. The stem of the vibrating tuning fork is placed on the mastoid process and the patient is asked to signal when sound is no longer heard. Then the tuning fork is inverted and the vibrating end held near the ear. A normal result is that the person will hear by both bone conduction and air conduction. (Courtesy Ivan Ellis)

© 1996 by Lippincott-Raven Publishers

Normal   Scoliosis   Examination position
                                    indicates scoliosis

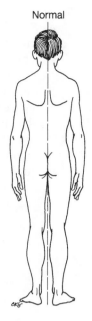
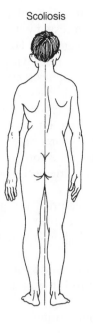
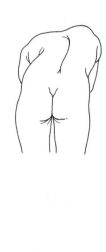

Figure 9–15. The nurse assesses the child for the presence of scoliosis by observing the symmetry of the spine from behind and the symmetry of the rib cage as the child bends forward.

(1) With either a male or female patient, observe the levels of the shoulders for equality while the patient is sitting and facing you. Inspect the pectoralis muscles of each side of the chest for symmetry as the patient presses the palms together and lifts the hands over the head. Note any abnormal dimpling, color, or discharge of the nipples.

(2) Ask the female patient to lie in the supine position. Examine each breast as previously described. A male patient should also have his breasts examined for lumps and masses.

c. *Heart*

(1) With the patient in the supine position, inspect the neck veins for normal filling.

(2) Auscultate the heart sounds as discussed earlier in this module, pp. 161–164. Replace the gown.

4. *Abdomen:* Keep the patient in the supine position for this assessment.

a. Observe the abdomen for general contour, distention, and asymmetry. Grasp the skin between the fingers to test for turgor. Auscultate for bowel sounds in all four quadrants.

b. Ask the patient about frequency of bowel movements, any recent changes in bowel habits, and when the last bowel movement occurred. Percuss and palpate for areas of tenderness, for the presence of fluid, and for the loss of normal dullness of tone, as discussed earlier in this module, pp. 167–169.

c. With the patient breathing deeply and with the knees flexed, palpate the abdomen for organs and masses. On expiration, feel for the position of abdominal structures.

5. *Legs, feet, ankles, and toes*

a. *Legs*

(1) With the patient still in the supine position, palpate each leg for muscle bulk.

(2) Observe for color, temperature, and skin condition. Skin integrity is particularly important in the feet and lower legs, especially if the patient is a diabetic.

b. *Feet*

(1) Dorsiflex each foot to check for calf pain (Homans' sign), which is a possible sign of thrombophlebitis.

(2) Palpate and compare pedal pulses on each foot.

c. *Ankles*

(1) Palpate the ankles with the fingers to assess for edema.

(2) Inspect the malleoli, the bones on each side of the ankle, for enlargement.

(3) Rotate the ankle to check for mobility.

d. *Toes*

(1) Inspect the toes for proper alignment. Also check for calluses and bunions.

(2) Inspect the nails, which should be without ridges. If thickening is present, it could be a sign of fungal infection of the toes.

e. Assess capillary refill bilaterally. Test the strength of the leg by having the patient press the sole of the foot against your palm.

6. *Reflexes:* Depending on the situation, you may test only a few of the more prominent reflexes or proceed with an abbreviated neurologic examina-

© 1996 by Lippincott-Raven Publishers

tion. Many of the measurements of neurologic functioning will have been tested when the other systems or areas were examined. For example, an examination of the optic discs with the ophthalmoscope can disclose a neurologic deficit or disease. If you want to check the cranial nerves, this can be accomplished during examination of the face by having the patient protrude the tongue, smile, and resist supraorbital pressure. (For a detailed description of a complete neurologic examination, refer to a medical-surgical text or a neurologic nursing text.)

Reflexes are usually recorded using the following symbols: 0 (no response), 1+ (hypoactive), 2+ (normal), 3+ (hyperactive), 4+ (very hyperactive).

a. *Corneal reflex (blink):* Touch the cornea with a soft, small wad of cotton; the patient should blink.

b. *Biceps reflex:* Place your thumb on the biceps tendon, which is located just above the antecubital fossa. Striking the thumb should cause flexion of the forearm (Fig. 9–16A).

c. *Triceps reflex:* Support the upper arm at a right angle to the body and allow the forearm to hang freely. Strike the triceps tendon with the reflex hammer (Fig. 9–16B) just above the elbow. Extension of the forearm should occur.

d. *Brachioradial reflex:* Strike the radius slightly above the wrist with the reflex hammer; this should cause flexion and supination of the forearm.

e. *Quadriceps reflex:* Ensure that the patient's lower leg is relaxed and hanging freely from the knee. Strike the patellar tendon, which is just below the knee, with the reflex hammer. Extension of the lower leg should occur (Fig. 9–16C&D).

f. *Achilles reflex:* Hold the foot in a position of dorsiflexion. Strike the Achilles tendon at the back of the ankle with the reflex hammer. This should cause plantar flexion of the foot (the toes bending downward) (Fig. 9–16E).

g. *Babinski reflex:* Using the end of the reflex hammer or the sharper edge of a tongue blade, stroke the sole of the foot from heel to toe. The negative response is plantar flexion. This is normal from the age of 6 months on (Fig. 9–16F).

h. *Skin sensation:* You may choose to test sensation by using a pinwheel that can be rolled over broad skin areas or by using a cotton-tipped applicator (Fig. 9–17). The patient is asked to state, without looking at the device, whether he or she can feel the sensation.

7. *Genitalia*

a. *Female patients:* Examine female patients in the lithotomy position with the knees flexed. Drape the patient as you would for catheterization (see Module 37, Catheterization), using a clean sheet or bath blanket. Cover both legs, exposing only the perineum. It is preferable to use an examination table with stirrups, but you can examine the patient in bed or on an examining table. Provide for adequate light.

(1) Put on clean gloves and lubricate the outside of a vaginal speculum. Do not lubricate the inside, because lubricating jelly interferes with the accuracy of the Papanicolaou (Pap) test. To perform this test, obtain secretions from the cervical os on a swab. Put the secretions on a glass slide, preserved with a fixative, and send it to the laboratory to be examined for the presence of abnormal cells. After inspecting the cervix with the speculum, withdraw the speculum.

(2) Next, lubricate the index and middle fingers of one hand. Insert these fingers into the vagina and push downward on the patient's abdomen with the other hand to palpate the uterus and ovaries. Assess these organs for location, size, outline, masses, and tenderness.

b. *Male patients:* Examine male patients in the standing position, if possible.

(1) Wearing clean gloves, palpate the inguinal ring to check for herniation.

(2) Retract the foreskin of the penis and inspect for irritation, ulceration, and lesions.

(3) Palpate the testes to assess for size, position, and masses.

8. *Rectum*

a. *Female patients:* This examination is usually done after the genital examination has been completed.

(1) Evaluate the anal area for the presence of external hemorrhoids.

(2) With your hand gloved and lubricated, insert your middle finger and palpate for size of lumen, masses, internal hemorrhoids, and tenderness.

b. *Male patients:* The same examination is performed on the male patient, with the patient either bending over the side of the bed or positioned in lithotomy with the penis and testes held aside. The knee–chest position can also be used.

© 1996 by Lippincott-Raven Publishers

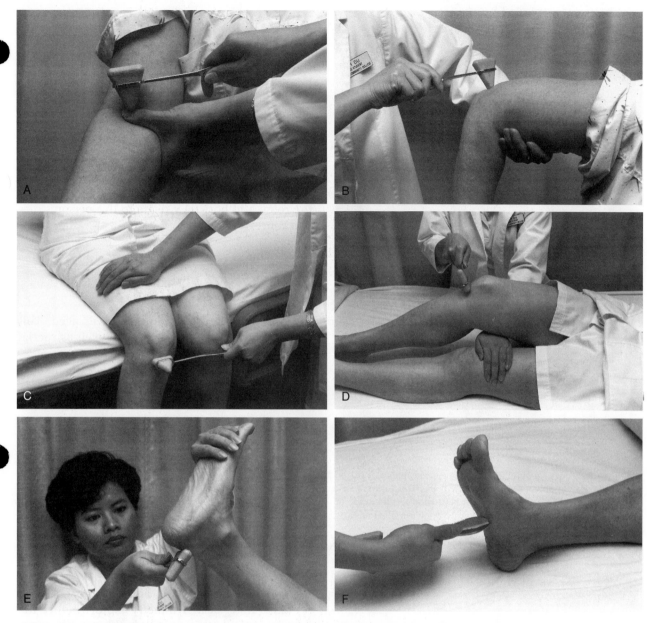

Figure 9–16. Many body reflexes can be tested using the reflex hammer. (**A**) *The biceps reflex.* Striking the thumb, placed on the biceps tendon, should cause flexion of the forearm. Note that the apex of the hammer is used for smaller sites (generally areas above the waist) and the base of the hammer is used for larger sites (generally those below the waist). (**B**) *The triceps reflex.* Extension of the forearm should occur when the triceps tendon is struck with the reflex hammer. (**C**) *The quadriceps reflex.* Extension of the lower leg should occur when the patellar tendon is struck with the reflex hammer. (**D**) *Testing the quadriceps reflex in the supine position.* The leg rests on the arm of the nurse. (**E**) *The Achilles reflex.* Plantar flexion of the foot should occur when the Achilles tendon is struck. (**F**) *The Babinski reflex.* The sole of the foot is stroked from heel to toe using the handle of the reflex hammer. A normal result in the adult patient is plantar flexion. (Courtesy Ivan Ellis)

(1) Inspect the anal area for the presence of external hemorrhoids.

(2) With your hand gloved and lubricated, insert your middle finger and palpate for size of lumen, masses, internal hemorrhoids, and tenderness.

(3) Assess the prostate gland for size and tenderness; this commonly is done by a physician performing a digital rectal examination.

© 1996 by Lippincott-Raven Publishers

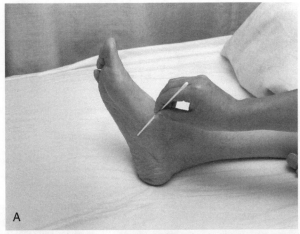

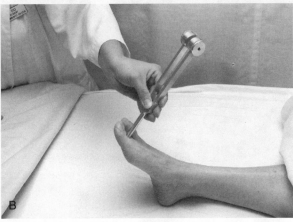

Figure 9–17. (**A.**) A pinwheel or cotton-tipped applicator can be used to test peripheral sensation of the body. (**B.**) A tuning fork placed over a bony prominence can be used to test for sense of vibration. The patient is asked to indicate when the vibation starts and stops. (Courtesy Ivan Ellis)

Regardless of the extent of the physical assessment you are doing, it is always a part of your responsibility to watch the patient carefully for signs of fatigue or other adverse responses and to stop the assessment if indicated. At the completion of the assessment, restore the patient to a comfortable position. Also, always care appropriately for all equipment and supplies used. Finally, document your findings as appropriate for your facility. Whatever you have learned during your examination should be documented in the patient's record, either on a flow sheet or on the progress notes. Report any abnormal findings to the appropriate person, such as your instructor, the registered nurse, or the physician.

THE "15-MINUTE HEAD-TO-TOE" ASSESSMENT[3]

At the beginning of a shift in an acute or chronic care facility, you will need to do a thorough, but abbreviated, physical assessment on each person for whom you will be providing care. This assessment will be focused toward the particular problems or concerns of each person. Each assessment can be individualized by omitting some parts or adding special techniques as necessary. Always include the environment in your assessment, noting all items in the room and how they relate to this person's care and concerns.

PROCEDURE FOR A "15-MINUTE HEAD-TO-TOE" ASSESSMENT

1. Assemble the equipment you will need. This may include a thermometer as well as special items related to individual needs.
2. Enter the room, identify and greet the patient, and introduce yourself and your role.
3. Meet any immediate needs of the patient before beginning the assessment.
4. Explain what you plan to do.
5. Measure the patient's temperature and blood pressure, assess the radial pulses bilaterally, and assess respirations. Compare with most recent assessments recorded and baseline.
6. Inspect and palpate the hands, noting the skin, nails, capillary refill, joints, and range of motion (ROM). Test grips bilaterally. If there is an intravenous (IV) line present, assess the site. Note cyanosis.
7. Inspect the head, face, and eyes. Assess facial skin. Note facial symmetry. Note whether the patient looks at you with both eyes and assess eye movement. Check sclerae and conjunctivae and corneal reflexes, as necessary. Check pupils for size as well as response to light and accommodation. Note visual acuity and any visual aids necessary.
8. Inspect the mouth and lips. Note the color and condition of the skin and mucous membranes. Note the presence or absence and condition of the teeth. Assess the gag reflex as necessary.

[3,4]"The 15-Minute Head-to-Toe Assessment" and "The 3-Minute Head-to-Toe Assessment" are adapted from "15-minute" and "3-minute" assessments conceptualized by Suzanna Johnson, MN, ARNP, Associate Faculty, Shoreline Community College, Seattle, Washington.

© 1996 by Lippincott-Raven Publishers

9. Assess the external ears. Note hearing acuity and use of any hearing aid(s).
10. Assess neck veins for distention.
11. Observe chest expansion and AP diameter. Auscultate anterior chest. Note whether the patient is a mouth breather, and assess for shortness of breath or dyspnea. Note presence and character of cough as well as presence, amount, and character of any sputum produced. If oxygen is in use, note route and liters per minute being delivered. Note whether an incentive spirometer is in use.
12. Auscultate the heart sounds and count the apical pulse. Compare the apical pulse with the radial pulse as well as with the most recent apical rate recorded and baseline.
13. Auscultate the posterior thorax. Note sacral edema.
14. Inspect, auscultate, and palpate the abdomen. Ask about any difficulty with urination and when the last bowel movement occurred.
15. Assess the perineal area as needed. Note presence of urinary catheter, condition of skin, odor.
16. Assess the lower extremities. Note condition, color, and temperature of skin, especially of heels, feet, and toes. Assess capillary refill, edema, sensation, pedal pulses, and mobility. Note presence and distribution of hair. Check Homans' sign and perform strength testing.

THE "3-MINUTE HEAD-TO-TOE" ASSESSMENT[4]

It will also be necessary for you to do "mini-assessments" or periodic assessments at times other than the beginning of the shift when you are caring for individuals in acute or chronic care facilities. In some situations this may be near the middle of the shift and in others more frequently as the circumstances indicate. Again, you will focus the assessment according to the individual needs and concerns of the patient.

PROCEDURE FOR A "3-MINUTE HEAD-TO-TOE" ASSESSMENT

1. *Vital Signs:* Measure vital signs as indicated.
2. *Upper Extremities:* Note color and temperature of extremities as well as capillary refill, radial pulses, and grips.
3. *Head:* Inspect skin and symmetry of face. Check conjunctivae, external ears, lip color, oral mucous membranes, JVD. If patient has altered level of consciousness (LOC), check pupil size and response to light and accommodation.
4. *Anterior Chest:* Auscultate heart and lung sounds. Check apical pulse and compare with radial pulse.
5. *Anterior Torso:* Auscultate bowel sounds in all four quadrants, palpate for tenderness and bladder distension.
6. *Posterior Chest:* Auscultate lung sounds and check for sacral edema.
7. *Lower Extremities:* Note color and temperature of extremities, capillary refill, pedal pulses, edema, Homans' sign, strength testing.

CRITICAL THINKING EXERCISES

You are caring for an 84-year-old woman in the nursing home. You heard in report that at 6:00 AM she had a temperature of 100.2°F, a pulse rate of 96 (irregularly irregular), and a respiration rate of 28 and shallow. You know she is scheduled to be taken for a chest x-ray at 8:00 AM; it is now 7:50 AM. Determine which areas of assessment are the *most* important for you to accomplish before she leaves to have the x-ray done. Justify your choices.

© 1996 by Lippincott-Raven Publishers

PERFORMANCE CHECKLIST

Assessing the Pupils	Needs More Practice	Satisfactory	Comments
1. Determine the need for examination of the pupils.			
2. Obtain a flashlight or penlight.			
3. Assess the patient's pupils. **a.** Inspect size, shape, and equality of pupils.			
b. Inspect the pupillary reaction to light. (1) Constriction and rate			
(2) Consensual response			
c. Test the pupillary reaction to accommodation. (1) Constriction			
(2) Convergence			
d. Observe for nystagmus.			
4. Document your observations on the patient's record.			
Assessing the Heart			
1. Determine the need for assessment of the heart.			
2. Obtain a stethoscope.			
3. Explain what you plan to do, ask the patient not to speak, and control the noise in the environment.			
4. Have the patient sit up, if able.			
5. Remove the patient's gown or pajama top.			
6. Auscultate the patient's heart. **a.** Warm the diaphragm of the stethoscope.			
b. Listen for the first and second heart sounds.			
c. Count the cardiac rate.			
d. Evaluate the cardiac rhythm.			
7. Document and report appropriately.			
Assessing the Lungs			
1. Determine the need for assessment of the lungs.			

(*continued*)

© 1996 by Lippincott-Raven Publishers

Assessing the Lungs *(Continued)*	Needs More Practice	Satisfactory	Comments
2. Obtain a stethoscope.			
3. Assist the patient to a sitting position or roll from side to side.			
4. Remove the patient's gown or pajama top if not already done.			
5. Assess the patient's lungs. **a.** Percuss the chest systematically.			
b. Ask the patient to breathe slowly in and out through an open mouth.			
c. Auscultate the anterior chest, comparing right and left sides.			
d. Auscultate the posterior chest, comparing right and left sides.			
e. If adventitious sounds are heard, ask the patient to cough and listen again.			
6. Document and report appropriately.			
Examining the Breasts			
1. Determine the need for examination of the breasts.			
2. Obtain a small pillow.			
3. Have the patient disrobe to the waist and be seated with hands in lap.			
4. Examine the breasts. **a.** Observe nipples for color, discharge, and dimpling.			
b. Observe breasts for size, symmetry, skin color, vascularity, and skin retraction. Ask patient to press hands against hips to bring out dimpling or retraction.			
c. Have patient raise hands above head, and observe for irregularities in skin texture and dimpling.			
d. Have patient lie down.			
e. Place a small pillow under patient's shoulder on side you are examining and have patient raise the arm over head.			
f. Palpate each breast systematically.			

(continued)

© 1996 by Lippincott-Raven Publishers

Examining the Breasts *(Continued)*	Needs More Practice	Satisfactory	Comments
5. Document and report appropriately.			
Assessing the Abdomen/Rectum			
1. Determine the need for assessment of the abdomen or rectum.			
2. Obtain a stethoscope to assess the abdomen. If a digital examination of the rectum is planned, include clean gloves, lubricant, and a bedpan.			
3. Place patient in supine position and arrange patient's gown or pajama top to cover chest and expose abdomen. Fanfold bed linen down to the symphysis pubis.			
4. Inspect the abdomen, noting scars, rashes, contour, symmetry, and visible masses or pulsations.			
5. Auscultate for bowel sounds and vascular sounds. **a.** Lightly place diaphragm of warmed stethoscope on abdomen.			
b. Auscultate all four quadrants systematically, starting with the right lower quadrant.			
c. With firmer pressure auscultate over the renal, iliac, and femoral arteries for bruits.			
6. Percuss each quadrant of the abdomen.			
7. Palpate each quadrant of the abdomen. **a.** Use the pads of your fingers.			
b. Ask the patient to breathe through the mouth.			
c. Systematically palpate for tone, swelling, tenderness, and rebound tenderness.			
8. Palpate for the liver. **a.** Ask patient to inhale.			
b. Standing on right side, place your left hand under rib cage and use your right hand to palpate just below right costal margin.			
9. Assess for ascites. **a.** With patient in supine position, place your hand against the lateral abdominal wall.			

(continued)

© 1996 by Lippincott-Raven Publishers

Assessing the Abdomen/Rectum *(Continued)*	Needs More Practice	Satisfactory	Comments
b. Tap the opposite abdominal wall with the other hand and check for fluid wave.			
c. Identify the area of greatest girth.			
d. Place marks at level of greatest girth on each side of patient's abdomen.			
e. Measure abdominal girth at the marks.			
10. Perform a digital examination of the rectum, if indicated. **a.** Assist patient to left lateral position.			
b. Drape to expose rectal area and provide warmth and privacy.			
c. Perform rectal examination. (1) Put on gloves.			
(2) Lubricate gloved index finger.			
(3) Spread patient's buttocks apart.			
(4) Ask patient to bear down while you gently insert your gloved index finger into rectum, pointing toward the umbilicus.			
(5) Ask patient to breathe in and out through the mouth.			
(6) Move examining finger in a circle, breaking up and removing any fecal material found.			
(7) Remove glove by turning inside out over soiled surface; discard in container outside patient's room.			
11. Document and report appropriately.			
Assessing the Neck Veins			
1. Obtain a centimeter ruler to measure any venous distention noted.			
2. Have patient lie flat on back.			
3. Assess neck veins. **a.** Identify jugular veins bilaterally.			
b. Gradually elevate head of bed to 45°.			

(continued)

© 1996 by Lippincott-Raven Publishers

Assessing the Neck Veins (*Continued*)	Needs More Practice	Satisfactory	Comments
c. If jugular veins are distended at 45°, measure vertical distance in centimeters from right atrium to upper level of distention.			
4. Document and report appropriately.			
Comprehensive Nursing Physical Assessment			
1. Arms, hands, and fingers **a.** Inspect arm musculature and range the arms, hands, and fingers.			
b. Inspect the skin for lesions, spotting, color, and temperature.			
c. Inspect hands and fingers for color and palpate for temperature.			
d. Inspect and palpate joints.			
e. Inspect nails for hardness; assess for capillary refill.			
f. Test each hand's grip.			
2. Head and neck **a.** Head (1) Palpate cranium.			
(2) Inspect hair.			
b. Neck (1) Palpate neck.			
(2) Perform range-of-motion.			
(3) Inspect neck veins.			
(4) Auscultate over carotid artery.			
c. Face (1) Inspect facial skin.			
(2) Note symmetry.			
(3) Note tongue deviation.			
(4) Note the presence of ptosis.			
d. Eyes (1) Observe pupillary response.			
(2) Inspect with ophthalmoscope.			

(continued)

© 1996 by Lippincott-Raven Publishers

Comprehensive Nursing Physical Assessment (*Continued*)	Needs More Practice	Satisfactory	Comments
(3) Assess conjunctivae.			
(4) Check visual acuity.			
e. Nose: inspect nares.			
f. Ears (1) Examine with otoscope.			
(2) Test hearing.			
(3) Check hearing aid(s), if used.			
g. Mouth (1) Inspect tongue, floor of mouth, back of throat, uvula, and tonsils.			
(2) Inspect teeth, oral mucosa, and lips.			
3. Thorax **a.** Back (1) Examine the skin.			
(2) Note spinal curvature.			
(3) Auscultate lungs.			
b. Chest (1) Observe shoulder symmetry and nipples.			
(2) Examine breasts.			
c. Heart (1) Inspect neck veins.			
(2) Auscultate heart sounds.			
4. Abdomen **a.** Observe contour, test for turgor, and auscultate bowel sounds.			
b. Ask patient about bowel habits and percuss and palpate for areas of tenderness.			
c. Palpate for organs and masses.			
5. Legs, feet, ankles, and toes **a.** Legs (1) Palpate muscles.			
(2) Observe color, temperature and skin condition.			

(continued)

© 1996 by Lippincott-Raven Publishers

Comprehensive Nursing Physical Assessment (*Continued*)	Needs More Practice	Satisfactory	Comments
b. Feet (1) Check Homans' sign.			
(2) Palpate and compare pedal pulses.			
c. Ankles (1) Palpate ankles.			
(2) Inspect malleoli for enlargement.			
(3) Rotate ankles to check for mobility.			
d. Toes (1) Inspect for proper alignment, calluses, and bunions.			
(2) Inspect nails			
e. Assess capillary refill and leg strength.			
6. Reflexes **a.** Corneal reflex			
b. Biceps reflex			
c. Triceps reflex			
d. Brachioradial reflex			
e. Quadriceps reflex			
f. Achilles reflex			
g. Babinski reflex			
h. Skin sensation			
7. Genitalia **a.** Female patients (1) Inspect and swab cervix for Pap test.			
(2) Palpate abdomen for uterus and ovaries.			
b. Male patients (1) Palpate inguinal ring.			
(2) Inspect penis.			
(3) Palpate testes.			
8. Rectum **a.** Female patients (1) Inspect externally.			
(2) Palpate internally.			

(continued)

© 1996 by Lippincott-Raven Publishers

Comprehensive Nursing Physical Assessment (*Continued*)	Needs More Practice	Satisfactory	Comments
b. Male patients (1) Inspect externally.			
(2) Palpate internally.			
(3) Assess prostate gland.			
15-Minute Head-To-Toe Assessment			
1. Assemble equipment.			
2. Identify and greet patient, introduce self and role.			
3. Meet immediate needs of patient.			
4. Explain plan.			
5. Measure temperature and blood pressure; assess radial pulses and respirations.			
6. Inspect and palpate hands; test grips.			
7. Inspect head, face, eyes, and visual acuity.			
8. Inspect mouth, lips, and teeth.			
9. Assess external ears and hearing acuity.			
10. Assess neck veins.			
11. Observe chest expansion and AP diameter; auscultate anterior chest; note presence of cough and oxygen use.			
12. Auscultate heart sounds; count apical pulse.			
13. Auscultate posterior thorax; assess sacral edema.			
14. Inspect, auscultate, and palpate abdomen.			
15. Assess perineal area.			
16. Assess lower extremities: note condition, color, and temperature of skin; assess capillary refill, edema, sensation, pedal pulses, mobility; check Homan's sign and perform strength testing.			
3-Minute Head-To-Toe Assessment			
1. Vital signs: Measure as indicated.			
2. Upper extremities: Note color, temperature, capillary refill, radial pulses, grips.			

(continued)

© 1996 by Lippincott-Raven Publishers

3-Minute Head-To-Toe Assessment (*Continued*)	Needs More Practice	Satisfactory	Comments
3. Head: Inspect skin and symmetry of face; check eyes, ears, mouth, JVD.			
4. Anterior chest: Ascultate heart and lung sounds.			
5. Anterior torso: Auscultate and palpate abdomen.			
6. Posterior chest: Auscultate lung sounds; assess sacral edema.			
7. Lower extremities: Note color, temperature, capillary refill, pedal pulses, edema, Homan's sign, strength testing.			

© 1996 by Lippincott-Raven Publishers

❓ Q U I Z

Short-Answer Questions

1. Before testing the pupillary reaction to light and accommodation, for what three things should the nurse inspect the pupils?

   a. _____

   b. _____

   c. _____

2. In what position are the jugular veins normally collapsed?
   in a position above 45°

3. Between what values is venous pressure considered normal?
   4 to 10 CM

4. Where is periorbital edema found? *around the eyes)*

5. Why should the nurse be aware of the patient's stage in the menstrual cycle when palpating the breasts of a female? *maybe tender*

6. When examining the abdomen, why should auscultation be done before percussion and palpation? *creates BT*

7. In what area is the first heart sound usually most easily heard?
   apical -apex

8. Name one situation in which breath sounds might be absent or decreased.
   broncial obstruction, Chronic lung disease, shallow breathing

9. Name one situation in which breath sounds might be louder or increased.
   Pneumonia

10. What is one way to differentiate between a pleural friction rub and a pericardial friction rub?
    lung   heart

© 1996 by Lippincott-Raven Publishers

MODULE

10

INTAKE AND OUTPUT

MODULE CONTENTS

RATIONALE FOR THE USE OF THIS
   SKILL
NURSING DIAGNOSES
ASSESSMENT FOR INITIATING
   MEASUREMENT OF INTAKE AND
   OUTPUT
ITEMS MEASURED
Intake
Output
DEVICES USED FOR MEASUREMENT
UNITS OF MEASUREMENT
PATIENT PARTICIPATION
RECORD KEEPING
Bedside Records
Permanent Records
PROCEDURE FOR MEASURING INTAKE
   AND OUTPUT
   Assessment
   Planning
   Implementation
   Evaluation
   Documentation
LONG-TERM CARE
HOME CARE
CRITICAL THINKING EXERCISES

PREREQUISITES

Successful completion of the following modules:

VOLUME 1
Module 1 An Approach to Nursing Skills
Module 2 Basic Infection Control
Module 3 Safety
Module 5 Documentation
Module 6 Introduction to Assessment Skills

© 1996 by Lippincott-Raven Publishers

OVERALL OBJECTIVE

To be able to measure correctly and keep accurate records of patients' fluid intake and output.

SPECIFIC LEARNING OBJECTIVES

Know Facts and Principles	Apply Facts and Principles	Demonstrate Ability	Evaluate Performance
1. Initiating measurement			
State who may initiate measurement and reasons for measurement.	Given a patient situation, state why measurement is important for that patient.	Determine relationship of amounts measured to the patient's medical status.	Evaluate with instructor.
2. What is measured			
State what items must be measured for intake and output.	Given a sample patient diet, identify items to be measured.	Measure intake accurately.	With instructor, evaluate choices of what to measure.
	Given a patient situation, identify intake, other than dietary, that must be measured.	Measure output accurately.	
	Given a patient situation, identify which excretions must be measured for output.		
3. Record-keeping forms			
List pertinent information that should be recorded at patient's bedside.	Given a listing of information about patient's intake and output, record it on correct form in proper place.	Record intake and output on proper forms.	With instructor, evaluate use of forms.
List pertinent information that should be recorded on patient's chart.			
4. Measurements used			
Identify when to add or subtract quantities to get correct totals.	Given a patient situation with amounts of intake and output, figure correct totals.	Total intake and output. Record totals on correct form.	Evaluate own performance using Performance Checklist.
5. Time periods for measurement			
Know variety of time periods that may be used for recording intake and output.	Given patient's amounts of intake and output, calculate total for 8-hour and 24-hour systems.	Calculate totals for 8- to 24-hour periods.	Evaluate own performance using Performance Checklist.

(continued)

© 1996 by Lippincott-Raven Publishers

SPECIFIC LEARNING OBJECTIVES (Continued)

Know Facts and Principles	Apply Facts and Principles	Demonstrate Ability	Evaluate Performance
6. *Fluid balance* Define fluid balance. Identify factors in addition to intake and output that must be considered in regard to fluid balance.	Given a patient situation, identify factors that relate to fluid balance. State additional data that may be needed for accurate assessment of fluid balance.	Determine whether patient is in fluid balance. Report instances of fluid imbalance to appropriate person.	Evaluate performance with instructor.
7. *Patient's participation* Identify ways of explaining to patient need for measurement of intake and output and method to be used.	Given a patient situation, devise plan for measuring intake and output that includes patient participation.	In the clinical setting, successfully maintain patient intake and output record from patient's list.	Compare own results with those of staff person also assigned to care of patient.

© 1996 by Lippincott-Raven Publishers

LEARNING ACTIVITIES

1. Review the Specific Learning Objectives.
2. Read the section on fluids in Ellis and Nowlis, *Nursing: A Human Needs Approach,* or comparable material in another textbook.
3. Look up the module vocabulary terms in the glossary.
4. Read through the module as though you were preparing to teach the content to another person.
5. In the practice setting: Practice accurately measuring liquids, using containers showing metric measurement.
6. In the clinical setting:
   a. Familiarize yourself with the various dietary fluid containers used in your facility and the fluid content of each.
   b. Check the form used by your facility for intake and output measurement.
   c. Identify three or four patients who are having their intake and output measured. Determine the rationale for this action. Prepare for teaching patients who are able to participate in intake and output measurement.
   d. Keep an intake–output record on one of your assigned patients for one meal and for the time you are on the unit. Have your instructor check your accuracy.
   e. For a patient in the clinical area who is on intake–output measurement, figure the last three 8-hour periods and total your figures for 24 hours.
   f. For the same patient, check the record and decide, based on recorded data, whether this patient is in fluid balance. Present your data and your decision to your instructor for verification.

VOCABULARY

catheter	diuretic	piggyback	tube feeding
diaphoresis	infusion	preformed water	water balance
diarrhea	minibottle	profuse	
diuresis	parenteral fluid	pureed — strained	

intravenous

diaphoresis — perspiration, especially copious or medically induced perspiration

Parenteral fluid — fluid given by infusion

infusion — intro. of a solution into a vein or vessel

catheter — slender flexible tube for inserting into a body cavity to distend or maintain an opening, used for drain or instill fluid

diuresis — inc. prod. & output of urine

diuretic — drug that inc. production & output of urine

Minibottle — a small container for

piggyback — an intravenous infusion set up in which a 2nd container is attached to the tubing of the primary container though a short tubing

preformed water — the water content of ingested foods

water balance — a state of the body in which O & I is equal

© 1996 by Lippincott-Raven Publishers

Intake and Output

Rationale for the Use of This Skill

Many illnesses cause changes in the body's ability to maintain fluid balance. Intake can be decreased as a result of anorexia, nausea, vomiting, and many other conditions. Output can be altered by various disease processes in the body, especially diabetes and kidney and heart problems. Infants, children, and older adults are particularly susceptible to fluid imbalance. A number of drugs in current use can cause kidney damage and alter urinary elimination.

A careful measurement of both intake and output is essential to total patient assessment. A record of this measurement is maintained for the use of all health team members.[1]

▼ NURSING DIAGNOSES

A variety of nursing diagnoses are useful for the patient placed on intake and output measurement by the physician or nurse. Some of these are appropriate because of the patient's medical condition, which may alter either intake or output. Medical conditions may also influence electrolyte balance, so that nursing diagnoses related to fluid volume are applicable. If the patient is on a medication that changes either intake or output, measurement should be initiated. Other nursing diagnoses are used when assessment shows data such as nausea, vomiting, constipation, or diarrhea.

The following are examples of nursing diagnoses related to intake and output measurement:

Altered Urinary Elimination
Constipation
Diarrhea
Fluid Volume Deficit
Fluid Volume Excess
Hyperthermia
Impaired Swallowing
Risk for Infection
These nursing diagnoses may also be used when the patient is at risk of the situation.

[1]Rationale for action is emphasized throughout the module by the use of italics.

ASSESSMENT FOR INITIATING MEASUREMENT OF INTAKE AND OUTPUT

Although a physician's order is commonly written for measurement of intake and output, usually referred to as I &O, you may also initiate this measurement if you determine that these data are important to your assessment. You may initiate measuring to assess whether a patient is receiving adequate fluids or to verify that the output is sufficient for optimum kidney function. In some facilities, patients receiving medications that have an effect on I &O, postoperative patients, and those who have intravenous fluids, indwelling urinary catheters, or feeding tubes are routinely placed on I &O to facilitate effective assessment.

Other considerations, such as medications and specific illnesses may also indicate the necessity for measuring I &O. Patients who are diabetic, have burns or draining wounds, or are on steroid therapy may be placed on I &O. A patient who has a debilitating disease may not have adequate oral fluid intake and would benefit from fluid measurement.

Age is also a factor. Infants, children, and the elderly are more fragile regarding fluid balance and need careful observation *to ensure effective hydration and elimination.* Many older patients are on diuretics or drugs that increase urinary elimination, causing them to become dehydrated.

The fluid intake should approximately equal the output. Report any ratio that is significantly unequal. Ideally, you should monitor intake for several days to get an accurate assessment of the patient's fluid status. If the total intake is substantially below the total output, the patient is at risk for fluid volume deficit. If the total fluid intake is substantially above the total output, the patient is at risk for fluid volume excess (Carpenito, 1993). A urine output of less than 30 mL/hr may indicate renal disease, inadequate blood flow to the kidneys, or dehydration, and should be reported. Some patients for whom fluid balance is important but not critical will have daily weights performed but not I &O measurement. For others whose water balance is crucial, I &O will be ordered along with daily weights. Daily weights are very important when I &O measurement is ordered. A change in daily weight indicates that the patient may be nutritionally deficient or in excess. It may also indicate fluid retention or dehydration. In some cases the measurement of I &O may be inaccurate, so that the patient's weight becomes important assessment data.

© 1996 by Lippincott-Raven Publishers

ITEMS MEASURED

Intake

Measure all dietary items that are naturally fluid at room temperature. These include water, milk, juice, and all other beverages, as well as ice cream, gelatin, and liquid content of soups.

Patients on I&O measurement receive a full water pitcher of 1,000 mL. When you change the water in the pitcher, measure the amount remaining in a container, discard this water, then "credit" the difference to the patient's intake because the patient actually took this amount. Occasionally a patient on restricted fluids will not have a water pitcher at the bedside. When very accurate measurement is needed, individual glasses are served and measured. For such a patient, calculate the small amount of water needed to take oral medications because this is usually a part of the individual glasses served or of the water pitcher measurement.

You should also add tube feedings to the intake. Occasionally, a patient will have a small-bore tube for feeding and also swallow oral fluids. Compute both of these. Do not measure pureed foods; *they are simply solids prepared in a different form.*

You must measure any solution that is infused intravenously (including blood products). The minuscule amount of solution used to ensure the patency of a peripheral access line or heparin lock is usually not computed. The larger amount of solution used to "flush" central lines may be figured into the intake if accurate measurement for the patient is crucial. The small amounts of fluid in intravenous antibiotic solutions (usually 50 mL or less) are sometimes overlooked, but may be a significant part of the daily total.

You must include in the intake irrigating solutions that are not returned. To do this, carefully measure the amount instilled and, at the end of the procedure, the amount returned. Then subtract the amount returned from the total amount.

Output

Urine is the major output item that is measured. In the healthy person, the volume of urine excreted is approximately equal to the volume of oral fluid ingested, and water derived from solid food and from chemical oxidation in the body approximately equals the normal loss of water through the lungs, skin, and stool. If the water losses through the skin and stool become excessive, measure them and add them to the output. For example, this measurement is appropriate if the patient has diarrhea or profuse diaphoresis.

Vomitus, drainage from suction devices, wound drainage, and bleeding are abnormal fluid losses. Always measure or estimate as well as describe these kinds of losses.

DEVICES USED FOR MEASUREMENT

A helpful device for measuring urine is a plastic collection "hat" which, when placed upside down, fits the seat of the toilet or commode so that urine can collect in it as the female patient urinates (Fig. 10–1). A male patient can use a urinal for collection.

Two methods can be used to measure the urine output of infants. Subtracting the weight of a dry diaper from a wet one will give you some idea of the output from a single voiding. This method is not completely accurate *because the diaper may also be soiled by stool and, even though the bulk of this is removed, the stool that is left adds to the weight.* The soiled diaper must be weighed promptly or evaporation will lessen the total weight. A more accurate method is to use an infant urine collection bag. These devices use a self-adhesive and are sealed over the perineum of either a female or male infant to collect urine. They can also be used to collect a urine specimen for examination (Fig. 10–2).

UNITS OF MEASUREMENT

Depending on the healthcare facility and the forms used, I&O are measured in either metric liquid units called milliliters (mL) or cubic centimeters (cc). The milliliter is a cubic centimeter equivalent. It is far

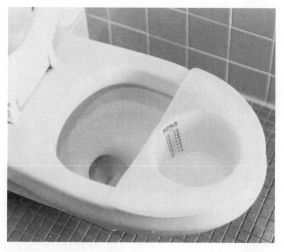

Figure 10–1. A "hat" used for urine collection. (Courtesy Ivan Ellis)

© 1996 by Lippincott-Raven Publishers

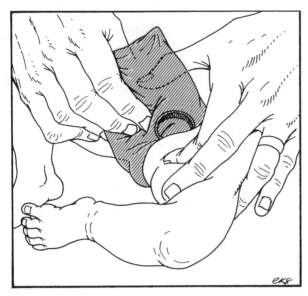

Figure 10–2. Applying a urinary collection device to an infant.

preferable to use the milliliter, which is the liquid unit, as a standard *because it lends itself more easily to calculations that require the conversion of liquid and weight measures. Intravenous fluids have been standardized in metric measurements for this reason also.*

PATIENT PARTICIPATION

Accurate I&O records are greatly facilitated when the patient is involved in the process. Patients can become highly motivated to participate when told the reasons for a procedure. First, make sure the patient knows which fluids of I&O are to be measured and the units of measurement. Explain the use of any devices for measuring either intake or output *so the patient is familiar with them.* Show the I&O records to the patient and demonstrate how to record items. Some patients may prefer to use paper and pencil at the bedside, which is a much simpler method of recording and which can be documented later. If the patient is on restricted or increased fluid intake, develop a plan that is the most acceptable and comfortable for that person. You and the patient may wish to plan water intake with the addition of juices throughout the day *to increase oral fluid intake.* Restricting oral fluids is very difficult for most patients. It is helpful to plan one-half or more of the total fluid intake for the day shift when the patient is more active and requires more hydration. One-third should be planned for the evening, with the remainder allocated for night hours. The patient will be more conscientious in complying with measurement of I&O if given this preparation and may even

assist with recording as well as alerting other healthcare workers concerning the need for measurement.

RECORD KEEPING

Bedside Records

First, a record must be kept at the patient's bedside or in the patient's room *so that measurements can be recorded immediately.* A form is often taped near the washbasin or on the door as a reminder to the healthcare team. Make a complete listing of the items measured and their quantities on this record. Many of these forms list the metric equivalents of the US standard units of liquid measurement (Fig. 10–3).

Permanent Records

There is a special form on the patient's chart for making a permanent record of the patient's I&O (Fig. 10–4).

Do not record individual items on this form, but do record totals for each 8-hour or 24-hour period (according to the facility's procedure) for each category. Thus, the intake record might include a figure for oral intake, one for intravenous fluid intake, one for miscellaneous intake (such as irrigating fluid), and a *total* intake figure. The output is recorded similarly, with totals for each category and then a comprehensive total for all outputs.

Parenteral fluids (those given by infusion) may be recorded on an independent record as well as on the overall record (Fig. 10–5).

PROCEDURE FOR MEASURING INTAKE AND OUTPUT

Assessment

1. Check the orders to learn whether the physician has ordered I&O to be measured.
2. If I&O has not been ordered, determine whether I&O should be initiated as a nursing action. Review the patient's status, including diagnosis, presence of intravenous infusions, medications being taken, the presence of an indwelling catheter, and other factors that would make the I&O measurement a helpful assessment tool for this patient. Be sure to write this on the plan of care *so that others on the team are aware of the need for measurement.*

© 1996 by Lippincott-Raven Publishers

SWEDISH HOSPITAL MEDICAL CENTER
747 Summit Avenue Seattle, WA 98104

B E D S I D E
I. & O.
W O R K S H E E T

PATIENT _George Dugan_

RM: _932_   BED: _W_

DATE: _3/16/99_

FLUID INTAKE FOR STANDARD SERVINGS

Juice glass 100	D'Zerta 100
Milk glass 180	Popsicle 80
Milk carton 240	Jello 150
Coffee pots (sm) 225 . . . . . . (lg). 300	Ice Cream, Sherbet 120
Coffee cup 150	
Coffee cream 15	Soup 180
Clear Disp. glass (sm) 150 . . (lg). 275	
Styrofoam cup 150	Cereal cream 120
Paper cup 180	
Plastic bowls . . . . 125 & 200	Ice cubes . . . . . . ½ of vol. . . . .
	Crushed ice . . . . ⅔ of vol. . . . .
	Pitcher c̄ or s̄ ice 900

SHIFT	TIME	INTAKE		OUTPUT				IRRIGATIONS		
		ORAL	TUBE	URINE	GASTRIC			IN	OUT	BALANCE
N I G H T S	2200-2300	240								
	2300-2400									
	2400-0100									
	0100-0200			400						
	0200-0300									
	0300-0400									
	0400-0500									
	0500-0600	75		120						
	TOTAL									
D A Y S	0600-0700									
	0700-0800	ᴮ445								
	0800-0900							100	100	———
	0900-1000	180		300						
	1000-1100									
	1100-1200									
	1200-1300	ᴸ470		360						
	1300-1400									
	TOTAL									
E V E N I N G S	1400-1500	100								
	1500-1600	ᴰ380								
	1600-1700									
	1700-1800									
	1800-1900									
	1900-2000	150						100	100	———
	2000-2100			300						
	2100-2200									
	TOTAL	1980		1480						

Figure 10–3. Intake–output worksheet.

© 1996 by Lippincott-Raven Publishers

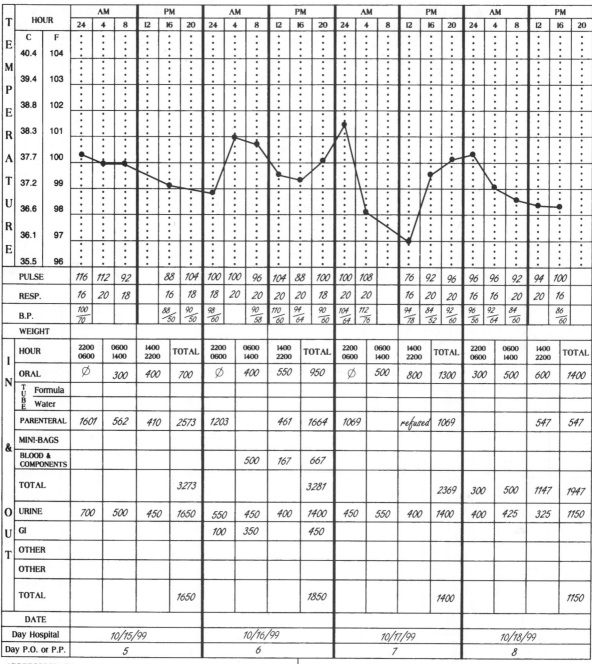

		AM			PM			AM			PM			AM			PM			AM			PM		
HOUR		24	4	8	12	16	20	24	4	8	12	16	20	24	4	8	12	16	20	24	4	8	12	16	20

T E M P E R A T U R E

C	F
40.4	104
39.4	103
38.8	102
38.3	101
37.7	100
37.2	99
36.6	98
36.1	97
35.5	96

	24	4	8	12	16	20	24	4	8	12	16	20	24	4	8	12	16	20	24	4	8	12	16	20
PULSE	116	112	92		88	104	100	100	96	104	88	100	100	108		76	92	96	96	96	92	94	100	
RESP.	16	20	18		16	18	18	20	20	20	20	18	20	20		16	20	20	16	16	20	20	16	
B.P.	100/70			88/50	90/50		98/60		90/58	110/60	94/64	90/60	104/64	112/76		94/78	84/52	92/60	96/56	92/64	84/60		86/60	
WEIGHT																								

I N &

HOUR	2200 0600	0600 1400	1400 2200	TOTAL	2200 0600	0600 1400	1400 2200	TOTAL	2200 0600	0600 1400	1400 2200	TOTAL	2200 0600	0600 1400	1400 2200	TOTAL
ORAL	Ø	300	400	700	Ø	400	550	950	Ø	500	800	1300	300	500	600	1400
TUBE Formula																
Water																
PARENTERAL	1601	562	410	2573	1203		461	1664	1069		refused	1069			547	547
MINI-BAGS																
BLOOD & COMPONENTS						500	167	667								
TOTAL				3273				3281				2369	300	500	1147	1947

O U T

URINE	700	500	450	1650	550	450	400	1400	450	550	400	1400	400	425	325	1150
GI					100	350		450								
OTHER																
OTHER																
TOTAL				1650				1850				1400				1150

DATE						
Day Hospital	10/15/99		10/16/99		10/17/99	10/18/99
Day P.O. or P.P.	5		6		7	8

ADDRESSOGRAPH:

Williams, Rosemary   F-52
201-56-4549
Dr. Connolly

THE SWEDISH HOSPITAL MEDICAL CENTER
SEATTLE, WASHINGTON

Figure 10–4. Intake–output record for patient's chart.

3. Assess the patient's knowledge base concerning the procedure and ability to participate in measuring I&O.

Planning

4. Locate the I&O worksheet. Familiarize yourself with the location at your facility.

5. Determine the extent to which the patient will participate in keeping records.

Implementation

6. Explain or reinforce the reasons for accurate measurement to the patient and encourage the patient to participate. Helping you compute the

© 1996 by Lippincott-Raven Publishers

Date and Time	TUBING CHANGE				DEVICE		Initials	AMOUNT-SOLUTION-ADDITIVES (number consecutively)	Rate	SHIFT TOTALS		Solu'	DC'd
	MACRO SET	MICRO SET	PUMP SET	BLOOD SET	PUMP	CONTR-OLLER				Time	Total	Time	Amount Absorb.
Date: 7/18 Time: 1430	✓		✓		✓		F.S.	D5 1/2 c̄ 20 meq KCl	125/hr	22	388	1640	1000
										06	372		
										14	240		
Date: 7/19 Time: 1900	✓		✓		✓		SA	HA# _9_ 1000 DEX _25_% A.A. _5_% NACL _30_ NA ACET___ KCL _25_ KPO4 _15_ CA GLU _8_ MG SO4 _8_ TR EL___ REG INS___ MVL _1_ VIT.K___	85/hr	22	381	0300	1025
										06	644		
Date: 7/20 Time: 1915	✓		✓		✓		SA	HA# _10_ 1000 DEX _25_% A.A. _5_% NACL _30_ NA ACET___ KCL _25_ KPO4 _15_ CA GLU _8_ MG SO4___ TR EL___ REG INS___ MVL _1_ VIT.K___	85/hr	22	377	0330	1119
										06	742		
Date: 7/21 Time: 0915	✓		✓		✓		F.S.	D5 1/2 c̄ 20 meq KCl	125/hr	22	108	2115	1008
										06	340		
										14	560		
Date: 7/22 Time: 2200	✓		✓		✓		K.R.	D5 1/2 c̄ 20 meq KCl	125/hr	22	124	0900	1034
										06	444		
										14	466		
Date: Time:													
Date: Time:													
Date: Time:													
Date: Time:													

Identify Initials with Signature:
1. Frank Shulz, RN
2. Shelly Atkinson, RN
3. Kerry Rollins, RN
4.
5.
6.
7.
8.
9.

ADDRESSOGRAPH:

Martinelli, Anita   F-67
288-39-5453
Dr. Ronderos

CODE: ★ see Nurses Progress Notes

SWEDISH HOSPITAL MEDICAL CENTER

SEATTLE, WASHINGTON

Figure 10–5. Parenteral fluid form.

© 1996 by Lippincott-Raven Publishers

values *makes some patients feel more involved in their own care.*

7. Measure intake. After a meal, record on the I&O sheet the amount of each fluid item taken. (Compute partial intake of any fluid item. This figure may have to be an estimate, except for a patient on very strict measurement for medical reasons.) Identify the fluid in any nourishment given between meals and note it on the worksheet.

8. Put on clean gloves *to protect yourself from contact with body fluids whenever measuring output of any kind,* then measure the patient's output. Note the amount on the work sheet after measuring it.

    a. With each voiding, use the measuring container to accurately measure the urine. Again, the patient may wish to do this for you and can be instructed to keep an accurate account. Remove any fecal material from the container for accuracy. Approximate toilet tissue displacement; the tissue is usually not removed. It is sometimes easier to pour off the urine from the bedpan to measure it.

    b. If the patient vomits, measure the vomitus before discarding.

    c. If the patient has an indwelling catheter, measure the contents of the drainage container at the end of the shift or earlier, if the container becomes full.

    d. Add any other output, including liquid stools, emesis, profuse diaphoresis, and any drainage of considerable volume. If there are other body fluids being collected (such as wound drainage or suction), measure each drainage source separately at the end of your shift.

    You will need to estimate the quantity of some of these items; even so, add them in.

9. Compute the intake at the end of your shift. Include all free water taken from the water pitcher or glasses of water. Add any water taken with medications if this is appropriate.

10. Compute any intravenous fluids infused. To do this, note the amount of fluid remaining in any intravenous container and compute the amount infused during your shift. Add any intravenous fluids given in the manner prescribed by your facility. Include "mini-bottles" of fluid given with intravenous medications as well as large bottles or bags infused (see Fig. 10–5).

11. Compute the output and record it on the I&O worksheet, using the proper column (see Fig. 10–3).

Documentation

12. Transfer the 8-hour totals from the I&O worksheet and the parenteral fluid sheet (see Fig. 10–4) to the permanent I&O record for the patient's chart.

Evaluation

13. Compare the I&O figures for the shift to obtain a general estimate of fluid balance. If there is a marked difference, review the I&O balance for the last several days and report any alarming trend to the physician.

14. Compare the I&O figures with the recommended norms for I&O for a person of that age and health status.

LONG-TERM CARE

Most residents in long-term care are elderly, and many cannot participate fully in a program that adequately provides sufficient oral fluid. As people get older, fluid intake decreases. Many of these residents take diuretic drugs and are *more susceptible to dehydration.* They incorrectly think they should decrease fluids because they are taking "water pills" to get rid of excess fluid. Your responsibility should include teaching residents and staff that older people, in general, need to consume sufficient fluid. The amount needed is guided by the person's medical condition. If urine output is much greater than fluid intake over several days, it should be reported. If the resident is incontinent, the best estimate is to record the number of times the person has been incontinent and whether, in your opinion, the amount has been small, moderate, or large.

It is important to remember that a variety of behavioral changes such as confusion can occur *because of dehydration.* Any resident on diuretic therapy in the long-term care setting should be on regular weight measurement, and if there is an unexplained weight gain, the resident should be placed on I&O *so that the nurse can accurately assess the patient's fluid status.*

© 1996 by Lippincott-Raven Publishers

HOME CARE

An increasing number of people are being cared for in the home, particularly elderly people and those with terminal or protracted illnesses. Family care providers may need to know how to monitor weight and, if it is not stable, how to measure I&O. Generally, a computation less rigid than the type done in the acute care setting is sufficient. Studies have shown that people being cared for in the home drink a greater variety and amount of fluids than do those in the long-term care setting. Despite this, a record is sometimes needed because of the debilitation or serious diagnosis of patients at home.

CRITICAL THINKING EXERCISE

• The physician has ordered measurement of I&O for your patient, Mr. Denner. Determine which food items should be included in these measurements. Then use the various containers given on the sample form in Fig. 10–3 to calculate the I&O for this patient.

On rising, Mr. Denner brushed his teeth. After rinsing his mouth, he drank half a glass (small) of water. He voided 250 mL urine. Breakfast arrived and was composed of:

Fruit juice, small glass

Cereal bowl of hot oatmeal with a pitcher of milk

Bacon and soft-boiled egg

Pot of black coffee

Glass of low-fat milk

Shortly after breakfast, Mr. Denner felt nauseated and vomited 75 mL semiliquid emesis. Throughout the morning, he voided two times: 50 mL and 225 mL.

By lunch, he was feeling much better, and a light diet was ordered. When it arrived, he ate a small bowl of broth and half of a small bowl of gelatin.

He voided once more after lunch: 125 mL.

He was given oral medications twice, each time with 1 oz. water.

At the end of the day shift, half of a 1,000-mL bottle of intravenous fluids had been absorbed.

Submit your calculations to your instructor for evaluation.

References

Carpenito, L. J. (1993). *Nursing Diagnosis: Application to Clinical Practice*. Philadelphia: J.B. Lippincott.

© 1996 by Lippincott-Raven Publishers

PERFORMANCE CHECKLIST

Procedure for Measuring Intake and Output	Needs More Practice	Satisfactory	Comments
Assessment			
1. Check physician's orders.			
2. Review patient's status and determine if I&O should be initiated as a nursing action.			
3. Assess patient's knowledge base.			
Planning			
4. Locate and familiarize yourself with I&O worksheet.			
5. Determine patient's willingness and ability to participate.			
Implementation			
6. Explain importance of measurement to the patient.			
7. Measure intake: fluids in diet, free water, fluids taken with medications.			
8. Put on clean gloves and measure output: urine, excessive diarrhea, diaphoresis, or drainage.			
9. Compute the intake at the end of your shift.			
10. Compute any intravenous fluids infused.			
11. Compute and record the output on the I&O worksheet.			
Documentation			
12. Transfer the 8-hour I&O totals for intake, parenteral fluids, and output to the permanent record.			
Evaluation			
13. Compare the intake figures with those of the output. If a marked difference exists, review record for last several days.			
14. Compare measurements with norms for patient's age and health status.			

© 1996 by Lippincott-Raven Publishers

? QUIZ

Multiple-Choice Questions

_____ **1.** I&O are measured in metric units because

    a. metric weights and measures lend themselves to easier conversion from one to another.
    b. metric measures are more accurate.
    c. intravenous fluids are measured in metric units.
    d. nursing is a science, and scientific disciplines use metric measures.

_____ **2.** The I&O worksheet is used primarily to

    a. show the patient his or her fluid status.
    b. total fluid intake and output.
    c. record the various items of fluid intake and output at the bedside.
    d. provide a permanent record of intake and output.

_____ **3.** The permanent record of I&O is usually kept

    a. on the worksheet.
    b. in the nurse's notes.
    c. on a special form in the chart.
    d. on the graphic record with temperature and vital signs.

_____ **4.** The following items should be included in the total measurement of intake: 1) dietary fluids; 2) irrigation fluids returned; 3) gelatin; 4) fluids at bedside; 5) cereal; 6) ice cream; 7) intravenous fluids; 8) pureed fruits and vegetables.

    a. 1, 4, 7, and 8
    b. 1, 3, 4, 6, and 7
    c. 1, 2, 4, 5, and 7
    d. All of these

_____ **5.** The following items should be included in the total measurement of output: 1) urine; 2) normal stools; 3) diarrheal stools; 4) vomitus; 5) normal perspiration; 6) excessive perspiration; 7) wound drainage.

    a. 1, 3, 4, 6, and 7
    b. 1, 4, 5, 6, and 7
    c. 1, 3, and 4
    d. All of these

_____ **6.** In checking the I&O sheet for a certain elderly patient, Jane Smith, RN, noted that the 8-hour intake total was recorded as 720 mL, which was larger than usual. She then checked the worksheet on which the exact items taken were recorded. The following items were listed.

Breakfast
cereal, 60 mL
half and half, 50 mL
apple juice, 100 mL
(water pitcher changed, 100 mL)

Snack
pureed peaches, 100 mL

Lunch
pureed peas, 60 mL
pureed meat, 50 mL
applesauce, 100 mL
milk, 100 mL

Jane Smith determined that an error had been made. The error resulted from

© 1996 by Lippincott-Raven Publishers

> **a.** incorrect addition.
> **b.** including in the morning shift water that had actually been taken from the pitcher during the previous 8-hour shift.
> **c.** including amounts for things that should not have been included.

_____ 7. A patient has taken the following amounts during the day shift (7:00 AM–3:00 PM). This hospital records all intake and output for 24-hour periods only. At the end of *your* shift, what will you record on the I&O record?

Breakfast
juice, 100 mL
milk, 90 mL
coffee, 150 mL

Lunch
milk, 240 mL
pureed peaches, 50 mL

Snack
gelatin, 50 mL

Water Pitcher
500 mL

> **a.** 1,080 mL
> **b.** 1,130 mL
> **c.** 1,180 mL
> **d.** Nothing should be recorded at that time.

_____ 8. Totals over 24-hour periods are helpful because

> **a.** I&O balance usually cannot be identified over shorter periods.
> **b.** they reduce the time needed for record keeping.
> **c.** physicians usually check them once every 24 hours.
> **d.** a 24-hour total is most accurate.

_____ 9. The following items were taken by Mr. Jones. What is his total intake for the day shift?

Water Pitcher Change, 7:00 AM
100 mL

Breakfast
coffee, 240 mL
juice, 90 mL

Snack
juice, 100 mL

Lunch
milk, 240 mL

Water Pitcher Change, 2:30 PM
300 mL

Dinner
coffee, 250 mL

Water Pitcher Change and Snack, 8:30 PM
150 mL
broth, 150 mL
water, 350 mL

> **a.** 980 mL
> **b.** 1,070 mL
> **c.** 1,220 mL
> **d.** 1,330 mL

_____ 10. If the facility in question 9 records intake every 8 hours, the total recorded by the nurse working from 3:00 PM to 11:00 PM would be

> **a.** 450 mL
> **b.** 750 mL
> **c.** 1,400 mL
> **d.** zero

_____ 11. Mr. Jones had an output of 400 mL for the two shifts. This might indicate

> **a.** that not enough data is given to identify the problem.
> **b.** water intoxication.
> **c.** edema formation.
> **d.** kidney malfunction.

© 1996 by Lippincott-Raven Publishers

_____ **12.** Mr. Ford is to have all I&O measured. He is 45 years old, a truck driver, father of four, and he has been admitted with a possible kidney infection. In planning for accurate measurement, you would

    a. measure all urine yourself because this is a critical concern.

    b. see that urine is measured by a staff person (aide, LPN, RN), to guarantee accuracy.

    c. have Mr. Ford measure his own urine and record it.

    d. ask Mr. Ford if he would prefer to measure his output himself or have a staff person do it.

© 1996 by Lippincott-Raven Publishers

MODULE

11

COLLECTING SPECIMENS AND PERFORMING COMMON LABORATORY TESTS

MODULE CONTENTS

RATIONALE FOR THE USE OF THESE
  SKILLS
ANALYZING TEST RESULTS
EQUIPMENT
COLLECTING SPECIMENS FOR TESTING
Urine Specimens
Blood Specimens
Stool Specimens
Sputum Specimens
Gastric Secretions
GENERAL PROCEDURE FOR
  COLLECTING AND TESTING
  SPECIMENS
Assessment
Planning
Implementation
Evaluation
Documentation
SPECIFIC PROCEDURES FOR
  COLLECTING AND TESTING
  SPECIMENS
SPECIFIC GRAVITY OF URINE
Procedure Using a Urinometer

Procedure Using a Urine Refractometer
URINE GLUCOSE
Supplies and Equipment
Specimen Collection
Procedure for Measuring Urine Glucose
KETONE BODIES IN URINE
Equipment
Procedure for Measuring Urine Ketones
TESTING URINE FOR OCCULT BLOOD
MULTIPURPOSE STRIP TESTS FOR URINE
Procedure for Measuring pH of Urine
BLOOD GLUCOSE
Procedure for Measuring Blood Glucose
BLOOD IN FECES
Procedure for Testing Feces for Occult
  Blood
CULTURES
Obtaining Cultures
Procedure for Obtaining a Culture
Urine Cultures
LONG-TERM CARE
HOME CARE
CRITICAL THINKING EXERCISES

PREREQUISITES

Successful completion of the following modules:

VOLUME 1
Module 1 An Approach to Nursing Skills
Module 2 Basic Infection Control
Module 3 Safety
Module 5 Documentation
Module 7 Temperature, Pulse, and
          Respiration
Module 8 Blood Pressure

The following modules may be needed for collecting specific specimens:

VOLUME 2
Module 33 Sterile Technique
Module 37 Catheterization
Module 43 Nasogastric Intubation

© 1996 by Lippincott-Raven Publishers

OVERALL OBJECTIVE

To collect and handle specimens correctly and perform common laboratory tests accurately.

SPECIFIC LEARNING OBJECTIVES

Know Facts and Principles	Apply Facts and Principles	Demonstrate Ability	Evaluate Performance
1. Check order			
State two reasons to check order for collection of specimen.	Given a patient situation, state rationale for laboratory test and nurse's involvement in securing specimen.	Check order, obtaining complete information. In the clinical setting, state rationale for test ordered. State information about nurse's responsibility in securing specimen.	Evaluate with instructor.
2. Review procedure for specimen collection, assess patient, and gather equipment			
State review of procedure and assessment of patient as integral part of activity.	Given a patient situation, describe equipment necessary for obtaining specimen, handling specimen, and observing patient's response.	In the clinical setting, review procedure involved, assess patient, and secure necessary equipment.	Evaluate with instructor.
3. Explain procedure to patient			
State two reasons for explanation to patient.	Given a patient situation, describe what would appropriately be included in explanation to patient.	In the clinical setting, prepare patient appropriately for obtaining laboratory specimen.	Evaluate with instructor.
4. Prepare environment			
List four aspects of preparation of environment.	Given a patient situation, state aspects of environmental preparation that would be appropriate.	In the clinical setting, perform appropriate aspects of environmental preparation for patient.	Evaluate with instructor.
5. Perform procedure			
State four "rights" of obtaining laboratory specimen.	Given a specific situation, state correct amount of given specimen and correct container.	In the clinical setting, secure right amount of specimen at right time in right container from right patient.	Evaluate with instructor using Performance Checklist.
6. Make the patient comfortable			
List examples of activities that might be included in making the patient comfortable.	Given a specific situation, state appropriate activities to make the patient comfortable.	In the clinical setting, make the patient comfortable as appropriate to the procedure.	Evaluate with instructor.

(continued)

© 1996 by Lippincott-Raven Publishers

Know Facts and Principles	Apply Facts and Principles	Demonstrate Ability	Evaluate Performance
7. *Care for equipment and specimen*			
State four aspects of caring for equipment and specimen.	Given a specific situation, state care of equipment and appropriate handling of specimen.	In the clinical setting, care for equipment, and handle specimen appropriately.	Evaluate with instructor.
8. *Test specimen*			
State information to be determined through laboratory testing.	Given a patient situation, describe how a specific laboratory test should be performed (specific gravity of urine, glucose in urine, ketone bodies in urine, occult blood in urine, blood glucose, or blood in feces).	In the clinical setting, test the specimen accurately.	Evaluate accuracy of testing with instructor.
9. *Evaluate patient's response and test results*			
State criteria to use in evaluation.	Given a patient situation, describe appropriate information included in evaluation.	In the clinical setting, evaluate appropriately.	Evaluate with instructor using Performance Checklist.
10. *Document*			
State data to be included in charting.	Given a patient situation, record appropriately.	In the clinical setting, record appropriately,	Evaluate with instructor using Performance Checklist.
11. *Special considerations* a. *Urine* b. *Blood* c. *Stool* d. *Sputum* e. *Gastric secretions*			
State special handling, preparation, and positioning of patient; role of nurse; special observations related to specific specimens.	Given a specific situation, identify special considerations related to situation.	In the clinical setting, secure laboratory specimens using special considerations as appropriate.	Evaluate with instructor.

© 1996 by Lippincott-Raven Publishers

LEARNING ACTIVITIES

1. Review the Specific Learning Objectives.
2. Read the section on performing treatments and the section on collecting urine specimens (in the chapter on elimination) in Ellis and Nowlis, *Nursing: A Human Needs Approach,* or comparable material in another textbook.
3. Look up the module vocabulary terms in the glossary.
4. Read through the module, and mentally practice the specific procedures. Study as though you were preparing to teach these skills to another person.
5. In the practice setting, do the following:
   a. Inspect and compare available laboratory requisitions. Note the information required for different types of tests.
   b. With a partner as a patient, give instructions for obtaining a clean catch specimen. Fill out a laboratory slip as if an actual specimen had been obtained, and document on the patient's record. Have your partner evaluate the clarity of your instruction.
6. In the clinical setting, do the following:
   a. Ask your instructor to help you obtain experience in filling out laboratory requisitions.
   b. Volunteer to obtain any specimen that can be secured by a nurse.
   c. Volunteer to perform specific laboratory tests in the clinical setting.

VOCABULARY

acetone	displacement	hydrometer	parasite
acid	exudate	incubate	pH
alkaline	feces	ketone body	protein
amoeba	gastric secretions	lancet	reagent
bilirubin	glucose	meniscus	specific gravity
culture and sensitivity	guaiac	occult	urine refractometer
cytology	hematuria	ova	urinometer

Collecting Specimens and Performing Common Laboratory Tests

Rationale for the Use of These Skills

Specimens obtained by the nurse, or with the assistance of the nurse, may be the key to the diagnoses and therapies of the patients concerned. To handle the task well, the nurse must know the rationale for the test(s) involved, necessary teaching and preparation of the patients, correct methods of obtaining and handling specimens, and how to care for patients after the test.

Laboratory tests are an important part of establishing a diagnosis. In addition, test results indicate a patient's progress and can be the basis for planning or altering therapy and nursing care.

Modern technology has made many laboratory tests simple to perform. Because no elaborate laboratory equipment is needed, the tests are commonly performed on the nursing unit, making the results immediately available.

Although they are not technically difficult, the tests must be done carefully and accurately. This places an additional burden on the nurse, who must know the purpose of the tests and the procedures to be followed.

In addition to conducting many laboratory tests yourself, you may also have to teach patients who will be returning home and their families or caregivers how to perform some tests. Diabetic patients, for example, test their urine or blood frequently for glucose content. You must master the skill before you are able to teach it.[1]

ANALYZING TEST RESULTS

The focus of this module is the technical skill of performing common laboratory tests. To function appropriately in the nursing role, you will need to analyze the results of any test through synthesizing information about the test itself, the patient's medical diagnosis and condition, and your assessment of the patient. You will need to identify the significance and the nursing implications for the patient. Your medical-surgical text and a text on clinical laboratory tests will provide the theoretical information for this analysis.

EQUIPMENT

Equipment for performing tests on the patient care unit is usually kept in the utility room. Patients who require frequent testing of one kind or another may

have individual equipment in the room or bathroom. The equipment for cultures is usually kept with other sterile supplies.

You should know how to order supplies used for laboratory tests in your facility. Reagent tablets and strips usually come from the pharmacy; glass urinometers, culture tubes, and swabs, are typically ordered from the central supply department. *However, facilities do vary,* so be familiar with the arrangement in your institution.

Tablets and strips have expiration dates that should be checked carefully. *Exposure to bright light or moisture may cause them to deteriorate.* Keep the brown glass bottles and the boxes used for these items tightly capped or closed. *To prevent errors,* keep all directions, packet inserts, and color charts with the appropriate products. Some reagent strips for testing urine have multiple areas on a single strip that can be used to measure a variety of components (Table 11–1).

COLLECTING SPECIMENS FOR TESTING

When collecting specimens, wear clean gloves *for protection from contact with body fluids, which can transmit microorganisms.* Specimen containers should be clearly labeled on the jar or tube (not on the lid), tightly sealed, and placed in plastic bags if being sent to a laboratory *to protect laboratory personnel from becoming exposed to microorganisms.* Some facilities double-bag all specimens for extra protection. Specimens to be tested in the laboratory should be sent promptly *so that time and temperature change do not alter the contents.* If you will be doing the testing, keep the specimen in an appropriate area, such as the utility room. If the test must be done in the patient's room, place a paper towel on the table *to prevent potential contamination of the table.* Refer to the specific procedures and Table 11–2 for further information.

Urine Specimens

Most urine specimens needed for routine analysis are obtained by having the patient void into a receptacle after cleaning the perineum. These specimens are considered clean, not sterile; however, they are used for urine cultures. See Table 11–2 for specific directions on obtaining a "clean catch" urine specimen.

Tests can identify specific abnormal components of the urine and the presence of abnormally large amounts of bacteria. Patients are infrequently

---

[1]Note that the rationale for action is emphasized throughout the module by the use of italics.

© 1996 by Lippincott-Raven Publishers

Table 11–1. Products Used for Testing Body Substances

Reagent	Type	Measures or Tests
Tests For Occult Blood Used on Feces, Gastric Contents, or Urine		
Hema-chek	Slide	Occult blood
Hemastix	Strip	Occult blood
Hematest	Tablet	Occult blood
Hemoccult	Folder	Occult blood
Tests For Blood Glucose Used on Blood Obtained Through a Finger Stick		
Chemstip bG	Strip	Blood glucose
Dextrostix	Strip	Blood glucose
Glucostix	Strip	Blood glucose
Tests For Urine Used on Freshly Voided Urine		
Acetest	Tablet	Ketones
Albustix	Strip	Albumin
Bili-Labstix	Strip	Bilirubin
Clinistix	Strip	Glucose
Clinitest	Tablet	All reducing substances (especially sugars)
Combistix	Strip	Glucose, protein, pH
Diastix	Strip	Glucose
Hema-combistix	Strip	pH, protein, glucose, blood
Hemastix	Strip	Blood
Ictotest	Tablet	Bilirubin
Keto-diastix	Strip	Glucose, ketones
Labstix	Strip	pH, protein, glucose, ketone, blood
Multistix	Strip	Produced in several configurations with 10 possible different tests: glucose, bilirubin, ketones, specific gravity, blood, pH, protein, urobilinogen, nitrite, leukocytes
Phenistix	Strip	Phenylketones
Uristix	Strip	Protein, glucose, nitrite, leukocytes

catheterized for the sole purpose of obtaining urine specimens *because of the risk of introducing microorganisms into the urinary tract.*

If the patient already has an indwelling catheter in place, obtain a sterile specimen by clamping the catheter briefly and using a sterile syringe and needle to extract a small amount of urine through the port designed for that purpose (Fig. 11–1). (Refer to Table 11–2 for the method of obtaining a urine sample when a catheter is in place.)

If a 24-hour specimen is ordered, it is timed to begin in the morning (check your facility for the exact time). Before you begin the timing, the patient should void and not save this urine *because it is urine that has been in the bladder for some time.* Then, all urine voided during the next 24 hours is collected in the type of container used in the facility. Some tests require the addition of a preservative to the container. If a preservative is used, *it may be a toxic substance* and should be treated with care. At the end of the 24-hour period, the patient voids a last specimen, which is added to the rest. The staff and the patient should know that a 24-hour specimen is being collected. A sign posted in the patient's bathroom is useful as a reminder. If the patient has a catheter, the urine is simply collected in one container for 24 hours.

If a voiding is inadvertently discarded, most laboratories can calculate an approximate value for the test based on the specimen that was obtained. *However, this lessens accuracy and should be avoided.* When a very precise measurement is needed, the test may need to be repeated if a specimen is discarded.

(text continues on page 220)

© 1996 by Lippincott-Raven Publishers

Table 11–2. Quick Reference for Collecting Specimens

Specimen	Preparing the Patient	Positioning the Patient	Role of the Nurse	Special Observations Concerning the Patient	Handling the Specimen
Urine a. Voided—"clean catch"	Instruct how to obtain clean voided specimen.	Up to bathroom or commode or use bedpan or urinal	Obtain specimen. Clean voided specimen: 1. Clean vulva or penis thoroughly with soap and water. 2. Hold vulva apart while voiding to decrease contamination of urine. 3. Initial part of voiding passed into commode, bedpan, or urinal; pass next part into clean or sterile container (disposable kits are available). 4. Do not allow container to touch body.	None	Specimen is clean. Done for routine urinalysis, and to check for presence of cells and for culture and sensitivity (C&S). If not sent immediately to laboratory, refrigerate.
b. Catheter in place	Inform patient of procedure.	Supine, with top linen draped back to expose catheter	To remove urine from indwelling catheter: 1. Obtain sterile 5-mL syringe with needle and alcohol swab. 2. Wipe entry port on tubing thoroughly with alcohol swab. 3. Insert needle into port and withdraw urine. If there is no urine in the catheter, clamp it off for 15–20 min before trying to obtain sample. 4. Remove syringe from catheter, and unclamp catheter if it was clamped. 5. Expel urine from syringe into sterile container. 6. Dispose of equipment safely in room receptacle.	None	Specimen is sterile. Often done for C&S.

(continued)

217

© 1996 by Lippincott-Raven Publishers

Table 11-2. Quick Reference for Collecting Specimens (Continued)

Specimen	Preparing the Patient	Positioning the Patient	Role of the Nurse	Special Observations Concerning the Patient	Handling the Specimen
c. Catheter to be inserted	Explain procedure.	See Module 37, Catheterization.	See Module 37, Catheterization, if urine from an indwelling catheter is needed.	See Module 37, Catheterization.	Specimen is sterile. Often done for C&S.
d. Infant	Infant may need to be restrained until specimen is collected.	Place infant in Fowler's position after urine collector is in place *to facilitate collection of urine by gravity.*	Obtain specimen. 1. Clean perianal area thoroughly. 2. Dry perianal area thoroughly *to ensure that urine collector will stay in place.* 3. Peel off protective paper and press adhesive material firmly against infant's skin 4. Check the bag at least every 15 minutes until an adequate amount of urine is collected. 5. The bag should be removed and cleansing repeated every hour until the specimen is collected. 6. Remove the bag gently. Transfer the specimen to an appropriate container.	If collecting bag is in place for a long period (24-hour urine specimen), skin care under adhesive should be given at least every 8 hours.	Specimen is clean. Done for routine urinalysis. If not sent immediately to laboratory, refrigerate.
Blood	Instruct as to what to expect and fasting directions if appropriate.	Babies may have to be mummied (see Module 19, Basic Infant Care).	Depending on setting, prepare patient and assist physician or laboratory technician, or prepare patient only.	Apply pressure to puncture site *to stop bleeding.* If blood is obtained from an artery, apply pressure for 5 min following procedure.	Procedure is sterile. For serology or chemical analysis, or if not immediately examined, refrigerate; for culture, incubate; for other tests, leave at room temperature.

© 1996 by Lippincott-Raven Publishers

Specimen	Patient preparation	Positioning/assistance	Procedure	Nursing considerations	Laboratory/evaluation
Stool	Provide commode or bedpan.		Obtain specimen. Transfer from commode or bedpan to specimen container with tongue blade.	Patient may be embarrassed. Be reassuring, and provide privacy.	Small amount usually adequate. If tests are for ova, parasites, or amoebas, send to laboratory immediately (while it is warm).
Sputum	Explain why specimen is needed, and show container in which to expectorate.	Usually patient will be sitting up; splinting may help. Postural drainage can be used (see Module 39, Respiratory Care Procedures).	Obtain specimen or assist respiratory therapist to obtain specimen. 1. Remind patient that saliva is not sputum, that sputum is coughed up from lungs. 2. Remind patient not to use mouthwash or toothpaste before sputum collection *because they may alter the specimen.*	Nausea may occur. Mouth care is indicated after a large amount of sputum is coughed up.	Specimen is clean for cytology; sterile for C&S. Best collected in morning. Send to laboratory as soon as possible.
Gastric secretions	Explain why specimen is needed, and tell patient how you plan to obtain it.	Patient with nasogastric (NG) tube will usually be in mid to high Fowler's.	Obtain specimen. 1. Turn off suction machine. 2. Disconnect distal portion of NG tube from adapter of suction tube. 3. Attach syringe with adapter to NG tube. 4. Gently withdraw secretions for specimen. 5. Turn on suction. 6. Reconnect tubes.	After obtaining specimen, check to be sure that suction is operating and secretions are draining.	Specimen is clean. Tests for blood and pH may be done on unit. If ordered, send to laboratory for other tests.

© 1996 by Lippincott-Raven Publishers

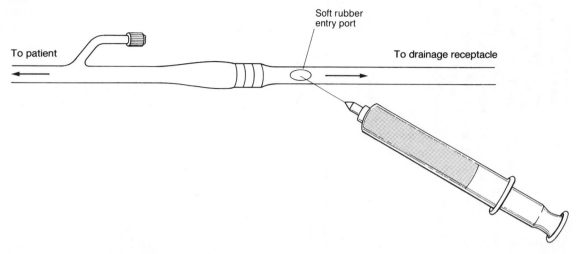

Soft rubber
entry port

To patient

To drainage receptacle

Figure 11–1. Obtaining a urine specimen through a port using a syringe.

Blood Specimens

Simple glucose testing may be done using a drop of blood obtained through a finger stick on an adult or a heel stick on an infant. Most routine blood specimens are obtained by the hospital laboratory technician or a certified healthcare provider. Venous blood is drawn for most tests, but arterial blood is drawn for blood gas measurement. See Table 11–2 for information on the nursing role in obtaining routine blood samples.

If a patient has a central intravenous catheter in place, check the hospital policy regarding drawing blood from the catheter. This is often a nursing responsibility. In some settings the nurse must be certified by the agency to perform this function. For the procedure on how to draw blood from a central line, see Module 54, Caring for Central Intravenous Catheters.

Arterial blood samples are commonly drawn by a laboratory technician or a respiratory therapy technician. In some settings, especially critical care and long-term care, nurses draw blood. The agency may certify nurses for this skill.

Procedures for blood drawing vary, but different color-coded tubes are used to indicate the type of preservative or anticoagulant that is in the tube. Using the correct tube is essential for accurate test results.

Stool Specimens

A single stool specimen may be ordered, or occasionally the physician may want specimens obtained from three subsequent and different defecations. Usually only a small amount of stool needs to be collected from a bedpan or "hat" container with a tongue blade. The tongue blade is then used to apply the stool to a disposable envelope type of container or to put the stool in a plastic specimen container (see Table 11–2).

Stool can be tested for blood, pus, ova, and parasites. More stool material is needed for ova and parasite determination than for other tests. The specimen for ova and parasite testing should go to the laboratory before it cools, *because cooling makes organisms less detectable*.

A simple test for the presence of occult (hidden) blood in stool may be done with only a smear of feces on a filter paper or special folder designed for this purpose.

Sputum Specimens

The examination of sputum is important in diagnosing a variety of conditions. Sputum arises from the tissue of the respiratory tract and should not be confused with saliva, which is excreted by the salivary and mucus glands in the mouth. Collecting a sputum specimen requires teaching the patient the difference.

Because secretions tend to accumulate during the night, the best time to obtain a sputum specimen is first thing in the morning. The amount needed varies with the type of test to be done. Tell the patient to take several very deep breaths and then cough forcefully. Sputum should be coughed directly into the specimen container *to decrease the chance of contamination of the specimen* (see Table 11–2).

When the patient cannot raise sputum, the respiratory therapist may use a mist treatment to induce sputum production. Suctioning may be needed to obtain a sputum specimen in some instances. (See

© 1996 by Lippincott-Raven Publishers

Module 40, Oral and Nasopharyngeal Suctioning, and Module 41, Tracheostomy Care and Suctioning.)

If the patient may have tuberculosis and is having a test for acid-fast bacillus, any healthcare provider working with the patient to obtain a specimen must wear a special high-efficiency particulate air filter mask *for personal protection from the organism (see Module 32, Isolation Technique).*

After the specimen has been collected in a sterile container, remove the container promptly, and send it to the laboratory. *The sight of a container of sputum can be offensive to the patient, visitors, and staff.*

Gastric Secretions

When a patient has a nasogastric (NG) tube in place, a specimen of gastric secretions may be obtained to assess the pH (the acid or alkaline status) and presence or absence of blood or other components. First, the suction should be interrupted. This is done by turning off the suction machine and then, with gloved hands, disconnecting the distal end of the NG tube from the adapter of the suction tube. Using a catheter tip syringe or a large, regular syringe with an adapter, gently aspirate the amount of gastric secretions needed for testing. Reinstate the suction by reconnecting the tubing and turning the suction back on. If a patient has a copious amount of drainage, a syringe may not be necessary. In this case, simply turn off the suction, disconnect the tubing, and place the end of the NG tube into a small container; only a short period of time is usually needed to collect the specimen (see Table 11–2).

GENERAL PROCEDURE FOR COLLECTING AND TESTING SPECIMENS

Assessment

1. Determine which tests are to be performed for the particular patient and the type of specimen required. Some of the tests below are done only with a physician's order. Others can be done either with a physician's order or when the nurse determines they are needed.
2. Review the procedure and equipment needed, carefully checking the following. (Some hospitals maintain a guide to specific laboratory tests that the nurse can use as a quick reference; Fig. 11–2).
   a. Whether a patient's written consent is needed
   b. The equipment needed for the test and for any monitoring of the patient (such as a blood pressure cuff)
   c. The type of specimen container required

SODIUM, SERUM

Fasting not required

Requisition: Chem III, order as Na (chemical symbol for sodium)
Specimen: Serum (red-top tube) or plasma (green-top tube)

Normal: 138–146

See also Sodium, urine

Turn-around time: Same day

May be stat

Figure 11–2. A sample of a laboratory test file that the nurse can use as a guide for tests.

   d. The specific procedure for obtaining the specimen
3. Assess the patient, focusing especially on the following:
   a. Factors present that might affect his or her ability to cooperate or to undergo the procedure
   b. Special needs that might require special equipment or extra help
   c. Knowledge base regarding the test

Planning
4. Wash your hands *for infection control.*
5. Obtain the necessary equipment to collect the specimen and carry out the test when indicated. Include clean gloves to wear while handling blood or body substances. *Gloves protect you from any contact with inadvertent spills.*

Implementation
6. Identify the patient *to be sure you are carrying out the procedure for the correct patient.*
7. Explain to the patient exactly what is going to happen to an extent that is appropriate and will enhance the patient's ability to cooperate. Allow the patient to express personal feelings and ask questions.
8. Prepare the environment. Depending on the procedure to be performed, provide for privacy, adjust the lighting, and assist in positioning and draping as appropriate.
9. Put on gloves; collect the specimen and send the specimen to the laboratory or perform the test as described in the specific procedures. Be certain that you obtain the right amount of specimen in the right container at the right time and

© 1996 by Lippincott-Raven Publishers

from the right patient. Do not get any of the specimen material on the outside of the container.

All of the above must be done while making observations of the patient that are appropriate to the procedure and offering support and reassurance as needed (see the column "Special Observations Concerning the Patient" in Table 11–2).

10. Properly dispose of gloves and specimens no longer needed and clean equipment as necessary. The care of the equipment is dictated by the type of equipment involved and the policies of your facility. Even with disposable equipment, you must be sure to dispose of particular items (needles, breakables) in appropriate ways.

11. Make the patient comfortable. This can include repositioning, changing or straightening the bedding, and administering medication for pain or discomfort. Again, this step depends on the procedure you have performed.

12. Wash your hands *for infection control.*

13. Record the result on paper of any test you have performed for future documentation, or send the specimen to the laboratory. Sometimes nurses attempt to remember test results in an effort to save time, only to have to repeat the procedures later when their recall is not accurate. It is better to record numbers when you first obtain them *to prevent having to repeat the procedure.*

An important aspect of the nurse's role is handling and labeling specimens correctly. You will place the specimen into a plastic bag (double-bagged if that is the facility policy). You must know whether the specimen should be kept warm or refrigerated, taken immediately to the laboratory, or handled in some other special way. In addition, labeling must be complete and accurate. Although each facility has its own procedure, the following information is often included: patient's name, identification number, age, room number (if in a healthcare facility), and physician's name. In most cases, a laboratory requisition will accompany the specimen and must also be completely and accurately filled out. The patient's identifying information, diagnosis, and the date and time of specimen collection are often included (Fig. 11–3). If the patient has an infectious disease, You must note this on the requisition slip and the specimen container to protect the laboratory personnel who may be handling the specimen.

Evaluation

14. Compare the results of this test with the normal values for such a test and any previous results for that patient. Identify any abnormalities.

15. Evaluate the patient's physical, psychosocial, and psychological responses to having the test done.

Documentation

16. Document appropriate data on a flow sheet. In some instances, you may need to make a note on the narrative. You may need to include the following:
    a. Date and time
    b. Results of any test you performed
    c. The amount, description, and disposition of the specimen obtained

Figure 11–3. A sample of a requisition the nurse can use to order blood chemistries by circling codes

© 1996 by Lippincott-Raven Publishers

DATE/TIME	
7/4/99	*Catheterized with #16 straight catheter without difficulty, 60 ml*
0800	*cloudy yellow urine obtained and sent to lab. Patient continues to*
	complain of burning on urination. —————— S. Prentice, NS

Example of Nursing Progress Notes Using Narrative Format.

c. The patient's emotional and physiologic response, if significant

17. Report abnormalities as directed in each specific procedure. Whether a test result is reported depends on the reason for the test and the patient's medical status.

SPECIFIC PROCEDURES FOR COLLECTING AND TESTING SPECIMENS

For each specific laboratory test discussed, some steps of the General Procedure may be modified. The modified steps and references to the steps of the General Procedure that remain the same follow.

SPECIFIC GRAVITY OF URINE

Specific gravity is a measurement of the concentration of urine. Overhydration, or any disease that affects the body's ability to concentrate particles in the urine, leads to a low specific-gravity figure. Conversely, dehydration, or any condition that increases water reabsorption in the kidney, results in a high specific-gravity figure. The numbers used to delineate the normal range vary slightly, depending on the facility in which you practice or the text that you consult. Generally, the normal specific gravity range for urine is approximately 1.010 to 1.025 g/mL.

Specific gravity can be measured using either a urinometer or a urine refractometer. The *urinometer,* which is more common, uses a displacement principle. The *refractometer* uses light refraction. Many hospitals have refractometers available, particularly for units (critical care, pediatrics, nurseries, and units for those with kidney disease) where accuracy of measurement is essential.

Procedure Using a Urinometer

Assessment

1.–3. Follow the steps of the General Procedure for Collecting and Testing Specimens.

Planning

4. Follow the General Procedure.
5. Obtain a urinometer (urine hydrometer), a urine container, and clean gloves *to protect yourself from contact with urine.* The urinometer (Fig. 11–4) measures the concentration of the urine by the simple principle of displacement. The particles in the urine displace or push the bulb of the urinometer upward. The specific gravity is read as the number at the meniscus of the urine. *Because a heavy concentration of particles in the urine pushes the bulb higher,* you will find a higher number at the meniscus as the specific gravity increases. Always test urine that is of room temperature because refrigerated urine condenses and therefore has a higher specific gravity (McConnell, 1991).

Implementation

6.–8. Follow the steps of the General Procedure.
9. Put on clean gloves, and measure the specific gravity with a urinometer.
   a. Collect at least 20 mL urine, and pour into a container. All containers must be clean *so that*

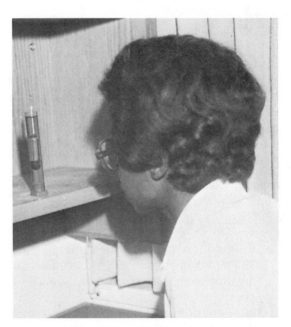

Figure 11–4. A urinometer (urine hydrometer) is viewed at eye level for accurate reading. (Courtesy Lawrence Cherkas, Urinometer courtesy of Francis Freas Glassworks.)

© 1996 by Lippincott-Raven Publishers

extraneous particles do not alter the true concentration of the urine.

b. Pour at least 20 mL urine into a urinometer so *that the base of the bulb floats and does not touch the bottom.*

c. Give the stem a slight spin so that the bulb floats freely and is not in contact with the sides.

d. Elevate the urinometer to eye level, or place it on a firm surface and read it at eye level.

e. Read the lowest point of the meniscus. If the meniscus falls directly between two lines, always read to the next higher number.

10. Dispose of materials and clean equipment.

a. Dispose of any urine not needed for a specimen in the toilet.

b. Place the urine container in an appropriate waste receptacle.

c. Clean the urinometer with soap and water.

d. Dispose of your gloves in a waste receptacle.

11.–13. Follow the steps of the General Procedure.

Evaluation

14.–15. Follow the steps of the General Procedure.

Documentation

16.–17. Follow the steps of the General Procedure.

Procedure Using a Urine Refractometer

Assessment

1. through 3. Follow the steps of the General Procedure for Collecting and Testing Specimens.

Planning

4. Follow the General Procedure.

5. Obtain the urine refractometer, a dropper, a urine container, and clean gloves. When the urine refractometer is used, a beam of light is refracted, or bent, according to the density of the urine and then projected onto a calibrated lens that looks somewhat like a simple microscope. The calibrations are read to give the density (Fig. 11–5).

Implementation

6.–8. Follow the steps of the General Procedure.

9. Put on clean gloves, and measure the specific gravity with a refractometer.

a. Collect a few drops of urine in the container. The refractometer can give an accurate reading from even a drop compressed from a wet diaper.

b. Place one drop on the horizontal glass slide at the top of the refractometer scope.

c. Close the cover over the slide.

d. Switch on the light.

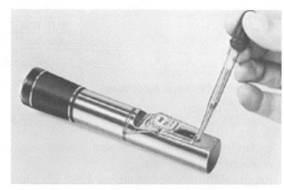

Figure 11–5. A urine refractometer measures specific gravity. (Courtesy AO Scientific Instruments, Buffalo, New York.)

e. With both eyes open, look with one eye through the scope.

f. Read the number at the line where the top black half and the lower white half of the circle meet.

10. Dispose of materials and clean equipment.

a. Dispose of any urine not needed for a specimen in the toilet.

b. Place the urine container in an appropriate waste receptacle.

c. Clean the slide with a dampened towel or gauze.

d. Dispose of your gloves in a waste receptacle.

11.–13. Follow the steps of the General Procedure.

Evaluation

14.–15. Follow the steps of the General Procedure.

Documentation

16.–17. Follow the steps of the General Procedure.

URINE GLUCOSE

Patients with elevated glucose levels in the blood will often have some glucose content in the urine. Testing the urine for glucose, using a variety of methods, has long been a nursing function. Sometimes this is done to compare with the blood glucose level to determine if a urine glucose measurement is an accurate reflection of the blood glucose level. It can also be used in other instances to avoid repeated finger sticks. Teaching these procedures to patients and families has been a part of the nursing role. Although urine tests have disadvantages because of variations in the filtering ability of the kidneys, urine testing may be important to determine the patient's medical status.

© 1996 by Lippincott-Raven Publishers

Supplies and Equipment

Many commercial products that test for glucose in the urine are available. Most people who are not in a healthcare facility will use reagent strips, but tablets and strips may be found within the institution. Most facilities routinely keep at least two products available. Among the most common are Clinistix, Clinitest, Dextrostix, Diastix, and Tes-tape.

Each has advantages and disadvantages. One problem is that certain medications can cause false readings on each product. Compare the literature regarding each product with the list of drugs the patient is taking *so that you can choose an appropriate product for the test* (Table 11–3).

Each product uses a color scale to reflect differences in glucose content. Each color scale is based on the reactions of the chemicals used in that product. Therefore, the color scales are *not* interchangeable.

Traditionally, products that tested for glucose in the urine had a scale that reported results as *negative, trace, one plus* (+ or 1+), *two plus* (++ or 2+), *three plus* (+++ or 3+), and so on. Each of these represented a specific percentage of glucose, from 0% to 5%. As new products have become available, their scales have also been set up with pluses. However, the pluses in one product do not correspond to the same percentage of glucose as the pluses in another product. For example, Clinitest (5-drop method) 2+ equals 0.75% glucose, whereas Testape 2+ equals 0.25% glucose.

Because a course of therapy such as diet and drugs is often based on the level of glucose in the urine, any confusion can be dangerous. Therefore, many facilities recommend that all glucose readings be reported as percentages, *which helps to eliminate one source of error.* Follow the policy in your facility, however. If pluses are used as a basis for prescribing therapy, it is your responsibility to clarify what product is to be used for testing. Be sure to consult further if you find that you must use a product other than the one recommended *because of drug interference with test accuracy.*

Once a product has been chosen, use it consistently for that patient. You will have a more reliable and consistent record if you always use the same product *because there are minor differences in each product.*

Specimen Collection

When collecting a urine specimen to test for glucose, timing is critical. *Urine that has accumulated in the bladder reflects conditions in the body at the time the urine was formed. Thus, the first specimen in the morning contains urine secreted throughout the night. It is impossible to know whether glucose in that specimen was secreted at midnight, 2:00 AM or 6:00 AM. This is true of any urine specimen obtained several hours after the last voiding.*

Therefore, use a second-voided (sometimes called a double-voided) specimen for glucose measurement. If you use this method, *you know you are testing freshly secreted urine.* Have the patient void 30

Table 11–3. Examples of Drug Interference With Urine Testing			
Drug	**Clinitest**	**Testape**	**Acetest**
Aldomet	False-positive		
Ascorbic acid (large doses)	False-positive	False-negative	
Benemid	False-positive		
Cancer metabolites		False-negative	
Cephalosporins (Keflex, Keflin, Loridine)	False-positive		
Chloral hydrate (large dose)	False-positive		
Chloromycetin	False-positive		
INH (isoniazid)	False-positive		
Levodopa (L-dopa)	False-positive	False-negative	False-positive
Paraldehyde			False-positive
Pyridium		False-positive or-negative	
Skelaxin	False-positive		
Sulfonamides	False-positive		
Tetracyclines	False-positive		

© 1996 by Lippincott-Raven Publishers

minutes before you want to test the urine. (This first specimen is saved *in case a further specimen is not obtained.*) Wait 30 minutes, and then ask the patient to void again. Use this second specimen for the test. Most patients have no difficulty voiding the amount required *because only 1 or 2 mL urine is needed for the test.*

If the patient cannot void again, test the first urine specimen. A negative reading can be recorded, *if no glucose was secreted at any time since the last voiding.* If, however, any glucose at all is present, you must test a second specimen for an accurate reading. In this case, you must wait until the patient is able to void.

Procedure for Measuring Urine Glucose

Assessment
1.–3. Follow the steps of the General Procedure for Collecting and Testing Specimens.

Planning
4. Follow the General Procedure.

5. Obtain correct product for measuring urine glucose, two specimen containers, and clean gloves.

Implementation
6.–8. Follow the steps of the General Procedure.

9. Put on clean gloves, and measure urine glucose.

a. Ask the patient to void and collect a specimen. Save this specimen in case the patient is unable to urinate again. Explain to the patient that he or she will be asked to urinate again in 30 minutes.

b. Return to the patient in 30 minutes and collect 1 to 2 mL urine in a second container. This is a second-voided specimen.

c. Review the directions on the product, and place the correct color scale where it is clearly visible.

d. Proceed with step (1) or (2), depending on the type of product you are using.

(1) *Clinitest:* One of the first simple tests for urine glucose was the Clinitest. It has three distinct advantages: It is easy to use; it is relatively precise (except for drug interference); and it tests for all reducing sugars, not glucose only. There are, however, several disadvantages. First, the tablets are poisonous, which could be a concern if the patient must carry out the test at home with small children present. Second, the tablets are caustic when moist and can burn fingers. Third, the tablets deteriorate when ex-

posed to moisture. Fourth, the method requires the use of test tubes and droppers and is slower than other methods. Finally, some drugs can cause false readings with the product.

There are two methods of using Clinitest. The 5-drop method is the most common; the 2-drop method is used to detect more exact percentages when high levels of glucose are found in the urine. Each has its own color scale.

(a) *5-drop method:*

(i) Obtain a clean glass test tube, a test tube holder, a dropper, and tablets.

(ii) Place the test tube in the holder. If necessary, you can hold the test tube carefully at the top edge. *Remember that the part of the test tube in contact with the solution will become hot enough to be uncomfortable to the touch.*

(iii) Using the dropper, place 5 drops of urine in the test tube. (Save the remainder of the specimen *in case you must repeat the test.*)

(iv) Rinse the dropper.

(v) Using the same dropper, add 10 drops of water to the test tube.

(vi) Using the container top, place one Clinitest tablet in the test tube.

(vii) Watch the tube carefully. *Pass-through* occurs if the color bubbles through orange and turns dark. Pass-through indicates a high percentage of glucose in the urine, so the 5-drop method will not be accurate. You should report this and usually do a 2-drop test. If the color does not turn dark, begin timing for 15 seconds when the bubbling stops.

(viii) After 15 seconds, shake the tube gently, and compare the color of the solution with the color chart.

(b) *2-drop method:* Follow the 5-drop directions, but use 2 drops of urine and 10 drops of water. Be sure to use the appropriate color chart for the method.

© 1996 by Lippincott-Raven Publishers

(2) *Reagent strip tests (Clinistix, Diastix, Testape):* These tests use a clinical reagent impregnated in paper strips. *The reagent strip tests are less often affected by drugs than Clinitest and therefore are commonly recommended.* The method of use for each is the same, although the timing and color charts are specific to the individual product.

  (a) Remove a reagent strip from the container. Do not touch the area of the strip where the reagent is present *because doing so may alter the reaction.*

  (b) Dip the strip into the urine, tapping it on the container *to remove excess urine.* For an incontinent patient or an infant, press the reagent strip onto the wet linen or wet diaper.

  (c) Begin timing according to directions.

  (d) At the end of the specified period, compare the color on the strip with the correct color chart.

10. Dispose of materials and clean equipment.

  a. Dispose of any unneeded urine in the toilet.

  b. Place the urine container and strip in an appropriate waste receptacle.

  c. Dispose of your gloves in a waste receptacle.

11.–13. Follow the steps of the General Procedure.

Evaluation

14.–15. Follow the steps of the General Procedure.

Documentation

16. Record the urine glucose results on the patient's chart. A flow sheet is usually used to keep a tabular account of urine glucose as either a percentage or pluses based on the policy of your facility.

17. Report any abnormally low or high glucose content.

KETONE BODIES IN URINE

Sometimes this test is called a test for *acetone.* Acetone is one of several ketones (ketone bodies) that can be produced in the body. Ketone bodies are a product of incomplete fat metabolism. They are present in urine only *when fat is being broken down rapidly and incompletely.* This can occur with rigid dieting or with uncontrolled diabetes. Most commonly, tests for ketone bodies are done with diabetic patients *to identify lack of control of the disease.* Test the urine for ketones at the same time that you test it for glucose.

Equipment

Tablets and reagent strips are available to test for ketones. The reagent strips are quicker and require less equipment. Most diabetic people testing the urine for ketones at home use reagent strips.

Procedure for Measuring Urine Ketones

Assessment

1.–3. Follow the steps of the General Procedure for Collecting and Testing Specimens.

Planning

4. Follow the General Procedure

5. Obtain the correct product (check for the expiration date), a urine specimen container, and clean gloves.

Implementation

6.–8. Follow the steps of the General Procedure.

9. Put on clean gloves and measure urine ketones.

  a. Place the color chart where it is clearly visible.

  b. Collect a fresh urine specimen. *If ketones are present in the urine, they will increase as the urine stands at room temperature. Therefore, old urine will give an incorrect result.*

  c. Proceed with step (1) or (2), depending on the product you are using.

    (1) *Acetest tablets:*

      (a) Place one tablet on a piece of filter paper or a paper towel.

      (b) Using a dropper, place 1 drop of urine on the tablet.

      (c) Begin timing for 15 seconds.

      (d) Compare the color of the tablet with the color chart.

    (2) *Reagent strips (Diastix, Ketostix, Uristix):*

      (a) Remove the strip from the bottle, being careful not to touch the area that is impregnated with the reagent *because doing so may alter the reaction.*

      (b) Dip the strip into the urine.

      (c) Tap the strip on the edge of the container *to remove excess urine.*

      (d) Begin timing for 60 seconds.

      (e) Compare the strip with the appropriate color chart.

10. Dispose of materials and clean equipment.

  a. Dispose of any unneeded urine in the toilet.

  b. Place the urine container and strip in an appropriate waste receptacle.

  c. Dispose of your gloves in a waste receptacle.

11.–13. Follow the steps of the General Procedure.

© 1996 by Lippincott-Raven Publishers

DATE/TIME	
9/10/99	
6:30 AM	Urine specimen: Neg/Neg. ————— J. Smith, RN

Example of Nursing Progress Notes Using Narrative Format.

Evaluation

14.–15. Follow the steps of the General Procedure.

Documentation

16. Document the information in the patient's record. Commonly, glucose and ketones are recorded together. The glucose result is given first, then the ketone result, for example, Neg/Neg, 2+/Pos, 1+/Neg. This may be entered on a flow sheet or recorded on the narrative.

17. Report any presence of ketones because this is considered abnormal.

TESTING URINE FOR OCCULT BLOOD

Normal urine is free of blood. Blood in the urine is called "hematuria" and can result from disease, trauma, or the menstrual flow. Blood can also be present in urine without being visible; for instance, the urine might have only a cloudy or hazy appearance. This is called *occult*, or hidden, blood. Urine can be tested for occult blood at the discretion of the nurse, or the physician may order this test to be done.

Hemastix reagent strips are used to test for occult blood. Collect a urine specimen, and follow the procedure for using urine glucose reagent strips. Read the product directions for timing and using the color chart.

MULTIPURPOSE STRIP TESTS FOR URINE

Although they are not widely used either in the healthcare facility or by people at home, combination or multipurpose reagent strips that test for several substances at the same time are available. These strips have a small area of reagent for each test being done. Common tests done using multipurpose strips are urine pH, urine ketone bodies, and occult blood.

Although multiple strips are convenient, they do create opportunities for error:

1. Confusion as to which area on the strip contains the reagent for which substance

2. Incorrect timing of the different areas

3. Comparison of the color of the area on the strip with the wrong color chart

When you use multipurpose reagent strips, be especially careful about these three points. Collect a urine specimen, and follow the steps bellow of the procedure for measuring pH when using multipurpose strips. Read the product directions for timing and color chart for each test.

Procedure for Measuring pH of Urine

To measure the pH of urine, use a multipurpose strip or a strip designed for measuring pH only, following the policy of your facility.

Assessment

1.–3. Follow the steps of the General Procedure for Collecting and Testing Specimens.

Planning

4. Follow the General Procedure.

5. Obtain the appropriate strip, container, and clean gloves.

Implementation

6.–8. Follow the steps of the General Procedure.

9. Put on clean gloves, and test for urine pH.
  a. Obtain a small amount of urine. *Only enough urine to moisten the reagent section of the strip is needed.*
  b. Dip strip into the urine. *The reagent strip must be thoroughly moistened to activate the chemical reaction.*
  c. Tap paper on container to remove excess urine *to prevent contaminating surfaces with urine.*
  d. Read strip, comparing it with the color chart on the container. *The color chart is specifically designed for the type of reagent used.*

10. Dispose of equipment and gloves in a waste container *to protect other staff from contaminated materials.*

11.–13. Follow the steps of the General Procedure.

Evaluation

14.–15. Follow the steps of the General Procedure.

© 1996 by Lippincott-Raven Publishers

Documentation

16.–17. Follow the steps of the General Procedure.

BLOOD GLUCOSE

The measurement of blood glucose is performed routinely on the nursing unit, particularly for insulin-dependent diabetics. If measurement of blood glucose is urgent or critical, the test may also be done as a laboratory procedure. Blood glucose tests are routinely done for diabetic patients and others for whom an accurate knowledge of glucose levels is important. Blood tests for glucose are much more reliable than urine tests. This test can be done by visually examining the color of a reagent strip, but in most instances, an electronic reflectance meter is used to identify more precisely the blood glucose level. Both methods for testing are described below. In addition to performing this procedure, you may also be teaching it to patients or their families *so that they can do it at home.*

Several meters have been developed to test blood glucose. Three commonly used brands are the Glucometer, the Glucoscan II, and the AccuChek bG. Blood glucose meters are now available with a computer memory that can store numerous test results (Kestel, 1994). These devices can be purchased for use in the home. Most patients in healthcare facilities and at home who are insulin dependent now use electronic glucose metering devices, although visually read reagent strips remain available for those who wish to use them. The meters determine glucose content by reading the color on the reagent strip prepared as described below. *Because the procedure for operating each meter varies in important ways,*check the manufacturer's directions carefully before proceeding.

Procedure for Measuring Blood Glucose

Assessment

1.–3. Follow the steps of the General Procedure for Collecting and Testing Specimens.

Planning

4. Follow the General Procedure.

5. Obtain a reagent strip for blood glucose (Chemstrip is a commonly used brand), and check the expiration date. Obtain tissues, clean gloves, and a sterile finger lancet. A sterile, disposable lancet is used each time the test is performed.

　　Most facilities use a special spring-loaded puncture device into which you fasten the lancet. One puncture device may be used for many patients, but each patient should have a separate

end platform that touches the patient's skin and a sterile lancet. This device provides a standardized force and depth of puncture. *Because each brand operates somewhat differently,* read the directions. You may want to practice loading and releasing the device before going to the bedside if it is new to you.

You will also need a glucose meter or a watch with a second hand (if using visual examination). Each brand of glucose meter is standardized and checked for accuracy using special techniques. Although students do not assume responsibility for this, you should know the policies regarding this procedure in the facility where you practice.

Implementation

6.–8. Follow the steps of the General Procedure.

9. Measure the blood glucose.

　　a. Have the patient wash hands with soap and warm water and dry the hands. *This cleans the skin and increases blood flow.* Soap and water are the preferred cleaning agents *because constant use of alcohol as a cleaning agent dries and toughens the skin.* Although it may be common practice to use an alcohol wipe to clean the finger, this is not a wise practice. If alcohol is used, it must be allowed to dry so that it does not compromise the test results.

　　b. Select location to pierce. Avoid the index finger, *because that causes the patient the most pain.* Slightly to the side of the pad on the tip of the finger is usually best. In succeeding punctures, rotate sites *to decrease chances of soreness.* Turn on the meter if one is being used.

　　c. Put on gloves. Hold the patient's hand in a dependent position and massage the base of the chosen finger *to increase blood flow.*

　　d. If you are using a puncture device, load the lancet. Remove the cover from the point of the lancet and set the spring. Place the device firmly against the side of the distal portion of the finger. *This location prevents soreness on the sensitive tip of the finger.* Release the spring to pierce the finger.

　　　With care, it is possible to do a simple finger stick without the device. Use the site described previously.

　　e. Allow a large drop of blood to form at the site. You may "milk" the base of the finger, but do not put pressure on the site *because doing so may alter the test results.*

　　f. Drop the blood onto the reagent portion of the strip, covering it completely with the rounded drop, and use a tissue to put pressure on the site.

© 1996 by Lippincott-Raven Publishers

g. If you are using *visual examination*, time the exact period specified by the reagent strip manufacturer with a watch. If you are using a *meter*, follow the directions for timing using the meter.

h. When the designated time has passed (indicated by an audible beep from the meter), wipe or blot the strip as directed.

i. If you are using *visual examination*, compare the color on the strip with the color chart on the package label to determine the blood glucose level, which is identified in mg/dL. If the strip is darker than any color on the first scale, wait for an additional 60 seconds, and compare it with the second color scale on the label.

If you are using a *meter*, place the strip in the meter as designated until the meter signals that it has read the strip. Read the blood glucose level from the meter.

10. Dispose of materials, and clean equipment.

a. Dispose of the strip and finger stick lancet in a "sharps" container.

b. Discard gloves in a waste receptacle.

c. If a meter was used, turn it off, and put it away.

d. If a spring-loaded lancet holder was used, clean all parts, and return them to their appropriate storage place.

11.–13. Follow the steps of the General Procedure.

Evaluation

14.–15. Follow the steps of the General Procedure.

Documentation

16. Results of blood glucose monitoring are usually recorded on a flow sheet. This flow sheet may contain other information, such as insulin administered, urine testing results, patient responses, and further nursing action taken.

17. Report any abnormal findings.

BLOOD IN FECES

Typically, blood is not as visible in feces as it is in other body tissues and fluids. Blood in feces is commonly occult blood. The undigested portions of oral iron preparations give the stool a black appearance that can be mistaken for blood or can mask the presence of occult blood. *Also, patients who have eaten rare red meat in the 3 days before the test may test positive for occult blood,* which is why some physicians restrict patients from eating red meat for 3 days before this test. Feces can be tested for blood at the discretion of the nurse if the materials are available on the unit.

If the stool must be sent to a laboratory for testing or the materials must be ordered and charged to the patient, a physician's order may be needed. After the patient has had a bowel movement, complete the testing as outlined below.

Procedure for Testing Feces for Occult Blood

Assessment

1.–3. Follow the steps of the General Procedure for Collecting and Testing Specimens.

Planning

4. Follow the General Procedure.

5. Obtain a tongue blade, a container for stool, a Hematest folder, a dropper bottle of Hematest reagent fluid or a Hematest tablet (or other brand of testing material), filter paper, dropper, and clean gloves. The supplies may be kept in a patient's bathroom *if there is frequent need for them.*

Implementation

6.–8. Follow the steps of the General Procedure.

9. Put on clean gloves, and test the stool.

a. Use a tongue blade to place a small amount of stool in a container.

b. Proceed with step (1), (2), or (3), depending on the product you are using.

(1) *Hematest tablet:*

(a) Smear a thin layer of fecal material on the filter paper provided. This can be done with a tongue depressor.

(b) Place a Hematest tablet in the center of the specimen.

(c) Place 1 drop of water on the tablet.

(d) Wait 10 seconds for the water to penetrate the tablet.

(e) Add a second drop of water to saturate the tablet and specimen thoroughly; the water should run down the side of the tablet.

(f) Wait an additional 20 seconds.

(g) Observe the paper for the presence of blue, which indicates occult blood (a positive test).

(2) *Hemoccult slide:* The Hemoccult slide is a small cardboard folder or envelope. It was originally designed for the visiting nurse or patient at home to mail in a specimen for testing. (The folder would be enclosed in a mailing envelope.) Because of its convenience, the Hemoccult slide is now widely used in healthcare facilities. The folder, with specimen enclosed (steps (a) and (b) below), can be

© 1996 by Lippincott-Raven Publishers

DATE/TIME	
2/9/99	D: Pt. experiencing abdominal cramping, Had three moderate-sized, loose, foul-smelling stools between 7:00 and 7:30 AM. Hemoccult test showed negative on all stools, P-88, BP-118/68, R-24.
	A: prn Lomotil given (see MAR).
	R: No stools since medication given.
	M. Roberts, RN

Example of Nursing Progress Notes Using Focus Format.

sent to the laboratory for the actual test. The procedure below is for processing on the unit.

(a) Open the folder flap.

(b) With an applicator, apply a thin smear of fecal material over the inside circle.

(c) Drop the reagent solution onto the fecal smear.

(d) Observe the paper for the appearance of blue, which indicates occult blood (a positive test).

(3) *Guaiac testing:* Guaiac is a gum resin that was once widely used for testing for occult blood in feces. Newer agents are now used, but the term has remained. Often a physician will write an order to "guaiac all stools." Rather than directing you to use the specific reagent guaiac, the physician is asking that the specimen be tested for occult blood. A few laboratories and facilities still use a guaiac solution, but most have changed to the more convenient strip or tablet method. If the guaiac test is used, the solutions must be refrigerated *because they deteriorate rapidly at room temperature.*

(a) Streak feces on filter paper or a paper towel.

(b) Drop reagents onto the smear, following the order in the directions.

(c) Observe for blue, which represents occult blood (a positive test).

10. Dispose of materials, and put test supplies away.

a. Dispose of slide or filter paper and your gloves in a waste receptacle.

b. Replace reagent containers in an appropriate place.

11.–13. Follow the steps of the General Procedure.

Evaluation

14.–15. Follow the steps of the General Procedure.

Documentation

16. Document the information in the patient's record. This is usually done on a flow sheet but may be placed in the narrative record if no flow sheet exists. It is simply recorded as negative (−) or positive (+).

17. Report any abnormal results.

CULTURES

Cultures can be obtained from almost any body surface or orifice using a wet or dry method. Usually, cultures are of fluids (secretions, exudates). All cultures should be sent to the laboratory promptly *so that the character of the specimen does not change with time and give a false reading.*

Obtaining Cultures

Wet cultures are often done using a Culturette. This is a plastic sealed tube that contains a transport medium (fluid) that is enclosed in an ampule in the bottom of the tube. A cotton swab is inside the tube and attached to the lid. Swab the area to be cultured by holding the lid. Place the swab and lid back on the tube, then break the ampule by crushing the tube between your fingers. *This releases the transport medium, which saturates the swab.* The purpose of the transport medium is *to prevent drying and to maintain the bacterial concentration.*

When a dry culture is ordered, use a sterile test tube and swab. Send the labeled culture to the laboratory immediately in a leak-proof plastic bag.

Procedure for Obtaining a Culture

Assessment

1.–3. Follow the steps of the General Procedure for Collecting and Testing Specimens.

© 1996 by Lippincott-Raven Publishers

Planning
4. Follow the General Procedure.

5. Obtain the appropriate culture tube and a pair of clean gloves.

   a. For a wet culture, use a commercially produced culture tube in which a swab attached to the tube lid can be immersed in the culture medium.

   b. For a dry culture, use a sterile cotton swab and a sterile dry test tube.

Implementation
6.–8. Follow the steps of the General Procedure.

9. Put on gloves, and perform either a wet or dry culture.

   a. *Wet cultures*:

     (1) Remove the tube from its package.

     (2) Remove the swab stick from the tube. *To prevent contamination with microorganisms,* do not touch the end of the swab against your fingers or any objects.

     (3) Collect the specimen to be cultured on the cotton end of the swab. Saturate the cotton.

     (4) Insert the swab in the tube (Fig. 11–6), and recap.

     (5) With the cap end down, crush the ampule at midpoint, releasing the transport medium.

     (6) Push the cap so that the swab moves down, making contact with the medium.

     (7) Note on the package in the places designated the patient's name, hospital number, and physician; date; time; and any antibiotics the patient is taking. *Some drugs affect the results.* Insert the culture tube, and discard gloves.

     (8) Send the culture to the laboratory immediately in a plastic bag. *Any bacterial content can change in number or character if left standing.*

   b. *Dry cultures*:

     (1) Using a sterile cotton swab stick, culture the area as described previously.

     (2) Place swab in test tube; recap, label, place in a plastic bag, and send to laboratory.

10.–13. Follow the steps of the General Procedure.

Evaluation
14. The culture must be evaluated after the microorganisms have had an opportunity to grow in the laboratory, usually 48 hours or more. Compare results of the culture with information on normal flora of the area being cultured and with information on sensitivity with the drugs being given. If previous cultures have been completed, compare results.

15. Evaluate the patient's response.

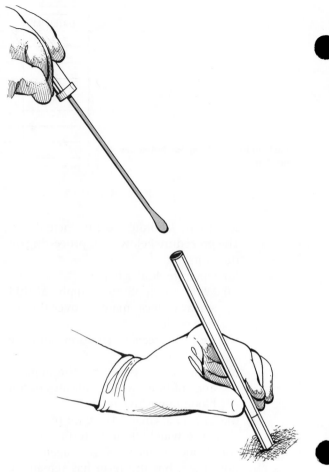

Figure 11–6. Placing the culture swab into the culture tube.

Documentation
16. Record that culture was completed and sent to the laboratory.

17. If a positive culture for pathogenic organisms is reported, notify the physician.

Urine Cultures

A clean catch specimen is usually sufficient for testing purposes. Use a sterile container, and wear clean gloves. *Because there is always a possibility of infection when a patient is catheterized,* the physician will usually not order a catheterized specimen for culture. *A clean-catch specimen and one obtained by catheterization are normally sterile so that either can be used when testing for bacterial content.*

© 1996 by Lippincott-Raven Publishers

LONG-TERM CARE

Long-term care facilities do not have laboratories. Therefore, when specimens must be sent to a laboratory, the nurse must usually make arrangements for transporting the specimen from the facility to the laboratory. This may require extra planning because of the time it will take to transport the specimen. Laboratories that are experienced in meeting the needs of long-term care facilities usually have specific directions to ensure that the specimen is useful when it arrives at the laboratory.

Nurses typically draw all blood samples in long-term care. If the nurses do not, the patient may be sent to a physician's office or clinic where there are laboratory facilities to have blood drawn.

HOME CARE

Some of these tests will be done by clients at home to monitor their own therapy and progress. The skill may be taught in a hospital or in a clinic situation. The client is asked to return the demonstration for evaluation. It is often useful to have clients redemonstrate such a skill on a subsequent outpatient or clinic visit to verify that their technique is correct. The home health nurse may be responsible for monitoring laboratory results, teaching clients, and evaluating their ability to perform tests independently.

CRITICAL THINKING EXERCISES

• You have noted that a patient being treated with large doses of prednisone (an adrenocorticosteroid) is complaining of gastric distress. This morning, the patient's stool is dark and odorous. Synthesize information about this drug, the characteristics of normal stool, and the assessment data you have gathered to identify a potential problem for this patient. Determine what further nursing assessment you should perform, and explain why.

• A resident with diabetes mellitus has been admitted to your unit in a long-term care facility. The medical orders include insulin daily, plus regular insulin coverage as needed. Identify which common laboratory tests you expect to perform for this resident, and explain why.

References

Kestel, F. (1994). Are you up-to-date on diabetes medications? *American Journal of Nursing*, 94(7), 48–52.

McConnell, E. A. (1991). How to use a urinometer. *Nursing '91*, 21(10), 28.

Melillo, K. D. (1993). Interpretation of laboratory values in older adults. *Nurse Practitioner, 18*(7), 59–67.

© 1996 by Lippincott-Raven Publishers

✔ PERFORMANCE CHECKLIST

General Procedure for Collecting and Testing Specimens	Needs More Practice	Satisfactory	Comments
Assessment			
1. Determine which tests are to be performed and type of specimen required.			
2. Review procedure and equipment needed, checking the following: a. Need for patient's written consent			
b. Testing and monitoring equipment needed			
c. Type of specimen container required			
d. Specific procedure			
3. Assess patient, focusing on the following: a. Ability to cooperate or undergo procedure			
b. Special needs			
c. Knowledge base			
Planning			
4. Wash your hands.			
5. Obtain equipment and clean gloves.			
Implementation			
6. Identify patient.			
7. Explain procedure to patient.			
8. Prepare the environment.			
9. Put on gloves, then collect the specimen or perform the specific test.			
10. Dispose of gloves and unneeded specimen; care for equipment.			
11. Make patient comfortable.			
12. Wash your hands.			
13. Record test results immediately on paper, or send specimen to laboratory.			
Evaluation			
14. Compare test results with normal values and patient's previous results; identify abnormalities.			
15. Evaluate patient response.			

(*continued*)

© 1996 by Lippincott-Raven Publishers

General Procedure for Collecting and Testing Specimens *(Continued)*	Needs More Practice	Satisfactory	Comments
Documentation			
16. Document data.			
17. Report abnormalities.			
Specific Gravity of Urine, Using Urinometer			
Assessment			
1.–3. Follow checklist steps 1–3 of the General Procedure for Collecting and Testing Specimens (determine test to be performed; review procedure and equipment; assess patient).			
Planning			
4. Wash your hands.			
5. Obtain urinometer, urine container, and clean gloves.			
Implementation			
6.–8. Follow checklist steps 6–8 of the General Procedure (identify patient; explain procedure; and prepare environment).			
9. Put on clean gloves, and measure the specific gravity with a urinometer. **a.** Collect at least 20 mL of urine.			
b. Pour urine into urinometer.			
c. Give stem slight spin so bulb floats freely.			
d. Elevate urinometer to eye level.			
e. Read number at lowest point of meniscus.			
10.–13. Follow checklist steps 10–13 of the General Procedure (dispose of gloves and unneeded specimen; care for equipment; make patient comfortable; wash your hands; record results immediately or send specimen to laboratory).			
Evaluation			
14.–15. Follow checklist steps 14 and 15 of the General Procedure (compare results with normal values and patient's previous results; identify abnormalities; and evaluate patient's response).			

(continued)

© 1996 by Lippincott-Raven Publishers

Specific Gravity of Urine, Using Urinometer *(Continued)*	Needs More Practice	Satisfactory	Comments
Documentation			
16.–17. Follow checklist steps 16 and 17 of the General Procedure (document data, and report abnormalities).			
Specific Gravity of Urine, Using Urine Refractometer			
Assessment			
1.–3. Follow checklist steps 1–3 of the General Procedure for Collecting and Testing Specimens (determine test to be performed; review procedure and equipment; assess patient).			
Planning			
4. Wash your hands.			
5. Obtain refractometer, dropper, container, and clean gloves.			
Implementation			
6.–8. Follow checklist steps 6–8 of the General Procedure (identify patient; explain procedure; and prepare environment).			
9. Put on clean gloves, and measure the specific gravity with a refractometer. **a.** Collect few drops of urine.			
b. Place one drop on slide at top of refractometer.			
c. Close cover over slide.			
d. Switch on light.			
e. With both eyes open, look through scope.			
f. Read number where halves of screen meet.			
10.–13. Follow checklist steps 10–13 of the General Procedure (dispose of gloves and unneeded specimen; care for equipment; make patient comfortable; wash your hands; record results immediately or send specimen to laboratory).			

(continued)

© 1996 by Lippincott-Raven Publishers

Specific Gravity of Urine, Using Urine Refractometer *(Continued)*	Needs More Practice	Satisfactory	Comments
Evaluation			
14.–15. Follow checklist steps 14 and 15 of the General Procedure (compare results with normal values and patient's previous results; identify abnormalities; and evaluate patient's response).			
Documentation			
16.–17. Follow checklist steps 16 and 17 of the General Procedure (document data, and report abnormalities).			
Urine Glucose			
Assessment			
1.–3. Follow checklist steps 1–3 of the General Procedure for Collecting and Testing Specimens (determine test to be performed; review procedure and equipment; assess patient).			
Planning			
4. Wash your hands.			
5. Obtain correct product, two containers, and clean gloves.			
Implementation			
6.–8. Follow checklist steps 6–8 of the General Procedure (identify patient; explain procedure; and prepare environment).			
9. Put on clean gloves and measure urine glucose. **a.** Ask patient to void; collect specimen and save.			
b. In 30 minutes, collect second specimen if possible.			
c. Review product directions, and place color chart where visible.			
d. Proceed with step (1) or (2) as described below, depending on the product used. (1) Clinitest: (a) Obtain test tube, holder, dropper, and tablets.			

(continued)

© 1996 by Lippincott-Raven Publishers

Urine Glucose (Continued)	Needs More Practice	Satisfactory	Comments
(b) Place test tube in holder.			
(c) For 5-drop method, place 5 drops of urine in test tube; for 2-drop method, use only 2 drops.			
(d) Rinse dropper.			
(e) Use dropper to place 10 drops of water in tube.			
(f) Using container top, place one Clinitest tablet in tube.			
(g) Watch reaction carefully for pass-through.			
(h) After 15 seconds, shake tube gently, and compare to the color chart.			
(2) Reagent strip tests (Clinistix, Diastix, Testape): (a) Remove reagent strip from container.			
(b) Dip strip into urine and tap on side of container to remove excess.			
(c) Begin timing according to directions.			
(d) At end of period, compare with correct color chart.			
10.–13. Follow checklist steps 10–13 of the General Procedure (dispose of gloves and unneeded specimen; care for equipment; make patient comfortable; wash your hands; record results immediately or send specimen to laboratory).			
Evaluation			
14.–15. Follow checklist steps 14 and 15 of the General Procedure (compare results with normal values and patient's previous results; identify abnormalities; and evaluate patient's response).			
Documentation			
16.–17. Follow checklist steps 16 and 17 of the General Procedure (document data, and report abnormalities).			

(continued)

© 1996 by Lippincott-Raven Publishers

Ketone Bodies in Urine	Needs More Practice	Satisfactory	Comments
Assessment			
1.–3. Follow checklist steps 1–3 of the General Procedure for Collecting and Testing Specimens (determine test to be performed; review procedure and equipment; assess patient).			
Planning			
4. Wash your hands.			
5. Obtain the correct product, specimen container, and clean gloves.			
Implementation			
6.–8. Follow checklist steps 6–8 of the General Procedure (identify patient; explain procedure; and prepare environment).			
9. Put on clean gloves, and measure urine ketones. **a.** Place color chart where it is visible.			
b. Collect urine specimen.			
c. Proceed with step (1) and (2) as described below, depending on product used. (1) Acetest tablets (a) Place one tablet on filter paper or paper towel.			
(b) Place 1 drop of urine on tablet.			
(c) Begin timing.			
(d) Time for 15 seconds.			
(e) Compare color with chart.			
(2) Reagent strips (a) Remove one strip from bottle.			
(b) Dip strip into urine.			
(c) Tap strip on edge of container.			
(d) Begin timing.			
(e) Time for 60 seconds.			
(f) Compare color with chart.			

(continued)

© 1996 by Lippincott-Raven Publishers

Ketone Bodies in Urine *(Continued)*	Needs More Practice	Satisfactory	Comments
10.–13. Follow checklist steps 10–13 of the General Procedure (dispose of gloves and unneeded specimen; care for equipment; make patient comfortable; wash your hands; record results immediately or send specimen to laboratory).			
Evaluation			
14.–15. Follow checklist steps 14 and 15 of the General Procedure (compare results with normal values and patient's previous results; identify abnormalities; and evaluate patient's response).			
Documentation			
16.–17. Follow checklist steps 16 and 17 of the General Procedure (document data, and report abnormalities).			
pH of Urine			
Assessment			
1.–3. Follow checklist steps 1–3 of the General Procedure for Collecting and Testing Specimens (determine test to be performed; review procedure and equipment; assess patient).			
Planning			
4. Wash your hands.			
5. Obtain the multipurpose strip, container, and clean gloves.			
Implementation			
6.–8. Follow checklist steps 6–8 of the General Procedure (identify patient; explain procedure; and prepare environment).			
9. Put on clean gloves, and test for urine pH. **a.** Obtain a small amount of urine.			
b. Dip strip into the urine.			
c. Tap paper on container to remove excess urine.			
d. Read strip, comparing it with color chart.			

(continued)

© 1996 by Lippincott-Raven Publishers

pH of Urine *(Continued)*	Needs More Practice	Satisfactory	Comments
10.–13. Follow checklist steps 10–13 of the General Procedure (dispose of gloves and unneeded specimen, care for equipment, make patient comfortable, wash your hands, record results immediately or send specimen to lab).			
Evaluation			
14.–15. Follow checklist steps 14 and 15 of the General Procedure (compare results with normal values and patient's previous results; identify abnormalities; and evaluate patient's response).			
Documentation			
16.–17. Follow checklist steps 16 and 17 of the General Procedure (document data, and report abnormalities).			
Blood Glucose			
Assessment			
1.–3. Follow checklist steps 1–3 of the General Procedure for Collecting and Testing Specimens (determine test to be performed; review procedure and equipment; assess patient).			
Planning			
4. Wash your hands.			
5. Obtain reagent strip, tissues, clean gloves, lancet, and a glucose meter or a watch with a second hand.			
Implementation			
6.–8. Follow checklist steps 6–8 of the General Procedure (identify patient; explain procedure; and prepare environment).			
9. Measure the blood glucose. **a.** Have patient wash hands.			
b. Select location to pierce.			
c. Put on clean gloves; place patient's hand in dependent position.			
d. Remove lancet cover, and pierce distal portion of finger.			

(continued)

© 1996 by Lippincott-Raven Publishers

Blood Glucose *(Continued)*	Needs More Practice	Satisfactory	Comments
e. Allow a drop of blood to form at site.			
f. Place blood on reagent portion of strip.			
g. If using visual examination, measure time recommended with a watch; if using a meter, follow directions on device for timing.			
h. After designated time, blot strip with tissues.			
i. If using visual examination, compare strip color with chart on package; if using a meter, place strip in meter, and read at time of signal.			
10.–13. Follow checklist steps 10–13 of the General Procedure (dispose of gloves and unneeded specimen; dispose of strip and lancet in "sharps" container; care for equipment; make patient comfortable; wash your hands; record results immediately or send specimen to laboratory).			
Evaluation			
14.–15. Follow checklist steps 14 and 15 of the General Procedure (compare results with normal values and patient's previous results; identify abnormalities; evaluate patient's response).			
Documentation			
16.–17. Follow checklist steps 16 and 17 of the General Procedure (document data, and report abnormalities).			
Blood in Feces			
Assessment			
1.–3. Follow checklist steps 1–3 of the General Procedure for Collecting and Testing Specimens (determine test to be performed; review procedure and equipment; assess patient).			
Planning			
4. Wash your hands.			
5. Obtain a tongue blade, container, Hematest folder or reagent fluid, filter paper, dropper, and clean gloves.			

(continued)

© 1996 by Lippincott-Raven Publishers

Blood in Feces *(Continued)*	Needs More Practice	Satisfactory	Comments
Implementation			
6.–8. Follow checklist steps 6–8 of the General Procedure (identify patient; explain procedure; prepare environment).			
9. Put on clean gloves, and test the stool. **a.** Place small amount of feces in the container.			
b. Proceed with step (1), (2), and (3) as described below, depending on product used. (1) Hematest tablet: (a) Using the tongue blade, lightly smear feces on paper.			
(b) Place Hematest tablet in center of specimen.			
(c) Place one drop of water on tablet.			
(d) Wait 10 seconds.			
(e) Add second drop of water.			
(f) Wait additional 20 seconds.			
(g) Observe specimen for color.			
(2) Hemoccult slide: (a) Open folder flap.			
(b) With applicator, apply feces to circle.			
(c) Drop reagent solution onto smear.			
(d) Observe specimen for color.			
(3) Guaiac: (a) Streak feces on filter paper or paper towel.			
(b) Apply reagents according to directions.			
(c) Observe specimen for color.			
10.–13. Follow checklist steps 10–13 of the General Procedure (dispose of gloves and unneeded specimen; care for equipment; make patient comfortable; wash your hands; record results immediately or send specimen to laboratory).			

(continued)

© 1996 by Lippincott-Raven Publishers

Blood in Feces *(Continued)*	Needs More Practice	Satisfactory	Comments
Evaluation			
14.–15. Follow checklist steps 14 and 15 of the General Procedure (compare results with normal values and patient's previous results; identify abnormalities; evaluate patient's response).			
Documentation			
16.–17. Follow checklist steps 16 and 17 of the General Procedure (document data, and report abnormalities).			
Procedure for Obtaining a Culture			
Assessment			
1.–3. Follow checklist steps 1–3 of the General Procedure for Collecting and Testing Specimens (determine test to be performed; review procedure and equipment; assess patient).			
Planning			
4. Wash your hands.			
5. Obtain the appropriate equipment for a wet or dry culture and clean gloves.			
Implementation			
6.–8. Follow checklist steps 6–8 of the General Procedure (identify patient; explain procedure; prepare environment).			
9. Put on gloves, and perform a wet or dry culture according to the following steps: **a.** Wet culture (1) Remove tube from package.			
(2) Remove the swab stick from the tube.			
(3) Obtain culture, saturating the cotton end of the stick.			
(4) Insert the swab stick into the tube.			
(5) With cap end down, release medium by crushing tube.			
(6) Push cap so swab is in contact with medium.			

(continued)

© 1996 by Lippincott-Raven Publishers

Procedure for Obtaining a Culture *(Continued)*	Needs More Practice	Satisfactory	Comments
(7) Label accurately.			
(8) Send culture to laboratory.			
b. Dry culture (1) Using a sterile cotton swab, culture as described previously.			
(2) Place swab in tube, cap, label, place container in plastic bag, and send to laboratory.			
10.–13. Follow checklist steps 10–13 of the General Procedure (dispose of gloves and unneeded specimen; care for equipment; make patient comfortable; wash your hands; record results immediately or send specimen to laboratory).			
Evaluation			
14. After results are available, compare culture and sensitivity with norms for area and medications being given; compare results with previous cultures, if any.			
15. Evaluate patient's response.			
Documentation			
16. Record that culture was completed and sent to the laboratory.			
17. If a positive culture for pathogenic organisms is reported, notify the physician.			

© 1996 by Lippincott-Raven Publishers

❓ Q U I Z

Short-Answer Questions

1. What is the nurse's responsibility when an abnormal laboratory test is identified?

   Report it to the physician, record the result
   ✓normal values, compare previous results, identify abnormal.

2. Where would you find information on how to perform a laboratory test in the hospital where you have clinical practice?

   _____

   _____

3. Identify four critical aspects of any laboratory testing performed by the nurse.

   a. *Need for Pts written consent (rationale for the test*

   b. *necessary teaching & preparation of Pt*

   c. _____

   d. _____

4. When should gloves be worn when collecting specimens?

   always —

   _____

5. How can you protect other staff when transporting laboratory specimens?

   wear gloves, double bag —
   tightly sealed containers) + ⌐

True-False Questions

True   6. Sputum specimens are best obtained first thing in the morning.

True — 7. When obtaining a 24-hour urine specimen, the last voiding is discarded.

True + false 8. Alcohol is recommended for cleansing a finger when performing a finger stick to measure blood glucose.

false   9. All urine glucose testing products are completely interchangeable.

_____ 10. To obtain a urine specimen from a catheterized patient, drain the specimen from the bottom of the drainage bag.

© 1996 by Lippincott-Raven Publishers

MODULE

12

ASSISTING WITH DIAGNOSTIC AND THERAPEUTIC PROCEDURES

MODULE CONTENTS

RATIONALE FOR THE USE OF THIS
   SKILL
NURSING DIAGNOSES
DIAGNOSTIC AND THERAPEUTIC
   PROCEDURES
GENERAL PROCEDURE FOR ASSISTING
   WITH DIAGNOSTIC AND
   THERAPEUTIC PROCEDURES
   Assessment
   Planning
   Implementation
   Evaluation
   Documentation

SPECIFIC PROCEDURES
Procedure for Assisting With Thoracentesis
Procedure for Assisting With Paracentesis
Procedure for Assisting With Spinal Tap
   (Lumbar Puncture)
Procedure for Assisting With Liver Biopsy
Procedure for Assisting With Bone Marrow
   Aspiration or Biopsy
Procedure for Assisting With Proctoscopy,
   Sigmoidoscopy, and Colonoscopy
CRITICAL THINKING EXERCISES

PREREQUISITES

Successful completion of the following modules:

VOLUME 1

Module 1 An Approach to Nursing Skills
Module 2 Basic Infection Control
Module 3 Safety
Module 5 Documentation
Module 6 Introduction to Assessment Skills

The following modules may be necessary for some selected situations:

Module 7   Temperature, Pulse, and Respiration
Module 8   Blood Pressure
Module 9   The Nursing Physical Assessment
Module 11 Collecting Specimens and Performing Common Laboratory Tests
Module 15 Moving the Patient in Bed and Positioning

VOLUME 2
Module 33 Sterile Technique

© 1996 by Lippincott-Raven Publishers

OVERALL OBJECTIVES

To assist with diagnostic and therapeutic procedures, with emphasis on the preparation and support of patients, and to handle properly specimens obtained.

SPECIFIC LEARNING OBJECTIVES

Know Facts and Principles	Apply Facts and Principles	Demonstrate Ability	Evaluate Performance
1. Equipment			
Name equipment needed for six procedures described.	Identify equipment needed for each of six procedures.	In the clinical setting, select appropriate equipment for procedure to be performed.	Evaluate own performance using Performance Checklist.
2. Nurse's role in assisting			
State the role of the nurse in each prcedure.			
3. Procedure			
a. Positioning			
b. Observation			
c. Specimen collection			
d. Recording			
With each of the procedures, describe procedure, including position, necessary observation, specimen collection, and recording.	In the practice setting, carry out nurse's role in simulated situation.	Under supervision in the clinical setting, assist examiner with any of six procedures. Collect specimens, and record correctly.	Evaluate performance with instructor.

© 1996 by Lippincott-Raven Publishers

LEARNING ACTIVITIES

1. Review the Specific Learning Objectives.
2. Read the section on performing treatments (in the chapter on direct care skills) in Ellis and Nowlis, *Nursing: A Human Needs Approach,* or comparable material in another textbook.
3. Look up the module vocabulary terms in the glossary.
4. Review the anatomy and physiology of the system being studied.
5. Read through the module as though you were preparing to teach these skills to another person. Mentally practice the skills.
6. Review what you might teach patients about these procedures.
7. Become familiar with the equipment available in the practice laboratory.
8. In the practice setting, do the following:
   a. Using your partner as the patient, practice positioning for a lumbar puncture, paracentesis, and thoracentesis. Have your instructor evaluate your performance.
   b. Form groups of three students, and take turns being the person performing the procedure, the patient, and the assisting nurse. Be sure to teach the patient appropriately, and identify the observations you would be making as you proceed. The student simulating the role of the physician will simply ask for equipment while standing in position as if to use it.
      (1) Set up for and perform a thoracentesis.
      (2) Set up for and perform a paracentesis.
      (3) Set up for and perform a lumbar puncture.
      (4) Set up for and perform a liver biopsy.
      (5) Set up for and perform a bone marrow aspiration or biopsy.
   c. For each of these procedures, discuss the things that made it easier for you as a patient, the concerns you felt, and how the nurse assisted with these concerns. Note how the equipment was set up. What made it convenient and what aspects were awkward? How could you reorganize the physical environment so that it would be more convenient?
   d. Using a practice manikin, set up for a sigmoidoscopy or proctoscopy, or both. Consider the same questions raised above.
9. In the clinical setting, consult with your instructor about opportunities to assist with a diagnostic or therapeutic procedure. Do this under supervision.

VOCABULARY

ascites	endoscopy	manometer	stylet
biopsy	endoscope	paracentesis	supine position
bone marrow	hypovolemic shock	proctoscope	thoracentesis
cerebrospinal fluid	liver biopsy	sigmoidoscope	trocar
cisternal	lumbar puncture	stab wound	
dorsal recumbent position	(spinal tap)	stopcock	

© 1996 by Lippincott-Raven Publishers

Assisting With Diagnostic and Therapeutic Procedures

Rationale for the Use of These Skills

A variety of diagnostic and therapeutic procedures are used to treat patients and to obtain specimens for laboratory testing. To assist effectively, the nurse must know the rationale for the procedure and test(s) involved, how the procedure is performed, the necessary teaching and preparation of the patient, appropriate methods of obtaining and handling specimens, and how to care for the patient after the procedure. Information obtained through these procedures may be the key to the diagnosis and therapeutic decisions for the patients concerned.[1]

▼ NURSING DIAGNOSES

When assisting with diagnostic and therapeutic procedures, one nursing diagnosis to keep in mind is Knowledge Deficit. Patients may need to receive information related to the rationale for the procedure, the risks involved, what to expect, or what they can do to facilitate the examination or procedure. Anxiety is a second nursing diagnosis to consider when assisting with diagnostic and therapeutic procedures. The anxiety can be related to lack of knowledge, the fear of an unwelcome diagnosis, or perceived necessary changes in lifestyle or events. Fear of pain or discomfort may also be present.

DIAGNOSTIC AND THERAPEUTIC PROCEDURES

Physicians provide the information needed for the patient to give informed consent and perform the procedures described. The nursing staff usually assumes responsibility for obtaining the patient's signature on a consent form, gathering the equipment, preparing the patient, supporting the patient during the procedure, and providing care needed after the procedure. In addition, the nurse may assist in collecting specimens and ensuring that they are sent for testing in the appropriate manner.

[1]Note that rationale for action is emphasized throughout the module by the use of italics.

© 1996 by Lippincott-Raven Publishers

GENERAL PROCEDURE FOR ASSISTING WITH DIAGNOSTIC AND THERAPEUTIC PROCEDURES

Assessment

1. Check the physician's order *to be sure of the exact procedure to be done and to identify the purpose of the procedure.*

2. Check to be sure that a permission form has been signed, if this is necessary. *A patient must give informed consent for any procedure, and when the procedure is invasive and has possible adverse consequences, most facilities require that a written form be signed and placed in the patient's record. Although informing the patient is the physician's responsibility, in many facilities the nurse obtains the signature on the form and witnesses it. This does not transfer the responsibility for informed consent from the physician to the nurse.* In other facilities, the nurse prepares the form for the physician to present to the patient when information is being given. Follow the procedure in your facility.

3. Assess the patient for the ability to assume and maintain the appropriate position for the procedure *to plan alternatives if necessary* and for the need for premedication for anxiety and pain. *Premedication may decrease the anxiety felt and the pain experienced by the patient during the procedure.*

Planning

4. Wash your hands *for infection control.*

5. Obtain the equipment available in your facility, and check the contents of any prepared tray *to identify what items must be obtained separately.* Obtain gloves if you will contact body secretions.

Implementation

6. Identify the patient *to be sure that you are performing the procedure on the correct patient.*

7. Discuss the procedure with the patient. At this time you will need to find out what the patient has been told by the physician and how well the patient understands the information provided. You will also clarify concerns and give explicit information about the way the procedure will affect the patient *to relieve anxiety and facilitate patient participation.* Do not increase the patient's anxiety with graphic descriptions of the procedure, but focus on how the patient will be positioned, what the patient will be asked to do, and what the patient will experience during the procedure. You might also emphasize that part of your role is to help the patient in whatever way is possible.

8. Prepare the unit:
  a. Provide for privacy.
  b. Set up a table for equipment. You may need to clean the surface of the table *for infection control.*
9. Prepare the patient:
  a. Premedicate the patient if indicated.
  b. Position the patient as needed to facilitate the procedure.
  c. Drape the patient as needed to provide privacy.
10. Assist with the procedure. (See the specific details for each procedure described below.)
  a. Assess the patient throughout the procedure. Observe the patient for adverse signs or reactions to the procedure. *Many times the physician is preoccupied with performing the procedure, and the nurse can see early signs of impending problems.* During any procedure, check the patient's pulse and respiration two or three times, and ask the patient to tell you about any feelings of distress or peculiar sensations. During some procedures, blood pressure may be monitored. Notify the physician promptly of any unusual signs.
  b. Reassure the patient, and strive to relieve anxiety throughout the procedure.
  c. Assist with the procedure, providing equipment as needed. Use gloves appropriately.
11. Conclude the procedure:
  a. Restore the patient to a comfortable position or to the ordered therapeutic position.
  b. Restore the unit by clearing away equipment and placing the call bell within reach.
  c. Label and properly care for any specimen obtained.
  d. Dispose of equipment.
  e. Wash your hands.

Evaluation

12. Establish specific criteria for evaluation based on the procedure. Include the following:
  a. Patient's comfort
  b. Patient's physiologic response, such as bleeding; temperature, pulse, and respiration; and blood pressure
  c. Patient's psychological response, such as anxiety, distress, or relaxation

Documentation

13. Although the physician will document that the procedure was performed, the nurse briefly documents the procedure, the patient's response, and the disposition of any specimen in the progress notes or appropriate flow sheet.
14. Report any abnormal findings to the appropriate person, such as your instructor or the registered nurse.

SPECIFIC PROCEDURES

For each procedure discussed, some steps in the General Procedure may be modified. The modified steps and references to the steps in the General Procedure that remain the same follow. Table 12–1 provides a quick overview of each of the procedures.

Procedure for Assisting With Thoracentesis

A thoracentesis is the insertion of a large-bore needle or a trocar (a large, sharp metal device) into the pleural space of the chest. This can be done to remove air or fluid from the pleural space, to enable a chest tube to be inserted, or to inject medication. You will need an understanding of sterile technique to assist appropriately with this procedure. When fluid is removed, it may be sent to the laboratory for analysis of content, examination for cells present, or culture and sensitivity.

Assessment

1.–2. Follow the steps of the General Procedure.
3. Assess whether the patient is able to sit upright during the procedure. *The patient must sit upright so that the pull of gravity will consolidate the chest fluid in the lower portion of the affected lung.* Also assess the need for premedication.

Planning

4. Follow the General Procedure.
5. Obtain the necessary equipment. A sterile thoracentesis set typically contains all needed equipment and is disposable. Read the label *to determine if any items are not included.* You may need to add sterile gloves in the size appropriate for the physician doing the procedure, a basin to receive large quantities of fluid being removed, and an injectable local anesthetic. If a chest tube is to be inserted, you will need a chest drainage set and a chest tube (see Module 42, Caring for Patients With Chest Drainage).

Implementation

6.–8. Follow the steps of the General Procedure.
9. Prepare the patient:
  a. Premedicate the patient if indicated.
  b. Assist the patient to an appropriate sitting position. The patient may sit on the edge of the bed leaning on an overbed table or may straddle a chair and lean on its back. Pad the back of the chair or the overbed table *for comfort.* Pillows on either side of the patient on the edge of the bed *may provide needed sup-*
(text continues on page 256)

© 1996 by Lippincott-Raven Publishers

Table 12-1. Overview of Common Diagnostic and Therapeutic Procedures

Test	Specimen	Preparing the Patient	Positioning the Patient	Role of the Nurse	Special Observations Concerning the Patient	Handling the Specimen
Thoracentesis	Fluid from pleural cavity	Explain. Warn patient not to cough or move suddenly during procedure or *needle may puncture lungs.*	Sitting position with arms over head or in front of chest (*The objective is to increase the size of the intercostal spaces.*)	Reassure patient. Assist physicians by setting up equipment, measuring fluid, and cleaning up.	Respiratory distress (cyanosis, dyspnea). Blood-tinged sputum. Monitor for 4–8 h after procedure for signs of respiratory distress or shock.	Specimen is sterile. Send to laboratory immediately.
Paracentesis	Ascitic fluid	Explain. Have patient void before procedure to prevent puncture of bladder.	Sitting position	Reassure patient. Assist physician by setting up equipment, measuring fluid, and cleaning up.	Signs of shock. Monitor vital signs for 4–8 h after procedure.	Specimen is sterile. Send to laboratory immediately.
Spinal tap	Cerebrospinal fluid (CSF)	Explain procedure.	On side with back near edge of bed, knees brought up, head forward on chest (see Fig. 12–1), or sitting on edge of bed	Assist patient to maintain position. Be reassuring. Assist physician by setting up equipment, holding and labeling tubes for specimens, and cleaning up.	Signs of shock, nausea, and vomiting. Headache occasionally. Physician may order patient to lie flat for 1–24 h after procedure. Observe for motion and sensation in lower extremities.	Specimen is sterile, usually in several tubes. Be sure to number tubes sequentially (tube 1, tube 2, and so on). Send to laboratory immediately.

© 1996 by Lippincott-Raven Publishers

Liver biopsy	Liver tissue	Explain. Patient must remain still during procedure.	Supine position	Reassure patient. Assist physically.	Bleeding is the most serious complication. The patient lies on the biopsy site to apply pressure and prevent bleeding. Observe blood pressure and pulse.	The core of tissue is placed in a container with a preservative and sent to the pathology department for examination.
Bone marrow aspiration or bone marrow biopsy	Bone Marrow tissue	Explain. The patient may hear a distressing noise. The procedure will include a local anesthetic but will still be uncomfortable.	Supine for sternal site; abdomen or side of iliac crest site	Reassure patient. Assist by providing supplies and equipment.	Bleeding is a major concern. Put pressure on the site for 5 min after the procedure. Check pulse and blood pressure.	The aspirated bone marrow or the core of bone marrow tissue is placed in a container with preservative and sent to the laboratory immediately.
Proctoscopy, sigmoidoscopy, or colonoscopy	The inside of the colon; biopsy may be done.	Explain. Assist physician.	Knee-chest position or left lateral position.	Reassure patient. Assist with equipment.	The patient may be somewhat weak and dizzy.	Any specimen is placed in a container with preservative and sent to the laboratory immediately.

© 1996 by Lippincott-Raven Publishers

port. If the patient is weak, you may need to have a person supporting the patient at all times.

c. Drape so that the patient's back is exposed *for access to the intercostal spaces.*

10. Assist with the procedure.

a. Set up for the procedure.

(1) Open the sterile set on a convenient table.

(2) Open the glove package in an accessible location.

b. Assess the patient especially for skin color, respirations, chest pain, and diaphoresis. *The sudden appearance of pallor (seen as a graying in those with dark skin), dyspnea, cough, chest pain, or diaphoresis may indicate that the needle is irritating or even puncturing the pleura.* Inform the physician immediately if these signs are identified.

c. Give the patient psychological support. If a patient is uncomfortable, reassure that the discomfort will only be for a short time. Let the patient know what is about to take place, and give clear instructions about ways to help. ("Please try not to move for the next few minutes so that we can get the test done quickly.") *All this adds to the patient's psychological comfort. Patients feel less anxious if they know what is going to happen and what they should do.* You may want to hold the patient's hand *for reassurance.*

d. Be prepared to hold the basin or set up the chest drainage if that is indicated. Because the equipment is sterile, the physician will handle it with sterile-gloved hands *to avoid contamination.* The physician will clean the insertion area with antiseptic, anesthetize the area using the local anesthetic, and insert a 16- or 17-gauge needle with a stylet into the pleural space at the level of the seventh intercostal space. The stylet is then removed, and a large syringe with a three-way stopcock is attached to the needle. This is used to aspirate fluid from the chest.

When all the fluid has been removed, the needle is withdrawn, and an impervious dressing is placed over the thoracentesis site. If a chest tube is being inserted, a large trocar is used; the chest tube is threaded through the trocar, the trocar is removed, and the chest drainage set is attached.

A specimen of fluid drained from the pleural cavity by thoracentesis can be used to determine the presence of abnormal cells or microorganisms. The specimen may be ob-

tained during the procedure, or a sample may be taken from the collecting container. Be careful that the fluid is not mistakenly discarded before a specimen is obtained.

11. Conclude the procedure.

a. Restore the patient to a comfortable position; semi-Fowler's position is usually used because *it will promote more effective chest expansion and ventilation.* In addition, plan for a period of undisturbed rest because *the removal of large amounts of fluid from the chest can result in weakness and fatigue caused by the shift in fluid distribution.*

b. Restore the unit.

c. Label the specimen, and care for it properly. Use gloves appropriately.

d. Dispose of equipment. Be sure that needles and trocar are discarded in a "sharps" container. The rest of the set is usually disposable.

e. Wash your hands.

Evaluation

12. Establish specific criteria to evaluate the patient's response, including the following:

a. Patient's comfort

b. Patient's physiologic response, especially respiratory status *because a thoracentesis is performed to facilitate effective respiration.* Evaluation of pulse and blood pressure also is important *because changes in chest pressures may affect cardiac function, especially in the person of advanced age or with existing cardiac disease.*

c. Patient's psychological response

Documentation

13.–14. Follow the steps of the General Procedure.

Procedure for Assisting With Paracentesis

A paracentesis is the insertion of a large-bore needle or a trocar through the wall of the abdomen into the abdominal cavity *to remove fluid or instill a solution.* You will need an understanding of sterile technique.

Assessment

1.–2. Follow the steps of the General Procedure.

3. Assess the patient's ability to sit upright and the need for premedication. The patient is often placed sitting on the edge of the bed for this procedure. Devising a back support from pillows may decrease tiring. If that is not possible, the patient may be able to remain in a supine position with the head of the bed elevated. *These positions consolidate the fluid in the lower portion of the abdomen.* If the patient is unable to be upright, con-

© 1996 by Lippincott-Raven Publishers

DATE/TIME	
7/6/99 0730	Interim note: Thoracentesis performed by Dr. Kraft. 450 ml serosanguinous fluid removed. Specimen to lab. Respiratory Status after procedure: S "I feel weak and shaky but I can take a deeper breath. I just want to sleep." O Breathing regular at 20/min. Site of thoracentesis clean and dry. P 1) Allow to rest for remainder of morning. 2) Assess respiratory status and wound site q15min × 4, then qh × 3, then q4h. See flow sheet. ———— D. Chaney, SN

Example of Nursing Progress Notes Using POR Format.

sult the physician about possible modifications of this position.

Planning

4. Follow the General Procedure.
5. Obtain the necessary equipment. A disposable paracentesis set is usually used for this procedure. You may need to add sterile gloves in the appropriate size for the physician, a large basin or container for any fluid removed, and a topical anesthetic agent.

Implementation

6.–8. Follow the steps of the General Procedure.
9. Prepare the patient:
   a. Premedicate the patient if indicated.
   b. Have the patient void before beginning the procedure *so that the bladder is empty and confined to the pelvis to prevent accidental bladder perforation during the procedure.*
   c. Position the patient sitting on the edge of the bed.
   d. Drape the patient's back and legs *to provide warmth and comfort.*
10. Assist with the procedure.
   a. Set up the equipment on a convenient overbed table, arranging the sterile field.
   b. Make sure that a straight chair is available. *The physician will sit facing the patient to perform the procedure.*
   c. Observe the patient particularly for pallor, dizziness, faintness, diaphoresis, and rapid pulse and respirations, *which could indicate an adverse response to the sudden removal of abdominal pressure from the fluid and the consequent movement of a large quantity of blood into the abdominal circulation. This change in blood flow may create a systemic lack of blood supply and a condition called hypovolemic shock.*

Ascitic fluid is usually tested for abnormal cells. Only 5 to 10 mL of the large amount of sterile fluid removed needs to be sent as a specimen. Some physicians will remove the specimen as the catheter drains, whereas others prefer the nurse to send a sample from the collecting container. Send the sample to the laboratory promptly *to prevent deterioration of the specimen or having it discarded unintentionally.* Use gloves appropriately.

   d. Reassure the patient, and strive to relieve anxiety throughout the procedure.
   e. Assist with the procedure, providing equipment as needed.
11. Conclude the procedure:
   a. Position the patient in bed, and allow a rest period *because the removal of large amounts of fluid from the abdomen can result in weakness and fatigue caused by the shift in body fluid distribution.*
   b. Restore the unit by clearing away equipment and placing the call bell within reach.
   c. Label and properly care for any specimen obtained.
   d. Dispose of equipment.
   e. Wash your hands.

Evaluation

12. Establish specific criteria to evaluate the patient's response, including the following:
   a. Patient's comfort
   b. Patient's physiologic response, especially respiratory status, pulse, and blood pressure; observe paracentesis site and abdominal girth and its changes.
   c. Patient's psychological response

Documentation

13.–14. Follow the steps of the General Procedure.

© 1996 by Lippincott-Raven Publishers

DATE/TIME	
7/6/99 7:30 AM	*Paracentesis performed by Dr. Kraft, 1200 ml cloudy fluid obtained. Specimen to lab. States no pain at site. Site clean and dry. Dry drsg. applied. Resting comfortably at this time. P-82, R-20, BP 126/84 ———————— D. Chaney, SN*

Example of Nursing Progress Notes Using Narrative Format.

Procedure for Assisting With Spinal Tap (Lumbar Puncture)

A spinal tap is the introduction of a long needle through the intervertebral space into the subarachnoid space of the spinal canal. This is done *to measure the pressure in the spinal fluid and to collect specimens of the cerebrospinal fluid (CSF).* The tap is most commonly performed in the lumbar area, but on occasion it is done at the top of the spinal canal in the cisternal space. A cisternal tap is performed more frequently on children.

Assessment

1.–2. Follow the steps of the General Procedure.

3. Assess the patient's ability to lie on his or her side in a flexed position and the need for premedication. If the patient has arthritis or some other condition that limits the ability to assume this position, consult with the physician regarding an alternative position.

Planning

4. Follow the General Procedure.

5. Obtain a disposable tray labeled "lumbar puncture" or "spinal" for this procedure. Sterile gloves in the size appropriate for the physician and a local anesthetic agent are provided in the set or may be obtained separately.

Implementation

6.–8. Follow the steps of the General Procedure.

9. Prepare the patient.

    a. Premedicate the patient if indicated.

    b. Position the patient on the side with a flat support under the head *so that the spinal column is in horizontal alignment and the flow of spinal fluid is not impeded.* Flex the legs and neck, bowing the back toward the side of the bed where the physician will sit. *This position of flexion widens the posterior intervertebral spaces.*

    c. Drape the patient so that the lower spine is exposed, but the rest of the patient is covered *for warmth and privacy* (Fig. 12–1).

10. Assist with the procedure.

    a. Assess the patient throughout the procedure. Pay particular attention to comments indicating pain radiating to a leg; sharp, severe back pain; or sudden numbness or tingling of the feet or legs. The puncture is usually performed below the area where the actual cord is located, but *irritation of spinal tissue may create adverse neurologic responses.*

    b. The physician will anesthetize the site and then introduce the spinal needle into the spinal subarachnoid space. You may need to assist the patient to remain still and in the proper position, because *the procedure is often uncomfortable.*

    c. When the physician attaches the manometer to the needle to measure the pressure, you may be asked to support the top of the manometer to maintain its alignment. If so, be sure you touch only the top *so that you do not contaminate the area that the physician must handle when disconnecting the manometer.*

    d. If specimens of fluid are needed, three separate specimens are usually obtained *because the first tube and even the second may be pink with blood* from the puncture itself. The third should be clear; if it is not, this may indicate that the patient's CSF contains blood. The physician performing the lumbar puncture may fill the three sterile collecting tubes, or you may be asked to hold the tubes while the physician manipulates the manometer. If you are collecting the fluid, you should wear

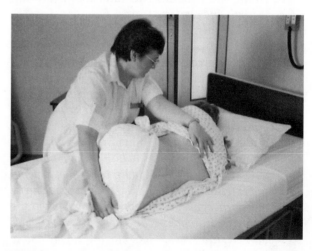

Figure 12–1. Nurse holding a patient in position for a lumbar puncture.

© 1996 by Lippincott-Raven Publishers

clean gloves *to protect yourself from potential contamination.* Keep your hands well away from any sterile area *to avoid introducing microbes to the patient.* You may also be responsible for correctly labeling the specimens as 1, 2, and 3 in the order they were collected. Be sure to send all three tubes to the laboratory. Be very careful with these specimens *because of the difficulty of obtaining them through the lumbar puncture procedure.*

11. Conclude the procedure.
    a. The patient may be advised to remain flat immediately after the procedure and for 4 to 8 hours, depending on the physician. *This is to allow the restoration of spinal fluid before the patient assumes an upright position. This may help to prevent postspinal headache, although recent data indicate that there is no significant difference in the incidence of postspinal headache based on the patient's postprocedure position.* Provide increased fluids *to help restore spinal fluid volume.*
    b. Restore the unit by clearing away equipment and placing the call bell within reach.
    c. Label and properly care for any specimen obtained.
    d. Dispose of equipment.
    e. Wash your hands.

Evaluation

12. Establish specific criteria to evaluate the patient's response, including the following:
    a. Patient's comfort, especially the presence of pain, numbness, or tingling in back and lower extremities and the presence of headache in the 24 hours postprocedure
    b. Patient's physiologic response, especially motion and sensation in lower extremities
    c. Patient's psychological response

Documentation

13.–14. Follow the steps of the General Procedure.

Procedure for Assisting With Liver Biopsy

A liver biopsy is the removal of a specimen of liver tissue for laboratory examination. A liver biopsy may be done during a surgical procedure when the abdominal cavity is open. The procedure discussed here is for a needle biopsy, in which a large-bore needle is inserted through the abdominal wall, and a core of tissue is obtained for examination. The local anesthetic agent numbs only surface tissue, and the entry of the needle into the liver and removal of the liver tissue cause pain. Acknowledging the discomfort and offering support and comfort measures are important.

Assessment

1. Check physician's order, and note whether preprocedure therapies were ordered to decrease the chance of bleeding.
   a. *Vitamin K enhances the body's clotting ability and decreases the chance of bleeding by facilitating the production of prothrombin, a clotting factor. Its effect does not occur immediately but after several days when the body has had an opportunity to produce the prothrombin from vitamin K.* If vitamin K was ordered and the drug was omitted for some reason, the physician may choose to postpone the procedure. Vitamin K may be given intramuscularly or intravenously.
   b. *When bleeding a serious concern, platelets may be infused to enhance clotting. These are given immediately before the procedure.* (See Module 56, Administering Blood and Blood Products.)
2. Follow the General Procedure.
3. Assess the need for premedication and the patient's ability to lie flat in a supine position. This position will *help flatten and expose the liver tissue.* If the patient cannot lie flat, consult the physician regarding an alternative position.

Planning

4. Follow the General Procedure.
5. Obtain the necessary equipment. A disposable liver biopsy tray is used for this procedure. Sterile gloves in the appropriate size for the physician and a local anesthetic agent may be obtained separately if they are not included in the set.

Implementation

6.–8. Follow the steps of the General Procedure.
9. Prepare the patient.
   a. Premedicate the patient if indicated.
   b. Position the patient supine.

DATE/TIME	
7/3/99	*Lumbar puncture performed by Dr. Kraft. Initial pressure 140 mm.*
7:20 AM	*Final pressure 90 mm. Three specimens of clear fluid sent to lab.*
	Resting comfortably c̄ bed flat. —————— D. Chaney, SN

Example of Nursing Progress Notes Using Narrative Format.

© 1996 by Lippincott-Raven Publishers

DATE/TIME	
7/3/99	*Interim note: Liver biopsy by Dr. Kraft. Spec to lab.*
0830	*S Expressed concern over pain and possible result of biopsy.*
	O BP 130/82, P 88, R 26
	A Anxiety related to procedure. Potential for bleeding.
	P Vitals q15min × 4 then q4h for 24 h.
	Encourage to voice concerns.
	D. Chaney, SN

Example of Nursing Progress Notes Using SOAP Format.

c. Drape so that the lower portion of the patient's chest and the abdomen are exposed. The patient's gown may be left in place if it is folded so that it cannot contaminate the work area during the procedure.

10. Assist with the procedure.

a. Assess the patient's vital signs before and after the procedure. Leave the blood pressure cuff in place during the procedure *to monitor patient response if bleeding is suspected.* The physician will anesthetize a small right subcostal area. The patient is instructed to take a deep breath, *which lowers the diaphragm and pushes the liver toward the abdomen,* then hold it while the actual biopsy is being done *to ensure that the liver does not move during insertion.* After insertion the needle is rotated *to create a core of tissue inside the biopsy needle,* which is then withdrawn.

b. Reassure the patient, and strive to relieve anxiety throughout the procedure.

c. Assist with the procedure, providing equipment as necessary.

d. Exert pressure over the site *to stop bleeding* if asked. Apply a small dressing. Use gloves.

11. Conclude the procedure.

a. Position the patient on the *right side so that the body weight provides continuing pressure to the site to prevent bleeding.* Bed rest may be advised for 2 to 8 hours.

b. Restore the unit by clearing away equipment and placing the call bell within reach.

c. Label and properly care for any specimen obtained. The specimen is placed in a preservative solution and sent to the laboratory.

d. Dispose of equipment.

e. Wash your hands.

Evaluation

12. Establish specific criteria to evaluate the patient's response to the procedure, including the following:

a. Patient's comfort

b. Patient's physiologic response, especially signs of internal bleeding. Establish a plan for observation and assessment of the patient for *this rare but potentially serious complication. The liver is a very vascular tissue, and internal bleeding may occur from the trauma of the biopsy.* Observation of pulse, respiration, blood pressure, and the biopsy site every 15 minutes for 1 hour is a wise practice. If your facility has a policy requiring a specified observation schedule, follow that policy.

c. Patient's psychological response

Documentation

13.–14. Follow the steps of the General Procedure.

DATE/TIME	
6/12/99	*D: Pt. expressed fear of pain from liver biopsy. States previous liver biopsy was "terrible," and she cannot face that again.*
	A: Physician contacted regarding pt. concern. Premedication ordered. Pt. notified of plan for premedication.
	R: Pt. expresses relief of fear.
	S. Mindoka, RN

Example of Nursing Progress Notes Using Focus Format.

© 1996 by Lippincott-Raven Publishers

Procedure for Assisting With Bone Marrow Aspiration or Biopsy

A specimen of bone marrow may be obtained by aspiration or needle biopsy. The specimen is sent to the laboratory to be examined *to establish a diagnosis or to evaluate the patient's response to treatment.* When a bone marrow aspiration is done, marrow is removed through a needle inserted into the marrow cavity of the bone. For a biopsy, a larger bore needle is inserted, and a small, solid core of marrow tissue is obtained. The anterior and posterior iliac crests and the sternum are the most common sites for bone marrow aspiration. The sternum is not usually used for a biopsy, however, *because it is small and close to vital organs.* The surface tissue is anesthetized, *but the patient does feel pressure and a "pulling" sensation when the marrow specimen is removed. In addition, the puncturing of the bone sounds distressing.* For these reasons, a sedative may be ordered to be given prior to a bone marrow biopsy. Acknowledging the discomfort, and not attempting to minimize or trivialize it, *provides support to the patient and sustains a trust relationship.* When bone marrow is aspirated from a donor for bone marrow transplantation, the marrow is aspirated by needle from multiple sites. This is done under anesthesia.

Assessment
1.–3. Follow the steps of the General Procedure.

Planning
4. Follow the steps of the General Procedure.
5. Obtain the necessary equipment. You will need a bone marrow aspiration or biopsy tray and sterile gloves. Most facilities use completely disposable equipment. In some facilities, a reusable metal bone marrow biopsy needle with stylet and a glass aspiration syringe are used. These are obtained separately.

Implementation
6.–8. Follow the steps of the General Procedure.
9. Prepare the patient.
  a. Premedicate the patient if indicated.
  b. Position the patient appropriately. If a sternal site is to be used, position the patient in a supine position with small pillows beneath the shoulders *to elevate the chest and lower the head.* If the anterior iliac crest site is to be used, the supine or side-lying position may be used. When the specimen is obtained from the posterior iliac crest, the patient is placed in either the side-lying or prone position.
  c. Drape the patient appropriately.
10. Assist with the procedure.

  a. Open the pack, and supply sterile gloves. You may be requested to pour antiseptic solution into a container.
  b. Assess the patient throughout the procedure. A small area in the midsternum or over the anterior or posterior iliac crest is anesthetized. A small incision may be made *to facilitate insertion of the needle.*
   (1) *Aspiration*: A short, large-gauge needle with a stylet is inserted. There may be a soft, crunching sound as it punctures the bone tissue. Warning the patient that this sound will occur will alleviate some anxiety. The stylet is removed, a syringe is attached, and 1 to 2 mL of bone marrow is aspirated.
   (2) *Biopsy*: A special needle with a sharp cutting edge and a hollow core is inserted, and a core of tissue removed.
  c. Reassure the patient, and strive to relieve anxiety throughout the procedure.
  d. Assist with the procedure, providing equipment as necessary.
  e. After the needle is removed, apply pressure for 5 minutes *to stop the bleeding that occurs.* If the patient has a bleeding disorder, you may be asked to apply pressure for 10 to 15 minutes. Use gloves appropriately.
  f. In some settings, you will need to apply a pressure dressing and ensure that the patient lies recumbent in bed for 60 minutes.
11. Conclude the procedure:
  a. Restore the patient to a comfortable position or to the ordered therapeutic position.
  b. Restore the unit by clearing away equipment and placing the call bell within reach.
  c. Label any specimen obtained. Place the specimen in a container with preservative, and send it to the laboratory immediately.
  d. Dispose of equipment.
  e. Wash your hands.

Evaluation
12. Establish specific criteria to evaluate the patient's response, including the following:
  a. Patient's comfort
  b. Patient's physiologic response, especially local bleeding at the site. If this occurs, apply pressure for 5 minutes, and apply a clean dressing. Take vital signs after the procedure is completed; there may be a policy regarding the schedule for postprocedure vital signs.
  c. Patient's psychological response

Documentation
13.–14. Follow the steps of the General Procedure.

© 1996 by Lippincott-Raven Publishers

DATE/TIME	
7/23/99 8:30 AM	*Bone marrow biopsy done by Dr. Kraft. Specimen sent to lab. Pressure applied for 5 min. Posterior iliac crest site covered by pressure dressing. Pt crying. States she is afraid of results. RN with pt for 15 min to provide reassurance. Currently resting quietly.* *D. Chaney, SN*

Example of Nursing Progress Notes Using Narrative Format.

Procedure for Assisting With Proctoscopy, Sigmoidoscopy, and Colonoscopy

A proctoscopy is the examination of the interior surface of the rectum, using a hollow tube with a light attached. A sigmoidoscopy uses the same principle to examine the interior surface of the bowel as high as the sigmoid colon. A colonoscopy involves examination of structures throughout the large intestine. During these examinations, small samples of tissue may be removed (biopsy) for laboratory examination, bleeding vessels may be cauterized, and the bowel can be visually examined for abnormalities. When only the rectum is being examined, a rigid metal tube is most commonly used (Fig. 12–2).

When high structures are to be examined, a flexible fiber-optic endoscope is used (Fig. 12–3). This permits the examiner to see higher bowel areas with less discomfort to the patient than would result from the use of a rigid endoscope.

Nevertheless, the procedure and position used are uncomfortable and both are considered embarrassing by most individuals. The more extensive examination, colonoscopy, is the most uncomfortable.

For all these procedures, thorough cleansing of the bowel is essential. If feces are present in the bowel, the examiner is unable to visualize the tissue.

See Module 28, Administering Enemas, and Module 49, Administering Medications by Alternative Routes, for information about the use of suppositories and other procedures frequently used to cleanse the bowel. Oral laxatives may also be used to help cleanse the bowel.

Assessment
1. Check the physician's order. Also check to see that the appropriate bowel cleansing plan has been completed. If it has not been completed or if it has been unsuccessful, notify the physician before proceeding. Some physicians prefer that the patient have a liquid diet the day before the examination. The patient is asked to remain NPO (have nothing by mouth) either for 8 hours before or from midnight until the examination *to decrease bowel activity.*
2.–3. Follow the steps of the General Procedure.

Planning
4. Follow the steps of the General Procedure.
5. Obtain the appropriate equipment, including an endoscope and a suction machine. Also obtain clean towels, water-soluble lubricant, long cotton-tipped swabs, and slides or containers for tissue specimens. Special drapes or draw sheets and examination gloves also are needed.

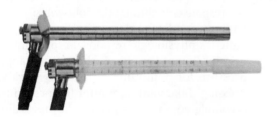

Figure 12–2. The sigmoidoscope is a hollow tube with a light attached that is used to examine the interior surface of the bowel as high as the sigmoid colon. (Courtesy Welch Allyn, Inc., Skaneateles Falls, New York, and American Hospital Supply Corp., McGaw Park, Illinois.)

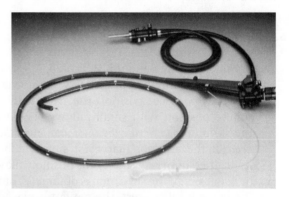

Figure 12–3. The flexible fiberoptic colonoscope permits the examiner to see higher bowel areas with less discomfort to the patient than would result from the use of a rigid scope. (Courtesy Olympus Corporation.)

© 1996 by Lippincott-Raven Publishers

DATE/TIME	
7/23/99 8:30 AM	*Proctoscopy performed by Dr. Kraft. Pt expressed relief that it was over and not as uncomfortable as feared. Late breakfast tray ordered and pt comfortable. — D. Chaney, SN*

Example of Nursing Progress Notes Using Narrative Format.

Implementation

6.–7. Follow the steps of the General Procedure.

8. Prepare the unit.

   a. Provide for the patient's privacy.

   b. *For convenience,* arrange the endoscope and other items on a clean towel placed on a table.

9. Prepare the patient.

   a. Premedicate the patient if indicated.

   b. Position the patient on a special examination table that "breaks" at the hips and has a kneeling platform at the end. This allows the patient to be placed in a knee-chest position, *which is best for visualization, and provides support to help the patient maintain the position.* If a special examination table is not available, the patient is placed in a knee-chest position, and pillows may be used *to help support the patient.* For a colonoscopy, the patient may be positioned on the left side and then turned several times to gain visualization of different areas of the bowel.

   c. Drape the patient *to expose the rectal area, but provide maximum protection of modesty. Anxiety often causes vasoconstriction and makes patients feel cold, and the drapes will help to minimize this.*

10. Assist with the procedure.

   a. Assess the patient throughout the procedure.

   b. Reassure the patient, and strive to relieve anxiety throughout the procedure.

   c. The physician lubricates the endoscope and inserts it through the anus. Encourage the patient to focus on breathing deeply through the mouth to *assist in relaxation of the anal sphincter.*

   d. If the physician requests suction, attach the tubing from the endoscope to the suction apparatus, and provide suction as needed.

   e. When the procedure is completed, assist in cleansing the patient's anal area of the lubricant. Use gloves as appropriate.

11. Conclude the procedure.

   a. Assist the patient to rise from the procedure table. *After such a procedure, a patient may feel weak and unsteady and need extra support.*

   b. Restore the unit by clearing away equipment and placing the call bell within reach.

   c. Label any specimen obtained. Place the specimen in a container with preservative, and send it to the laboratory immediately.

   d. Dispose of equipment.

   e. Wash your hands.

Evaluation

12. Establish specific criteria to evaluate the patient's response to the procedure, including the following:

   a. Patient's comfort; discomfort is common but is not usually acute.

   b. Patient's physiologic response, such as sudden, acute abdominal pain, which may indicate the rare complication of perforated colon

   c. Patient's psychological response

Documentation

13. and 14. Follow the steps of the General Procedure.

CRITICAL THINKING EXERCISES

• Ben Jamerson, 58, has a family history of colon cancer. His physician has decided that he should have a colonoscopy. As the nurse in the physician's office, you are responsible to schedule the procedure, provide instructions to the patient regarding the procedure, and assist with the procedure when it is performed. Identify what concerns Mr. Jamerson might have, and determine what information he needs. Tell what advice you might give this patient about driving to the office for this procedure.

© 1996 by Lippincott-Raven Publishers

PERFORMANCE CHECKLIST

General Procedure for Assisting With Diagnostic and Therapeutic Procedures	Needs More Practice	Satisfactory	Comments
Assessment			
1. Check the physician's order.			
2. Check for signed permission form.			
3. Assess patient's physical abilities and need for premedication.			
Planning			
4. Wash your hands.			
5. Obtain equipment.			
Implementation			
6. Identify patient.			
7. Discuss procedure with patient.			
8. Prepare unit. a. Privacy			
b. Equipment			
9. Prepare patient. a. Premedicate if indicated.			
b. Positioning			
c. Draping			
10. Assist with procedure. a. Assess.			
b. Reassure and support.			
c. Provide equipment and assist.			
11. Conclude the procedure. a. Restore the patient to a comfortable or therapeutic position.			
b. Restore the unit.			
c. Label and care for specimen.			
d. Dispose of equipment.			
e. Wash your hands.			

(continued)

© 1996 by Lippincott-Raven Publishers

Procedure for Assisting With Diagnostic and Therapeutic Procedures *(Continued)*	Needs More Practice	Satisfactory	Comments
Evaluation			
12. Establish specific criteria. **a.** Comfort			
b. Physiologic response			
c. Psychological response			
Documentation			
13. Record the procedure, and include the following: **a.** Patient's response			
b. Disposition of specimen			
14. Report abnormal findings to the appropriate person.			
Procedure for Assisting With Thoracentesis			
Assessment			
1.–2. Follow Checklist steps 1 and 2 of the General Procedure for Assisting With Diagnostic and Therapeutic Procedures (check order and check signed permission).			
3. Assess patient's ability to sit upright and need for premedication.			
Planning			
4. Wash your hands.			
5. Obtain thoracentesis set and sterile gloves, large basin, if indicated; injectable local anesthetic; chest tube and chest drainage set, if indicated.			
Implementation			
6.–8. Follow Checklist steps 6–8 of the General Procedure (identify patient, discuss procedure with patient, and prepare unit).			
9. Prepare patient **a.** Premedicate if indicated.			
b. Positioning: sitting leaning over table			
c. Draping			

(continued)

© 1996 by Lippincott-Raven Publishers

Procedure for Assisting With Thoracentesis *(Continued)*	Needs More Practice	Satisfactory	Comments
10. Assist with procedure. **a.** Set up for the procedure.			
b. Assess for skin color, diaphoresis, respiratory status, chest pain.			
c. Reassure and support.			
d. Provide equipment.			
11. Follow Checklist Step 11 of the General Procedure (restore position of comfort, plan for rest period, restore unit, label and care for specimen, dispose of equipment, and wash hands).			
Evaluation			
12. Establish specific criteria. **a.** Comfort			
b. Physiologic response, especially respiratory status, pulse, and blood pressure			
c. Psychological response			
Documentation			
13.–14. Follow Checklist steps 13 and 14 of the General Procedure (record procedure and report abnormal findings).			
Procedure for Assisting With Paracentesis			
Assessment			
1.–2. Follow Checklist Steps 1 and 2 of the General Procedure for Assisting With Therapeutic and Diagnostic Procedures (check order and check signed permission).			
3. Assess patient's ability to sit upright and need for premedication			
Planning			
4. Wash your hands.			
5. Obtain paracentesis set and sterile gloves; large basin, if indicated; and topical anesthetic.			

(continued)

© 1996 by Lippincott-Raven Publishers

Procedure for Assisting With Paracentesis *(Continued)*	Needs More Practice	Satisfactory	Comments
Implementation			
6.–8. Follow Checklist steps 6–8 of the General Procedure (identify patient, discuss procedure with patient, and prepare unit).			
9. Prepare patient. **a.** Premedicate, if indicated.			
b. Have patient void.			
c. Position sitting on edge of bed.			
d. Drape.			
10. Assist with procedure. **a.** Set up equipment.			
b. Ensure a straight chair is available.			
c. Assess for pallor, dizziness, faintness, diaphoresis, rapid pulse, rapid respirations.			
d. Reassure and support.			
e. Provide equipment.			
11. Follow Checklist step 11 of the General Procedure (restore position of comfort, plan for rest period, restore unit, label and care for specimen, and wash hands).			
Evaluation			
12. Establish specific criteria. **a.** Comfort			
b. Physiologic response, especially respiratory status, pulse, and blood pressure and observation of paracentesis site and changes in abdominal girth			
c. Psychological response			
Documentation			
13–14. Follow Checklist steps 13 and 14 of the General Procedure (record procedure and report abnormal findings).			

(continued)

the puncture of a cavity w/removal of fluid as in pleural effusion or ascites.

© 1996 by Lippincott-Raven Publishers

Procedure for Assisting With Spinal Tap	Needs More Practice	Satisfactory	Comments
Assessment			
1.–2. Follow Checklist steps 1 and 2 of the General Procedure for Assisting with Diagnostic and Therapeutic Procedures (check order and check signed permission).			
3. Assess patient's ability to lie in flexed position and need for premedication.			
Planning			
4. Wash your hands.			
5. Obtain equipment (disposable set, sterile gloves, local anesthetic).			
Implementation			
6.–8. Follow Checklist steps 6–8 of the General Procedure (identify patient, discuss procedure with patient, and prepare unit).			
9. Prepare patient. **a.** Premedicate if indicated.			
b. Position on side in flexed position.			
c. Drape.			
10. Assist with procedure. **a.** Assess.			
b. Reassure patient, and support in position.			
c. Hold manometer.			
d. Don clean gloves; hold tubes for specimen if asked.			
11. Follow Checklist step 11 of the General Procedure (restore position of comfort, plan for rest period, restore unit, label and care for specimen, dispose of equipment, and wash hands).			
Evaluation			
12. Establish specific criteria. **a.** Comfort, especially pain in back and lower extremities or headache			

device for determining liquid or gaseous pressure.

(*continued*)

© 1996 by Lippincott-Raven Publishers

Procedure for Assisting With Spinal Tap *(Continued)*	Needs More Practice	Satisfactory	Comments
b. Physiologic response, especially abnormal neurologic response in lower extremities			
c. Psychological response			
Documentation			
13–14. Follow Checklist steps 13 and 14 of the General Procedure (record procedure and report abnormal findings).			
Procedure for Assisting With Liver Biopsy			
Assessment			
1. Check physician's order, or note whether vitamin K or platelets were ordered and given previously.			
2. Check for signed permission form.			
3. Assess patient's ability to lie flat and need for premedication.			
Planning			
4. Wash your hands.			
5. Obtain liver biopsy tray, sterile gloves, and local anesthetic.			
Implementation			
6.–8. Follow Checklist steps 6–8 of the General Procedure (identify patient, discuss procedure with patient, and prepare unit).			
9. Prepare patient. **a.** Premedicate if indicated.			
b. Position patient supine.			
c. Drape with upper right abdomen exposed.			
10. Assist with procedure. **a.** Assess.			
b. Reassure and support.			
c. Provide equipment.			
d. Exert pressure over site; apply dressing.			

(continued)

© 1996 by Lippincott-Raven Publishers

Procedure for Assisting With Liver Biopsy *(Continued)*	Needs More Practice	Satisfactory	Comments
11. Follow Checklist Step 11 of the General Procedure (restore position of comfort, plan for rest period, restore unit, label and care for specimen, dispose of equipment, and wash hands).			
Evaluation			
12. Establish specific criteria. **a.** Comfort			
b. Physiologic response, especially signs of internal bleeding (ie, pulse, blood pressure, skin color, respiratory rate)			
c. Psychological response			
Documentation			
13.–14. Follow Checklist steps 13 and 14 of the General Procedure (record procedure and report abnormal findings).			
Procedure for Assisting With Bone Marrow Aspiration/Biopsy			
Assessment			
1.–2. Follow Checklist steps 1 and 2 of the General Procedure for Assisting with Diagnostic and Therapeutic Procedures (check order and check signed permission).			
3. Assess patient's physical abilities and need for premedication			
Planning			
4. Wash your hands.			
5. Obtain bone marrow aspiration or biopsy tray and sterile gloves.			
Implementation			
6.–8. Follow Checklist steps 6–8 of the General Procedure (identify patient, discuss procedure with patient, and prepare unit).			
9. Prepare patient. **a.** Premedicate if indicated.			
b. Position for sternal or anterior or posterior iliac crest biopsy.			
c. Drape.			

(continued)

© 1996 by Lippincott-Raven Publishers

Procedure for Assisting With Bone Marrow Aspiration/Biopsy *(Continued)*	Needs More Practice	Satisfactory	Comments
10. Assist with procedure. a. Open the pack, and supply sterile gloves.			
b. Assess.			
c. Reassure and support patient.			
d. Provide equipment.			
e. Apply pressure after needle is withdrawn.			
f. Apply pressure dressing.			
11. Follow Checklist step 11 of the General Procedure (restore position of comfort, plan for rest period, restore unit, label and care for specimen, dispose of equipment and wash hands).			
Evaluation			
12. Establish specific criteria. a. Comfort			
b. Physiologic response, especially local bleeding at site			
c. Psychological response			
Documentation			
13.–14. Follow Checklist steps 13 and 14 of the General Procedure (record procedure and report abnormal findings).			
Procedure for Assisting With Proctoscopy, Sigmoidoscopy, and Colonoscopy			
Assessment			
1. Check physician's order regarding bowel cleaning, intake status, and procedure to be done.			
2. Check for signed permission form.			
3. Assess patient's physical abilities and need for premedication.			
Planning			
4. Wash your hands.			
5. Obtain scope, suction machine, towels, lubricating jelly, long swabs, slides or containers, examination gloves.			

(continued)

© 1996 by Lippincott-Raven Publishers

Procedures for Assisting With Proctoscopy, Sigmoidoscopy, and Colonoscopy *(Continued)*	Needs More Practice	Satisfactory	Comments
Implementation			
6.–8. Follow Checklist steps 6–8 of the General Procedure (identify patient, discuss procedure with patient, and prepare unit).			
9. Prepare patient. **a.** Premedicate if indicated.			
b. Position on special table, in knee-chest position or on left side, as indicated.			
c. Drape with anus exposed.			
10. Assist with procedure. **a.** Assess.			
b. Reassure and support.			
c. Encourage patient to deep breathe.			
d. Provide suction if needed.			
e. Cleanse patient's anal area.			
11. Follow Checklist step 11 of the General Procedure (restore position of comfort, plan for rest period, restore unit, label and care for specimen, dispose of equipment and wash hands).			
Evaluation			
12. Establish specific criteria. **a.** Comfort			
b. Physiologic response, especially acute abdominal discomfort			
c. Psychological response			
Documentation			
13.–14. Follow Checklist steps 13 and 14 of the General Procedure (record procedure and report abnormal findings).			

© 1996 by Lippincott-Raven Publishers

? QUIZ

Short-Answer Questions

1. What are two important functions of the nurse when assisting with a diagnostic procedure?

a. *reassure & support pt*

b. *prepare pt (physically & mentally)*

2. During a thoracentesis, the patient should be observed carefully for such signs as *skin color, diaphoresis* *chest pain*, or *respiration status*

3. Vitamin K is sometimes given to the patient who is to have a liver biopsy to

improve clotting of blood

4. List four aspects that might be included in the preparation of the environment for performing a diagnostic procedure.

a. *check physician's orders*

b. *✓ for permission form*

c. *assess pt physical abilities & need for premed.*

d. _____

True-False Questions

True **5.** It is important for the patient to void prior to a thoracentesis. *(so it isn't procedure is irrupted nervous)*

False **6.** The specimen from a paracentesis is often examined for the presence of abnormal cells. *—fluid*

True **7.** Headache is a common complication of a lumbar puncture.

Multiple-Choice Questions

_____ **8.** The signs listed in Question 2 could indicate

a. infection.
b. respiratory arrest.
c. pleural irritation or puncture.
d. all of the above.

_____ **9.** The patient about to undergo a paracentesis should be instructed to void first so that

a. there will be no discomfort from distention.
b. the urine can be tested.
c. the bladder will not be punctured.
d. the bladder will not be in the way of the intestines.

_____ **10.** The reason for positioning the patient having a lumbar puncture in the flexed position is to

a. widen the intervertebral spaces to allow entrance of the needle.
b. attain a position of comfort.
c. gain exposure of the back.
d. relax the musculature.

© 1996 by Lippincott-Raven Publishers

MODULE

13

ADMISSION, TRANSFER, AND DISCHARGE

MODULE CONTENTS

RATIONALE FOR THE USE OF THIS
 SKILL
PLACEMENT OF PATIENTS ADMITTED
ADMISSION
Immediate Needs
Introductions and Orientation
Baseline Assessment
Personal Property
Documentation
TRANSFER
Order for Transfer
Notifying Appropriate Persons
Interacting With the Patient
Caring for Personal Property
Completing or Duplicating Records
Completing Assessment Data and Care
 Plan

Arranging Transportation
Giving Report
DISCHARGE
Order for Discharge
Patient Teaching
Continuity of Care
Final Assessment
Personal Property
Business Matters
Record Keeping
DELEGATING TASKS
LONG-TERM CARE
HOME CARE
CRITICAL THINKING EXERCISES

PREREQUISITES

Successful completion of the following modules:

VOLUME 1

Module 1 An Approach to Nursing Skills
Module 2 Basic Infection Control
Module 3 Safety
Module 5 Documentation
Module 6 Introduction to Assessment Skills
Module 7 Temperature, Pulse, and Respiration
Module 8 Blood Pressure

Module 11, Collecting Specimens and Performing Common Laboratory Tests, may be needed.
Module 20, Transfer, and Module 21, Ambulation, may be essential for admitting some incapacitated patients.

© 1996 by Lippincott-Raven Publishers

OVERALL OBJECTIVE

To admit, transfer, and discharge patients, taking into consideration both the needs of individual patients and the needs of the healthcare agency.

SPECIFIC LEARNING OBJECTIVES

Know Facts and Principles	Apply Facts and Principles	Demonstrate Ability	Evaluate Performance
ADMISSION			
1. Immediate needs			
a. *Physical*			
b. *Psychosocial*			
Discuss various physical needs patient may have on admission.	Given a patient situation, identify physical needs that take priority.	When admitting a patient, take action to meet immediate needs, both physical and emotional.	Check patient for evidence of comfort and relaxation.
Discuss various psychosocial needs patient may have on admission.	Given a patient situation, identify psychosocial needs that take priority.		
2. Introduction and orientation			
a. *Staff*			
b. *Environment*			
c. *Expectations and role*			
State rationale for introducing patient to staff and environment.	List information specific patient would need on admission.	When admitting a patient, introduce staff present and environment, and discuss expectations for patient's behavior.	Elicit patient's evaluation of adequacy of introductions and orientation.
State rationale for orienting patient to expectations and role and discussing patient's expectations.			
3. Baseline assessment			
a. *Observation*			
b. *Physical assessment*			
c. *Interview and history taking*			
List initial observations that must be made.	Given data on a new patient, identify observations needed for patient.	When admitting a patient, make appropriate observations.	Use the Basic Data Gathering Guide in Module 6, General Assessment Overview, to evaluate completeness of assessment.
List information that should be obtained.	Given data on a new patient, outline interview to be done.	Obtain needed information through interview.	
4. Care of personal property			
Discuss nurse's responsibility toward patient's property.	State usual disposition of personal effects in own facility.	Arrange for safekeeping of patient's property.	

(continued)

© 1996 by Lippincott-Raven Publishers

SPECIFIC LEARNING OBJECTIVES (Continued)

Know Facts and Principles	Apply Facts and Principles	Demonstrate Ability	Evaluate Performance
5. Documentation			
State rationale for maintaining accurate patient records.	List records required in own facility.	Document observations, interview, disposition of personal property.	Evaluate own performance using list of forms in Performance Checklist.
TRANSFER			
1. Notify appropriate persons			
List persons who should be made aware of transfer.	Within the facility, note names and departments that should be contacted.	Under the supervision of a staff nurse, make necessary calls.	Check calls made against written hospital policy.
2. Interaction with patient			
Explore reason for visit and topics that might be discussed.	Given a situation, discuss topics that may be discussed with patient before time of transfer.	Vist a patient being transferred and identify information needed.	Validate your assessment of needs with primary nurse.
3. Care of personal property			
State procedure for transfer of property with patient.	Consult policy manual for places personal effects are stored.	Review forms used in your facility for logging personal effects.	Assess patient's completed forms before transfer.
4. Communication to receiving staff			
Discuss written and verbal communications to be transmitted to those who will be caring for the patient.	List kinds of forms and other verbal information that should be communicated to receiving staff.	Review policy of your facility regarding communicating patient data to receiving staff.	Elicit primary nurse's evaluation of information you have communicated to receiving staff.
DISCHARGE			
1. Planning for continuity of care			
State rationale for continuity of care. List resources for continuing care.	Given a situation, identify resources that would be needed for continued care.	For a patient in the clinical area, plan appropriately for care after discharge from unit.	Evaluate comprehensiveness of planning with instructor.
2. Patient teaching			
List common learning needs for patients being discharged.	Given a situation, identify learning needs.	Teach patient in clinical area before discharge within limits of own ability.	Evaluate effectiveness of teaching with instructor.
3. Final assessment			
Explain why final assessment is needed.	Given a situation, list appropriate final assessment information for patient.	Make complete final assessment of patient.	Evaluate own performance using the Basic Data Gathering guide in Module 5, General Assessment Overview.

(continued)

© 1996 by Lippincott-Raven Publishers

SPECIFIC LEARNING OBJECTIVES (Continued)

Know Facts and Principles	Apply Facts and Principles	Demonstrate Ability	Evaluate Performance
4. Care of personal property			
List places personal effects may be kept.	List forms for own facility that must be completed at discharge regarding patient's belongings.	Retrieve all of patient's personal effects and see that they accompany patient.	Use Performance Checklist to see that all items are completed.
5. Business functions			
Discuss usual business functions for which nurse is responsible.	List business functions required in facility.	When discharging patient, see that financial arrangements are completed. Obtain medications and supplies if needed.	Evaluate completion of business functions with instructor.
6. Documentation			
Discuss usual records to be filled out.	List discharge records required in facility.	Document data on entire discharge procedure.	Evaluate own performance using list of forms in Performance Checklist.

© 1996 by Lippincott-Raven Publishers

LEARNING ACTIVITIES

1. Review the Specific Learning Objectives.
2. Read the section on threats to the patient's mental health (in the chapter on mental health) in Ellis and Nowlis, *Nursing: A Human Needs Approach,* or comparable material in another textbook.
3. Look up the module vocabulary terms in the glossary.
4. Read through the module contents and mentally practice completing the process with a patient. Study the material as though you were planning to teach it to someone else.
4. Check the procedure book at your facility for the forms and processes required for admission, transfer, and discharge.

5. Assist a staff member or more experienced student with the admission of a patient. Discuss the procedure:
   a. Were all steps included?
   b. Did more than one person participate in the process?
6. With the supervision of your instructor, admit a patient. Evaluate your own performance using the Performance Checklist. Consult with your instructor regarding your performance.
7. Repeat steps 5 and 6 for the transfer of a patient.
8. Repeat steps 5 and 6 for the discharge of a patient.

VOCABULARY

acuity	nursing history
AMA	referral
assessment	urinalysis
chart	

© 1996 by Lippincott-Raven Publishers

Admission, Transfer, and Discharge

Rationale for the Use of This Skill

Nursing has moved to a focus on continuity of care, wherever that care occurs. This means assuring that as the patient moves between home, acute care, and long-term care, healthcare needs are identified, nursing care is appropriately planned, and support services are continued. To effectively assure this smooth progression, the nurse must give careful attention to the processes involved in admission, transfer, and discharge. Many facilities have developed plans for continuous progress called "care pathways" or "critical paths." These provide guidelines for all staff in monitoring the patient's progress.

For most people, entering a healthcare facility is a major crisis. Individuals have many needs and concerns that must be identified and for which action must be taken. In addition, each healthcare facility must maintain certain routine procedures and gather specific information about incoming patients that will help it perform its functions. Identifying and meeting both sets of needs is a challenging task for the nurse. The person entering the hospital may be coming from either a long-term care facility or home. The person entering long-term care may likewise be moving from home or from an acute care hospital. Admission information must be complete and accurate. A care provider in the family or a home care nurse is often appropriately involved in this transition; their perceptions may provide valuable information.

Units within the hospital may be specialized, and this means that a patient may sometimes need to be transferred from one unit to another within the facility. Also, since the passage of the 1983 Medicare prospective reimbursement system, which limited the funding available for acute hospitalization for those on Medicare and Medicaid and changes in health insurance benefits that restrict the number of acute care hospital days, patients are being transferred to long-term care facilities or home for continued treatment and convalescence. Consequently, the transfer procedure is of growing importance. If it is done carefully, the relocation will have minimal impact on the patient, and the receiving staff or family caregivers will be provided with adequate knowledge on which to base comprehensive nursing care.

Whenever a patient enters any healthcare facility, the nurse should always keep that person's possible transfer and eventual discharge in mind. For most patients, the nurse should begin planning for eventual transfer or discharge at the time the patient is admitted (Fig. 13–1).

When people are ready to leave the healthcare facility for home, the nurse has a similar responsibility. You should instruct the patient in any aspect of care that will be done on a continuing basis and that involves the patient or family. Answer any questions to decrease anxiety and share any resources that may be useful. [1]

PLACEMENT OF PATIENTS ADMITTED

The placement of patients who are admitted into the facility is usually a cooperative effort between the admitting department and the individual unit. The individual unit must assure that there is adequate staffing for the number of patients who will be on the unit and that the staff members have the expertise to meet the patient's needs. Placement also depends on the condition of the patient and the size of the facility and whether it has specialty units.

In larger hospitals, patients are admitted to units that specialize in treatment of their condition. For example, surgical patients are admitted to a surgical unit. A hospital may be large enough that there is even specialization within the units; patients having abdominal surgery are admitted to one unit and patients having facial surgery are admitted to another. In smaller hospitals, rather than being admitted to specialized units, patients may be admitted strictly on the basis of empty beds. Acuity (the seriousness of the patient's condition) is another factor determining where patients are placed. *Very ill patients need a higher staff ratio than patients who are more convalescent.* If the room is not private, efforts are made to choose an appropriate roommate for the new patient.

ADMISSION

When admitting a person to a healthcare facility, the patient should be your primary source of information if at all possible. However, the family or caregiver may provide useful information that will help you carry out your assessment. As the nurse, you have many responsibilities, which include:

1. Reviewing the physician's orders
2. Meeting the person's immediate needs
   a. Physical
   b. Psychosocial
3. Providing introductions and orientation
4. Performing a baseline assessment
   a. Observations and physical examination
   b. Interview and history taking
5. Caring for personal property
6. Documentation

---

[1] Rationale for action is emphasized throughout the module by the use of italics.

© 1996 by Lippincott-Raven Publishers

These activities will not always be done in the same order. For example, an item from baseline assessment may conveniently be done at the same time that you begin documentation. The needs of the individual patient and your own convenience will guide you.

Reviewing the Physician's Orders

A review of the physician's orders will identify the reason for admission and the plans for medical care that the nurse will assure are initiated. Some of these tasks may require immediate communication to other departments or implementation by the nurse. Some of these tasks may be delegated to a unit secretary or clerk in order for the nurse to move quickly to assessment of the patient.

Meeting the Person's Immediate Needs

A brief general assessment of a new patient *to ascertain immediate needs* is essential. This should be your first concern. *A person does not enter a hospital unless a healthcare problem is present.* This problem may not be causing any immediate distress, or it may be acute. A well-founded criticism of some healthcare workers is that they are so concerned about routines and forms that the patients' primary problems remain uncared for.

Immediate needs can be either physical or psychosocial. If a patient is in acute pain, contact the physician immediately regarding orders for medication and care; meanwhile, institute nursing measures to relieve pain. If a patient is upset or distraught, spend time listening and talking to the patient; *this can facilitate the transition to the hospital environment. If patients believe that those around are concerned about their immediate needs and are taking action to meet them, a relationship of trust may well have begun.*

Providing Introductions and Orientation

When you deem it appropriate, it is your responsibility to introduce the patient and family members to people in the environment. This may be the very first thing you do, but it can wait until more immediate needs have been met. Here you must use your judgment.

Your greeting should convey interest in and concern for patients. Patients just entering a healthcare facility are really not concerned about your problems of staffing or time except as they directly affect their own care. If it is necessary for patients to wait, an explanation is appreciated.

Although you should not expect a patient to remember the names of all staff members initially, *introducing yourself and others by both name and position helps the patient to become oriented to what is happening.* Other patients in the same room should also be introduced using the desired name.

Explain what will occur during the admitting process. *This relieves the anxiety created by fear of the unknown.*

A thorough orientation to the unit includes an explanation of all items for the patient's use which areas are for personal belongings, and the location of the bathroom. Especially important are directions on how to operate the bed and TV and how to call a nurse.

Explain in detail anything you expect a patient to do, from exactly what to wear under the hospital gown to what activity is ordered. *A patient will be better able to participate in care if expectations are clearly defined.*

Performing a Baseline Assessment

The information to be gathered in baseline assessment varies from one facility to another based on the common needs and problems of the patients. In some facilities, the nurse does a complete physical examination. In others, the nurse may do a thorough nursing assessment that does not encompass the traditional physical examination. In long-term care facilities, the federally mandated Minimum Data Set (MDS) guides admission assessment.

Admission assessment almost always includes temperature, pulse, and respiration (TPR) and blood pressure (Fig. 13–2).

(For guidelines on taking TPR, see Module 7, and for taking blood pressure, Module 8.) Height and weight are also measured. If the patient cannot stand, estimate his or her height or ask the patient or family for this information. You can measure weight using one of several types of scales. A regular balanced scale may be used, but many hospitals now use electronic scales. Bed and chair scales are also available. Scales often have wheels *to facilitate moving them to the bedside.* Both bed and chair scales have the directions printed on them.

Laboratory values often are a part of the baseline assessment. Depending on the diagnosis, some patients now have needed laboratory work done the day before admission to decrease costs and length of stay in the hospital. Much of the routine admitting laboratory work done in the past is now viewed as unnecessary; therefore, many patients enter the hospital with little or no laboratory work complet-

© 1996 by Lippincott-Raven Publishers

HEALTH CARE TEAM MEMBERS

Primary Nurse: *Beth Jordan, R.N.*

Associate Nurse: *Ann Strong, R.N.*

Consultants:
Nurse: ——

Physician: *Wm. Hawkins, M.D.*

Resident: *Tom Andrews, M.D.*

Chaplain: ——

Other: *Donna Nunn,*   Old Charts Ord.:
Resp. Therapy

Sacrament of Sick:

Code Status: *Full*   Per MD:

Date: *4/16/99*   Initials:

Diagnosis:
Asthma/pneumonia

Surgical Procedures:
∅

ADDRESSOGRAPH:
Jordan, Ellen C.   F-53
278-16-4351
Dr. Radford

DISCHARGE NEEDS:

Patient's plans for care after discharge: *Temporary conval. center placement*

Obstacles in living environment: *Lives in rural area, husband works.*

Need for discharge care referral/services: NO/(YES) Equipment/Supplies
(ECF)/VNS/Sustaining Care/Support Services
Patient Services Coordinator/Maternal Newborn Coordinator Notified:
NO/(YES)

4/16 Contact Blaine Conval. Center.
prior to discharge per Wm. Hawkins, M.D.

Discharge plans discussed with
family, B.J.

Postop day:
——

Hospital day:
1

SWEDISH HOSPITAL MEDICAL CENTER
Seattle, WA 98104

Figure 13–1. Discharge planning may be recorded at the time of admission.

ed. In some facilities, patients are taken to the laboratory area on the way to the unit for any necessary testing.

A nursing history is usually obtained. Even if a formalized nursing history is not used, information relating to allergies, current medications, and the patient's perception of the entering problem (often called the *chief complaint*) is gathered. An interview is used to gather subjective information regarding the patient. A variety of forms are available for recording both subjective and objective data (Figs. 13–1 through 13–3). These data are necessary to evaluate future observations and other data gathered.

Caring for Personal Property

One of the more difficult problems in an institution, large or small, is keeping track of a patient's personal property. *The loss of valued items is upsetting to patients and can be costly to an institution.*

Most facilities have a routine for checking and noting all personal items a patient brings or wears to the facility. Items that are not needed can be sent home with family members. This is perhaps the best safeguard. Large sums of money and valuable items are usually kept in a safe in the business office with proper documents attesting to their location and their value. The amount of money a patient should keep at the bedside depends on the policy of the facility and the patient's personal wishes and needs.

Items kept with the patient are less likely to get lost if they are marked with the patient's name, but this is not always possible in an acute care environment. In long-term care facilities, the staff arranges to have personal belongings, including all clothing, marked. Arrange to keep these possessions together in a place accessible to the patient. A printed list of clothing and personal effects that you can quickly check off is often used to make an exact inventory. Fig. 13–4 is an example of a clothing and personal effects list.

Documentation

Documenting all parts of the admission process is essential for legal records. The baseline assessment serves as a reference throughout the period of care, and fre-

© 1996 by Lippincott-Raven Publishers

NURSING ADMISSION DATA

Patient arrived via: Amb. (WC) Cart		TPR 98² - 88 - 24		BP 142/82		WT. 163	HT. 6'

From: (Home) ECF ER Other

Emergency Notification: *Eileen (wife)*
Phone No. *(714) 283 6140*

Allergies: (drug, food, other) — *NKA*
Reaction (describe):

VALUABLES: DESCRIPTION	LOCATION	Medications	Dose	Frequency	Last Dose	Location
(Glasses)(Contacts):	on pt.	*Theophyllin p.o.*	200 mg.	q. 6. h.	0600 4/16	
Hearing Aid:	Ø	*Imipenem i.v.*	500 mg.	q. 6. h.	1200 4/15	
Mobility Aid:	cane	*Prednisone p.o.*	10 mg.	B.I.D.	0900 4/16	
Prosthesis:	Ø	*Colace p.o.*	100 mg.	B.I.D.	—	
Dentures(Upper)(Lower) Partial	in place	*Hycodan Syrup p.o.*	5 ml.	q 4 h PRN for cough	—	
Wallet:	wife					
Money:	pt. $9.40					
Watch: ✓	wearing silver colored					
Jewelry: ✓	wedding ring					
Camera:	Ø					

ORIENTATION TO HOSPITAL: Visiting Hours ☑ Chaplaincy Service ☑ Hospital Educational TV ☑
Info Booklet ☐ Call System ☑ Bed Controls ☑ Bathroom ☑ Storage ☐ TV ☑ Telephone ☑

Date: 4/13/99   Time: 1300   Signature: *S. Martin, R.N.*

Williams, Thomas   **NURSING DATA BASE**

Significant Past Health History: NO (YES) Cardiac/Respiratory/Neurological/Muscular-skeletal/Endocrine/G.I./G.U./Liver Disease/Skin/Past Surgeries: Pregnancies/At risk for hepatitis B: (NO)YES HBS_A +/−

Present Illness and Patient's Expectation of Hospitalization: *Recurrence of Asthma/pneumonia*

Figure 13–2. A form used to record baseline information gained from a nursing history.

quently the record of care of personal effects must be consulted. In addition, you may be responsible for a variety of other records (notification of the dietary department, starting a Kardex card and medication record, filling out census forms, and so forth). Consult the procedure book at each facility to determine which forms are your responsibility.

TRANSFER

A patient may be transferred within the unit. This may be at the request of the physician, nurse, or the patient. The physician or nurse may request a change to a private room because of a deterioration in the patient's condition. The patient or family may also request a change, usually to a private room, because of excessive talking by a roommate or disturbances in the environment that interfere with the patient's rest. In either event, efforts are made to accommodate the request on a vacancy basis.

You are responsible to document in the record that the change has been made and the reason. Inform the admitting department and information desk of the room and bed change. Make sure that all forms and lists correctly note the patient's new location.

When you transfer a patient to another unit or to another facility, you are responsible for carrying out certain procedures that will make the transition as smooth and nonstressful as possible for the patient and the receiving staff. These include:

1. Obtaining the order for transfer
2. Notifying appropriate persons
3. Interacting with the patient, including reinforcing any health teaching
4. Caring for the patient's personal property
5. Completing and duplicating records, assessment data, and care plan
6. Arranging transportation
7. Giving report

Obtaining the Order for Transfer

A physician usually writes the order transferring a patient within the hospital or to another facility. If there is some nursing reason for transfer, such as inability to provide a room or equipment for a special patient need, notify the physician, who will then write the order. In an emergency, such as when a patient must be moved to a critical care unit, the transfer is made and the physician writes the order later. A physician's order must be obtained for transferring a patient.

Notifying Appropriate Persons

You are responsible to notify all persons involved of the transfer. These include the nursing supervisor, admitting department personnel, the patient's family, and the unit or facility that is receiving the patient. The discharge planner may already have made these contacts for you.

<table>
<tr><td>

SLEEP/COMFORT

PAIN: NO/(YES) Location _breathing_
Duration _____ Type _Sharp_
Pain Tolerance 1 2 3 4 (5) 6 7 8 9 10
Usual bedtime _____ 2200 _____
Usual awakening _____ 0600 _____
Nap during day: ☐ Yes ☒ No

</td><td>

NEUROSENSORY

LEVEL OF CONSCIOUSNESS: Alert/Lethargic/Restless/
Agitated/Coma/Seizure Disorder _Ø_
PUPIL STATUS (when indicated) _N.A._
ORIENTATION: Person/Place/Time/Situation _oriented_

SENSORY DISABILITY:(NO)/YES

DTR'S: RA | LA Clonus (NO)/YES _____
       RL | LL

Headache/Visual Disturbances:(NO)/YES

</td></tr>
</table>

COMMUNICATION

PRIMARY LANGUAGE: (If not English) _____
Interpreter _N.A._
Phone Number _____
Deficit of Speech/Hearing/Vision/(None)

SKIN

SENSITIVITIES: Soap/Tape/Lotion/Iodine/Other _none_
CONDITION: Normal/Dry/Bruises/Abrasions/Open Wounds/
Ulcers/Rash
Describe _____

SOCIAL/EMOTIONAL

AFFECT: Within normal limits/Angry/Anxious/
Depressed/Flat/Hostile

LIVES: Alone/With family/With friends – _with wife_

SUPPORT SYSTEMS: Describe _minimal – wife anxious,_
close to couple from church
OCCUPATION:
Last Date Worked: _____
Length of Maternity Leave _N.A._

NUTRITION

Pre-Pregnant Weight
RECENT WEIGHT CHANGE: Gain/Loss _none_ Pounds
INTAKE: Normal/Nausea/Vomiting/Malnourished/Indigestion
Other _____

SPECIAL DIET: NO/(YES) Type _4 small meals until breathing improves_

ALCOHOL: Type and amount _occasional_

RESPIRATORY

QUALITY: Normal/Labored/Shallow/SOB/SOB c̄
exertion/Orthopnea/Other _____
COUGH: Absent/Non-productive/Productive _mod. amt –_
LUNG SOUNDS: _dull in ↓ lobes, wheezes_   _clear mucus_
TOBACCO USE:(NO)/YES Type and amount _____

GI/GU

ABDOMEN: Normal/Tender/Rigid/Distended/Gravid

EPIGASTRIC PAIN:(NO)/YES
BOWEL TONES: Normal/Hypo-active/Hyper-active/Absent
BOWELS: Usual Pattern _qod_ Last BM _4/12_
Laxatives/Enemas: NO/YES
Diarrhea/Constipation/Hemorrhoids/Other
URINARY: No difficulty/Frequency/Urgency/Pain/Burning/
Hematuria

Proteinuria/Glucosuria _Ø_

CIRCULATORY

HEART RHYTHM: Regular/Irregular

PERIPHERAL PULSES (When Indicated) _present_

Edema/(NO)/YES Periorbital/Facial/Hands/Lower
Extremities

Dehydration (NO)/YES

SKIN COLOR: Normal/Cyanotic/Dusky/Jaundice _mild_
SKIN TEMPERATURE: Normal/Cold/Hot/Diaphoretic
PREVIOUS TRANSFUSIONS:(NO)/YES

ACTIVITY LEVEL _bedrest – up as tolerated_
LIMITATIONS IN MOVEMENT:(NO)/YES

REPRODUCTION/SEXUALITY

LAST MENSTRUAL PERIOD _N.A._ EDC _____

Discharge/Bleeding/Pain _N.A._

SEXUALLY TRANSMITTED DISEASES:(NO)/YES Chlamydia/
Yeast/Trich/GC/Syphilis/B. Strep/Others _____
Herpes NO/YES Site _____
Last Culture _____ Current Status _____

Date: _4/13/98_   Time: _1300_   RN Signature _S. Martin, R.N._

ROOM # _1402_   NAME: _Williams, Thomas_   _Dr. Bernie Schiff_   CATEGORY: _Medical_

Figure 13–3. A form used to record both subjective and objective information related to functional areas.

Interacting with the Patient

Any patient has the right to know of the transfer plans. This principle is most often violated with the elderly. Transferring frail, sick, older people without their knowledge takes away their right to decision-making about their own healthcare. Transfers from a familiar long-term care setting to the hospital and from an acute care setting to long-term care may each be upsetting. You can clarify the transfer and answer any questions the patient or family may have regarding the new environment. If you note any signs of anxiety about the transfer, spend time with the patient and the family, allowing them to talk about their concerns.

Caring for Personal Property

Make sure that all personal property is checked and accompanies the patient being transferred when appropriate. The resident of a long-term care facility

© 1996 by Lippincott-Raven Publishers

Northwest Hospital
SEATTLE, WASHINGTON 98133

**PATIENT'S VALUABLE
ENVELOPE**

Nolan, Christine   F-47
276-89-3796
Dr. Stewart

CONTENTS OF ENVELOPE DEPOSITED WITH HOSPITAL	ARTICLES RETAINED BY PATIENT OR RESPONSIBLE PARTY
☑ CASH *$50.00*	☑ CASH *$11.20*
☐ WATCH	☑ WATCH
☐ RINGS	☑ RINGS *wedding (1)*
☐ WALLET	☐ WALLET
☐ OTHER EXPLAIN	☐ OTHER EXPLAIN
☐ OTHER EXPLAIN	☑ DENTURES PARTIAL *lower / partial*
☐ OTHER EXPLAIN	☑ GLASSES
☐ OTHER EXPLAIN	☐ RAZOR
☐ OTHER EXPLAIN	☐ OTHER EXPLAIN
☐ OTHER EXPLAIN	☐ OTHER EXPLAIN

NEITHER NORTHWEST HOSPITAL NOR THE MEMBERS OF ITS STAFF SHALL BE
RESPONSIBLE FOR VALUABLES NOT DEPOSITED IN THE BUSINESS OFFICE.

I, THE PATIENT, OR RESPONSIBLE PARTY ASSUME FULL RESPONSIBILITY FOR
THOSE ITEMS RETAINED IN MY POSSESSION DURING MY HOSPITALIZATION.
I HAVE CHECKED THE ABOVE AND ACKNOWLEDGE THE LISTS TO BE CORRECT.

DATE: *4/16/98*   PATIENT'S SIGNATURE OR RESPONSIBLE PARTY: *Bella Sutherland*

TIME: *0845*   HOSPITAL EMPLOYEE: *Al Feldon, N.A.*

RECEIVED BY BUSINESS OFFICE: *Karen Jornis, Sec.*

RELEASE OF VALUABLES:

ORIGINAL — PATIENT
YELLOW — CHART
ENVELOPE— BUSINESS OFFICE
NWH A-50 8/74

Released By: _____ Date __/__/__

Patient or Responsible Party: _____

Figure 13–4. An example of a list of valuables and their disposition.

may be returning to that facility to reside after an acute hospitalization.

Completing or Duplicating Records, Assessment Data, and Care Plan

If the patient is being transferred *within the facility,* gather all assessment forms and care plans, bedside equipment, and plastic identification card. Review the assessment and care plan for completeness and accuracy. Make an appropriate entry in the record concerning the move. Although you can begin preparing the documents that will accompany the patient a day or so before transfer, it is essential to update the data and care plan just before the patient leaves. This provides the receiving staff with a cur-

rent assessment and identification of any unresolved patient problems. Remember that these documents are confidential and should be given only to authorized persons (Fig. 13–5).

Arranging Transportation

When the patient is being transferred from an acute care hospital to a nursing home or another facility, the business office or discharge planner often makes arrangements for an ambulance or Cab-ambulance (a specially fitted van that can transport patients who do not need close monitoring). When critical care is needed, the nurse may make arrangements, particularly when the patient needs special equipment, such as oxygen or maintenance of intravenous therapy, or specialized personnel, such as a

© 1996 by Lippincott-Raven Publishers

Original Copy Goes To Receiving Facility — Xerox Copy To Be Retained In Patient Record — **Attach Xerox Copy Of Patient Admittance Sheet.**

Patient's Last Name	First Name	MI
Hogan	*Susan*	*T*

Address, City, State, Zip Code		Phone
1018 Alder St., Blaine, OR 87453		*(503) 788-1011*

Date of Birth	Age	Sex	Marital Status	Church
1-18-59	*36*	*F*	S (M) W D Sep.	*C*

Relative or Guardian (specify relationship) name, address		Phone
Jeff	*husb.*	*same*

Name and Address of Facility Transferring:

From: *Mountain View Hospital*

To: *Coast Conval. Center*   Pt. Hosp. No. *6402573*

Family Informed Of Transfer   Yes ☑ No ☐
Does patient know diagnosis   Yes ☑ No ☐
Does family know diagnosis   Yes ☑ No ☐
Date of telephone referral: *5/19* Adm. Date: *4/16* Discharge Date: *5/21/99*
Previous Hospitalization and/or Nursing Home Stay (Within last 90 days):
   none

Health Insurance Info: Soc. Sec. No. *462-51-8717*
   Medicare ———   Medicaid ———
   Other *Loggers Int.*

PHYSICIANS ORDERS

Attending Physician: *Wm. Hawkins, M.D.*
Consulting Physician(s): *Tom Andrews, M.D.*
Physician after transfer: *Donna Wilson, M.D.*
Admitting Diagnosis:
Discharge Diagnosis:
   Primary: *Multiple Sclerosis*

   Secondary: *Infected (R) hip decubitus*

Course of Treatment: attach copy of Physician's Discharge Summary.
   see attached

Any significant changes from initial H & P   ☐ Yes   ☑ No
   If Yes, changes are:

MEDICATION ORDER FOR RECEIVING FACILITY (If PRN, state reason for giving and max, amt. to be given. List discontinuation date, if any, on all medications ordered) Note: Any brand or form of drug identical in form and content may be dispensed unless checked here: ☐

   Ibuprofen 200 mg. PRN for pain.
   Multivit. ī q. d.
   Colace 100 mg. B.I.D.

DIET ☑ Regular ☐ Sodium Restriction, _____ gm. ☐ Salt Substitute _____ ☐ Diabetic, ___ calories ☐ Low Residue ☐ Bland
☐ Mechanical ☐ Soft ☐ Tube, ___ cc per _____ hr ☐ Dietary Supplement _____ ☑ Other *added fiber*

ALLERGIES ☑ No ☐ Yes   Type: _____

SPECIAL TREATMENTS (Including Physical Therapy, Speech, O.T., etc.) Specify frequency.
   ↑ oral fluids to 2600 ml./day   *Dressing - OpSite over decubiti p̄ warm*
   special air mattress   *saline soaks q. d.*
   assist pt. to turn frequently when in bed.

ACTIVITY ORDERS (List activity level, restrictions and/or precautions, etc.) Note: If ordering restraints indicate reason for use.

   Increase activity level - assist with cane walking.

REHABILITATION POTENTIAL (Describe the highest level of independent, functioning the patient can be expected to achieve.)
   ☐ **Independent**   **Semi-Independent:** ☑ Assistance for few activities   ☐ Assistance for most activities
ADDITIONAL COMMENTS: *Outcomes — Maintain skin integrity, possible remission of M.S.*

Certification ☑ I certify that post hospital skilled nursing care is medically necessary on a continuing basis for any of the conditions for which he/she received care during this hospitalization. ☐ I certify that my above orders regarding home health services (skilled nursing care, therapy, or others as defined) are medically necessary because my patient is confined to home. These services are related to the condition(s) for which he/she received inpatient hospital or SNF care.

Signature of Physician *Wm. A. Hawkins* _____ MD   Phone: *732-8077*   Date: *5/20/99*
This form has been approved by the Seattle Area Hospital Council and the Washington State Health Facilities Association. To re-order, call (206) 281-8989
Revised Date September 1981   **PATIENT TRANSFER FORM**   Seattle Area Hospital Council

Figure 13–5. An example of a patient's transfer form.

© 1996 by Lippincott-Raven Publishers

respiratory therapist or critical care nurse. If the patient is going to another unit of the facility, you may decide whether the patient can be transferred by wheelchair or stretcher.

Giving Report

When the patient is going to another unit of the same facility, call the new unit and go with the patient *so that you can give the nursing staff a verbal report and answer any questions.* When the patient is being transferred to another hospital or to another facility, duplicate the records and make a telephone call to the receiving staff, giving them a comprehensive report regarding the patient. Records also may be faxed.

DISCHARGE

When you are planning for a patient's discharge home, your responsibilities are similar to those in transfer to another unit and include the following:

1. Obtaining order for discharge
2. Planning for continuity of care
3. Providing patient teaching
4. Performing a final assessment
5. Caring for personal property
6. Performing business functions
7. Documentation

Obtaining Order for Discharge

An order is needed for the patient to be discharged. Although the nurse begins planning for the patient's discharge as early as admission, no business documents or final papers are started until the precise time of discharge is determined. However, if you have been told verbally that a patient is to be discharged but the order has not yet been written, you may sometimes complete such tasks as ordering take-home medications and making patient assessments before the actual discharge order is written *so that the patient's departure is not delayed.*

Occasionally, a patient becomes disgruntled or impatient and demands to leave the facility without the physician's order for discharge. Efforts are made to contact and notify the physician when this occurs. An AMA (against medical advice) form is completed and signed by the patient before leaving, releasing the facility of any responsibility. Some facilities are no longer using the AMA form but instead request the nurse on duty to document the patient's leaving without an order on the record.

Planning for Continuity of Care

Your nursing responsibility does not end when the patient leaves the area in which you work. You are responsible to see that plans are made for continuing care as needed. Because of current regulations regarding increasing healthcare costs both in the private sector (insurance) and Medicare, more patients are being discharged to either long-term care or home earlier than they used to be. You as the nurse often identify an ongoing patient need that could be addressed by a community agency. You should be knowledgeable regarding the many agencies in your area. Making referrals to agencies that provide a variety of home services is becoming a vital extension of nursing care. As a member of the healthcare team, always include the physician, discharge planner, and others in deciding on a referral. Some agencies require a physician's order, and others do not. Both the patient and the family should be informed of the availability of the service before the contact actually takes place. Share confidential and appropriate information with the agency involved. Fill in the name of the agency on the discharge form or make an addendum (Fig. 13–6).

Many nurses encourage patients to call the unit after discharge if they have any concerns. On some acute care and long-term care units, it is the nurse's responsibility to call patients after discharge to ask about their progress and answer any questions.

When a postdischarge call is made, it is documented for legal purposes.

Providing Patient Teaching

Talk with the patient regarding the planned time of departure and how you might be useful in the discharge. Explain what will happen and when it will happen. The patient may need information about medications, treatments, activity, diet, and continued health supervision. You may need to plan to obtain medications that will be taken home to facilitate teaching about them. Ideally, teaching will have begun earlier so the patient is not overwhelmed with stimuli and information at the time of discharge. Occasionally, however, teaching is not done in advance and must be done on the day of discharge. Often the family is also included in the teaching.

A form detailing home care instructions may be given to the patient being discharged. These forms may give only general guidelines or they may be very specific, for example, postdischarge care after a certain type of illness or surgery (Fig. 13–6). Either verbally or by written order, physicians will sometimes request that you make appointments for pa-

© 1996 by Lippincott-Raven Publishers

HOME CARE INSTRUCTIONS AFTER SURGERY

1. **DISCHARGE PLAN:** (Please Circle)   ECF   Home Health Agency   Sustaining Care   Other
   Follow-up plan not indicated because: (independent)   (family and/or friends will assist)   refused

2. **DIET:** *Regular*   , Fluid, fiber and fruits in your diet will help prevent constipation. Food rich in protein will aid in wound healing.

3. **ACTIVITY:**   Follow your doctor's instructions regarding activity.
   a.   Avoid pushing, pulling, lifting, prolonged standing or sitting until advised by your physician.
   b.   Take an hour rest period in the morning and afternoon.
   c.   Contact physician prior to driving a car.

4. **MEDICATIONS:**   (OWN MEDICATIONS)   PHARMACY: (PRESCRIPTION)
   Review Pharmacy handout regarding discharge medications.

   Tylox one – two every four hours if needed for pain.
   Conjugated estrogen 0.625 mg. q. d. (daily)

5. **TREATMENTS/EQUIPMENT AND SUPPLIES:**

   none
   May shower, resume walking to tolerance.

6. **SYMPTOMS TO REPORT TO YOUR DOCTOR:**   Call your doctor with any questions.
   a.   Bleeding, drainage, redness or swelling from incisional area.
   b.   If feeling chilled or feverish, take temperature and report if over 100.5 degrees.
   c.   Nausea and vomiting or abdominal distention.
   d.   Pain not relieved by pain medication or rest should be reported to your doctor.
   e.   Difficulty with urination - frequency and/or burning.

7. **OTHER INSTRUCTIONS:**
   a.   As you increase your activity you may experience some discomfort or moderate pain.
   b.   Showers may be taken. Do not tub bathe before checking with doctor.
   c.   After gynecological or bladder repairs check with physician prior to resuming intercourse.
   d.   Consult with physician if any change from normal bowel functions.

8. **APPOINTMENTS:**   Please call to make appointment.
   With: *Dr. Sue Hancock*   When: *one week*

I have received and understand the above instructions:

DATE: *7/2/99*   PATIENT: *Martha Cheavers*

WITNESS: *Jim Peters, RN*

PATIENT'S AGENT OR REPRESENTATIVE

ADDRESSOGRAPH	SWEDISH HOSPITAL MEDICAL CENTER Seattle, Washington

Figure 13–6. A form containing home care instructions may be given to a patient on discharge.

© 1996 by Lippincott-Raven Publishers

tients for an office visit after discharge. Always include this information on the discharge form if one is given to the patient or write it down and give it to the patient so that it will not be forgotten.

Preparing a Final Assessment

Before a patient leaves your unit, you must prepare a final assessment. Include the patient's physical status, psychosocial status, and ability to continue or participate in care.

If data indicate that the patient is not ready for discharge (if the patient has an elevated temperature, for example), report the information to the physician immediately for evaluation.

Caring for Personal Property

Be sure that all personal belongings accompany the patient. Especially critical are dentures, glasses, and special appliances such as crutches. Referring to the list of personal effects that was made on admission may be helpful, but remember that items brought in after admission may not be on the list. Check your list with the patient. Do not forget that there may be items in the safe or in the medicine room.

The patient may also take home items that were purchased in the hospital and are billed to the patient. These might include an egg-crate mattress, a sheepskin mattress pad, or an admission kit.

Performing Business Functions

Before a patient leaves a healthcare facility, it is customary for either the patient or the family to consult with the business office regarding financial matters. This may have been taken care of on admission through identification of an insurance company or a third-party payer. Be sure you know the usual routine in your facility. You may have to get drugs from the pharmacy or supplies from somewhere else for the patient to take home. You should plan for these items when you consider continuity of care and patient teaching.

Documentation

Again, forms vary from facility to facility. Document your plans for continuity of care, patient teaching, final assessment, disposition of personal items, and completion of business functions. Some facilities use a chart with a section that should help to remind you of all these points.

DELEGATING TASKS

If a nursing assistant, a volunteer, or anyone else is able to assist with a patient's admission, transfer, or discharge, you must carefully evaluate which tasks require greater skill and judgment. For example, decision-making and assessment are nursing functions that do not lend themselves to delegation to non-nursing personnel. A routine task such as orientation to the physical unit can be delegated.

LONG-TERM CARE

The procedures of admission, transfer, and discharge are very important to nurses practicing in long-term care settings. Along with direct admissions from home, many transfers take place between long-term and acute care. Residents whose condition requires hospitalization are transferred to hospitals, and chronically ill or recovering patients are transferred to long-term care. More patients are using long-term care facilities for rehabilitation purposes with home as the eventual destination.

Follow the same principles as those discussed earlier in this module. In the long-term care setting, however, it is essential that you include family members in planning. Clearly communicate information concerning special needs of residents so that the receiving facility is prepared to meet these needs. Close interaction and cooperation between the nursing staffs of the facilities leads to safe and effective care.

HOME CARE

As with long-term care, one of your responsibilities as a nurse is coordinating care between the home and the receiving or discharging facility. Your assessments and sharing of information is crucial to a smoother transition from one setting to another. You may also be a resource to family members in determining what is important to the patient. If going to the hospital or long-term care facility, the patient needs information on what clothing and possessions are appropriate to include. If coming home from a care setting, you can discuss what arrangements need to be made in the home, including adaptations that will aid the patient.

© 1996 by Lippincott-Raven Publishers

CRITICAL THINKING EXERCISES

• Mr. Robert Wagner is scheduled for discharge on the third morning after his cholecystectomy. His wound has an open draining area. He will have a prescription for pain medication and an oral antibiotic to take at home. He is to make an appointment to see his physician at the beginning of the next week. Identify the major concerns for this man's self-care at home. Describe the nursing responsibilities in managing his discharge.

• Margaret Wilson has resided in a special care unit for those with Alzheimer's disease for almost one year. This morning she collapsed and was found to have paralysis on her left side. The physician has ordered her transfer via ambulance to the hospital for diagnosis and treatment of a possible cerebral vascular accident. What unique problems might this transfer present? What are the special concerns that the nurse should communicate to the admitting hospital? What steps should the nurse take to ensure a smooth transition in this transfer?

© 1996 by Lippincott-Raven Publishers

✔ PERFORMANCE CHECKLIST

Admission	Needs More Practice	Satisfactory	Comments
1. Check for orders.			
2. Meet immediate needs. **a.** Physical			
b. Emotional			
3. Make introductions and orient patient. **a.** Greet patient.			
b. Introduce self.			
c. Explain admission routine			
d. Orient patient to individual unit: bed, bathroom, call light, supplies, and belongings.			
e. Orient patient to entire unit: location of nurses' station and day room or lounge.			
f. Explain expected behavior.			
g. Introduce other staff and roommates.			

4. Perform baseline assessment.
  a. Observation and physical examination
    (1) TPR			

(2) BP			
(3) Weight and height			
(4) Physical assessment			
b. Interview and history (1) Medications			
(2) Allergies			
(3) Entering complaints and concerns			
5. Take care of personal property. **a.** Items to be kept at bedside			
b. Items to be put in safe or medicine room			
c. Items to be sent home			
6. Document appropriately. **a.** All data recorded.			
b. Special forms for facility completed (add your own list of forms)			

(continued)

© 1996 by Lippincott-Raven Publishers

Transfer	Needs More Practice	Satisfactory	Comments
1. Check for orders.			
2. Notify appropriate persons. a. Nursing supervisor			
b. Admitting office			
c. Unit or facility receiving the patient			
d. Family members			
3. Visit the patient. a. Answer any questions about the transfer.			
b. Allay anxiety by spending time with the patient.			
4. Take care of personal property. a. Items kept at bedside			
b. Items in safe or medicine room			
5. Complete or duplicate records. a. Complete basic assessment.			
b. Complete or duplicate care plan.			
6. If not already arranged, obtain transportation; within hospital, wheelchair or stretcher.			
7. Give report. a. If transferring to another unit in the hospital, accompany patient and give report.			
b. If transferring to another facility, call and give report by phone.			
Discharge			
1. Check for orders.			
2. Plan for continuing care. a. Referrals as needed			
b. Information for new persons involved in care			
c. Contacting family or significant others if needed			
d. Transportation			
3. Teach patient. a. What to expect			
b. Medications			
c. Treatments			

(*continued*)

© 1996 by Lippincott-Raven Publishers

Discharge *(Continued)*	Needs More Practice	Satisfactory	Comments
d. Activity			
e. Diet			
f. Needs for continued health supervision			
4. Perform final assessment. **a.** Physical status			
b. Emotional status			
c. Ability to continue own care			
5. Check and return personal property. **a.** Personal items on unit			
b. Items from safe or medicine room			
6. Perform business functions. **a.** Financial matters			
b. Obtaining supplies			
7. Document appropriately. **a.** Discharge note			
b. Special forms for facility (add your own list of forms)			

© 1996 by Lippincott-Raven Publishers

? QUIZ

Multiple-Choice Questions

_____ **1.** The first thing you should do when admitting a patient is

    a. orient the patient to the unit.
    b. ascertain and meet the patient's immediate needs.
    c. take TPR and BP.
    d. make a baseline assessment.

_____ **2.** When orienting a patient to the environment, which of the following is not necessary?

    a. The location of the utility room and kitchenette
    b. How to call a nurse
    c. The location of the bathroom
    d. How to operate the bed

_____ **3.** If a patient is very distraught on admission, you should

    a. hurry as quickly as possible.
    b. go slowly to provide calm as you follow the usual routine.
    c. temporarily omit routine items.
    d. continue with the regular admission procedure as usual.

_____ **4.** If a volunteer is available to assist with admission, which task would it be most appropriate to delegate to him or her?

    a. Baseline assessment
    b. Ascertaining immediate needs
    c. Orientation to the unit
    d. Charting data

_____ **5.** Which of the following should you consider if you are transferring a patient to another unit? 1) continuing care; 2) patient teaching; 3) care of belongings; 4) final assessment

    a. 1, 2, and 4
    b. 2, 3, and 4
    c. 1 and 2 only
    d. All of these

_____ **6.** A patient has a very valuable jeweled ring. You would suggest

    a. that the patient wear it.
    b. that the patient hide it well in the suitcase.
    c. keeping it at the nursing station.
    d. putting it in the office safe.

_____ **7.** Which of the following are usually nursing responsibilities related to transfer? 1) equipment for transfer; 2) teaching the patient about medications; 3) making a final assessment; 4) making sure the patient's property is also transferred

    a. 2 and 3
    b. 1 and 4
    c. 1, 3, and 4
    d. All of these

© 1996 by Lippincott-Raven Publishers

_____ 8. Which of the following are usually nursing responsibilities related to discharge? 1) planning for transportation; 2) teaching the patient about medications; 3) making a final assessment; 4) making sure that the patient's personal property is sent along

    a. 1, 2, and 3
    b. 2, 3, and 4
    c. 1, 3, and 4
    d. All of these

_____ 9. Which of the following patients are most likely to need a referral to provide continuing care after discharge? 1) one who had a routine appendectomy; 2) one who had a stroke and has right-sided paralysis; 3) one who had acute pneumonia; 4) one with a new colostomy

    a. 1 and 3
    b. 2 and 4
    c. 3 and 4
    d. All of these

Short-Answer Questions

10. The person within some facilities whose task it is to facilitate discharge is called

_____

11. One patient situation that may delay discharge and should be reported to the physician is

_____

12. Health teaching the patient and family before discharge is important because

_____

13. Two functions you may fulfill for the patient at home who is being transferred to a healthcare facility are

    a. _____

    b. _____

© 1996 by Lippincott-Raven Publishers

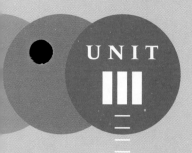

UNIT III

Fundamental Personal Care Skills

MODULE 14
Bedmaking

MODULE 15
Moving the Patient in Bed and Positioning

MODULE 16
Feeding Adult Patients

MODULE 17
Assisting With Elimination and Perineal Care

MODULE 18
Hygiene

MODULE 19
Basic Infant Care

MODULE

14

BEDMAKING

MODULE CONTENTS

RATIONALE FOR THE USE OF THIS
   SKILL
NURSING DIAGNOSES
INFECTION CONTROL IN BEDMAKING
BODY MECHANICS IN BEDMAKING
PROCEDURE FOR MAKING THE
   UNOCCUPIED BED
Assessment
Planning
Implementation
Evaluation
Documentation
PROCEDURE FOR MAKING THE POSTOP,
   OR SURGICAL, BED
Assessment
Planning
Implementation

Evaluation
Documentation
PROCEDURE FOR MAKING THE
   OCCUPIED BED
Assessment
Planning
Implementation
Evaluation
Documentation
ACCESSORIES FOR THE BED
Bedboards
Footboards
Special Mattresses
Cradles
LONG-TERM CARE
HOME CARE
CRITICAL THINKING EXERCISES

PREREQUISITES

Successful completion of the following modules:

VOLUME 1
Module 1   An Approach to Nursing Skills
Module 2   Basic Infection Control
Module 3   Safety
Module 4   Basic Body Mechanics
Module 25 Special Mattresses and Therapeutic Frames and Beds

© 1996 by Lippincott-Raven Publishers

OVERALL OBJECTIVE

To make beds that are both safe and comfortable for patients in healthcare settings.

SPECIFIC LEARNING OBJECTIVES

Know Facts and Principles	Apply Facts and Principles	Demonstrate Ability	Evaluate Performance

1. Related principles
  a. Infection control
  b. Body melchanics
State principles of infection control and body mechanics related to bedmaking.
	Apply principles of infection control and body mechanics when making beds.	Use principles of infection control and body mechanics in making hospital beds.	Evaluate own performance with instructor.

2. Types of beds
  a. Closed (unoccupied)
  b. Open
  c. Occupied
  d. Postop
Describe type of beds.
	Given a patient situation, identify appropriate type of bed to be made.	In the clinical setting, identify type of bed to be made for particular patient.	Evaluate own performance with instructor.

3. Linen Identify individual pieces of linen used in making hospital beds.	Given a patient situation, identify appropriate pieces of linen to use in correct order.	In the clinical setting, identify appropriate pieces of linen to use in correct order for particular patient.	Evaluate own performance with instructor.

4. Procedures
  a. Closed (unoccupied)
  b. Open
  c. Occupied
  d. Postop
Describe correct procedures for making closed (unoccupied), open, occupied, and postop beds.
Describe modifications to bedmaking procedure that might exist in a long-term care facility.
	Initiate appropriate bedmaking activities in patient settings.	Demonstrate ability to correctly make closed (unoccupied), open, occupied, and postop beds.
		Make appropriate modifications when making beds in long-term care facilities.
			Evaluate own bedmaking ability with instructor using Performance Checklist and facility policies and procedures.

(continued)

© 1996 by Lippincott-Raven Publishers

SPECIFIC LEARNING OBJECTIVES (Continued)

Know Facts and Principles	Apply Facts and Principles	Demonstrate Ability	Evaluate Performance

5. Accessory devices
  a. Cradle
  b. Footboard
  c. Bedboard
  d. Special mattresses
Identify cradle, footboard, bedboard, and special mattresses.
	Given a patient situation, identify appropriate accessory device to use.	Initiate use of accessory devices in appropriate situations.	Evaluate appropriateness of choice with instructor.

© 1996 by Lippincott-Raven Publishers

LEARNING ACTIVITIES

1. Review the Specific Learning Objectives.
2. Read the section on care of the patient's bed (in the chapter on hygiene) in Ellis and Nowlis, *Nursing: A Human Needs Approach,* or comparable material in another textbook.
3. Look up the module vocabulary terms in the glossary.
4. Read through the module as though you were preparing to teach the procedures to another person and mentally practice the skills.
5. In the practice setting:
   a. Identify the various pieces of linen used in making beds in the facility to which you are assigned.
   b. Make an unoccupied, closed bed, using the Performance Checklist as a guide. When you are satisfied with your performance, have a fellow student evaluate you. Compare your own evaluation with that of the other student. Perfect your technique. Have your instructor evaluate your performance.
   c. Demonstrate how to convert a closed bed to an open bed.
   d. Demonstrate how to convert a closed bed to a postoperative bed.
   e. Make an occupied bed, using a fellow student as a patient. Pretend that it is a real situation, complete with patient communication. Have the student comment on comfort. When you are satisfied with your performance, have your instructor evaluate you.
   f. Demonstrate the use of a footboard and cradle when making an unoccupied bed.
6. In the clinical setting: Make an unoccupied bed, an occupied bed, and a postop bed to your instructor's satisfaction.

VOCABULARY

cradle	footboard	plantar flexion
edema	footdrop	toe pleat
fanfold	mitered corner	trochanter roll

© 1996 by Lippincott-Raven Publishers

Bedmaking

Rationale for the Use of This Skill

The bed is one of the most important parts of the patient's environment in the healthcare setting. Knowing how to make various types of beds and how to modify them for special situations is of paramount importance for the nurse. A clean, wrinkle-free bed that remains intact when a patient moves does a great deal for the patient's physical and psychological comfort.[1]

▼ NURSING DIAGNOSES

A nursing diagnosis that is important when making beds is Risk for Impaired Skin Integrity. Skin integrity can be placed at risk because of wrinkled or soiled linen and the manner in which patients are moved. Food crumbs or other small articles inadvertently dropped in the bed can also place the skin at risk.

A second nursing diagnosis related to bedmaking is Risk for Infection related to linen soiled with urine, stool, or wound drainage, especially in the presence of an open wound or in the case of an immunocompromised patient.

INFECTION CONTROL IN BEDMAKING

Apply these principles of basic infection control to all bedmaking procedures:

1. *Microorganisms move through space on air currents;* therefore, handle linen carefully. Avoid shaking it or tossing it into the laundry hamper (it should be *placed* in the hamper).
2. *Microorganisms are transferred from one surface to another whenever one object touches another.* Therefore, hold both soiled and clean linen away from your uniform *to prevent contamination of the clean linen by the uniform and contamination of the uniform by the soiled linen.* In addition, avoid placing it on the floor *to prevent the spread of any bacteria present either on the linen or on the floor.*
3. *Proper handwashing removes many of the microorganisms that would be transferred by the hands from one item to another.* Therefore, wash your hands before you begin and after you finish bedmaking.

[1]Rationale for action is emphasized throughout the module by the use of italics.

BODY MECHANICS IN BEDMAKING

Apply these principles of body mechanics to all bedmaking procedures:

1. *A person or an object is more stable if the center of gravity is close to the base of support.* Therefore, when you must bend, bend your knees, not your back, *to keep the center of gravity directly above and close to the base of support and to help prevent fatigue* (Fig. 14–1).
2. *Facing in the direction of the task to be performed and turning the entire body in one plane (rather than twisting) lessens the susceptibility of the back to injury.* Therefore, face your entire body in the direction that you are moving and avoid twisting to prevent back strain or injury.
3. *Smooth, rhythmical movements at moderate speed require less energy.* Therefore, organize your work. Conserve steps by making as few trips around the bed as possible.
4. *It takes less energy to work on a surface at an appropriate height (usually waist level) than it does to stoop or stretch to reach the surface.* Therefore, raise the

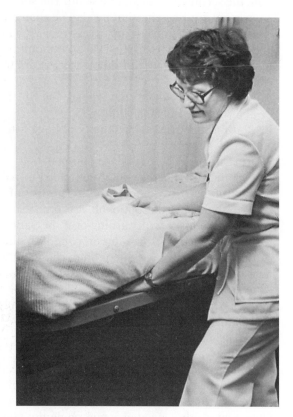

Figure 14–1. Correct posture for bedmaking. The nurse bends at the knees, not the back, to keep the center of gravity directly above and close to the base of support. (Courtesy Ivan Ellis)

© 1996 by Lippincott-Raven Publishers

bed to an appropriate height for maximum working comfort for yourself *to prevent fatigue.*

PROCEDURE FOR MAKING THE UNOCCUPIED BED

Assessment

1. Check the activity order for the patient *to determine if it is possible for the patient to be out of bed during the bedmaking procedure.*
2. Assess the patient *to determine whether there are factors present (fatigue or pain, for example) that might affect the patient's ability to be out of bed during the bedmaking procedure.*
3. Check the condition of the linen on the bed to *determine which items need to be replaced or added to complete the bedmaking procedure.*
4. Check for any of the patient's special needs that might require extra linen or special equipment.

Planning

5. Wash your hands *for infection control.*
6. Obtain a laundry bag or hamper.
7. Gather the linen to be used and place it in order, so that the first item to be used will be on the bottom, the second item next, and so on. You should choose only those items that need to be changed. Remember that preventing excessive purchase and laundry costs is part of cost containment in the healthcare environment. Items can include:
   a. Mattress pad, which may already be on the bed (not used in all facilities)
   b. Bottom sheet (many facilities will have fitted bottom sheets)
   c. 1 plastic drawsheet (may be optional)
   d. 1 cloth drawsheet (A top sheet folded in half may be used in some settings. The use of a drawsheet may be optional; use one if it is needed to assist with turning or if the patient has drainage or some other condition that may require more frequent linen changing. It is much easier to change a drawsheet than an entire bottom sheet.)
   e. 1 top sheet
   f. 1 blanket
   g. 1 bedspread (optional)
   h. 1 pillowcase for each pillow on the bed
      If linen is stacked in this order, the stack need merely be turned over for it to be *in the correct order for use.*
8. Obtain any other needed items or equipment. You will need clean gloves if you will be handling linen soiled with body secretions.

Implementation

9. Raise the bed to an appropriate working height to *help prevent fatigue.* Be certain the wheels are locked *to keep the bed from moving.*
10. Remove attached equipment (call light, waste bag, personal items). Place side rails in the down position. Put on gloves before handling linen soiled with body secretions.
11. Remove cases from pillows and place the pillows on a chair or bedside table.
12. Loosen the top and the bottom linen from the mattress, moving around the bed from head to foot on one side and from foot to head on the opposite side.
13. Remove any clean items to be reused (spread, blankets, sheets) one at a time. Fold each in quarters and place across the back of a chair.
14. Remove the remaining linen and place it in a laundry hamper. If you put on gloves to handle linen soiled with body secretions, remove them and wash your hands before touching any clean items.
15. If the mattress is to be turned, do so at this point by grasping it, pulling it toward you, and turning it.
16. Move the mattress to the head of the bed.
17. Wash your hands after handling the soiled bed linens.
18. Place a mattress pad on the mattress and secure it smoothly.
19. Place a bottom sheet on the bed, with the center fold at the center of the bed, the lower hem even with the edge of the mattress at the foot of the bed, and the seam toward the mattress. Spread the sheet, tucking it under at the head of the bed, if it is a flat sheet.
20. If your facility uses fitted sheets, first fit diagonal corners over the mattress. If your facility does not use fitted sheets, use mitered or square corners. Sheets with either mitered or square corners *remain tucked better and appear neater* than sheets that are simply tucked under the mattress.
    To make a mitered corner:
    a. Pick up the side edge of the sheet approximately 12 inches from the corner of the mattress. Hold it straight up and down, parallel to the side of the mattress (Fig. 14–2**A**).
    b. Lay the upper part of the sheet on the bed (Fig. 14–2**B**).
    c. Tuck the part of the sheet that is hanging below the mattress smoothly under the mattress (Fig. 14–2**C**).
    d. Holding the sheet in place against the mattress with one hand, use your other hand to

© 1996 by Lippincott-Raven Publishers

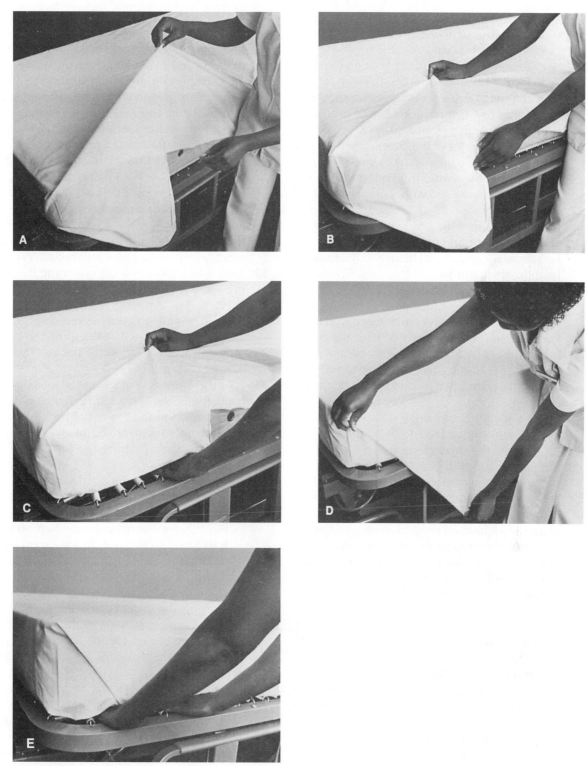

Figure 14–2. Mitering a corner. (**A** and **B**) Pull sheet up at corner and fold back. (**C**) Tuck sheet under at corner. (**D** and **E**) Fold rest of sheet down and tuck under. (Courtesy Ivan Ellis)

© 1996 by Lippincott-Raven Publishers

lift the folded part of the sheet lying on the bed and bring it down. Tuck it under the mattress (Fig. 14–2**D** and 14–2**E**).

To make a square corner, pick up the sheet to form a 45° angle (in step a [above]), so that when the folded edge is placed on the top of the mattress before tucking, it is even with the bottom edge of the mattress.

21. Tuck the remainder of the sheet under the side of the mattress all the way to the foot of the bed, pulling it tightly toward the bottom of the bed as you go *to create a smooth surface.*

22. If a plastic drawsheet is to be used, place it over the middle part of the bed, with the center fold at the center. Unfold the drawsheet toward the far side of the bed. Tuck the near edge smoothly under the mattress.

23. Place the cloth drawsheet over the plastic drawsheet, and place it on the bed, making sure that the plastic drawsheet is completely covered.

24. Place the top sheet on the bed with the center fold at the center of the bed, seam side up. Align the top edge of the sheet with the top edge of the mattress. Unfold it toward the far side of the bed.

25. Make a toe pleat (optional—follow the procedure at your clinical facility) by folding a 2-inch pleat across the sheet about 6 to 8 inches from the foot of the bed. Then tuck the end of the sheet under the mattress. This is more comfortable for the patient in that *it prevents impingement of the top linen on the patient's toes.*

26. Place the blanket on the bed, center fold at the center of the bed, so that the top edge of the blanket is about 6 inches from the top of the mattress. Unfold the blanket toward the far side of the bed. Tuck it under the foot of the mattress, making a toe pleat if necessary. In warm weather, or at the patient's request, omit the blanket, or, if the patient is cold, use additional blankets.

27. Place the bedspread on the bed, with the center fold at the center of the bed. The top edge of the spread should be about 6 inches from the top of the mattress. Unfold the remainder of the spread toward the far side of the bed. Tuck it under at the foot of the mattress, making a toe pleat if necessary. Some nurses prefer to tuck all three— top sheet, blanket, and spread—together.

28. Miter the corner of the top linen at the foot of the bed. Do not tuck in the upper portion; allow it to hang down smoothly and freely.

29. Move to the other side of the bed. It is easier to make one entire side of the bed (both bottom and top linen) before moving to the other side *to save time and energy.* Pull the bottom linen smoothly and tightly across the mattress and tuck the bottom sheet under the head of the mattress and make a mitered or square corner.

30. Tuck the bottom sheet along the side of the bed, pulling toward you and slightly toward the bottom of the bed to make the sheet tight as you move toward the foot of the bed. *This creates a smooth, comfortable surface for the patient.*

31. Pull the center of the plastic drawsheet (if present) toward you. With palms down, tuck it under the mattress, as snugly as possible. Grasp the top corner of the drawsheet, pull it diagonally, and tuck it under the mattress snugly. Repeat this activity with the lower corner of the drawsheet *to obtain an absolutely wrinkle-free surface.*

32. Tuck the cloth drawsheet under the mattress in the same way you tucked in the plastic drawsheet.

33. Straighten and smooth the top sheet, blanket, and spread starting at the top of the bed and moving toward the foot of the bed. Miter the bottom corner.

34. Fold the top sheet back over the top edge of the blanket and the spread. If there is more spread than blanket at the top of the bed, fold the excess spread back over the blanket to form an even line. Then fold the top sheet over as described.

    a. Closed Bed: The upper edge of the spread is left even with the upper edge of the mattress to designate a *closed* bed. In healthcare facilities this may only be done when no patient is assigned to the bed. In long-term care facilities, the bed is usually closed during the day.

    b. Open Bed: Opening a bed is usually done by grasping the upper edge of the top linen with both hands, bringing it all the way to the foot of the bed, then folding it back toward the center of the bed. This is known as fanfolding (Fig. 14–3).

    If beds are left open, it is easier to assist patients back to bed when they are ready. Open beds are usually made when patients are up for a brief period in the room or out of the unit, perhaps for x-ray or laboratory procedures, but are expected to spend much of the time in bed.

35. Put a pillowcase on the pillow. One way to do this is as follows:

    a. Grasp the pillowcase at the center of the closed end of the case (Fig. 14–4).

    b. Gather the case up over that hand and grasp the zipper, or open end of the pillow cover,

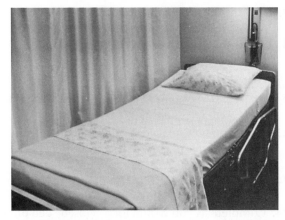

Figure 14–3. The open bed, with the top linen fanfolded back, is ready for the patient. (Courtesy Ivan Ellis)

with the same hand, pulling the case down over the pillow with the other hand.

c. Straighten and smooth the case over the pillow and place it at the head of the bed with the open end away from the door (*for neater appearance*).

d. Keep the pillow and case away from your uniform as you apply the case.

36. Replace the call light in an appropriate place and leave the bed in low position, *ready for the patient who will be returning to bed from a chair or a walk*.

When a patient is to be transferred from a stretcher to the bed, the bed is usually placed in the high position *to allow for easier transfer*.

Evaluation

37. Evaluate the unoccupied bed, using the following criteria:
    a. Smooth, wrinkle-free surface
    b. Tight corners
    c. Correct position (high or low) for the patient's needs.
    d. Call light attached in appropriate place

Documentation

38. Linen changes are not routinely documented but the tolerance of the patient's being out-of-bed might be recorded.

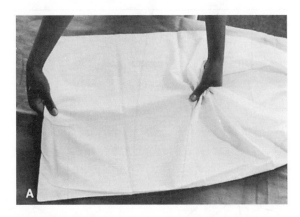

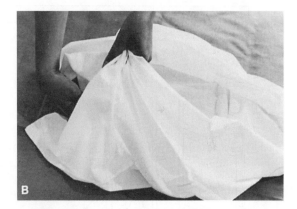

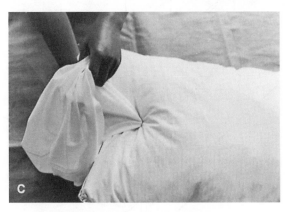

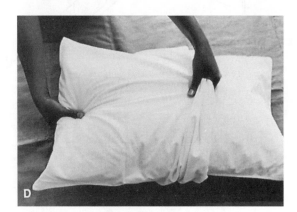

Figure 14–4. Putting a case on a pillow. (**A**) Hold pillowcase at closed end, from outside. (**B**) Gather pillowcase over your hand, inside out. (**C**) With pillowcase in hand, grasp pillow at center of one end. (**D**) Holding pillow, pull case over pillow, right side out.

© 1996 by Lippincott-Raven Publishers

PROCEDURE FOR MAKING THE POSTOP, OR SURGICAL, BED

The postop bed is also called the anesthetic or surgical bed. It is made *so that the patient can be transferred from a stretcher to the bed with a minimum of motion and discomfort, then covered with the top linen, including the blanket, which is easily within reach, to prevent chilling* (Fig. 14–5).

Assessment

1. Follow the Procedure for Making the Unoccupied Bed.
2. Assess the type of surgery the patient is having performed to determine the length of time the patient will have to be confined to bed.
3.–4. Follow the steps of the Procedure for Making the Unoccupied Bed.

Planning

5.–6. Follow the steps of the Procedure for Making the Unoccupied Bed.

7. Discard all used linen. You may retain the mattress pad which is on the bed.
8. Follow the Procedure for Making the Unoccupied Bed.

Implementation

9.–22. Follow the steps of the Procedure for Making the Unoccupied Bed.
23. After you have placed the drawsheet on the bed, add a bath blanket over the drawsheet. *This is sometimes done to provide extra warmth.*
24.–33. Follow the steps of the Procedure for Making the Unoccupied Bed.
34. Complete as you would for a "closed" bed but *do not* tuck at bottom. Fold back top linen toward head or foot of bed as policy directs. Fanfold top linen to the far side of the bed or to the foot of the bed, as indicated by facility policy.
35. Place each pillow in a pillowcase. Place pillow(s) on a table or chair, or on top of the fanfolded top linen.
36. Leave the bed in high position to receive the pa-

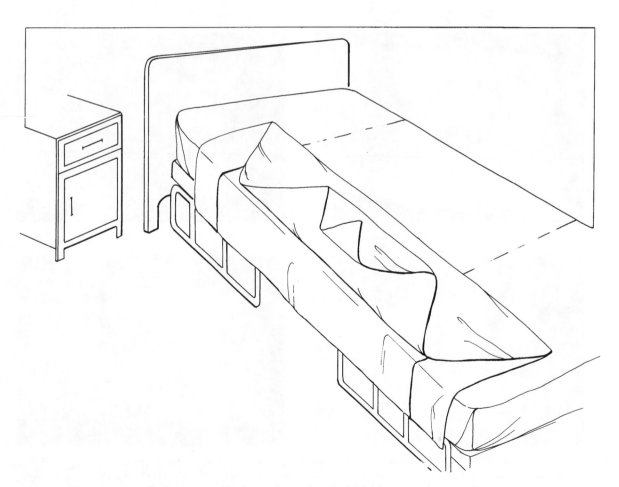

Figure 14–5. Postoperative bed. Top sheet, blanket, and spread are fanfolded for convenient transfer of patient from stretcher to bed.

© 1996 by Lippincott-Raven Publishers

tient. Place emesis basin, tissues, IV stand, call light, and any other necessary items conveniently in the unit.

Evaluation

37. Evaluate, using the following criteria:
    a. Smooth, wrinkle-free surface
    b. Top covers folded back out of the way
    c. Necessary items at bedside
    d. Bed in high position *to receive patient more easily from the stretcher.*

Documentation

38. Follow the Procedure for Making the Unoccupied Bed.

PROCEDURE FOR MAKING THE OCCUPIED BED

There are many instances in which a bed must be wholly or partially made with a patient in it. In most cases this is *because the patient is too ill or disabled to get out of bed.*

Practice making an occupied bed, keeping the patient's safety and comfort foremost in your mind, and taking care to avoid bumping the bed or exposing the patient. If the patient cannot participate, you may need another staff member to assist you. The order of activities remains the same; the procedure differs from making an unoccupied bed only *because a patient is in the bed* (Fig. 14–6).

Assessment

1. Check activity orders *to be sure that the patient must stay in bed* as well as orders for any restrictions related to position. Also check for any position that *must* be maintained (for example, head of bed elevated 30°).
2. Assess the patient *to determine whether there are any factors (such as fatigue, shortness of breath, or pain, for example) that might affect the ability of the patient to undergo the bedmaking activity at that time.*
3.–4. Follow the steps of the Procedure for Making the Unoccupied Bed.

Planning

5.–8. Follow the steps of the Procedure for Making the Unoccupied Bed.

Implementation

9. Explain what you plan to do. *The patient's cooperation will greatly help you.* Provide for the patient's privacy by closing the door to the room or pulling the curtain around the patient.
10. Raise the bed to an appropriate height for you *to help prevent fatigue.* Be certain the wheels are locked.

11. Remove the call light and other equipment, spread, and blanket from the bed. If the spread and the blanket are to be reused, fold them and place over a chair. Put on gloves before handling linen soiled with body secretions.
12. Before removing the top sheet, place a bath blanket over the sheet. The bath blanket will remain in place as you remove the sheet *to provide privacy and warmth for the patient.* Ask the patient, if able, to hold the top edge of the bath blanket while you pull the sheet out from under it. Discard the top sheet if you will not be reusing it.
13. If the mattress must be moved toward the head of the bed, get assistance from another person.
14. Elicit the patient's help and roll the patient to the far side of the bed, making sure that the pillow is moved also. If possible, the patient should be side-lying, facing away from you. The side rail on the far side of the bed should be up *for safety and comfort.*
15. Loosen the foundation (bottom linen) of the bed on the near side, leaving the mattress pad in place unless it is wet or soiled.
16. Fanfold each piece of linen toward the center of the bed, with the last fold toward the opposite side of the bed and tucked under the patient's back and buttocks *to make it easier to reach later.* If you put on gloves to handle linen soiled with body secretions, remove them and wash your hands before touching any clean items.
17. Straighten the mattress pad. If you must replace the mattress pad, use the process in Step 16.
18. Lay the bottom sheet lengthwise on the bed and unfold it so that the center fold of the sheet is at the center of the bed, the bottom hem is at the bottom edge of the mattress, and the top hem of the sheet is over the top of the mattress. Fanfold half the sheet lengthwise toward the center of the bed, allowing the other half to drape over the side toward you.
19. Place the fanfolded sheet under the patient as far as possible, tucking it under the soiled bottom sheet *so that it is not against the soiled upper surface.*
20. Tuck the sheet under at the top, miter the top corner, and tuck it in along the side of the mattress to the foot of the bed.
21. If a plastic drawsheet is in use, unfold it at this point, pull it over the folded bottom sheets, and tuck it in snugly and smoothly.
22. If a plastic drawsheet is used, always cover it with a cloth drawsheet as well. If only a cloth drawsheet is used, place it so that the center fold is at the center of the bed.
23. Tuck the near side under the mattress. Fanfold

© 1996 by Lippincott-Raven Publishers

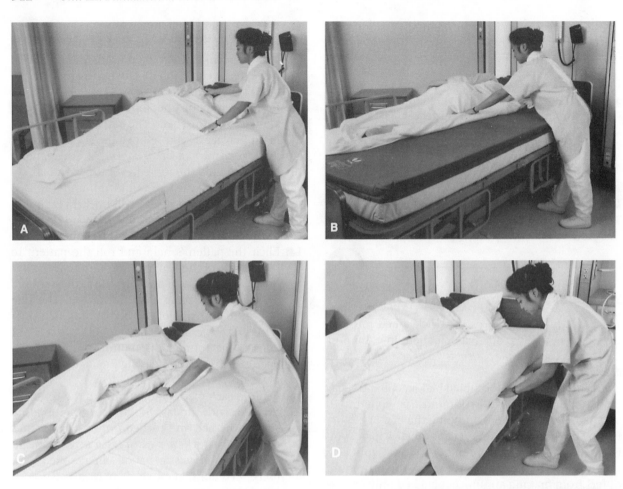

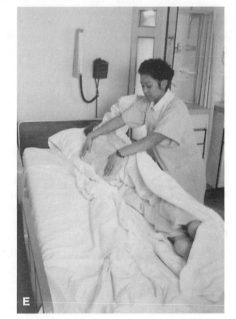

Figure 14–6. Occupied bed. (**A**) Move the patient to the far side of the bed, facing away from you. (**B**) Each piece of linen is fanfolded toward the center of the bed, with the last fold toward the opposite side of the bed. (**C**) Place the fanfolded sheet under the patient as far as possible, tucking it under the soiled bottom sheet so that it is not against the soiled upper surface. (**D**) Pull the draw sheet over the folded bottom sheets and tuck in. (**E**) Help the patient roll over the folded linen onto the clean linen.

© 1996 by Lippincott-Raven Publishers

the other half toward the center of the bed, tucking it under the patient's back and buttocks.

24. Help the patient roll over the folded linen toward you and onto the clean linen. Adjust the pillow. Put up the side rail *for safety and comfort.*

25. Move to the other side of the bed. Lower the side rail.

26. Loosen the bottom linen. Put on gloves *if the linen is soiled with body secretions.* Remove the soiled linen (bottom sheet and cloth drawsheet) and place it in a laundry hamper or bag. Remove gloves and wash your hands before touching any clean items.

27. Straighten the mattress pad. Pull the fanfolded bottom sheet, and any drawsheet (if used) out from under the patient. Straighten, pull, and tuck the bottom sheet as if making an unoccupied bed. Pull the sheet tight by bracing against the bed and pulling with both hands *to make the sheet smooth and tight under the patient before tucking it.*

28. If a drawsheet is being used, pull and tuck it as you did previously.

29. Now move the patient to the center of the bed in a comfortable position.

30. Place the top sheet on the bed over the bath blanket. Remove the bath blanket, instructing the patient to hold the sheet as you pull the blanket from the top to the bottom. Place the bath blanket in the laundry hamper or (if it is unsoiled and dry) fold it and leave it in the patient's unit *for future use.*

31. Add the blanket and the spread as in the Procedure for Making the Unoccupied Bed. Instead of making a toe pleat, you may have the patient point the toes up while you are tucking in the foot of the bed; *this allows room for the toes after the bed has been made.*

32. Remove the pillow and put on a clean pillowcase.

33. Reattach the call light and any other equipment you removed.

34. Place the bed in the low position, adjusting the side rails according to your facility's policies and the individual situation.

Evaluation

35. Evaluate the occupied bed using the following criteria:
   a. Patient comfort
   b. Smooth, wrinkle-free surface
   c. Tight corners
   d. Bed and side rails in correct position
   e. Bed in the low position *for safety*
   f. Call light and other personal items within patient's reach.

Documentation

36. Document any assessment data or change in the patient's clinical status.

ACCESSORIES FOR THE BED

Among the devices often added to the bed are the bedboard, the footboard, and the cradle. These devices may be ordered by a physician, but in many facilities they are added at the nurse's discretion.

Bedboards

A bedboard may be used directly under a mattress *when the patient needs an especially firm bed.* Bedboards are often used for orthopedic patients or for those who have a history of back problems. Some patients are simply more comfortable sleeping on a firm surface. Most modern beds in healthcare facilities do not need a bedboard to create a firm surface.

Footboards

A footboard may be placed on the bed *to keep the feet at right angles to the legs when the patient is in the supine position (lying flat on the back) in bed and prevent prolonged plantar flexion.* The feet are positioned to rest firmly against the footboard (Fig. 14–7).

Linen is tucked in around the footboard and is held up off the patient's feet. This prevents the top sheet, blanket, and spread from forcing the feet into plantar flexion. Trochanter rolls may be used *to keep the hips from externally rotating.*

Not all footboards are alike. Some are merely boards that fit at the foot of the mattress. Some require that a box or "block" be added, *so that the feet*

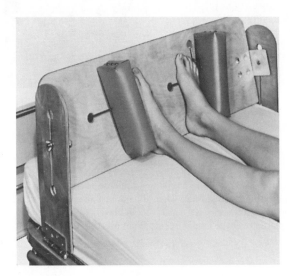

Figure 14–7. The footboard provides a firm surface to hold the feet at a right angle. Footboards are usually padded.

© 1996 by Lippincott-Raven Publishers

of a shorter patient can reach the board. Other footboards fit under the mattress and slide up to the appropriate point on the bed.

Only footboards that allow the patient's feet to rest flat against them help *to prevent footdrop. Footdrop* is an abnormal shortening of the Achilles tendon from a prolonged period of plantar flexion. Footdrop results in the patient's inability to walk normally and requires extensive physical therapy to correct. A footboard is only effective if the patient's feet are resting firmly against it.

High-topped tennis shoes are also used *to prevent plantar flexion.* Evidence indicates that they are more effective than a footboard. Foot and ankle splints to prevent plantar flexion are available, but these are costly and must be specially ordered for the individual patient.

Special Mattresses

A variety of special mattresses have been manufactured *to diminish pressure on the patient's skin and thus help prevent the formation of pressure ulcers (decubitus ulcers).* These include egg-crate, inflatable, and alternating-pressure mattresses. (A more detailed description of these special mattresses is given in Module 25, Special Mattresses and Therapeutic Frames and Beds.) When making a bed that has one of these mattresses, do not tuck the linen tightly under the mattress, *because this does not allow the mattress to expand and defeats the purpose of the special mattress.* The manufacturers of many of these special mattresses recommend that drawsheets and incontinent pads not be used with their products *because the sheet or pad interferes with the purpose of the mattress.*

Cradles

A bed cradle is a device designed specifically *to keep linen up off the feet and lower legs of patients when necessary, as in cases of edema, leg ulcers, and burns.* Place the device on the bed over the patient's legs and feet. Arrange the top linen over the device and pin or clip it in place. Some facilities do not allow pinning *because it can tear the linen.* In these situations, linen must simply be tucked as securely as possible around the frame.

There are several kinds of bed cradles, including one called the Anderson frame, which is a simple rod that arches over the bed and is held in place by the mattress (Fig. 14–8), and a lattice-work affair that is also arch-shaped.

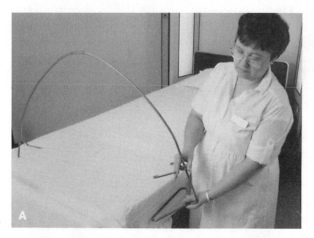
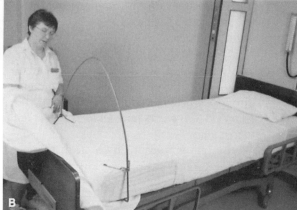
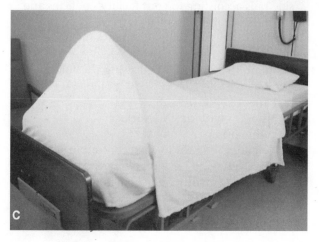

Figure 14–8. (**A**) The triangles at the base of the cradle slide under the mattress; the V-shaped parts just above fit over the top of the mattress. (**B**) The cradle in place. (**C**) The top linen is placed over the cradle to keep linen off the feet and legs.

© 1996 by Lippincott-Raven Publishers

If your facility has no cradle, you can make one by simply cutting one side out of a strong cardboard box.

LONG-TERM CARE

The resident in a long-term care facility usually spends far less time in bed than does the hospitalized patient. For this reason, beds in long-term care facilities are changed less frequently, usually once or twice a week, often on "bath day," and as needed. Other differences between hospital and long-term care facility bedmaking may include all or some of the following:

1. A mattress pad may not be used. Instead, you may find that the mattress is protected by a moisture-proof cover.
2. Plastic drawsheets may not be used. Often cloth drawsheets are not used either. Instead, cloth or disposable moisture-proof pads are used *to protect the bed from spills and incontinence.*
3. More than one blanket may be needed, because many elderly residents complain of feeling chilled. In addition, a blanket may be placed folded at the foot of the bed *so that it is available to cover the resident during daytime rest periods.*
4. The bedspread may belong to the individual resident and not to the facility and therefore not be a standard size or shape. You will need to adapt your bedmaking skills accordingly.

HOME CARE

If the client being cared for at home spends a large amount of time in bed or is severely disabled, the family may need to make arrangements to rent or buy equipment to facilitate caregiving. Hospital beds, side rails, overbed tables, and other equipment are available for rental or purchase. A bedboard, an egg-crate mattress, and disposable moisture-proof pads are other items that might be desirable. If a cradle is needed, you can make one by cutting one side out of a strong cardboard box.

CRITICAL THINKING EXERCISES

The long-term care resident you are caring for is an alert, 86-year-old woman with chronic arthritis. You are assigned to change her bed. She reports that she is very tired, it is painful to move, and the bed "isn't dirty anyway." Explain what assessment you should make before proceeding with bedmaking. Formulate the kinds of questions you will ask the client and what information you will give. What type of bed should you make? Describe your rationale.

© 1996 by Lippincott-Raven Publishers

PERFORMANCE CHECKLIST

Infection Control in Bedmaking	Needs More Practice	Satisfactory	Comments
1. Handle linen carefully; do not shake; place in hamper.			
2. Hold both soiled and clean linen away from your uniform.			
3. Wash hands before and after bedmaking.			
Body Mechanics			
1. When you must bend, bend your knees, not your back.			
2. Face your entire body in the direction in which you are moving and avoid twisting.			
3. Organize your work and conserve steps.			
4. Raise the bed to an appropriate height.			
Procedure for Making the Unoccupied Bed			
Assessment			
1. Check activity order for patient.			
2. Assess patient.			
3. Check condition of linen on bed.			
4. Check for patient's special needs.			
Planning			
5. Wash your hands.			
6. Obtain laundry bag or hamper.			
7. Gather linen to be used.			
8. Obtain other needed items or equipment, including gloves if linen soiled with body secretions.			
Implementation			
9. Raise bed to appropriate working height. Be certain wheels are locked.			
10. Remove attached equipment. Put on gloves before handling linen soiled with body secretions.			
11. Remove cases from pillows.			
12. Loosen top and bottom linen from mattress.			

(continued)

© 1996 by Lippincott-Raven Publishers

Procedure for Making the Unoccupied Bed *(Continued)*	Needs More Practice	Satisfactory	Comments
13. Remove clean items to be reused, fold, and place across back of chair.			
14. Remove remaining linen and place in hamper. If you put on gloves, remove them and wash your hands before touching clean items.			
15. Turn mattress if necessary.			
16. Move mattress to head of bed.			
17. Wash your hands.			
18. Place mattress pad on mattress.			
19. Place bottom sheet on bed.			
20. Miter top corners of bottom sheet or, if fitted sheet, tuck diagonally.			
21. Tuck remainder of sheet under.			
22. Place plastic drawsheet (if used) on bed, using center fold as guide. Tuck near edge.			
23. Place cloth drawsheet over plastic drawsheet. Tuck near edge.			
24. Place and unfold top sheet on bed.			
25. Make toe pleat (optional).			
26. Place blanket on bed, using center fold as guide.			
27. Place bedspread on bed; tuck all three together or separately.			
28. Miter corner of top linen at foot of bed.			
29. Move to other side of bed.			
30. Tuck bottom sheet.			
31. Tuck plastic drawsheet (if used) snugly under mattress.			
32. Tuck cloth drawsheet.			
33. Smooth top sheet, blanket, and spread; miter bottom corner.			
34. Fold top sheet back over top edge of blanket and spread.			
35. Apply pillowcase, keeping pillow and case away from uniform.			

(continued)

© 1996 by Lippincott-Raven Publishers

Procedure for Making the Unoccupied Bed *(Continued)*	Needs More Practice	Satisfactory	Comments
36. Replace call light and leave bed in appropriate position.			
Evaluation			
37. Evaluate using the following criteria: **a.** Smooth, wrinkle-free surface			
b. Tight corners			
c. Low position			
d. Call light attached in appropriate place			
Documentation			
38. Document linen change according to policy at your facility.			
Procedure for Making the Postop or Surgical Bed			
Assessment			
1. Follow Checklist step 1 of the Procedure for Making the Unoccupied Bed.			
2. Assess the type of surgery the patient is to have and length of time in bed.			
3. Follow Checklist steps 3 and 4 of the Procedure for Making the Unoccupied Bed.			
Planning			
5.–6. Follow Checklist steps 5 and 6 of the Procedure for Making the Unoccupied Bed.			
7. Discard all used linen except the mattress pad.			
8. Follow Checklist step 8 of the Procedure for Making the Unoccupied Bed.			
Implementation			
9.–22. Follow Checklist steps 9–22 of the Procedure for Making the Unoccupied Bed.			
23. Place a bath blanket over the draw sheet.			
24.–33. Follow Checklist steps 24–33 of the Procedure for Making the Unoccupied Bed.			

(continued)

© 1996 by Lippincott-Raven Publishers

Procedure for Making the Postop or Surgical Bed *(Continued)*	Needs More Practice	Satisfactory	Comments
34. Complete as for "closed" bed but *do not* tuck at bottom. Fold top linen toward head or foot of bed as policy requires. Fanfold as facility policy requires.			
35. Place pillowcases on each pillow and put pillows on table, chair, or on top of fanfolded linen.			
36. Leave bed in high position; obtain emesis basin, tissues, intravenous stand, call light, and other necessary items.			
Evaluation			
37. Evaluate using following criteria: **a.** Smooth, wrinkle-free surface			
b. Top linen folded out of way			
c. Necessary items at bedside			
d. Bed in high position			
Documentation			
38. Follow the Procedure for Making the Unoccupied Bed.			
Procedure for Making the Occupied Bed			
Assessment			
1. Check activity order for patient and orders for position restrictions.			
2.–4. Follow Checklist steps 2–4 of the Procedure for Making the Unoccupied Bed.			
Planning			
5.–8. Follow Checklist steps 5–8 of the Procedure for Making the Unoccupied Bed.			
Implementation			
9. Explain what you plan to do and provide for privacy of patients.			
10. Raise bed to appropriate height and lock wheels.			

(continued)

Procedure for Making the Occupied Bed *(Continued)*	Needs More Practice	Satisfactory	Comments
11. Remove attached equipment, spread, and blanket from bed. Fold if to be reused. Put on gloves if linen is soiled with body secretions.			
12. Place bath blanket over top sheet, pull sheet from under it.			
13. If mattress needs repositioning, get assistance.			
14. Elicit patient's help, roll patient to other side with side rail up.			
15. Loosen bed linen.			
16. Fanfold each linen item to be used toward center of bed, tucking under patient's back.			
17. Straighten mattress pad.			
18. Lay clean bottom sheet lengthwise. Fanfold far side toward patient.			
19. Tuck clean sheet so that it does not touch used soiled bottom sheet.			
20. Miter top corner and tuck length under mattress.			
21. If plastic drawsheet is used, pull over folded bottom sheets and tuck.			
22. Cover plastic drawsheet (if used) with cloth drawsheet.			
23. Tuck nearest side, fanfold other portion toward patient's back.			
24. Raising side rail, assist patient in rolling toward you over linen, raising side rail.			
25. Move to the other side of bed and lower rail.			
26. Remove soiled linen and place in hamper. Remove gloves and wash hands.			
27. Straighten mattress pad.			
28. Pull and tuck drawsheets, if used.			
29. Move patient to center of bed.			
30. Place top sheet on bed, removing bath blanket.			
31. Add blanket and spread, make toe pleat if appropriate, and miter bottom corners.			

(continued)

© 1996 by Lippincott-Raven Publishers

Procedure for Making the Occupied Bed *(Continued)*	Needs More Practice	Satisfactory	Comments
32. Put clean case on pillow.			
33. Reattach cell light and reinstate equipment.			
34. Place bed in low position.			
Evaluation			
35. Evaluate using the following criteria: **a.** Patient comfort			
b. Smooth, wrinkle-free surface			
c. Tight corners			
d. Bed and side rails in correct position			
e. Bed in low position			
f. Call light and other items within patient's reach			
Documentation			
36. Document any assessment data or change in patient's clinical status.			

© 1996 by Lippincott-Raven Publishers

? **QUIZ**

Short-Answer Questions

1. Because the bed is the bedridden patient's environment, beds should be made with two goals, which are _____

_____ and _____

2. The reason for completely finishing one side of the unoccupied bed and then moving to the other side is that this _____

_____

3. Two important differences between the postop bed and the unoccupied bed are

_____

and _____

_____

4. The most important safety step when making an occupied bed is to remember to

_____

5. Linen is never tucked tightly over special mattresses because doing this

_____

_____

Multiple-Choice Questions

_____ **6.** Mr Green is to be up in a chair each morning for 30 minutes. Given this information, what type of bed would be most appropriate for you to make for him?

    a. Closed bed
    b. Open bed
    c. Occupied bed
    d. Postop bed

_____ **7.** Mrs. Pine is going to x-ray for some special tests. She will arrive back on the floor via stretcher. Under these circumstances, what type of bed would be most appropriate for you to make?

    a. Closed bed
    b. Open bed
    c. Occupied bed
    d. Postop bed

_____ **8.** A patient who has severe edema of the lower legs should be provided with which accessory device?

    a. Cradle
    b. Bedboard
    c. Footboard
    d. Mattress pad

© 1996 by Lippincott-Raven Publishers

————— 9. Patients who are confined to bed should be provided with which accessory device to help prevent footdrop?

    a. Cradle
    b. Bedboard
    c. Footboard
    d. Mattress pad

————— 10. Which of the following beds may be left in the high position on completion: 1) closed bed; 2) open bed; 3) occupied bed; 4) postop bed?

    a. 1 only
    b. 4 only
    c. 2 and 3
    d. 1 and 4

Short-Answer Question

————— 11. Number the following pieces of linen in the order in which they would be used in the usual unoccupied hospital bed.

————— Blanket

————— Pillowcase

————— Top sheet

————— Bottom sheet

————— Mattress pad

————— Cloth drawsheet

————— Spread

————— Plastic drawsheet

© 1996 by Lippincott-Raven Publishers

15

MOVING THE PATIENT IN BED AND POSITIONING

MODULE CONTENTS

RATIONALE FOR THE USE OF THIS
  SKILL
NURSING DIAGNOSES
GENERAL PROCEDURE FOR MOVING
  THE PATIENT IN BED AND
  POSITIONING
  Assessment
  Planning
  Implementation
  Evaluation
  Documentation
SPECIFIC PROCEDURES FOR MOVING
  PATIENTS
Moving a Patient Closer to One Side of the
  Bed
Moving a Patient Up in Bed: One-Person
  Assist
Moving a Patient Up in Bed: Two- or
  Three-Person Assist
Turning a Patient in Bed: Back to Side
Turning a Patient in Bed: Back to
  Abdomen
Turning a Patient in Bed: Logrolling

Moving a Patient in Bed: Using a Turn
  Sheet or Pull Sheet
POSITIONING A PATIENT IN BED
PROCEDURES FOR POSITIONING A
  PATIENT IN BED
Supine Position
Side-Lying Position
Prone Position
POSITIONING A PATIENT IN A CHAIR
THERAPEUTIC POSITIONS
Fowler's Position
High Fowler's Position
Semi-Fowler's Position
Orthopneic Position
Dorsal Recumbent Position
Lithotomy Position
Sims' Position
Knee–Chest Position (Genupectoral)
Trendelenburg Position
LONG-TERM CARE
HOME CARE
CRITICAL THINKING EXERCISES

PREREQUISITES

Successful completion of the following modules:

VOLUME 1
Module 1 An Approach to Nursing Skills
Module 2 Basic Infection Control
Module 3 Safety
Module 4 Basic Body Mechanics
Module 5 Documentation
Module 6 Introduction to Assessment Skills
Module 9 Performing a Nursing Physical Assessment

© 1996 by Lippincott-Raven Publishers

OVERALL OBJECTIVES

To move patients in bed, using good body mechanics; to place patients in positions that are anatomically correct as well as comfortable; and to place patients in the special positions required for examination and therapy.

SPECIFIC LEARNING OBJECTIVES

Know Facts and Principles	Apply Facts and Principles	Demonstrate Ability	Evaluate Performance
MOVING THE PATIENT IN BED			
1. General procedure			
Give assessment factors and safety precautions for both nurse and patient.	State rationale for assessment and safety.	Adapt procedure to individual patient.	Evaluate own performance with instructor.
2. Moving patient closer to one side of bed			
3. Moving patient up in bed: one-person assist			
4. Moving patient up in bed: two- or three-person assist			
5. Turning patient in bed: back to side			
6. Turning patient in bed: back to abdomen			
7. Turning patient: logrolling			
8. Using turn sheet with any of above			
Describe each move in detail.	Choose best movement procedure for particular patient.	In clinical setting, perform each move with patient if possible.	Using the Performance Checklist, evaluate moves performed with help of instructor.
DOCUMENTATION		Document plan for turning on care plan. Chart on record.	
POSITIONING			
1. Reasons for frequent and proper positioning			
Give three reasons for frequent and proper positioning.	State rationale underlying each reason.	Make adaptations for individual patients.	Evaluate adaptations with instructor.
2. Positioning aids			
List available aids that are used for positioning.	From list, select appropriate aids for each body position.	In clinical setting, use aids correctly for patient situation.	Evaluate own performance with help of instructor.
3. Supine position			
4. Side-lying position			
5. Prone position			
6. Sitting position			
7. Fowler's position			
8. High Fowler's position			
9. Semi-Fowler's position			

(continued)

© 1996 by Lippincott-Raven Publishers

SPECIFIC LEARNING OBJECTIVES (Continued)

Know Facts and Principles	Apply Facts and Principles	Demonstrate Ability	Evaluate Performance
10. *Orthopneic position* 11. *Dorsal recumbent position* 12. *Lithotomy position* Describe each.	Choose best position for particular patient.	In clinical setting, place at least one patient in each position if possible.	Using the Performance Checklist, critically evaluate patient's body alignment and comfort.
13. *Sims' position* 14. *Knee–chest position* 15. *Trendelenburg position* Describe each.	Choose best position for particular patient.	In clinical setting, place at least one patient in each position if possible.	Using the Performance Checklist, critically evaluate patient's body alignment and comfort.
DOCUMENTATION		Document plan for positioning in Nursing Care Plan, stating rationale. Chart on record, using proper format.	

© 1996 by Lippincott-Raven Publishers

LEARNING ACTIVITIES

1. Review the Specific Learning Objectives.
2. Read the section on the effects of immobility (in the chapters on Mobility and Activity and Rest and Sleep) in Ellis and Nowlis, *Nursing: A Human Needs Approach,* or comparable material in another textbook.
3. Look up the module vocabulary terms in the glossary.
4. Read through the module and mentally practice the techniques described. Study so that you would be able to teach these skills to another person.
5. In the practice setting, select three other students and form a group of four.
   a. Changing so that each has the opportunity to play the role of the patient, perform each of the following procedures for moving the patient in bed. Use the Performance Checklist for guidance. Those who are not participating at a given time can observe and evaluate the performances of the others.
      (1) Move the "patient" closer to one side of the bed.
      (2) Move the "patient" up in bed: one-person assist.
      (3) Move the "patient" up in bed: two- or three-person assist.
      (4) Turn the "patient" in bed: back to side.
      (5) Turn the "patient" in bed: back to abdomen.
      (6) Turn the "patient" in bed: logrolling.
      (7) Perform two of the above using a pull sheet. Does this make the task easier? How? Why?
   b. With the same group, change roles as you did before and position the "patient" in the following ways:
      (1) Supine position
      (2) Side-lying position
      (3) Prone position
      (4) Sitting position (in a chair)
      (5) Fowler's position
      (6) High Fowler's position
      (7) Semi-Fowler's position
      (8) Orthopneic position
      (9) Dorsal recumbent position
      (10) Lithotomy position
      (11) Sims' position
      (12) Knee–chest position
      (13) Trendelenburg position
   c. Note the different positions you assume during a normal night's sleep. Is one particular position more comfortable for you than others? How often do you estimate you change your position during the night?
6. In the clinical setting:
   a. Consult with your instructor regarding the opportunity to move patients using a variety of techniques. Evaluate your performance with the instructor.
   b. Consult with your instructor regarding the opportunity to position patients in a variety of appropriate positions. Evaluate your performance with the instructor.

VOCABULARY

alignment	extension	gravity	plantar flexion
anatomic position	external rotation	increased intracranial	pronation
axilla	flaccid	pressure	thoracentesis
dorsiflexion	flexion	orthopneic	trapeze
dyspnea	footdrop	paralysis	trochanter

© 1996 by Lippincott-Raven Publishers

Moving the Patient in Bed and Positioning

Rationale for the Use of This Skill

Maintaining the correct position of the body while at rest contributes to comfort and rest and prevents strain on muscles. A regimen of good positioning prevents pressure sores (decubitus ulcers) and joint contractures. Frequent movement also improves muscle tone, respiration, and circulation. To position the patient properly, the nurse must have a knowledge of anatomy and good body alignment. The nurse should learn a number of positions, so that patients can be repositioned approximately every 2 hours.

Many examinations and procedures use special positions to improve visibility. It is usually the nurse's responsibility to assist patients into these positions and to make them as comfortable as possible.

When you must move a patient in bed, correct body mechanics are essential for both you and the patient. If you do not use correct body mechanics and moving techniques, you may injure your back. You may also put excessive stress on a patient's joints and cause the patient severe discomfort.

The aim in moving the patient is to put the least possible stress on the patient's joints and skin. Patient positioning is designed to maintain body parts in correct alignment so that they remain functional and unstressed.

Because more persons with limited mobility are residing in the long-term care setting or in the home, these skills are becoming increasingly important in these settings. Teaching others on the staff of a facility and the care providers in the home are added responsibilities of your nursing role. [1]

▼ NURSING DIAGNOSES

Patients who cannot move themselves in bed or need assistance in getting out of bed have a variety of nursing diagnoses concerning activity. Examples are:

Impaired Physical Mobility: Unable to turn self in bed related to immediate postoperative state

Activity Intolerance: Unsteadiness in getting out of bed related to anemia

Bathing/Hygiene Self-Care Deficit related to inability to move self

Dressing/Grooming Self-Care Deficit related to inability to maintain upright position

[1]Rationale for action is emphasized throughout the module by the use of italics.

GENERAL PROCEDURE FOR MOVING A PATIENT IN BED AND POSITIONING

Assessment
1. Assess the patient's need to move.
2. Assess the patient's ability to move unaided.
3. Check on the available assistive devices.

Planning
4. Plan the moving technique.
5. Wash your hands.
6. Obtain any needed supportive devices or assistance.

Implementation
7. Identify the patient *to be sure you are carrying out the procedure for the correct patient.*
8. Raise the bed to the high position. *This lets you use correct body mechanics and protects you from back injury.*
9. Put the bed in the flat position, if possible. In this way *you will not be working against gravity.* If the patient is medically unable to lie flat, you will have to adjust to the altered position, possibly with the help of an assistant.
10. Move the patient according to one of the specific procedures described in the following pages. Remember to use smooth, coordinated movements.
11. Correctly position the patient, using one of the specific positions described in the following pages.
12. Make sure all safety devices (side rails, pillows, protective restraints, call light) are in place *to protect the patient.*
13. Wash your hands.

Evaluation
14. Examine the patient's position for correct alignment.
15. If the patient is able to respond, ask about comfort.

Documentation
16. Document the patient's activity as required by your facility. Usually position changes from side to side or from back to abdomen are noted on a flow sheet. If your facility does not use a flow sheet, document this activity in the narrative nurses' notes. Simply assisting a patient to move up in bed is not usually recorded.
17. *To help other nursing personnel,* you may note the techniques used for moving the patient on a nursing care plan. If the patient's ability to move is a significant part of the general assessment, you may have to write a progress note about the patient's activity.

© 1996 by Lippincott-Raven Publishers

SPECIFIC PROCEDURES FOR MOVING PATIENTS

For each procedure discussed, some steps in the General Procedure may be modified. We have included completely the modified steps as well as references to the steps of the General Procedure that remain the same.

Moving a Patient Closer to One Side of the Bed

This activity is needed in many other moves; therefore, it is being presented separately. Most of the time, you will use this technique in conjunction with another type of movement.

Assessment
1.–3. Follow the steps of the General Procedure.

Planning
4.–6. Follow the steps of the General Procedure.

Implementation
7.–9. Follow the steps of the General Procedure.
10. Move the patient as follows:
   a. Slide your hands and arms under the patient's head and shoulders, and pull that section of the body toward you. Keep your back straight and your hips and knees flexed. Keep one foot forward to give you a broad base of support that can withstand a shift in weight as the patient is pulled toward the side of the bed.
   b. Move your hands and arms down under the patient's hips, and pull that section of the body toward you. Use the body mechanics described in 10.a.
   c. Slide your hands and arms under the patient's legs, and pull them toward you. Again using the body mechanics described in 10.a.
   d. Repeat steps a through c above in sequence until the patient is in the desired location on the bed. If two people are available, the same general technique is used, but two sections of the body are moved at the same time. One nurse slides hands and arms under the patient's shoulders; the other nurse slides hands and arms under the patient's hips. *To make sure they work together,* one of the nurses signals the move by saying, "One, two, three, *pull!*" (Fig. 15–1)
11.–13. Follow the steps of the General Procedure.

Evaluation
14.–15. Follow the steps of the General Procedure.

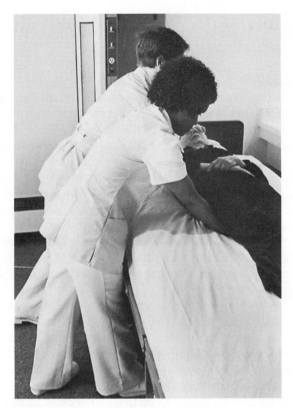

Figure 15–1. Moving a patient to one side of a bed: Two-person assist. The nurses slide their arms under the patient (one at the shoulders, one at the hips) and pull toward themselves. (Courtesy Ivan Ellis)

Documentation
16.–17. Follow the steps of the General Procedure.

Moving a Patient Up in Bed: One-Person Assist

The following technique is used for the patient who is alert and able to cooperate and help. Encourage independence, *both to benefit the patient's physical progress and to support feelings of self-esteem.*

Assessment
1.–3. Follow the steps of the General Procedure.

Planning
4.–6. Follow the steps of the General Procedure.

Implementation
7.–9. Follow the steps of the General Procedure.
10. Move the patient as follows:
   a. Have the patient bend the knees and place the soles of the feet firmly on the surface of the bed. *This reduces the drag of the legs.* The patient may need some assistance with this procedure.
   b. Have the patient grasp the overhead trapeze, if one is in place, or the side rails at shoulder

© 1996 by Lippincott-Raven Publishers

level. Some patients may be able to grasp the headboard and pull themselves up.

c. Slide your hands and arms under the patient's hips. You should be turned slightly toward the foot of the bed with your outside foot slightly ahead of your inside foot (Fig. 15–2). Keep your back straight, bend at the hips and the knees, and keep your elbows bent *so that you are using your strong leg muscles to pull.*

d. Instruct the patient to move with you on the count "One, two, three, *up!*" All effort should be simultaneous *to supply the most combined energy to the task.*

e. Count, "One, two, three, *up!*" The patient should pull with the arms and push with the feet. From your position, you will *pull* the patient up in bed. *In pulling, you use your strong flexor muscles most effectively.* Many people car-

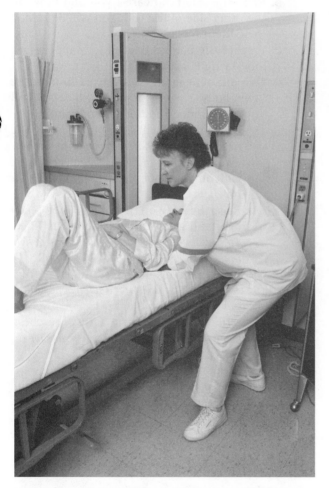

Figure 15–2. Moving a patient up in bed: One-person assist. The patient pushes with feet flat on the bed. The side rails and trapeze have been omitted to clarify the nurse's position. If they are not available, the patient pushes on the bed with the palms of the hands to further assist in moving. (Courtesy Ivan Ellis)

ry out this maneuver facing the head of the bed, pushing the patient up. This method has two drawbacks: first, *you cannot move as much weight this way; second, you meet greater resistance from the bed surface in pushing along it than in pulling along it.*

11.–13. Follow the steps of the General Procedure.

Evaluation

14.–15. Follow the steps of the General Procedure.

Documentation

16.–17. Follow the steps of the General Procedure.

Moving a Patient Up in Bed: Two- or Three-Person Assist

When you must move a heavy patient or one who is unable to help, you will find an assistant useful. Two people are sufficient for most patients, but for exceptionally heavy patients, three people may be necessary.

Assessment

1.–3. Follow the steps of the General Procedure.

Planning

4.–6. Follow the steps of the General Procedure.

Implementation

7.–9. Follow the steps of the General Procedure.

10. Move the patient as follows:
    a. Move the patient close to one side of the bed.
    b. If possible, have the patient bend the knees and plant the soles of the feet firmly on the bed. Even if the patient is unable to push with the feet and legs, *this positioning of the knees and soles eliminates the need to drag the weight of the legs as well as the weight of the trunk.*
    c. The first nurse (nurse 1) slides his or her arms under the patient's head and shoulders. This nurse faces the foot of the bed. *This puts nurse 1 in a position to pull strongly.*
    d. The second nurse (nurse 2) slides his or her arms under the patient's hips from the same side of the bed. This nurse also faces the foot of the bed (Fig. 15–3).
    e. The nurse with the heavier burden (usually nurse 2) counts, "One, two, three, *up!*" *so that both pull the patient up in bed at the same time.* This procedure can be repeated several times until the patient is in the correct position.

If a third nurse is needed, all three should position themselves on the same side of the bed, distributing the weight among them. Because the patient is close to the side of the bed where the nurses are standing, it is possible for each *to maintain firm support with the*

© 1996 by Lippincott-Raven Publishers

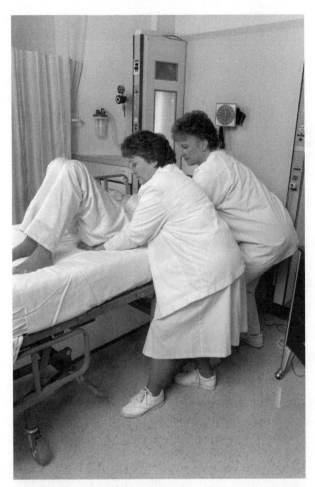

Figure 15–3. Moving a patient up in bed: Two-person assist. The nurses face toward the foot of the bed. The outside foot (left, in this instance) is placed more toward the foot of the bed to provide a wide stance. The back is straight and knees and hips are slightly bent. (Courtesy Ivan Ellis)

legs, keeping the center of gravity over that base of support and working close to the body. This is an efficient way to use muscles. On occasion, it will be necessary to leave a patient in the middle of the bed. In that case, the lifters should position themselves on each side of the bed, paying close attention to their body mechanics. *It is very easy to bend from the waist and put strain on the back.*

Under no circumstances should a nurse pull a patient up in bed by grasping the patient under the axillae and pulling. This may work well for the nurse, but it is very uncomfortable for the patient and can cause a shoulder dislocation, especially for a person with extremely weak muscles or paralysis.

11.–13. Follow the steps of the General Procedure.

Evaluation

14.–15. Follow the steps of the General Procedure.

Documentation

16.–17. Follow the steps of the General Procedure.

Turning a Patient in Bed: Back to Side

Assessment

1.–3. Follow the steps of the General Procedure.

Planning

4.–6. Follow the steps of the General Procedure.

Implementation

7.–9. Follow the steps of the General Procedure.
10. Move the patient as follows:

  a. Move the patient so that the side the patient is to lie on is close to the center of the bed. *This will help the patient to end up in the correct place in the bed and will also help to prevent falls from the bed.*

  b. Raise the side rail nearest you and move to the other side of the bed. You will be rolling the patient toward you.

  c. Prepare the pillows needed for support (see Side-Lying Position, page 336).

  d. Two different methods are used to turn the lower body. The one you use will depend on your preference and the patient's ability.

    (1) Cross the patient's far ankle over the near ankle *so that the weight of the legs will help to turn the body.* Then grasp the patient with one hand behind the far hip.

    (2) Raise the knee on the far leg. Then reach over and grasp the far side of the knee. *This also allows the weight of the legs to help in the turn.*

  e. Move the patient's near arm out away from the patient's body, *so that it is not trapped under the body.*

  f. Place the patient's far arm across the chest. *This allows the arm to be used as leverage for the body.*

  g. Grasp the patient behind the far shoulder.

  h. Roll the patient toward you (the hips and shoulders may be turned as one unit) (Fig. 15–4).

  i. Adjust the patient until he or she is in the correct side-lying position.

11.–13. Follow the steps of the General Procedure.

Evaluation

14.–15. Follow the steps of the General Procedure.

Documentation

16.–17. Follow the steps of the General Procedure.

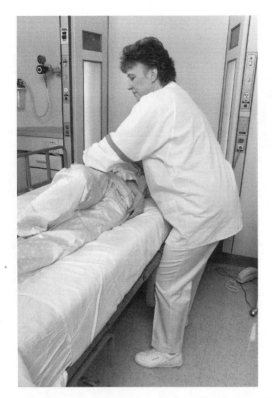

Figure 15–4. Turning a patient from back to side: The nurse uses a wide base of support with back straight and knees slightly bent. The nurse rocks backward, using the entire weight of the body to turn the patient. (Side rails have been omitted for clarity.) (Courtesy Ivan Ellis)

Turning a Patient in Bed: Back to Abdomen

Assessment
1.–3. Follow the steps of the General Procedure.

Planning
4.–6. Follow the steps of the General Procedure.

Implementation
7.–9. Follow the steps of the General Procedure.
10. Move the patient as follows:
    a. Move the patient to the extreme edge of the bed.
    b. Raise the side rail on that side and move to the other side of the bed.
    c. Prepare the pillows needed for support. *Frequently, a heavy-breasted patient will need a pillow under the abdomen for comfort. A very thin patient might be more comfortable with a small pillow under the iliac crests.*
    d. Place the patient's near arm over the head *so that it is out of the way as the patient rolls.*
    e. Turn the patient's face away from you *so that the patient will not roll onto his or her face during the turning procedure* (Fig. 15–5).
    f. Roll the patient onto the side, using the tech-

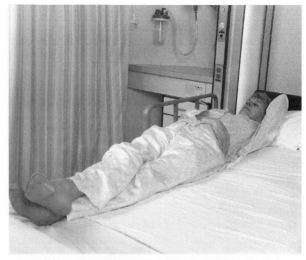

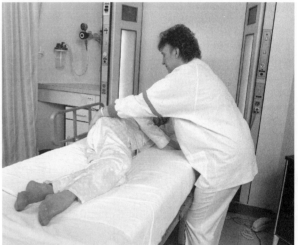

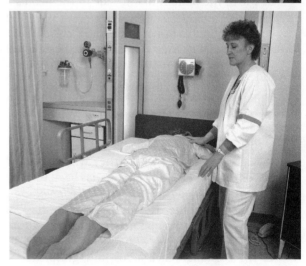

Figure 15–5. Turning a patient to the abdomen. (**A**) Patient positioned for turn. (**B**) Turning the patient. (**C**) Patient positioned on the abdomen. (Courtesy Ivan Ellis)

© 1996 by Lippincott-Raven Publishers

nique described under Turning a Patient in Bed: Back to Side.

g. Once the patient is on the side, check the arm and face carefully *to see that they are correctly positioned.*

h. Roll the patient over onto the abdomen.

i. Adjust the patient until he or she is in a correct abdominal position.

11.–13. Follow the steps of the General Procedure.

Evaluation

14.–15. Follow the steps of the General Procedure.

Documentation

16.–17. Follow the steps of the General Procedure.

Turning a Patient in Bed: Logrolling

Patients who must maintain a straight alignment at all times are turned by a technique called *logrolling.* The technique requires at least two nurses, and sometimes three if the patient is very large.

Assessment

1.–3. Follow the steps of the General Procedure.

Planning

4.–6. Follow the steps of the General Procedure.

Implementation

7.–9. Follow the steps of the General Procedure.
10. Move the patient as follows:

a. Move the patient to one side of the bed as a single unit. Each person assisting with the turn slides his or her arms under the patient. At a signal ("One, two, three, *move!*"), all pull the patient, making sure that the patient's body stays correctly aligned at all times.

b. Raise the side rail on that side of the bed *for safety.*

c. All assistants move to the other side of the bed.

d. Place the pillows where they will be needed for support after the patient has been turned. One is needed *to support the head with the spine straight.* Another is needed between the legs (in fact, two may be needed here) *to support the legs and prevent twisting of the hips.*

e. All assistants reach across and grasp the far side of the patient's body.

f. At the signal ("One, two, three, *turn!*"), all turn the patient smoothly, keeping the patient's body perfectly straight, like a log (Fig. 15–6).

11.–13. Follow the steps of the General Procedure.

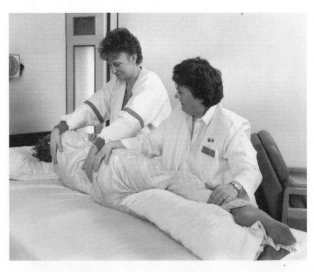

Figure 15–6. Logrolling: The patient is rolled as a unit. The legs remain parallel and a pillow is placed between them to keep the upper leg from dropping and twisting the spine. A pillow is placed to support the head. At least two nurses are essential for this procedure. (Courtesy Ivan Ellis)

Evaluation

14.–15. Follow the steps of the General Procedure.

Documentation

16.–17. Follow the steps of the General Procedure.

Moving a Patient in Bed: Using a Turn or Pull Sheet

A sheet can be used as an aid in turning and moving a patient in bed. One advantage of using a turn or pull sheet is that *the movement takes place between two layers of dry cloth, which produces less friction than does skin on cloth. Another advantage is that it is much easier to grasp a sheet firmly than it is to hold a patient's body. Your hands can slip off the patient if you do not grasp hard enough; and if you grasp too hard, you can cause discomfort or even bruising. A third advantage is that the turn sheet supports the patient's entire body and makes it easier to keep the patient straight.*

A draw sheet or a flat sheet folded in half may be used as a turn or pull sheet. Place the turn sheet under the patient's trunk, with the bottom edge below the patient's buttocks and the top edge at the top of the patient's shoulders. *The sheet will then support the heaviest part of the patient's body.* Do not tuck in the sides; fan fold or roll them along the patient on each side. To move the patient up in bed or to turn the patient, grasp the fan-folded edges of the sheet instead of the patient's body and move the patient up as depicted in Fig. 15–7. Do not lift the patient with

© 1996 by Lippincott-Raven Publishers

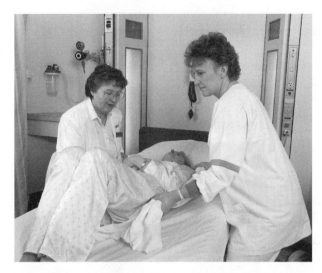

Figure 15–7. Moving a patient up in bed using a turn sheet. Both nurses face the foot of the bed. Knees and hips are slightly bent and backs are straight. Feet are spread to form a wide base of support. (Courtesy Ivan Ellis)

the pull sheet; always slide the patient *to lessen strain on your back.*

POSITIONING A PATIENT IN BED

Positioning patients in bed in proper body alignment and changing their positions frequently are important nursing functions. Many alert patients automatically reposition themselves and readily move about in bed. They may not need special attention, but they often need a reminder that comfort and good body alignment are sometimes not the same. For example, two large pillows under the head may be comfortable, *but when the neck is in constant flexion, it can develop spasms and even contracture.* Patients' bodies must be repositioned during the night as well. Keep in mind that healthy people turn many times and adopt many positions during sleep. Repositioning is usually done every 2 hours. For some patients more frequent turning is needed *to prevent skin breakdown. Without a 24-hour repositioning schedule, positioning may be inadvertently omitted. Patients will develop pressure sores readily if pressure on bony prominences is not relieved.* It is helpful to give range-of-motion exercises (ROM) to patients when they are repositioned *to maintain joint flexibility.* (See Module 22, Range-of-Motion Exercises.)

Positioning aids are devices used to maintain the patient in the correct position. You can make positioning aids easily from ordinary items found in your facility. Pillows, towels, washcloths, blankets, sandbags, footboards, and strong cardboard cartons can all be used to help maintain a position (Fig. 15–8).

PROCEDURES FOR POSITIONING A PATIENT IN BED

Use the following directions to position the patient as indicated in step 11 of the General Procedure for Moving a Patient in Bed and Positioning (page 000):

Supine Position

Assessment
1.–3. Follow the steps of the General Procedure.

Planning
4.–6. Follow the steps of the General Procedure.

Implementation
7.–10. Follow the steps of the General Procedure.
11. Position the patient on his or her back.
  a. Check that the spine is in straight alignment.
  b. Place a low pillow under the head *to prevent neck extension.*
  c. Place the patient's arms at the patient's side with the hands pronated. The forearms can also be elevated on pillows.
  d. If the patient's hands are paralyzed, use handrolls to maintain the hands in functional positions. Handrolls can be made of several washcloths (or other linen) that have been rolled and taped. Place the handroll in the palm of the patient's hand. The fingers and thumb should be flexed around it. The roll should be large enough so that the fingers are only slightly flexed. A handroll may have to be secured to the hand with paper tape (Fig. 15–9).
  e. Position the legs so that external rotation does not occur. Externally rotated hips become less functional and do not support a patient who is trying to regain function. *A trochanter roll provides support to the hip joint to maintain its position and is effective in preventing external hip rotation.* (This roll can be made from a sheet, bath towel, or pad.) Place one end flat under the patient's hip (*trochanter*) and roll the linen under to form a roll *that stabilizes the leg and prevents it from turning outward.* An ankle roll, which is made in the same way but is smaller than a trochanter roll, can accomplish the same purpose. If

© 1996 by Lippincott-Raven Publishers

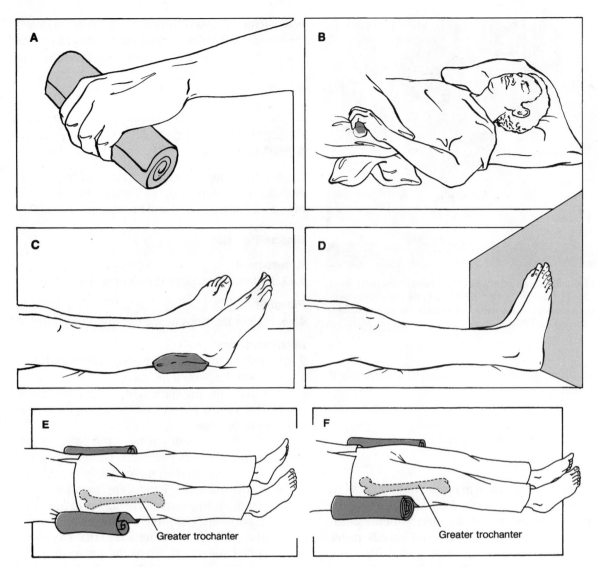

Figure 15–8. Positioning aids. (**A**) A rolled washcloth is used as a handroll. (**B**) Pillows support the extremities. (**C**) A sandbag supports the ankles. (**D**) A firm footboard prevents foot extension. (**E**) A rolled blanket is placed for use as a trochanter roll. (**F**) The blanket is rolled tightly to provide support to the hip.

both legs are paralyzed, place a roll on either side at the hip or the ankle.

f. Support the foot so that the toes point up- ward in anatomic position and do not fall into plantar flexion. *When plantar flexion is maintained for a long time, a permanent deformi- ty called footdrop develops. The foot becomes un- able to dorsiflex and ceases to be functional.* High- topped athletic shoes are very effective in preventing footdrop. Special splints may also be used to maintain position. Although a manufactured footboard, sandbags, or a strong cardboard carton can be used *to main- tain the feet at right angles to the legs, these are less*

effective because the feet slip out of their right- angle position.

12.–13. Follow the steps of the General Procedure.

Evaluation

14.–15. Follow the steps of the General Procedure.

Documentation

16.–17. Follow the steps of the General Procedure.

Side-Lying Position

The side-lying position can be particularly comfort- able for the patient when attention is given to good body alignment (Fig. 15–10).

© 1996 by Lippincott-Raven Publishers

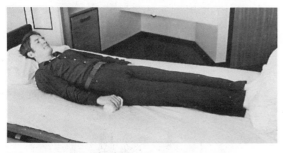

Figure 15–9. Supine position. A small pillow and a footboard help put the patient in correct supine position. Handrolls are used for patients whose hands are paralyzed. (Courtesy Ivan Ellis)

A patient who is paralyzed on one side can be placed on that side as well as on the unaffected side. Pain of the affected joints due to muscle relaxation may lead to dislocation of the joints; therefore, special consideration should be taken when moving or positioning these persons. To avoid dislocation, never pull on the affected extremities. Any pain in the joint should always be reported to the team leader or physician.

Assessment
1.–3. Follow the steps of the General Procedure.

Planning
4.–6. Follow the steps of the General Procedure.

Implementation
7.–10. Follow the steps of the General Procedure.
11. Position the patient on the side with the head supported on a low pillow.
   a. Tuck a pillow along the patient's back *to both support the back and hold the position.*
   b. Bring the underlying arm forward and flex it onto the pillow used for the head.
   c. Bring the top arm forward, flex it, and rest it on a pillow in front of the body.
   d. Put handrolls in place if needed.
   e. Flex the top leg and bring it slightly forward *to help provide balance.*

   f. Place a pillow lengthwise under the top leg *to keep the legs separated and support the top leg.*
   g. Support the feet at right angles to prevent plantar flexion and footdrop.
12.–13. Follow the steps of the General Procedure.

Evaluation
14.–15. Follow the steps of the General Procedure.

Documentation
16.–17. Follow the steps of the General Procedure.

Prone Position

The prone position (Fig. 15–11) is used infrequently by nurses *because respirations of some patients may be compromised in this position.* However, if it is done properly, a great number of patients can tolerate it. The position can be used very effectively with a patient who has pressure sores because it *relieves the pressure on the buttocks and both hips.*

Assessment
1.–3. Follow the steps of the General Procedure.

Planning
4.–6. Follow the steps of the General Procedure.

Implementation
7.–10. Follow the steps of the General Procedure.
11. Position the patient by turning him or her onto the abdomen. You will often need two people to allow you to do this with ease.
   a. Turn the head to one side. Usually you do not use a pillow, but sometimes a small pillow or a folded bath towel *may provide added comfort for the patient.* Be sure that the spine is straight.
   b. Place supports as needed for the trunk. A folded towel under each shoulder prevents slumping of the shoulders. A flat pillow under the abdomen of a female patient who has large breasts *adds to her comfort without defeating the principles of good alignment.*
   c. Position the arms so that they are comfort-

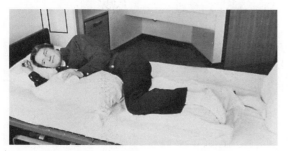

Figure 15–10. Side-lying position. Two pillows support the upper leg and arm; the lower leg lies straight. (Courtesy Ivan Ellis)

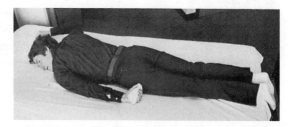

Figure 15–11. Prone position. A small pillow supports the patients' ankles. The patient's arms bend upward toward the shoulders or remain at the sides. A small pillow may be used under the head. (Courtesy Ivan Ellis)

© 1996 by Lippincott-Raven Publishers

able. The arms may be flat at the patient's side or flexed at the elbow with the hands near the patient's head.

d. Place handrolls if needed.

e. Position the feet in dorsiflexion. With tall patients, the feet should extend beyond the end of the mattress, so that they are pointing down in the space between the mattress and the footboard. With shorter patients, place a roll under the ankles. *This will keep the feet in proper alignment, preventing plantar flexion.*

12.–13. Follow the steps of the General Procedure.

Evaluation

14.–15. Follow the steps of the General Procedure.

Documentation

16.–17. Follow the steps of the General Procedure.

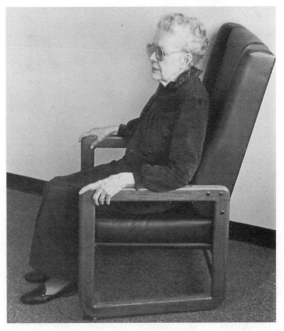

Figure 15–12. Positioning a patient in a chair. The patient's buttocks should fit well back into the seat of the chair. The back is straight, the knees are bent, and the feet are flat on the floor. The elbows are supported by armrests. (Courtesy Ivan Ellis)

POSITIONING A PATIENT IN A CHAIR

The following discussion will guide you in assisting the patient into a correct sitting position in the chair. Remember that the patient who is physically able to change positions may sit in what would be an uncomfortable position for a short time and will then move. The incapacitated patient must rely on your careful judgment to be in a seated position that provides comfort.

1. To move a patient into a chair, follow the directions in Module 20, Transfer.

2. Then place the patient's feet flat against the floor.

3. Position the knees and hips at 90- to 110-degree angles. The patient will be upright and the joints in a comfortable position.

4. Ensure that the buttocks rest firmly against the back of the chair and that the spine is in straight alignment *to provide proper support and comfort* (Fig. 15–12).

　　In most cases you should avoid placing pillows at the back *because they may interfere with proper alignment.* In some chairs, pillows at the back are needed because the seat is deep and the patient will lean backward at an uncomfortable angle if no pillows are used. Support the patient's elbows with arm rests.

5. If needed, place handrolls in the patient's hands. A footrest of some type may be needed for shorter patients. Foam bolsters or pillows are sometimes needed beside the patient to prevent falling toward the side.

THERAPEUTIC POSITIONS

In addition to the resting positions described above, a variety of special positions are used for therapeutic reasons. The reasons for their use can be found in a medical-surgical text.

Fowler's Position

1. Place the patient in the supine position.

2. Elevate the head of the bed 18 to 20 inches, or approximately 45° (Fig. 15–13). *The Fowler's position promotes lung expansion. This position also decreases intracranial pressure for the patient with neurologic problems. It can be used to perform certain procedures such as oral care and the insertion of a nasogastric tube and is a comfortable position for*

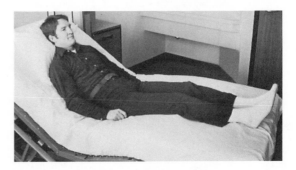

Figure 15–13. In Fowler's position, the head is up approximately 45°. The knees are not elevated to avoid putting pressure on the popliteal areas. (Courtesy Ivan Ellis)

© 1996 by Lippincott-Raven Publishers

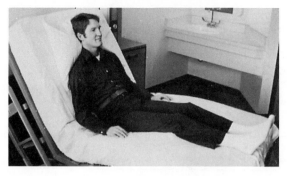

Figure 15–14. High Fowler's position. (Courtesy Ivan Ellis)

eating. Always make a careful assessment of the needs and toleration of the individual patient.

High Fowler's Position

1. Place the patient in the supine position.
2. Elevate the head of the bed to an angle of more than 45° (Fig. 15–14).

Semi-Fowler's Position

1. Place the patient in the supine position.
2. Elevate the head of the bed to an angle of less than 45° (often 20–30°).

Orthopneic Position

1. Have the patient sit up in or at the edge of the bed with an overbed table across the lap.
2. Pad the table with a pillow and elevate to a comfortable height.

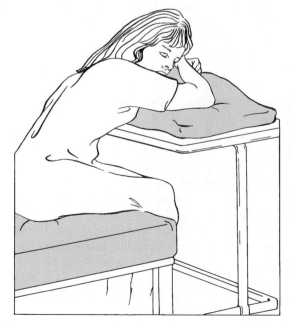

Figure 15–15. In the orthopneic position, the patient rests the elbows on a pillow on the overbed table.

© 1996 by Lippincott-Raven Publishers

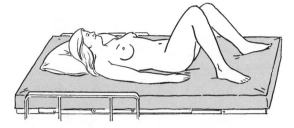

Figure 15–16. Dorsal recumbent position. (Draping omitted for clarity.)

3. Have the patient lean forward and rest head and arms on the table *for support* (Fig. 15–15).

This position is used to promote lung expansion for the patient who has extreme difficulty breathing and who is unable to lie flat or with the head only moderately elevated. It is also used to perform a thoracentesis. (See Module 12, Assisting with Diagnostic and Therapeutic Procedures.)

Dorsal Recumbent Position

1. Position the patient in the supine position.
2. Raise the patient's knees and separate the legs (Fig. 15–16). *The dorsal recumbent position is often used as a position of comfort for patients with backstrain.*

Lithotomy Position

1. Place the patient in the supine position.
2. Flex both knees simultaneously so that the feet are brought close to the hips. Separate the legs widely, maintaining the flexed position.

   If the patient is on an examining table, place the feet in stirrups. Then drape the patient *to provide for visibility of the perineal area for purposes of examination* while the legs and body remain covered *for warmth and modesty* (Fig. 15–17). *The lithotomy position is used for perineal and vaginal examinations as well as for procedures such as the vaginal douche.*

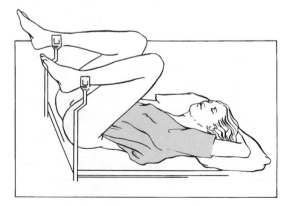

Figure 15–17. Lithotomy position. (Draping omitted for clarity.)

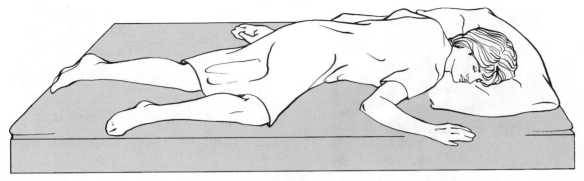

Figure 15–18. Sims' position. (Draping omitted for clarity.)

Sims' Position

1. Place the patient in a side-lying position using only a single supporting pillow under the head.
2. Turn the patient far enough onto the abdomen so that the lower arm is extended behind the back and both knees are slightly flexed. The upper leg is flexed farther forward than the lower leg and rests on the bed.

   The Sims' position is used for the administration of enemas or for examination of the rectal area (Fig. 15–18). It may also be used for catheterization in the patient who is unable to be in the lithotomy position.

Knee–Chest Position (Genupectoral)

1. Have the patient kneel on the bed or table, then lean forward with the hips in the air and the chest and arms on the bed or table. A pillow can be placed under the patient's head (Fig. 15–19).
2. If a special examination table is available, have the patient kneel on a platform and lean on the table. The patient is draped *to allow visibility of the rectal area and coverage of the rest of the body for warmth and modesty.* The knee–chest position is used for rectal procedures such as sigmoidoscopy.

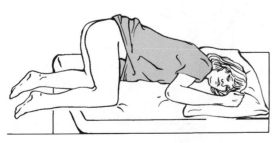

Figure 15–19. Knee–chest position. (Draping omitted for clarity.)

Trendelenburg Position

1. Place the patient in the supine position with the head of the bed down and the entire bed frame tilted downward with the head approximately 30° below horizontal level.
2. Use a pillow *to protect the head from the bed's headboard. This position is sometimes used for postural drainage, which is a procedure for draining secretions from certain segments of the lungs. The Trendelenburg position is also used to promote venous return in patients with problems in tissue perfusion (Fig. 15–20).*

LONG-TERM CARE

Moving the patient in bed and positioning is a frequent and essential task for staff persons in long-term care settings. *This is because many of the residents cannot adequately move themselves because of physical limitations.* It is essential that you have knowledge of these skills because the registered nurse or licensed practical nurse is always in the position of team leading or supervising others in the long-term care setting.

Assessment of the resident in the facility is crucial *so that proper and safe positioning and transfer takes place.* Knowing the physical effects of diseases (such as stroke and Parkinson's disease) as well as the more normal changes brought on by the aging process is an essential part of the knowledge base for assessment of the physically limited resident. Maintaining good body alignment at all times and avoiding undue pressure on the body parts and limbs of elderly patients are important parts of safety.

© 1996 by Lippincott-Raven Publishers

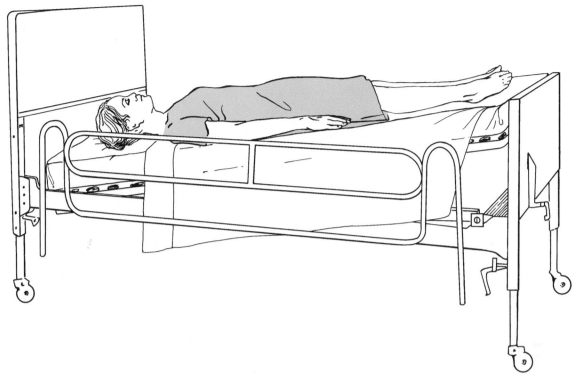

Figure 15–20. Trendelenburg position.

HOME CARE

More persons who have problems that require assistance in moving and changing position are being cared for in the home. One of the roles you have in this setting may be health teaching. Family members will want to become proficient using these skills *so they can provide better care for the family member involved.* Assisting the caregivers in learning these techniques may require a teaching plan with demonstration on your part, followed by a return demonstration and feedback. At first, positioning and moving a loved one with physical limitations may be awkward and may create anxiety. With repetition and your encouragement and praise, this will soon become more comfortable for both the client and the family.

CRITICAL THINKING EXERCISES

Martha Smith, a resident in a long-term care facility, has had a stroke that left her left arm weakened and her left leg paralyzed. The plan is for her to be up in a chair three times a day. Considering what you know of the results of stroke, identify the concerns you have. Devise several alternative strategies for making her comfortable in a chair.

© 1996 by Lippincott-Raven Publishers

PERFORMANCE CHECKLIST

General Procedure for Moving a Patient in Bed	Needs More Practice	Satisfactory	Comments
Assessment			
1. Assess patient's need.			
2. Assess patient's ability.			
3. Check on assistive devices available.			
Planning			
4. Plan moving technique.			
5. Wash your hands.			
6. Obtain assistive devices.			
Implementation			
7. Identify patient.			
8. Raise bed to high position.			
9. Put bed in flat position.			
10. Move patient according to specific procedure.			
11. Position patient correctly.			
12. Make sure safety devices are in place.			
13. Wash your hands.			
Evaluation			
14. Evaluate position for alignment.			
15. Evaluate patient comfort.			
Documentation			
16. Record time and position on flow sheet or nurses' notes.			
17. Record technique for moving on Nursing Care Plan.			
Moving a Patient Closer to One Side of a Bed			
Assessment			
1.–3. Follow Checklist steps 1–3 of the General Procedure for Moving a Patient in Bed (assess patient's need to move and ability to move unaided, and check on available assistive devices).			

(continued)

© 1996 by Lippincott-Raven Publishers

Moving a Patient Closer to One Side of a Bed *(Continued)*	Needs More Practice	Satisfactory	Comments
Planning			
4.–6. Follow Checklist steps 4–6 of the General Procedure (plan moving technique, wash your hands, and obtain assistive devices or assistance).			
Implementation			
7.–9. Follow Checklist steps 7–9 of the General Procedure (identify patient, raise bed, and put bed in flat position).			
10. Move the patient as follows: **a.** Slide your hands and arms under patient's head and shoulders, and pull toward you.			
b. Move your hands and arms under patient's hips, and pull toward you.			
c. Slide your hands and arms under patient's legs, and pull toward you.			
d. Repeat in sequence until patient is in correct position.			
11.–13. Follow Checklist steps 11–13 of the General Procedure (correctly position patient, have safety devices in place, and wash your hands).			
Evaluation			
14.–15. Follow Checklist steps 14 and 15 of the General Procedure (assess for correct alignment and ask patient about comfort).			
Documentation			
16.–17. Follow Checklist steps 16 and 17 of the General Procedure (record as required by your facility and add to care plan if appropriate).			
Moving a Patient Up in Bed: One-Person Assist			
Assessment			
1.–3. Follow Checklist steps 1–3 of the General Procedure for Moving a Patient in Bed (assess patient's need to move and ability to move unaided, and check on available assistive devices).			

(continued)

© 1996 by Lippincott-Raven Publishers

Moving a Patient Up in Bed: One-Person Assist *(Continued)*	Needs More Practice	Satisfactory	Comments
Planning			
4.–6. Follow Checklist steps 4–6 of the General Procedure (plan moving technique, wash your hands, and obtain assistive devices or assistance).			
Implementation			
7.–9. Follow Checklist steps 7–9 of the General Procedure (identify patient, raise bed, and put bed in flat position).			
10. Move the patient as follows: **a.** Have patient bend knees and place soles firmly on bed.			
b. Have patient grasp overhead trapeze, side rails, or headboard.			
c. Slide your hands and arms under patient's hips, facing foot of bed, with outside foot ahead of inside foot.			
d. Instruct patient to move with you at count.			
e. On count, patient pulls with arms and pushes with feet as you pull.			
11.–13. Follow Checklist steps 11–13 of the General Procedure (correctly position patient, have safety devices in place, and wash your hands).			
Evaluation			
14.–15. Follow Checklist steps 14 and 15 of the General Procedure (assess for correct alignment and ask patient about comfort).			
Documentation			
16.–17. Follow Checklist steps 16 and 17 of the General Procedure (record as required by your facility and add to care plan if appropriate).			

(continued)

© 1996 by Lippincott-Raven Publishers

Moving a Patient Up in Bed: Two- or Three-Person Assist	Needs More Practice	Satisfactory	Comments
Assessment			
1.–3. Follow Checklist steps 1–3 of the General Procedure for Moving a Patient in Bed (assess patient's need to move and ability to move unaided, and check on available assistive devices).			
Planning			
4.–6. Follow Checklist steps 4–6 of the General Procedure (plan moving technique, wash your hands, and obtain assistive devices or assistance).			
Implementation			
7.–9. Follow Checklist steps 7–9 of the General Procedure (identify patient, raise bed, and put bed in flat position).			
10. Move the patient as follows: **a.** Move patient close to one side of bed.			
b. If possible, have patient's knees bent and soles firmly on bed.			
c. Nurse 1 slides arms under patient's head and shoulders.			
d. Nurse 2 slides arms under patient's hips.			
e. Nurse 2 counts, and both move patient.			
11.–13. Follow Checklist steps 11–13 of the General Procedure (correctly position patient, have safety devices in place, and wash your hands).			
Evaluation			
14.–15. Follow Checklist steps 14 and 15 of the General Procedure (assess for correct alignment and ask patient about comfort).			
Documentation			
16.–17. Follow Checklist steps 16 and 17 of the General Procedure (record as required by your facility and add to care plan if appropriate).			

(continued)

© 1996 by Lippincott-Raven Publishers

Turning a Patient in Bed: Back to Side	Needs More Practice	Satisfactory	Comments
Assessment			
1.–3. Follow Checklist steps 1–3 of the General Procedure for Moving a Patient in Bed (assess patient's need to move and ability to move unaided, and check on available assistive devices).			
Planning			
4.–6. Follow Checklist steps 4–6 of the General Procedure (plan moving technique, wash your hands, and obtain assistive devices or assistance).			
Implementation			
7.–9. Follow Checklist steps 7–9 of the General Procedure (identify patient, raise bed, and put bed in flat position).			
10. Move the patient as follows: **a.** Move patient to one side of bed.			
b. Raise rail and move to other side.			
c. Prepare pillows for support.			
d. Turn lower body, using one of two methods described.			
e. Move patient's near arm out of patient's way.			
f. Place patient's far arm across chest.			
g. Grasp patient behind far shoulder.			
h. Roll patient toward you.			
i. Adjust position as needed.			
11.–13. Follow Checklist steps 11–13 of the General Procedure (correctly position patient, have safety devices in place, and wash your hands).			
Evaluation			
14.–15. Follow Checklist steps 14 and 15 of the General Procedure (assess for correct alignment and ask patient about comfort).			
Documentation			
16.–17. Follow Checklist steps 16 and 17 of the General Procedure (record as required by your facility and add to care plan if appropriate).			

© 1996 by Lippincott-Raven Publishers

(*continued*)

Turning a Patient in Bed: Back to Abdomen	Needs More Practice	Satisfactory	Comments
Assessment			
1.–3. Follow Checklist steps 1–3 of the General Procedure for Moving a Patient in Bed (assess patient's need to move and ability to move unaided, and check on available assistive devices).			
Planning			
4.–6. Follow Checklist steps 4–6 of the General Procedure (plan moving technique, wash your hands, and obtain assistive devices or assistance).			
Implementation			
7.–9. Follow Checklist steps 7–9 of the General Procedure (identify patient, raise bed, and put bed in flat position).			
10. Move the patient as follows: **a.** Move patient to edge of bed.			
b. Raise side rail and move to other side of bed.			
c. Prepare pillows for support.			
d. Place patient's near arm close to body.			
e. Turn patient's face away from you.			
f. Roll patient onto side.			
g. Check arm and face positioning.			
h. Roll patient further onto abdomen.			
i. Adjust position as needed.			
11.–13. Follow Checklist steps 11–13 of the General Procedure (correctly position patient, have safety devices in place, and wash your hands).			
Evaluation			
14.–15. Follow Checklist steps 14 and 15 of the General Procedure (assess for correct alignment and ask patient about comfort).			
Documentation			
16.–17. Follow Checklist steps 16 and 17 of the General Procedure (record as required by your facility and add to care plan if appropriate).			

© 1996 by Lippincott-Raven Publishers

(continued)

Turning a Patient: Logrolling	Needs More Practice	Satisfactory	Comments
Assessment			
1.–3. Follow Checklist steps 1–3 of the General Procedure for Moving a Patient in Bed (assess patient's need to move and ability to move unaided, and check on available assistive devices).			
Planning			
4.–6. Follow Checklist steps 4–6 of the General Procedure (plan moving technique, wash your hands, and obtain assistive devices or assistance).			
Implementation			
7.–9. Follow Checklist steps 7–9 of the General Procedure (identify patient, raise bed, and put bed in flat position).			
10. Move the patient as follows: **a.** With help, move patient to side of bed in one unit.			
b. Raise side rail on that side of bed.			
c. All assistants move to other side of bed.			
d. Place pillows correctly.			
e. Assistants reach across and grasp patient's body.			
f. At count, all turn patient in one unit.			
11.–13. Follow Checklist steps 11–13 of the General Procedure (correctly position patient, have safety devices in place, and wash your hands).			
Evaluation			
14.–15. Follow Checklist steps 14 and 15 of the General Procedure (assess for correct alignment and ask patient about comfort).			
Documentation			
16.–17. Follow Checklist steps 16 and 17 of the General Procedure (record as required by your facility and add to care plan if appropriate).			
Note: All the movements described can be facilitated by using a turn or pull sheet (see page 334).			

© 1996 by Lippincott-Raven Publishers

(*continued*)

Positioning a Patient in Bed: Supine Position	Needs More Practice	Satisfactory	Comments
Assessment			
1.–3. Follow Checklist steps 1–3 of the General Procedure for Moving a Patient in Bed (assess patient's need to and ability to move, and check on available assistive devices).			
Planning			
4.–6. Follow Checklist steps 4–6 of the General Procedure (plan moving technique, wash your hands, obtain assistive devices or assistance).			
Implementation			
7.–10. Follow Checklist steps 7–10 of the General Procedure (identify patient, raise bed, put bed in flat position, move patient according to specific procedure).			
11. Position patient on back. **a.** Check spine for straight alignment.			
b. Place low pillow under head.			
c. Place arms at side or elevated on pillow, with hands prone.			
d. Place handrolls if needed.			
e. Keep legs straight and prevent external rotation.			
f. Position feet with toes pointed up, and support with footboards, sandbags, or carton.			
12.–13. Follow Checklist steps 12 and 13 of the General Procedure (have safety devices in place and wash your hands).			
Evaluation			
14.–15. Follow Checklist steps 14 and 15 of the General Procedure (assess for correct alignment and ask patient about comfort).			
Documentation			
16.–17. Follow Checklist steps 16 and 17 of the General Procedure (record as required by your facility and add to care plan if appropriate).			

(continued)

© 1996 by Lippincott-Raven Publishers

Positioning a Patient in Bed: Side-Lying Position

	Needs More Practice	Satisfactory	Comments
Assessment			
1.–3. Follow Checklist steps 1–3 of the General Procedure for Moving a Patient in Bed (assess patient's need to and ability to move, and check on available assistive devices).			
Planning			
4.–6. Follow Checklist steps 4–6 of the General Procedure (plan moving technique, wash your hands, obtain assistive devices or assistance).			
Implementation			
7.–10. Follow Checklist steps 7–10 of the General Procedure (identify patient, raise bed, put bed in flat position, move patient according to specific procedure).			
11. Position patient on side with head on pillow. **a.** Tuck pillow along back.			
b. Place lower arm forward of body and flex and support lower arm on pillow used for head.			
c. Flex top arm and rest on pillow in front of body.			
d. Place handrolls if needed.			
e. Flex top leg and bring slightly forward.			
f. Place pillow lengthwise between legs.			
g. Support feet with positioning aids to prevent plantar flexion.			
12.–13. Follow Checklist steps 12 and 13 of the General Procedure (have safety devices in place and wash your hands).			
Evaluation			
14.–15. Follow Checklist steps 14 and 15 of the General Procedure (assess for correct alignment and ask patient about comfort).			
Documentation			
16.–17. Follow Checklist steps 16 and 17 of the General Procedure (record as required by your facility and add to care plan if appropriate).			

© 1996 by Lippincott-Raven Publishers

(continued)

Positioning a Patient in Bed: Prone Position	Needs More Practice	Satisfactory	Comments
Assessment			
1.–3. Follow Checklist steps 1–3 of the General Procedure for Moving a Patient in Bed (assess patient's need to and ability to move, and check on available assistive devices).			
Planning			
4.–6. Follow Checklist steps 4–6 of the General Procedure (plan moving technique, wash your hands, obtain assistive devices or assistance).			
Implementation			
7.–10. Follow Checklist steps 7–10 of the General Procedure (identify patient, raise bed, put bed in flat position, move patient according to specific procedure).			
11. Position patient on abdomen. **a.** Turn patient's head to one side with spine straight.			
b. Place folded towel under each shoulder.			
c. Place arms flat at side or flexed at elbow near patient's head.			
d. Place handrolls if needed.			
e. Position patient's feet in space between mattress and footboard or use roll under ankles.			
12.–13. Follow Checklist steps 12 and 13 of the General Procedure (have safety devices in place and wash your hands).			
Evaluation			
14.–15. Follow Checklist steps 14 and 15 of the General Procedure (assess for correct alignment and ask patient about comfort).			
Documentation			
16.–17. Follow Checklist steps 16 and 17 of the General Procedure (record as required by your facility and add to care plan if appropriate).			

(*continued*)

© 1996 by Lippincott-Raven Publishers

Positioning a Patient in a Chair	Needs More Practice	Satisfactory	Comments
1. Move patient into chair, following directions in Module 20, Transfer.			
2. Place feet flat against floor.			
3. Position knees and hips at right angle.			
4. Straighten spine.			
5. Support elbows on armrests.			
6. Place handrolls, footrest, or bolsters if needed.			
Fowler's Position			
1. Place patient in supine position.			
2. Elevate head of bed 18–20 inches (approximately 45°).			
High Fowler's Position			
1. Place patient in supine position.			
2. Elevate head of bed to angle of over 45°			
Semi-Fowler's Position			
1. Place patient in supine position.			
2. Elevate head of bed to angle of less than 45° (usually 20°–30°).			
Orthopneic Position			
1. Have patient sit up in bed with overbed table across lap.			
2. Pad table with pillows and elevate to comfortable height.			
3. Have patient lean forward with head and arms resting on table.			
Dorsal Recumbent Position			
1. Position patient on back.			
2. Raise knees and separate legs.			
3. Feet remain in position on bed.			

(continued)

© 1996 by Lippincott-Raven Publishers

	Needs More Practice	Satisfactory	Comments
Lithotomy Position			
1. Position patient on back.			
2. Raise knees and separate legs.			
3. If on table, place feet in stirrups.			
Sims' Position			
1. Use side-lying position, with single pillow only under head.			
2. Turn far enough onto abdomen so lower arm extends behind patient's back.			
Knee–Chest Position (Genupectoral)			
1. Have patient kneel on bed or table with hips in air and chest on bed or table.			
2. If special table is available, have patient kneel on platform with head and chest on table.			
Trendelenburg Position			
1. Place patient in supine position with head of bed lowered. Tilt entire bed frame downward with head approximately 30° below horizontal level.			
2. Use a pillow to protect the patient's head.			

© 1996 by Lippincott-Raven Publishers

? QUIZ

Short-Answer Questions

1. What is the primary reason for having the bed in the flat position when moving a patient?

   _____

2. What two important functions are fulfilled by having the patient assist you whenever possible?

   a. _____

   b. _____

3. If the nurse attempts to move a patient by grasping him or her under the axillae, a(n) _____ may occur.

4. A turn sheet should be placed under which part of a patient's body?

   _____

5. List two reasons why patients should be checked after moving.

   a. _____

   b. _____

6. List three reasons for proper and frequent positioning of a patient in bed.

   a. _____

   b. _____

   c. _____

7. To prevent external rotation of the leg when a patient is in the supine position, you might use

   _____

8. When a patient is in a side-lying position, the top leg is _____ over the lower leg.

9. When a patient is in the prone position, two methods can be used to keep the feet from plantar flexion and possible development of footdrop. What are these two methods?

   a. _____

   b. _____

10. When working in long-term care or home care, how could you facilitate the proper moving and positioning of patients by staff and families?

    _____

    _____

Multiple-Choice Questions

_____ 11. In all positions the spine should be

   a. slightly flexed.
   b. straight.
   c. slightly extended.
   d. curved.

© 1996 by Lippincott-Raven Publishers

_____   **12.** A patient's position should usually be changed

        a. every hour.
        b. every 2 hours.
        c. every 4 hours.
        d. once per shift.

_____   **13.** Sims' position is one in which the patient

        a. has the feet and legs elevated.
        b. has the head elevated at a 30° angle.
        c. is on the left side with both knees flexed, the right higher than the left.
        d. is in a kneeling position.

© 1996 by Lippincott-Raven Publishers

FEEDING ADULT PATIENTS

MODULE CONTENTS

RATIONALE FOR THE USE OF THIS
   SKILL
NURSING DIAGNOSES
GENERAL CONSIDERATIONS
Factors That Affect Eating Habits
Psychosocial Considerations
Physical Problems
The Patient With Dysphagia
PROCEDURE FOR FEEDING ADULT
   PATIENTS
   Assessment
   Planning
   Implementation
   Evaluation
   Documentation
LONG-TERM CARE
HOME CARE
CRITICAL THINKING EXERCISES

PREREQUISITES

Successful completion of the following modules:

VOLUME 1

Module 1   An Approach to Nursing Skills
Module 2   Basic Infection Control
Module 3   Safety
Module 5   Documentation
Module 6   Introduction to Assessment Skills
Module 10 Intake and Output

Familiarity with the basic diets used in most institutions.
Knowledge of the food guide pyramid.

© 1996 by Lippincott-Raven Publishers

OVERALL OBJECTIVE

To assist patients in feeding themselves or to feed those who are unable to feed themselves independently.

SPECIFIC LEARNING OBJECTIVES

Know Facts and Principles	Apply Facts and Principles	Demonstrate Ability	Evaluate Performance

1. Preparation
    a. Environment
    b. Patient (physical and psychosocial)
 List factors in environment that might affect appetite.
 	
 Describe optimum position for comfort and ease of eating, and discuss possible modifications.
 	
 Discuss emotional needs and responses related to eating.
	In a specific patient situation, state what needs to be done to prepare patient and environment for meal.	In clinical setting, carry out preparation appropriately.	Evaluate with instructor.

2. Adaptations of procedure List factors that often make adaptations to procedure necessary. List easy to swallow and difficult to swallow foods. List actions that help the dysphagic patient swallow.	Assess muscular and other physical difficulties, including swallowing problems and emotional reactions. Check patient's tray for appropriate foods.	When feeding patient in the clinical setting, vary the procedure appropriately in light of a particular patient's difficulties. Teach patient how to facilitate swallowing.	Review performance with instructor and patient. Evaluate with your instructor.
3. Retention and tolerance List adverse reactions toward eating or being fed.	Know problems most commonly experienced by patients being cared for.	In the clinical setting, assess for specific responses unique to patient.	Share problems with instructor.
4. Documentation State importance of monitoring patient's food intake.	Be familiar with portions of food items and terms used. Describe amount of food taken and patient's responses.	After feeding an individual patient, appropriately record amounts taken and pertinent observations.	Evaluate with instructor.

© 1996 by Lippincott-Raven Publishers

LEARNING ACTIVITIES

1. Review the Specific Learning Objectives.
2. Read the section on nutrition (in the chapter on nutrition) in Ellis and Nowlis, *Nursing: A Human Needs Approach,* or comparable material in another textbook.
3. Look up the module vocabulary terms in the glossary.
4. Read through the module as though you were preparing to teach these concepts and skills to another person.
5. Review the steps of the procedure in the Performance Checklist and mentally practice the techniques.
6. In the practice setting:
   a. Have a classmate feed you lunch. Try eating half in a recumbent position (lying down) and half in a sitting position in bed. Close your eyes for 3 minutes while being fed. At this point, have your classmate describe the food to you. Eat a part of the meal with your eyes closed, as though you were blind. Have your classmate assist you by telling you where various foods are located. Now answer the following questions:
      (1) What was pleasant about the experience?
      (2) What was unpleasant?
      (3) What did you learn?
   b. Repeat a, but this time reverse roles. Discuss the questions from your point of view as the one administering the feeding.

   c. Examine the pictures of feeding aids on page 364. These aids can be purchased commercially or made by the patient's family members or by staff members in the occupational or physical therapy departments.
7. In the clinical setting:
   a. Observe a patient being fed. What was done that was helpful to the patient? What might you have done differently?
   b. Feed a patient an entire meal. Note the time when you begin and end the procedure. Answer the following questions for your own learning or discuss them with your instructor.
      (1) How long did the feeding procedure take?
      (2) What conclusions can you draw from the timing?
      (3) What were some of the blocks to effective feeding that you encountered?
      (4) What went well?
      (5) Were you uncomfortable at any point?
      (6) Did the patient appear to be uncomfortable at any point?
      (7) Did you use all the steps of the procedure?
      (8) Did you make adaptations? If so, what were they and why did you make them?
   c. Record, on a piece of paper, observations you made regarding the amount of food taken and the patient's response. Share your notes with your instructor.

VOCABULARY

antiemetic	condiments	ingestion	stereotype
aspiration	dexterity	malnutrition	tremor
anorexia	digestion	NPO	
body language	dysphagia	reflux	
cachexia	ethnic	regurgitate	

© 1996 by Lippincott-Raven Publishers

Feeding Adult Patients

Rationale for the Use of This Skill

During illness, trauma, or wound healing, the body needs more nutrients than usual. However, many patients, because of weakness, immobility, or inability to use one or both of the upper extremities, are unable to feed themselves all or part of a meal. To be sure the patient receives adequate nutrition, the nurse must be knowledgeable, sensitive, and skillful in carrying out the feeding procedure. To promote the patient's well-being, the nurse must also consider the patient's psychological response to being fed.

Feeding patients is considered a less than professional skill and is often delegated to nursing assistants or volunteers. Frequently this may be both necessary and appropriate. However, when it is essential for you to assist patients with eating, you should welcome this opportunity for an extended interaction. When feeding patients has been delegated to assistive personnel, you should carefully supervise the activity.[1]

▼ NURSING DIAGNOSES

> Examples of some nursing diagnoses related to nutrition include:
>
> Altered Nutrition: Less than Body Requirements related to, for example, nausea and vomiting
>
> Altered Nutrition: More than Body Requirements related to, for example, excessive intake
>
> Feeding Self-Care Deficit related to, for example, right upper extremity paralysis
>
> Knowledge Deficit related to, for example, normal nutrition or "special" diet
>
> Impaired Swallowing related to, for example, muscle paralysis

GENERAL CONSIDERATIONS

Factors That Affect Eating Habits

Many factors influence eating. For example, eating habits have been affected by escalating food prices during the last few years. Although you must recognize individual differences and not contrive stereotypes, ethnic background also must be considered. For example, keep in mind that people may enjoy eating the foods that are commonly consumed by their family or ethnic group, but this is not necessarily so in all cases.

Age is another important factor. Watching a teenager devour two large hamburgers, fries, and a large shake and then rush off to other activities is a totally different experience from observing an elderly couple who linger before a TV set with prepackaged dinners on trays.

Within an institution, various factors may influence how well the patient eats. The serving portions may be unduly large for a light eater or too small for a person with a large appetite. Some facilities give patients the opportunity to select serving sizes, usually small, medium, or large. Altered mealtimes, unfamiliar foods, or the desire for customary foods may also lead to anorexia or lack of appetite. Neuromuscular disturbances can also contribute to eating difficulties.

The nature of the patient's illness is also important. Remember that illness interferes with both body and mind, and that *most illnesses produce a degree of anxiety within the individual* that may cause a diminished appetite, an increased appetite, or erratic eating. An understanding attitude on your part, taking into account all of these factors, *promotes a more satisfactory outcome to the mealtime experience.* Being with the patient during a meal and participating in this significant activity also gives you time for several of your most basic and important functions: assessing, planning, implementing, and evaluating.

Psychosocial Considerations

To human beings, eating is ultimately more than taking in nutrients to maintain vital bodily functions and metabolism. Meals can be times of relaxation, celebration, and, importantly, times for sharing.

The psychosocial aspects of feeding an adult patient can be quite challenging. Supplying food for someone is a satisfying experience for most people. Many mothers and fathers enjoy providing healthful, attractive diets for their young children. Preparing a festive meal for guests or for a special family occasion is a delight to most people. In the same way, helping a patient eat a meal can be equally challenging and satisfying for you.

To the institutionalized person, the meal may take on new meaning. It may well be the high point of the day, often punctuating an otherwise long, weary day of immobilization. The patient may have the nurse at the bedside for a longer time during mealtime than at any other period in the day. However, it is crucial to remember that being fed can be degrading to some patients and may give them a feeling that they are now dependent, unable to carry

---

[1]Rationale for action is emphasized throughout the module by the use of italics.

© 1996 by Lippincott-Raven Publishers

out the simple task of feeding themselves. The person who is having difficulty eating—someone who dislikes the food, is experiencing nausea and vomiting, or is having other difficulties—may dread mealtime.

As with all skills and procedures, whether performed by the professional or the paraprofessional, time and caring are essential components.

Physical Problems

Physical problems that may affect a person's ability to feed himself or herself include those in which neuromuscular control is impaired, such as stroke or head injury. These individuals may need to be fed for a period and then may be assisted with eating as they gradually relearn skills. People with movement limited by traction, casts, and special positioning may need assistance with some aspects of a meal, although they may be able to do some things for themselves. A careful assessment of the precise abilities of each individual patient with regard to self-feeding is important to ensuring adequate nutrition.

The Patient With Dysphagia

Dysphagia is difficulty in swallowing. Typically, strokes or other neuromuscular disorders can cause dysphagia. The patient with dysphagia chokes and aspirates (inhales into the lungs) food easily. The techniques of assisting the dysphagic patient focus on maintaining safety.

Symptoms of dysphagia include coughing and choking while attempting to eat. However, some less obvious symptoms may also indicate dysphagia. The patient may drool, spill food, or "pocket" food in the cheek. Some people aspirate liquids with no symptoms at all.

Speech therapists are experts on the muscles of the mouth and throat and on techniques for facilitating swallowing. The physician may make a referral to a speech therapist for an evaluation and treatment plan for a dysphagic patient. The nurse who has assessed the patient may bring the need for a referral to the physician's attention.

You can assist the dysphagic patient by providing the appropriate foods. The goal is to provide foods that stimulate the swallowing reflex, do not move too rapidly through the mouth for the muscles to adapt, and are easy for the muscles of the mouth to move. Table 16–1 lists foods and fluids that are usually easy to swallow and those that may cause choking.

You can also assist by providing directions on positioning and swallowing techniques. The mouth

Table 16–1. Foods for the Dysphagic Patient

Easily Swallowed Food and Fluids	Foods That May Cause Choking
Thickened liquids (milkshakes, slushes)	Thin, watery liquids (water, tea, coffee, soda)
Hot or cold temperature foods or fluids (hot cream soup, iced fruit)	Neutral temperature foods and fluids (room temperature water)
Easily chewed foods (cooked vegetables, ground meat)	Tough, stringy, or hard foods (roast beef, nuts, dry crackers)
Soft, smooth foods (pureed fruits, pudding)	Sticky foods (peanut butter and thick mashed potatoes)

and throat are in the optimum position when the patient is sitting up straight with the head tilted forward. Figure 16–1 shows how head position can prevent choking and aspiration.

Instruct the patient to observe the following precautions. If staff or family members will be feeding the person, they should also observe these precautions.

1. Maintain a relaxed pace. *Hurrying increases the likelihood of choking.*
2. Do not try to talk until a few seconds after swallowing. *When you talk, the epiglottis must open for air to exit and small amounts of food may be aspirated if they are still in the mouth.*
3. Take small bites of food. *Small bites are easier for the mouth to control.*
4. If you are weak or paralyzed on one side, place the fork or spoon on the unaffected side of the tongue. *The muscles and nerves of the unaffected side are better able to control the movement of food through the mouth and pharynx.*
5. Use a rocking motion of the utensil on the tongue when placing the food. *This provides greater stimulation to the tongue and will help you to clearly feel the presence of the food.*
6. Swallow twice after each bite. *The second swallow may prevent food from being left in the mouth.*
7. Check for food left in the cheek of the affected side. You can check your mouth with a mirror or by slipping a forefinger into the cheek to feel for food left there. *Food "pocketed" in a paralyzed side may not be felt and therefore can cause ongoing potential for choking and aspiration as well as becoming a*

© 1996 by Lippincott-Raven Publishers

Correct swallowing position

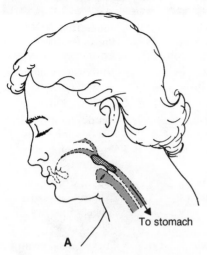

To stomach

A

Incorrect swallowing position

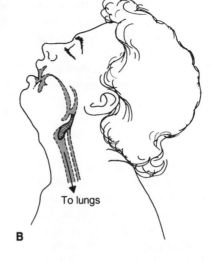

To lungs

B

Figure 16–1. (**A** and **B**) The effect of head position.

source of mouth odor. If you are not able to check independently, have someone check for you.

8. Do not "wash down" food with liquids. Thin liquids such as water, tea, coffee, and the like often cause choking. *The liquids may increase the speed with which material moves to the back of the pharynx and increase the chance for aspiration.*

9. *Sit up for 15 minutes after completing the meal.* This prevents reflux of stomach contents and aspiration.

PROCEDURE FOR FEEDING ADULT PATIENTS

Assessment

1. Identify the type of diet ordered *to determine whether the diet is appropriate for the patient in his or her present condition and to determine whether any special feeding utensils will be needed.* If a patient has just developed a high fever and nausea or is in pain, you may wish to change to a lighter meal *that the patient can digest more easily* or to delay the meal *until medications can be given to alleviate the patient's problem.* If you are aware that there is potential for nausea, vomiting, or pain with a particular patient, it is wise to see that the ordered medication is given 20 to 30 minutes before the meal *to enhance the potential for adequate food intake.*

2. Check to see whether there is any reason why the patient's meal should be delayed or omitted. Scheduled laboratory tests, radiologic examinations, and surgery may mean that the patient must be kept "NPO" (nothing by mouth) for a period before the test or surgery.

3. Check the nursing care plan, nursing history, or nursing record *to identify any previous need for assistance or use of modified eating utensils.* At the same time, note information about allergies, cultural or religious preferences, and specific dietary likes and dislikes. Do your own assessment as well, because the patient's condition may have changed or the previous assessment may have been incomplete.

4. Note any nursing diagnoses related to eating or feeding. Knowledge of these, along with the related plans of care, can do a lot to *make feeding easier and more pleasant for both you and the patient.*

Planning

5. When planning care, consider the time food trays arrive on the unit *so that tasks and procedures may be scheduled away from mealtime and so that you or the patient are not in the middle of a task or treatment at that time.*

6. Allow enough time for feeding so that you are free of other tasks and can spend uninterrupted time with the patient. This is important *to prevent food from getting cold and the patient from feeling unattended.*

7. Set a tentative goal for how much of the diet the patient will consume, based on physiologic status and past intake.

8. Wash your hands *for infection control.* As the food handler, your hands must be meticulously clean.

Implementation

9. Identify the patient *to be sure you are carrying out the procedure for the correct patient.*

10. Greet the patient and explain what you are going to do. Communication is a skill that is basic

© 1996 by Lippincott-Raven Publishers

to all interaction with patients, and feeding is no exception. Telling patients that they *must* eat to get well is not helpful and seldom elicits cooperation. It is better to approach the meal as an enjoyable experience both for yourself, as a sharer of time and conversation, and for the patient, for whom it should be a respite from painful experiences that may take place during the day. Approach with the expectation that the patient will join in the procedure willingly and benefit from it.

11. Offer the bedpan or urinal *for patient comfort and so that the meal will not have to be interrupted for reasons of elimination.*

12. Assist in washing the patient's hands and face and providing mouth care as indicated *to add to comfort and cleanliness.*

13. Prepare the patient's room by removing all unsightly equipment, replacing soiled linens, and arranging the bedside table to receive the tray. Unpleasant odors can be controlled by using an air freshener or opening a window. *A restful, neat, and odor-free environment makes eating more pleasant and aids digestion.*

14. Position the patient comfortably in mid- or high-Fowler's, if possible. *The higher position makes swallowing easier and lessens the risk of choking and aspiration.*

15. If the patient wears eyeglasses or dentures, be sure they are in place *so that the patient can see and chew properly.*

16. Protect the bed linen by using a suitable protective cover. Avoid using the word "bib," *which may be a humiliating term to the patient.* Place a colorful napkin, if available, over the protecting linen *for attractiveness.*

17. Obtain any special modified eating utensils that you have planned to use. Utensils such as those shown in Figure 16–2 *foster self-esteem by allowing patients who are partially disabled to feed themselves.*

18. Check to be sure that the name on the tray corresponds with the name on the patient's identification bracelet and that the food choices marked on the menu correspond with the food on the tray.

19. Assist the patient to prepare the food on the tray as needed. For example, cut food into bite-sized pieces, open milk cartons and cereal boxes, and butter toast. Encourage independence appropriately. Discard all wrappings and clutter before the patient begins to eat.

20. Position yourself at the patient's eye level by sitting if at all possible. *This establishes an unhurried atmosphere* (Fig. 16–3).

21. Involve the patient as much as possible. You can do this most effectively if you work from the unaffected side (the side of the patient least affected by the disease process). *In this way, the patient gains a sense of participation.* Place the tray so that the patient can see the food that is being offered. If the patient is sightless, describing what is on the meal tray is both necessary and helpful. Many such patients can manage with very little assistance if they know where food items are located. Often a clock format is used to assist the sightless patient, for example, "The milk is at 2 o'clock and the potatoes are at 6 o'clock." Many disabled patients can hold and enjoy feeding themselves pieces of bread or toast during the meal. Managing their own napkins also *offers them some degree of independence.*

22. Allow choices. Many individuals may believe they have few choices available when they are in healthcare facilities. If a patient indicates particular preferences (likes and dislikes) on the menu or displays an interest in having something *not* on the menu, communicate this information to the dietitian. To someone who is in good health, this may appear unimportant; but to the incapacitated person, it says, "I am still a person," "This nurse cares what I think," "I still have some control."

    When possible, find out from the patient what food sequence is preferred. If this is not possible, feed the items in the order in which you would choose to eat them. Provide fluids between bites of solids. This is good practice *because it affords the patient a variety of tastes,* which is usually the most pleasant way to eat a meal. If the patient does not respond to being given a choice, feed the more nutritious items of the diet first, *in case the patient's intake capacity is limited.* For example, if the choice is between broth and tea, broth, which is high in protein, is preferable.

    The elderly patient who has difficulty eating because of poorly fitting dentures may prefer to mix eggs, fruit, cereal, and toast together. Although this may strike you as unappetizing, affably feeding this mixture to the patient *serves to develop a good nurse–patient relationship.* Do not feel compelled to change long-standing eating habits, although you may adopt as a long-term goal, for example, arranging for the patient to be fit with comfortable dentures.

23. Continue assessment as you feed the patient. You can easily and accurately assess the patient's muscular dexterity, mental status, and feelings

© 1996 by Lippincott-Raven Publishers

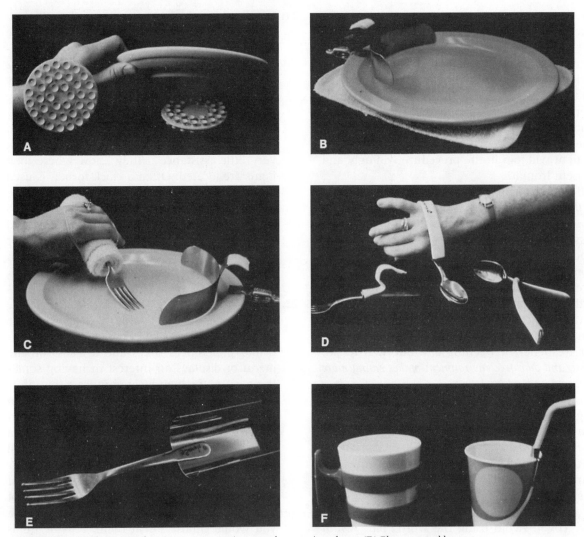

Figure 16–2. Feeding utensils. (**A**) Octopus suction cups for securing plates. (**B**) Plate secured by wet washcloth, with metal food guard attached to keep food on plate. (**C**) Fork in handroll for easy grip. (**D** and **E**) Modified handles. (**F**) Cup handle and straw secured with pen clip. (Courtesy Florence E. Smith)

at this time. Signs such as skin color, respiratory rate, and the presence or absence of tremor can also be assessed.

24. Do not discuss stressful events at mealtime. *It has been shown that digestion is better when a patient*

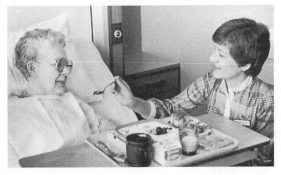

Figure 16–3. Feeding the older patient.

is not emotionally upset. Try to maintain an open and congenial atmosphere.

25. Never hurry a patient's eating. *This not only can cause the patient to feel uncomfortable and fearful of taking up too much of your time, but it can also be dangerous if it causes the patient to choke in an attempt to finish eating quickly.*

26. Allow the patient to determine when enough has been eaten *as a way of providing control.*

27. Remove the tray, offer the bedpan or assist to the bathroom as indicated, and provide hygiene as needed.

28. Reposition the patient. If there have been problems with digestion or vomiting, keep the patient in the high position *so that gravity can help the retention of food in the stomach.* Turning the head to one side *can prevent aspiration if vomiting does occur.*

© 1996 by Lippincott-Raven Publishers

DATE/TIME	
11/12/98 1800	Ate 75% chopped diet with some difficulty swallowing solid food. Feeding facilitated by providing small bites followed by sips of liquids. Left in high Fowler's position. No emesis. ———— *Dave Martin, SN*

(A) Example of Nursing Progress Notes Using Narrative Format.

DATE/TIME	
11/12/98 1800	4. *Dysphagia:* ——— S *"The meat seems to stick in my throat."* ——— O *Appears to swallow solid foods with difficulty. Fluids taken without difficulty.* ——— A *Dysphagia with solid food.* ——— P *Give small bites of solid food alternated with fluids.* ——— *Dave Martin, SN*

(B) Example of Nursing Progress Notes Using SOAP Format.

29. Provide quiet *so that the patient may relax after the meal, which also promotes good digestion.*

30. Wash your hands *for infection control.*

Evaluation

31. Evaluate using the following criteria:
  a. The patient is satisfied and comfortable.
  b. The amount of food and fluid consumed has been observed, as well as measured and recorded, if necessary.
  c. Any problems or helpful techniques have been noted for later documentation.

Documentation

32. Document the food consumed, either by using the checklist the institution provides or by charting in more detail on the progress notes (depending on the situation), as well as the patient's response. If food intake has previously presented problems, chart the individual food items and the amounts taken for greater accuracy. Document other appropriate information, such as difficulty swallowing or changes in the patient's ability or behavior.

Add to the nursing care plan any new information related to the patient's likes and dislikes or methods of assisting that you have noted *to enhance continuity of care.*

LONG-TERM CARE

In the long-term care setting, the residents may have many self-care deficits; a feeding self-care deficit is common. These residents often eat in a dining room rather than in their rooms and are grouped at tables with others with whom they can interact. Having residents dressed in day clothing and helping them to be attractively groomed is important for everyone's feelings about the meal. As you plan for feeding assistance, remember that it should be as unobtrusive as possible so as not to interfere with interactions. In addition, you will be working toward developing independence in the resident whenever that is possible. Sometimes encouragement and "cuing" an individual as to the next step are all that are needed to promote independence in eating.

Nursing assistants often do most of the feeding in long-term care settings. The nurse is often involved in teaching them feeding techniques and serving as a role model of how appropriate feeding techniques may contribute to increased intake and nutritional well-being.

HOME CARE

Before a patient is discharged, discuss with the patient and his or her caregiver the potential for any difficulties related to eating that might occur at home. As part of your plan you may help the family obtain assistive devices and teach family members how to assist with feed-ing. You should also be aware of problems related to shopping, storage, refrigeration, and cooking practices. It may be necessary for you to ask for a referral to a community agency to assist the patient and family.

CRITICAL THINKING EXERCISES

• A hospitalized patient for whom you are providing care has just returned from having a diagnostic study done. He appears upset and tells you he is nauseated and just wants to rest. You are disappointed because the two of you spent considerable time this morning discussing his poor nutritional status and, with the help of the dietitian, ordered special foods from the Dietary Department to encourage optimum intake. His tray has just arrived, and it looks appetizing. In light of the current situation, describe how you will proceed.

• The 82-year-old woman you have been caring for in the nursing home is going home after rehabilitation following a stroke. She is still having some difficulty with a mild swallowing problem. Identify at least three strategies you will teach her and her primary caregiver to help prevent choking and aspiration.

© 1996 by Lippincott-Raven Publishers

✔ **PERFORMANCE CHECKLIST**

Procedure for Feeding Adult Patients	Needs More Practice	Satisfactory	Comments
Assessment			
1. Identify type of diet ordered.			
2. Check to see whether there is any reason why patient's meal should be delayed or omitted.			
3. Check on patient's previous need for assistance.			
4. Note any nursing diagnoses related to eating or feeding.			
Planning			
5. When planning care, consider the time food trays arrive on the unit.			
6. Plan time for feeding.			
7. Set tentative goal.			
8. Wash your hands.			
Implementation			
9. Identify patient.			
10. Greet patient and explain what you are going to do.			
11. Offer bedpan or urinal.			
12. Assist in washing patient's hands and face.			
13. Prepare patient's room.			
14. Position patient comfortably, preferably in mid- to high-Fowler's.			
15. Provide eyeglasses or dentures if worn.			
16. Protect bed linen.			
17. Obtain any special utensils needed.			
18. Check to be sure that name on tray matches that of patient and that food on tray is consistent with ordered diet and special needs.			
19. Assist patient to prepare food on tray.			
20. Position yourself at patient's eye level.			
21. Involve patient as much as possible.			

(continued)

© 1996 by Lippincott-Raven Publishers

Procedure for Feeding Adult Patients *(Continued)*	Needs More Practice	Satisfactory	Comments
22. Allow choices.			
23. Continually assess patient.			
24. Do not discuss stressful events.			
25. Never hurry the patient's eating.			
26. Allow the patient to determine when enough has been consumed.			
27. Remove tray, offer opportunity for elimination, and provide hygiene.			
28. Reposition the patient.			
29. Provide a quiet atmosphere.			
30. Wash your hands.			
Evaluation			
31. Evaluate using the following criteria: **a.** Patient is satisfied and comfortable.			
b. Amount taken was observed and measured or recorded, if necessary.			
c. Problems encountered noted.			
Documentation			
32. Document the type and amount of food taken and patient response. Add new information to the nursing care plan.			

© 1996 by Lippincott-Raven Publishers

? **Q U I Z**

Short-Answer Questions

1. List four factors that can influence a patient's eating abilities.

a. _____

b. _____

c. _____

d. _____

2. List four easily swallowed foods.

a. _____

b. _____

c. _____

d. _____

3. List four foods that may cause choking.

a. _____

b. _____

c. _____

d. _____

Multiple-Choice Questions

_____ **4.** Every feeding situation presents which of the following opportunities for the nurse?

a. Time for health teaching
b. Determination of the medical diagnosis
c. Time for nursing assessments to be made
d. Repositioning of the patient

Situation: Mr. Swenson, a 63-year-old Scandinavian with a right-sided hemiplegia (paralysis on the right side of the body), has been in the hospital for 10 days. The patient's chart states that a soft diet has been ordered and that he is allowed up in a chair q.d. (once daily).

Lunch trays will be arriving in 20 minutes, and you have been assigned to feed Mr. Swenson. As you enter his room, you see a denture cup on the bedside table and glasses on the overbed table. A urinal is on the floor. Questions 5–10 refer to Mr. Swenson.

_____ **5.** From the data given, you determine that Mr. Swenson's feeding problem is

a. lack of ability to swallow food.
b. not evident from the information available.
c. lack of ability to use small-muscle groups to feed himself.
d. depression brought on by dependency.

© 1996 by Lippincott-Raven Publishers

_____ **6.** Your *first* action in the above situation should be to

    a. introduce yourself and give the reason for your presence.
    b. empty and put away the urinal.
    c. encourage Mr. Swenson to discuss his feelings about being dependent.
    d. reposition Mr. Swenson in a high Fowler's position for lunch.

True-False Questions

_____ **7.** Mr. Swenson should be encouraged to talk about his anxieties while you are at the bedside feeding him.

_____ **8.** Because Mr. Swenson is Scandinavian, he will certainly enjoy the fish on the menu.

_____ **9.** The goal for Mr. Swenson in regard to self-feeding this meal should be established only after you check to see what his previous ability has been.

_____ **10.** Mr. Swenson ate only half his meal. This means your feeding plan was unsuccessful.

© 1996 by Lippincott-Raven Publishers

MODULE

17

ASSISTING WITH ELIMINATION AND PERINEAL CARE

MODULE CONTENTS

RATIONALE FOR THE USE OF THIS SKILL
NURSING DIAGNOSES
PRINCIPLES
EQUIPMENT
Bedpans
Urinals
Commodes
COMFORT CONSIDERATIONS
ASSISTING WITH ELIMINATION
PROCEDURE FOR ASSISTING WITH A BEDPAN
Assessment
Planning
Implementation
Evaluation
Documentation
PROCEDURE FOR ASSISTING WITH A URINAL
Assessment
Planning

Implementation
Evaluation
Documentation
PROCEDURE FOR ASSISTING WITH A COMMODE
Assessment
Planning
Implementation
Evaluation
Documentation
GIVING PERINEAL CARE
PROCEDURE FOR GIVING PERINEAL CARE
Assessment
Planning
Implementation
Evaluation
Documentation
LONG-TERM CARE
HOME CARE
CRITICAL THINKING EXERCISES

PREREQUISITES

Successful completion of the following modules:

VOLUME 1

Module 1 An Approach to Nursing Skills
Module 2 Basic Infection Control
Module 3 Safety
Module 5 Documentation
Module 6 Introduction to Assessment Skills

© 1996 by Lippincott-Raven Publishers

OVERALL OBJECTIVE

To assist patients with the use of bedpans, urinals, or commodes in a hygienic manner, taking into account psychological factors; and to provide perineal care according to individual needs.

SPECIFIC LEARNING OBJECTIVES

Know Facts and Principles	Apply Facts and Principles	Demonstrate Ability	Evaluate Performance
ASSISTING WITH ELIMINATION			
1. Equipment			
Describe equipment needed.	Given a patient situation, list appropriate equipment.	When caring for patient, select correct equipment.	Evaluate own performance with instructor.
2. Assisting with bedpan, urinal, or commode			
State three principles for carrying out procedures.	Given a patient situation, explain and discuss infection control, psychological needs, and normal conditions of elimination.	In the clinical setting, carry out infection control, provide psychologic comfort, and approximate normal conditions of elimination.	Evaluate own performance with instructor.
3. Procedure			
a. Positioning			
Describe positions used for individual patients.	Given a patient situation, plan particular procedure correctly.	In the clinical setting, individualize procedure to particular patient and carry out plan.	Evaluate with instructor using Performance Checklist.
b. Privacy			
State measures to ensure privacy.	Given a patient situation, plan privacy measures.	In the clinical setting, provide privacy for patient.	Evaluate own performance with instructor.
c. Providing bedpan or urinal			
Describe several techniques used in providing bedpan, urinal, or commode.	Given a patient situation, plan appropriate technique for providing bedpan, urinal, or commode.	In the clinical setting, demonstrate individual technique for providing bedpan, urinal, or commode.	Evaluate own performance with instructor.
d. Cleaning patient			
Recognize need for cleanliness.	Demonstrate correct cleaning of patient.	In the clinical setting, provide cleanliness for patient after use of bedpan, urinal, or commode.	

(*continued*)

© 1996 by Lippincott-Raven Publishers

SPECIFIC LEARNING OBJECTIVES (Continued)

Know Facts and Principles	Apply Facts and Principles	Demonstrate Ability	Evaluate Performance
4. Documentation State what should be recorded.	Given a hypothetical situation, record as if on chart.	In the clinical setting, record complete observations in correct format.	Evaluate recording with instructor.
GIVING PERINEAL CARE **1. Equipment** Describe various pieces of equipment used to provide perineal care.	Given a patient situation, simulate correct method for postpartum patient and for patient with a catheter.	In the clinical setting, give perineal care to postpartum patient, nonsurgical patient, and catheterized patient, adapting equipment and procedure correctly.	Evaluate with instructor using Performance Checklist.
2. Psychological comfort Explain why giving psychological support is important.	Given a patient situation, discern possible causes of psychologic discomfort.	In the clinical setting, provide psychologic support to patient.	

3. Procedure
  a. *Postpartum patient*
  b. *Nonsurgical patient*
  c. *Patient with catheter*
Describe appropriate adaptations in procedure related to particular patient condition.
	Given a patient situation, adapt procedure appropriately for a particular patient.	In the clinical setting, carry out procedure for postpartum patient, nonsurgical patient, and catheterized patient safely and correctly.	Evaluate own performance with instructor.

4. Documentation List what should be recorded.	Given a patient situation, record as if on chart.	In the clinical setting, record observations correctly.	Evaluate documentation with instructor.

© 1996 by Lippincott-Raven Publishers

LEARNING ACTIVITIES

1. Review the Specific Learning Objectives.
2. Read the chapter on elimination in Ellis and Nowlis, *Nursing: A Human Needs Approach,* or a comparable chapter in another textbook.
3. Look up the module vocabulary terms in the glossary.
4. Read through the module as though you were going to teach the module contents to another person and mentally practice the techniques described.
5. In the practice setting:
   a. Become familiar with the various pieces of available equipment (different types of bedpans, urinals, commodes, perineal packs).
   b. Select a partner and perform the following:
      (1) Act as if you are an incapacitated patient. Without disrobing, have your partner place you on a bedpan.
      (2) Remain on the bedpan for 3 minutes in a flat position, then for another 3 minutes in a sitting position.
      (3) Have your partner remove the bedpan as though you were incapacitated.
      (4) Describe your feelings about the experience.
      (5) Reverse the roles, repeating (1), (2), (3), and (4).
   c. Using a manikin, go through the specific procedure for giving perineal care to each of the following:
      (1) A postpartum or perineal surgical patient
      (2) A nonsurgical patient
      (3) A patient with a catheter
6. In the clinical setting, with your instructor's supervision:
   a. Place a patient on a bedpan using both a lifting and a rolling method.
   b. Give a urinal to a male patient.
   c. Assist a patient to a commode.
   d. Administer perineal care to a postpartum patient, a nonsurgical patient, and a catheterized patient.
7. Using the Performance Checklist, evaluate yourself with the help of your instructor.

VOCABULARY

ADLs *activities of daily living*	fracture pan *smaller than bedpan*	recumbent	urinal
bedpan	genital area	renal calculi *kidney stones*	urination
catheter	labia	smegma	void
commode *BSC*	lumbosacral *lumbar & sacral region*	sutures *stitches*	vulva *part female genitalia*
defecation *excretion*	penis	trapeze *overhang on bed*	
foreskin	perineum	urethral meatus *the opening of the urethra through which pass urine*	

emesis basin - kidney shaped

BSC - bedside commode

smegma an odorous collection of disquamated epithelial cells & mucus.

void to empty any body cavity usually bladder

recumbent - lying down position

© 1996 by Lippincott-Raven Publishers

Assisting With Elimination and Perineal Care

Rationale for the Use of This Skill

Illness, physical disability, and weakness may make it impossible for an individual to go to a bathroom for toileting. Because elimination is a private function in our society and individuals learn to manage this need independently at a very young age, those who require assistance with toileting and perineal care are often distressed and embarrassed. In addition, special techniques are required to avoid strain to either the patient or the nurse, to maintain safety, and to prevent soiling of the bed. Whether the need for assistance is temporary or permanent, the nurse provides support and reassurance by responding promptly and competently to this care need.[1]

▼ NURSING DIAGNOSES

> The primary nursing diagnosis for which the skills in this module are needed is Toileting Self-Care Deficit which may be due to a lack of neuromuscular control, fatigue and weakness, shortness of breath, or a wide variety of other disabilities. Special perineal care may be needed when a nursing diagnosis of Bathing/Hygiene Self-Care Deficit is present.

PRINCIPLES

Keep several principles in mind. First, observe infection control throughout *for your own protection as well as the patient's. When performing these procedures, your hands may come in contact with mucous membrane, which is receptive to infection. It is even more important to protect the patient from the dangers of cross-contamination (contamination from other patients). For practical as well as aesthetic reasons, you must use good aseptic technique.* The Centers for Disease Control and Prevention (CDC) requires the use of clean gloves whenever body substances may be contacted. Wearing gloves when performing any tasks involving the perineum and when cleaning bedpans is a prudent practice and conforms to body substance precautions.

Second, the procedure can be embarrassing to you and to the patient. It is important to recognize these feelings in yourself and to know that with experience, assisting with intimate procedures will become less

personal and more routine to you. *To lessen a patient's embarrassment or discomfort,* maintain a straightforward attitude and respect the patient's privacy, keeping exposure to a minimum.

Third, when you help a patient with any substitution or adaptation of the usual activities of daily living (ADLs), it is important—in terms of efficiency and patient comfort—that you approximate the normal as closely as possible. For a female patient the normal position for urination or defecation is sitting; a male commonly stands to urinate and sits to defecate. Therefore, *having a patient assume these positions* when using a bedpan or urinal is very helpful and *may,* in some cases, *be a strong factor in whether the patient will be able to eliminate.* Let patients have as much control as possible, for example, by giving them privacy, allowing them to use tissue by themselves, and allowing them to wash their own hands afterward. If patients are unable to perform these activities, you should perform them for the patients.

EQUIPMENT

The type of equipment used depends on the health status of the patient. For the patient on strict bed rest, a bedpan is used. The urinal is used by the male for voiding urine. If the activity status permits, a bedside commode offers a more relaxed and convenient option. It is best to keep in mind that equipment that most closely corresponds to what is normal is the better choice.

Bedpans

Bedpans are made of either metal (Fig. 17–1) or plastic and come in two sizes, the smaller designed for pediatric patients.

For reasons of infection control, each patient has a personal bedpan that is kept in a storage unit in the patient's room. Generally, it is stored with a bedpan

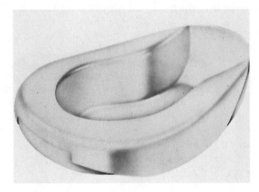

Figure 17–1. Bedpan.

---

[1] Rationale for action is emphasized throughout the module by the use of italics.

© 1996 by Lippincott-Raven Publishers

cover over it. The cover, which is made of heavy fabric or paper, may be in the form of a loose square or large envelope that slips easily over the bedpan. The paper cover is disposable. A cover should be used *for aesthetic reasons, to conceal the sight of the contents, and to decrease odor after the patient has used the bedpan.*

A *fracture pan* is a type of bedpan that was originally designed to be used by patients in casts, who could not use a pan with a high lip. It is smaller and easier to get onto than a standard bedpan. There is a handle at the front to facilitate placement and removal. Fracture pans also come in two sizes, in plastic or metal, and with a handle for easier placement (Fig. 17–2).

An *emesis basin* (Fig. 17–3) can be used for voiding in place of a bedpan for the female patient who, *because of extreme pain or for a medical reason,* should not be raised to bedpan height except for defecation.

Because the use of an emesis basin is uncommon, you can use the following procedure: After placing a waterproof pad under the patient *to protect the linen,* hold the emesis basin lengthwise between the legs and firmly against the perineum. Instruct the patient to void. At first a patient may be hesitant, *fearing that she will soil the bed.* Encourage the patient to void freely. Usually the urine flows into the pan with only a drop or so on the pad, and the patient will be very grateful for this easy, more comfortable way to urinate.

Urinals

A *urinal* is used by the male patient for urination. It is made of plastic or metal with a bottle-like configuration (Fig. 17–4).

A flat side allows it to rest without tipping. Urinals are available with or without attached tops or lids. Female urinals are also available.

Commodes

A commode is a portable toileting device. It resembles a movable chair with wheels, back, and arms. The seat lifts up to reveal an opening with a sliding

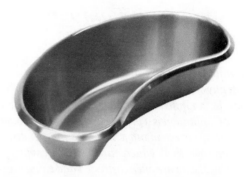

Figure 17–3. Emesis basin (kidney basin) can be used by the immobile female patient for urine elimination.

tray beneath, which is used as a receptacle for urine or feces. The patient uses the seat as a back rest (Fig. 17–5).

This device is useful for the patient who is able to get out of bed but unable to walk the distance to the bathroom because of weakness or partial immobilization. Most facilities supply commodes without an order. However, the care plan may read "BSC," which stands for "bedside commode." The same considerations are given to this procedure as are given for getting a patient out of bed or walking a patient to the toilet. (Consult Module 15, Moving the Patient in Bed and Positioning, and Module 20, Transfer, for the proper procedures for getting the patient out of bed and to the chairlike commode.) Have sufficient help if the patient requires transfer.

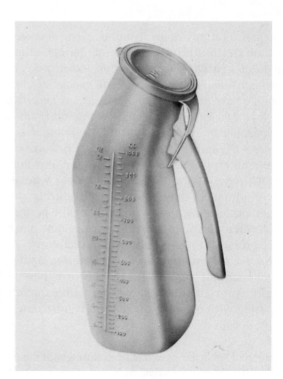

Figure 17–4. A urinal for use by the male patient.

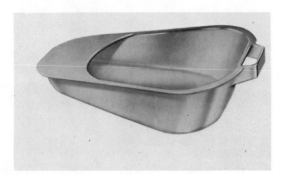

Figure 17–2. Fracture pan.

© 1996 by Lippincott-Raven Publishers

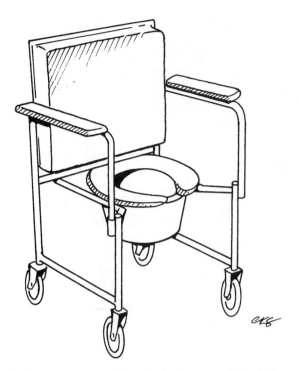

Figure 17–5. A commode for elimination use at the bedside.

Be sure the wheels of the bed and commode are locked *for safety*.

COMFORT CONSIDERATIONS

Although often unavoidable, using any of these devices is not a pleasant experience. A thin, fragile patient may even feel pain from the pressure of the hard surfaces. Fold a soft pad or small towel over the edges of the pan *to lessen this discomfort*. With metal pans, another source of discomfort is cold. Warm metal pans by holding them under running warm water and then drying them. These simple measures can make the experience less disagreeable. You may also wish to place padding over the edges of a commode *for the patient's comfort*.

ASSISTING WITH ELIMINATION

The following procedures are designed to guide you in assisting patients with the use of bedpans, urinals, or commodes.

PROCEDURE FOR ASSISTING WITH A BEDPAN

Assessment

1. Check the patient's activity order and physical status to determine whether a bedpan is necessary.

2. Review the patient's past use of such equipment and note any problems encountered.

Planning

3. Decide how much assistance the patient currently needs and get the help needed.
4. Plan for the specific procedure or technique to be used (see step 10 for options).
5. Wash your hands and put on clean gloves *to protect both the patient and yourself*. Use the principles of infection control throughout.

Implementation

6. Explain in general how you plan to proceed. Of course, if a patient verbalizes the need to eliminate, do not go into detail.
7. Close the door *to provide privacy*.
8. Raise the bed to the high position *for your convenience*. *For the patient's safety*, put up the side rail on the opposite side of the bed from where you plan to stand.
9. Take the bedpan, cover, and toilet tissue out of the bedside storage unit. Set the cover and tissue aside. A fracture pan or emesis basin, as previously mentioned, can be used in the same way as a conventional bedpan. (Figs. 17–6 and 17–7).
10. Put the patient on the bedpan, using one of the following methods, depending on the patient's condition and ability to assist you:
    a. With the patient in a recumbent position and your hand under the small (lumbosacral area) of the back *for support*, ask the patient to raise the buttocks by raising up with the feet as you push the pan into position under the patient.
    b. Ask the patient who is able to assume the sitting position to simply lift the body by pushing down with the hands and feet as you place the pan in position.
    c. Roll a more immobilized patient onto the pan. For this maneuver, elicit the patient's cooperation. Ask the patient to grasp the side rail on the opposite side of the bed (across from where you are standing) *for stability* as you roll the patient away from you in one plane. Place the pan against the patient, in position. (You may want to pad the pan with a towel *to relieve pressure on the patient's buttocks*.) Now, hold the pan firmly in place as you roll the patient back. Finally, check the position of the pan. If the patient must remain flat, you may want to place a small pillow above the bedpan under the patient's back for support. Note: If the patient's bed has a trapeze, make use of this device for placing and removing the bedpan. Have the patient use the trapeze to lift the hips.

© 1996 by Lippincott-Raven Publishers

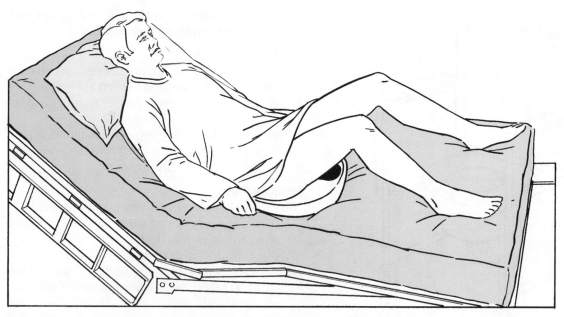

Figure 17–6. The bedpan is placed under the patient with the flat side under the buttocks.

11. Raise the side rail nearest you *for safety.*

12. Elevate the head of the bed to mid- or high-Fowler's position, if not contraindicated, as the patient grasps the rails. *This provides a position that approximates what is normal for elimination.*

13. Place the toilet tissue and the call bell within the patient's reach.

14. Leave the patient. *Because our culture emphasizes privacy during elimination*, it is very difficult for some patients to eliminate with a nurse in attendance. If the patient is safe, it is best to leave the patient for a time; if this is not possible,

you might step just outside to be within calling distance if the patient suddenly needs assistance.

15. When the patient signals, return promptly. *It can be very irritating and uncomfortable for a patient to sit for unnecessarily extended periods on a bedpan* because a nurse is inattentive. If a patient does not signal you within a reasonable amount of time, return to the patient *to ensure safety and comfort.*

16. Put on clean gloves *for infection control.*

17. If necessary, clean the genital area with toilet tissue. Most alert patients will be able to clean

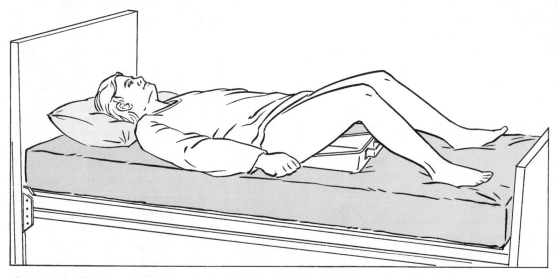

Figure 17–7. The fracture pan is placed under the patient with the handle toward the legs and the low, flat side under the buttocks.

© 1996 by Lippincott-Raven Publishers

themselves adequately. Some who are incapacitated may need further assistance. Always clean with fresh tissue from the anterior (urinary) region to the posterior (rectal) region. Cleaning in this direction minimizes the chance of contaminating the urinary tract with fecal microorganisms.

18. Remove the bedpan, reversing the method that you used when you placed the patient on the bedpan. If you used the rolling technique, hold onto the pan firmly or get help, *so that the contents do not spill.*

19. Cover the pan.

20. Carry the pan to the bathroom and, if ordered, measure the urine. If a patient is on intake and output, a measuring container is usually kept in the bathroom. You must estimate as accurately as possible, taking into account the amount of toilet tissue used *because the tissue can displace the urine and make measurement inaccurate* (see Module 10, Intake and Output).

21. Collect a specimen of urine or feces, if ordered (see Module 11, Collecting Specimens and Performing Common Laboratory Tests).

    Even when precise measurements or specimens are not ordered, note the amount, color, consistency, and odor, as well as the presence of blood, mucus, or foreign material. These are important data to convey that *may affect the diagnosis.* A patient who is being observed for renal calculi (kidney stones) may have an order to have all urine strained *so that the small stones or particles can be retained and examined.* If you even suspect that a patient's urine or feces contain blood, in most facilities you can independently test a specimen *to verify your suspicion* (see Module 11).

22. Empty the contents into the toilet and flush.

23. Thoroughly clean the pan with cold water, *which subdues odors and combines with the contents more effectively than hot water.* Health regulations require that a container of disinfectant solution and a long-handled brush be kept in the bathroom *for cleaning bedpans.* Wash and rinse the pan thoroughly. Use paper towels for drying. Then return the pan to the patient's storage unit.

24. Remove and dispose of gloves.

25. Give the patient a basin of warm water, a washcloth, soap, and a towel, or a packaged moist towelette so that hygiene can be carried out. Allow the patient to wash the hands and perineal area, if desired. Nurses usually remember to wash their own hands after assisting a patient with a bedpan but sometimes forget that the patient would also like to wash.

26. Place the bed back in the low position *for safety* and lower the rail on the stand side, if appropriate. Make the patient comfortable.

27. Dispose of the equipment.

28. Wash your hands *for infection control.*

Evaluation

29. Note the efficiency of the technique used and how suitable it was for that patient.

30. Identify any specific problems and possible improvements and note them on the nursing care plan.

Documentation

31. Record any problems or unusual observations. Routine elimination is usually recorded on a checklist or output sheet.

PROCEDURE FOR ASSISTING WITH A URINAL

The steps used to assist a male patient in using the urinal are essentially the same as those for a bedpan (see the Performance Checklist), except for a few adaptations.

DATE/TIME	
1/5/99 1630	*Impaired Skin Integrity: Scrotal irritation related to urinary incontinence*
	S "It hurts between my legs."
	O Scrotum reddened and warm to touch.
	A Irritation of scrotal area possibly due to intermittent incontinence.
	P Offer urinal q2h when awake and follow with good perineal care.
	L. Kenny, NS

Example of Nursing Progress Notes Using SOAP Format.

© 1996 by Lippincott-Raven Publishers

If a male patient is able to stand alone, he will usually be more successful if he is allowed to stand to urinate. If the patient is unable to stand alone, have him lean on the edge of the bed *for stability* with his feet on the floor. Always check the patient's activity order and activity tolerance before undertaking this action.

Never place a urinal between a patient's legs for long periods of time in an effort to control incontinence. *This can irritate and erode the skin of the penis.* If a patient is unable to use the urinal himself, protect the linen with a waterproof pad, place the head of the penis into the opening, and tell the patient he can now urinate without soiling the bed linen.

PROCEDURE FOR ASSISTING WITH A COMMODE

Assessment
1. Check the patient's activity order and physical status to determine whether a commode is necessary.
2. If patient has been using a commode, note any problems with using the equipment.

Planning
3. Decide how much assistance is needed and get help if appropriate.
4. Plan a specific procedure for getting the patient out of bed using the guidelines described in Module 20, Transfer.
5. Wash your hands to *protect the patient.*

Implementation
6. Explain in general how you plan to proceed. Elicit the patient's help or get assistance.
7. Provide privacy.
8. Help the patient out of the bed.
9. Place the call light within the patient's reach.
10. Leave the patient, allowing adequate time for elimination.
11. Put on clean gloves *for infection control.*
12. Return and clean the perineal area, if necessary.
13. Help the patient back to bed.
14. Remove the sliding container and measure or properly dispose of contents.

Evaluation
15. Assess how well the patient tolerated getting out of bed and using the commode. This is particu-

larly important if it is the first time the patient has used a commode.
16. Note any problems encountered. Problems might include dizziness, a drop in blood pressure, or discomfort from sitting on the hard surface.

Documentation
17. Document any problems. Record output if necessary. Indicate bowel movement on correct flow sheet. Describe stool if abnormal.

GIVING PERINEAL CARE

In the clinical setting, this procedure is sometimes called "pericare." People who are immobilized or ill may have an increased need for perineal care or will need assistance with it. *When ill, the body's defenses against infection may be weakened or impaired,* and unless perineal hygiene is meticulous, urinary tract infections can occur. This is especially true if the patient is incontinent or has an indwelling urinary catheter. *If not promptly removed, urine or feces on the skin of the incontinent patient can result in skin breakdown and infection.* The incontinent patient should have perineal care given after each voiding and defecation. If the patient has a catheter in place, *the catheter itself can be a means for microorganisms to travel upward into the bladder and cause a urinary tract infection.* For this reason, patients who have an indwelling catheter should have meticulous perineal care at least every 8 hours. The CDC no longer recommends special "cath care" for these patients but, more appropriately, frequent and good perineal hygiene. The nurse may provide perineal care to any patient who is assessed as needing it without a physician's order.

PROCEDURE FOR GIVING PERINEAL CARE

Assessment
1. Determine the condition of the patient's skin and the extent of soiling of the perineal area.
2. Identify the patient's capabilities.

Planning
3. Plan the equipment that will be needed (see step 7, page 381, for options).
4. Decide whether you will need assistance.
5. Wash your hands and put on clean gloves. *It has been shown that infections can be transmitted through minor breaks in the skin.*

© 1996 by Lippincott-Raven Publishers

Implementation

6. Explain what you are about to do. Use words the patient understands: "washing your genital area" or "washing between your legs." Again, *the patient may be embarrassed,* so proceed in a professional manner.

7. Select the appropriate equipment. The equipment used will vary with the type of patient receiving care. Gloves are used for all patients.

   a. *Postpartum or surgical patient*
   (1) Bedpan
   (2) Waterproof pad
   (3) Pitcher
   (4) Tap water or antiseptic solution
   (5) Cotton balls, gauze squares, or "wipes"
   (6) Clean pad or dressing

   b. *Nonsurgical patient*
   (1) Waterproof pad
   (2) Washcloth and towel
   (3) Basin of warm water
   (4) Mild soap or cleansing agent

   c. *Patient with a catheter:* Research has shown that washing around the catheter insertion site and rinsing thoroughly is sufficient care. The CDC has recommended that special cleaning procedures not be done because they are not associated with decreased incidence of infection.

8. Provide privacy.

9. *For purposes of convenience and privacy,* place the patient in the dorsal recumbent position and drape with a bath blanket as you would to catheterize a patient (see Module 37, Catheterization).

10. Put on gloves and proceed as follows:

    a. *Postpartum or surgical patient:* Remove dressing or pads. After placing a waterproof pad under the patient, position the bedpan following step 10 of the Procedure for Assisting with a Bedpan, page 377. Pour tepid tap water or the solution used in your facility over the perineum (Fig. 17–8). Do not spread the labia; this may *allow solution to enter the vagina and might cause infection.* Rinse with clear water. Using cotton balls or gauze, wipe from anterior to posterior *because wiping in this direction lessens the possibility of contamination of the urinary tract from the anal area.* Always clean gently, *to prevent pain and avoid pressure on sutures (stitches).* Use extra gauze squares or cotton balls, if needed, but use each only one time and then discard into waste bag (not bedpan) *to prevent contamination.* Replace any pads or dressings, *for infection control.* Remove the bedpan, make any necessary observations, and discard the contents. This proce-

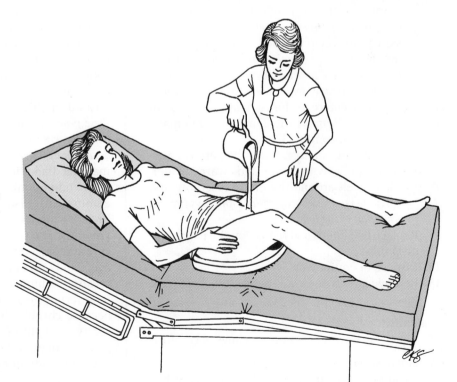

Figure 17–8. Giving perineal care by pouring water over the perineum.

© 1996 by Lippincott-Raven Publishers

DATE/TIME	
1/3/99 8 AM	*Pericare given. Vulva appears reddened. Small am't clear vaginal drainage.* *J. Adams, NS*

Example of Nursing Progress Notes Using Narrative Format.

DATE/TIME	
5/19/99 0930	*D:* *Patient able to stand unassisted but ambulation is unsteady. Reluctant to use bedpan.*
	A: *Beside commode obtained. Patient encouraged to use commode.*
	R: *Patient uses commode without difficulty.*
	B. Bulliet, RN

Example of Nursing Progress Notes Using Focus Format.

dure can also be done with the patient sitting on a toilet.

b. *Nonsurgical patient:* After placing a waterproof pad under the patient, wash the perineum, using warm water and mild soap. Gently separate the labia of the female patient as you clean, to remove secretions and smegma (an odorous collection of desquamated epithelial cells and mucus). Clean the male patient beginning with the penile head and moving downward along the shaft. Retract the foreskin of the uncircumcised male gently *to avoid causing irritation or pain, so that the underlying tissue can be cleaned.* All patients should be rinsed, *to remove soap residue,* and dried thoroughly. Replace the foreskin over the head of the penis. Remove the damp pads and make the patient comfortable.

c. *Patient with a catheter:* Wash the perineal area thoroughly with soap and warm water. Clean well around the entire insertion site. Rinse *to remove all soap residue and thus prevent irritation of the mucosa.*

11. Replace bed linens and reposition the patient *for comfort.*

12. Dispose of equipment.

13. Remove gloves and wash hands *for infection control.*

Evaluation

14. Check back with patient for feelings of comfort.

Documentation

15. Good perineal care is assumed as a part of hygiene. Record any pertinent observations such as residual redness or tenderness of the area or difficulties with performance.

LONG-TERM CARE

Depending on the limitations of the resident in the long-term care facility, you may have to meet his or her elimination needs by supplying and being able to help with a bedpan, urinal, or bedside commode. Urinary incontinence is often observed in older women and may be in response to problems with decreased mobility (Sherman, 1993). *Because these people are often thin with bony prominences near the skin surface, sharp and hard edges of these devices may have to be padded.* Older residents may need additional time to urinate or defecate, and you must provide this for successful elimination. Persons of advanced age may also be more modest than are younger people, so you must also take this into consideration. Accurately assessing the resident, regardless of age, and providing the most appropriate means for elimination is a nursing challenge in long-term care. Perineal care is very important because chronically ill persons may have less reserve to fight off urinary tract infections. A great number of these infections could be prevented with frequent and meticulous perineal care.

© 1996 by Lippincott-Raven Publishers

HOME CARE

The person being cared for in the home may temporarily or permanently use either a bedpan, urinal, or commode. Bedpans and urinals are inexpensive to buy or may be covered by health insurance; some home care agencies supply either or both free of charge. Commodes can be purchased or rented from a medical supply company. Regardless of the device used, your role may be that of teaching the care provider in the home the proper procedure and the adaptations that should be made on an individual basis. Giving perineal care may be seen as an invasion of privacy, so your instruction and support in having the care provider carry out this procedure are essential.

CRITICAL THINKING EXERCISES

Your patient, 89-year-old Robert Aston, has been somewhat confused at times. This afternoon when you answer his call light, you find him with his lower leg draped over the side rail and his safety device untied. He calls out, "Help me! I have to use the commode, and I can't get out of bed!" Analyze the situation. Identify further assessment that is needed immediately. Outline your nursing actions, including the priority order in which you would undertake them. Predict future care needs, and develop a plan to meet this patient's elimination needs.

References

Guidelines for Handwashing and Hospital Environmental Control. (1985). Atlanta: Centers for Disease Control.

Guidelines for Prevention of Catheter-Associated Urinary Tract Infections. (1983). Atlanta: Centers for Disease Control.

Sherman, A. M. V. (1993). An introduction to urinary incontinence. *Orthopedic Nursing, 12*(6), 27–30.

© 1996 by Lippincott-Raven Publishers

✔ PERFORMANCE CHECKLIST

Assisting With a Bedpan or Urinal	Needs More Practice	Satisfactory	Comments
Assessment			
1. Check patient's activity order.			
2. Check for past use of bedpan or urinal and problems.			
Planning			
3. Determine assistance needed.			
4. Plan technique to be used.			
5. Wash your hands and put on clean gloves.			
Implementation			
6. Explain to patient how you plan to proceed.			
7. Provide privacy.			
8. Raise both bed and rail on opposite side.			
9. Obtain bedpan or urinal and other items needed.			
10. Place patient on the bedpan using one of the following: a. Have patient lift up from recumbent position.			
b. Have patient lift up from sitting position.			
c. Roll patient onto the pan.			
11. Raise side rail nearest you.			
12. Elevate patient to sitting position.			
13. Place tissue and call bell within reach.			
14. Leave patient for privacy.			
15. Return when patient signals.			
16. Put on clean gloves.			
17. Clean perineum if necessary.			
18. Remove bedpan or urinal.			
19. Place cover on pan.			
20. Carry pan or urinal to bathroom; observe and measure any contents as ordered.			
21. Collect any specimens ordered.			

(continued)

© 1996 by Lippincott-Raven Publishers

Assisting With a Bedpan or Urinal *(Continued)*	Needs More Practice	Satisfactory	Comments
22. Empty contents into bowl and flush.			
23. Clean equipment with cold water.			
24. Remove and dispose of gloves.			
25. Return to patient and offer hygiene items.			
26. Reposition bed and patient for comfort.			
27. Dispose of equipment.			
28. Wash your hands.			
Evaluation			
29. Note efficiency of procedure and results.			
30. Identify any problems encountered.			
Documentation			
31. Record any unusual observations or problems.			
Assisting With a Commode			
Assessment			
1. Check the patient's activity order and physical status.			
2. Note any past problems using the equipment.			
Planning			
3. Determine assistance needed.			
4. Plan procedure for getting patient out of bed.			
5. Wash your hands.			
Implementation			
6. Explain to patient how you plan to proceed.			
7. Provide privacy.			
8. Help patient out of bed.			
9. Place call light within reach.			
10. Leave patient for privacy.			
11. Put on clean gloves.			
12. Return and clean perineal area, if necessary.			
13. Help patient back to bed.			

(continued)

© 1996 by Lippincott-Raven Publishers

Assisting With a Commode *(Continued)*	Needs More Practice	Satisfactory	Comments
14. Remove sliding container and measure or dispose of contents.			
Evaluation			
15. Note tolerance of the procedure.			
16. Identify any problems.			
Documentation			
17. Document any problems. Measure output if necessary. Indicate bowel movement on correct flow sheet and describe stool if abnormal or pertinent to patient's condition.			
Giving Perineal Care			
Assessment			
1. Determine the extent of soiling.			
2. Identify patient's capabilities.			
Planning			
3. Plan equipment needed.			
4. Decide if you will need assistance.			
5. Wash your hands. Put on clean gloves.			
Implementation			
6. Explain what you are about to do.			
7. Select appropriate equipment for: a. Postpartum or surgical patient			
b. Nonsurgical patient			
c. Patient with a catheter			
8. Provide privacy.			
9. Drape as appropriate.			
10. Put on gloves and follow appropriate procedure for particular patient.			
11. Replace bed linens and reposition patient.			
12. Dispose of equipment.			
13. Remove gloves and wash your hands.			

(continued)

© 1996 by Lippincott-Raven Publishers

Giving Perineal Care *(Continued)*	Needs More Practice	Satisfactory	Comments
Evaluation			
14. Check back with patient for comfort.			
Documentation			
15. Document any pertinent observations or difficulties.			

© 1996 by Lippincott-Raven Publishers

? QUIZ

Short-Answer Questions

1. List three principles to be followed when assisting a patient with a bedpan or urinal.

    a. _____

    b. _____

    c. _____

2. Name four pieces of equipment that are used to help the bed patient to eliminate.

    a. _____

    b. _____

    c. _____

    d. _____

3. Which two comfort measures should you take for a thin elderly patient who must use a bedpan?

    a. _____

    b. _____

4. Describe two methods for placing a patient on a bedpan.

    a. _____

    b. _____

5. You would need which two skills for assisting a patient to a commode?

    a. _____

    b. _____

6. List five of the seven observations that you might make about a patient's urine or feces.

    a. _____

    b. _____

    c. _____

    d. _____

    e. _____

7. Identify three categories of patients who may need special pericare.

    a. _____

    b. _____

    c. _____

8. Describe the procedure for one of the three categories in question 7.

    _____

9. Why is a cover used over a bedpan? _____

    _____

10. Where should specific methods of assisting a patient with using a bedpan be noted?

_____

_____

11. Why is all cleansing on the female patient's perineum done from front to back?

_____

_____

HYGIENE

MODULE CONTENTS

RATIONALE FOR THE USE OF THIS
  SKILL
NURSING DIAGNOSIS
GENERAL PROCEDURE FOR HYGIENE
  Assessment
  Planning
  Implementation
  Evaluation
  Documentation
SPECIFIC PROCEDURES FOR HYGIENE
BATHING PROCEDURES
Complete Bedbath
Partial Bedbath
Self-Bedbath
Tub Bath
Shower
BACK RUB
ORAL CARE
Toothbrushing
Flossing
Oral Care for Unconscious Patients
CARE OF DENTURES
HAIR CARE

Brushing and Combing
Shampooing
EYE CARE
  Assessment
  Planning
  Implementation
  Evaluation
  Documentation
Contact Lens Care, Removal, and Insertion
  Assessment
  Planning
  Implementation
  Evaluation
  Documentation
Care of Glasses
CARE OF HEARING AIDS
Cleaning the Hearing Aid
Protecting the Hearing Aid
AM and PM Care
LONG-TERM CARE
HOME CARE
CRITICAL THINKING EXERCISES

PREREQUISITES

Successful completion of the following modules:

VOLUME 1
Module 1   An Approach to Nursing Skills
Module 2   Basic Infection Control
Module 3   Safety
Module 4   Basic Body Mechanics
Module 5   Documentation
Module 6   Introduction to Assessment Skills
Module 14 Bedmaking
Module 17 Assisting with Elimination and Perineal Care

© 1996 by Lippincott-Raven Publishers

OVERALL OBJECTIVE

To provide each patient with hygiene according to individual needs, conditions, and preferences.

SPECIFIC LEARNING OBJECTIVES

Know Facts and Principles	Apply Facts and Principles	Demonstrate Ability	Evaluate Performance
1. Providing hygiene a. Baths b. Back rubs c. Oral care d. Hair care e. Eye care f. AM and PM care Describe several aspects of hygiene, including baths, back rubs, oral care, hair care, eye care, AM and PM care.	Given a patient situation, identify type of bath that should be given and appropriate type of oral and hair care. Explain rationale for types of baths, oral care, hair care, eye care, AM and PM care.	In the clinical setting, identify the appropriate hygiene for an individual patient.	Evaluate choice of hygiene with instructor.
2. Procedures Describe procedures.	Given a patient situation, state what should be done according to procedures.	Demonstrate ability to perform several aspects of hygiene, including baths, back rubs, oral care, and hair care, according to patient's needs. Initiate performance of several aspects of hygiene independently, according to patient's needs.	Evaluate own performance with instructor, using Performance Checklist.
3. Documenting hygiene measures State items to be documented.	Given a patient situation, document appropriate information regarding hygiene.	Document hygiene procedures according to facility's procedure.	Evaluate own performance with instructor.

© 1996 by Lippincott-Raven Publishers

LEARNING ACTIVITIES

1. Review the Specific Learning Objectives.
2. Read the chapter on hygiene in Ellis and Nowlis, *Nursing: A Human Needs Approach,* or a comparable chapter in another textbook.
3. Look up the module vocabulary terms in the glossary.
4. Read through the module and mentally practice the techniques.
5. At home, give yourself a complete sponge bath using the technique for giving bedbaths. This can be done at the bathroom sink, but you should use a basin filled with water (not running water) to simulate the bedside situation. Pay special attention to the following:
   a. The water temperature that feels comfortable to you
   b. Possible chilling due to exposure
   c. The amount of pressure or friction that is comfortable
   d. How easily soap can be rinsed off and how much soap should be used
   e. The effect of "trailing" ends of a washcloth
   f. The need for thorough drying
6. In the practice setting:
   a. Practice giving a complete bedbath, back rub, oral care, hair care, and eye care, using another student as your patient. Communicate as you would with a real patient. Have the student comment on his or her comfort and the communication skills you demonstrated. Use the Performance Checklist to evaluate yourself. When you are satisfied with your performance, have your instructor evaluate you.
   b. Describe to your instructor what you would do differently to provide a partial bedbath or a self-bedbath with assistance.
   c. Describe the necessary safety measures for the patient receiving a shower or a tub bath.
   d. Practice denture care if dentures are provided in the practice setting. Use the Performance Checklist to evaluate yourself. When you are satisfied with your performance, have your instructor evaluate you.
   e. Practice care of glasses, hearing aids, and contact lenses if they are provided in the practice setting. Use the Performance Checklist to evaluate yourself. When you are satisfied with your performance, have your instructor evaluate you.
7. In the clinical setting:
   a. Assist a patient with a tub bath or shower and morning care.
   b. Give a complete bedbath and morning care to a patient.
   c. Provide AM and PM care.

VOCABULARY

- asepto syringe
- aspirate
- axilla
- canthus
- cariogenic
- expectorate
- Fowler's position
- genital
- semi-Fowler's position
- sordes
- supine
- umbilicus

© 1996 by Lippincott-Raven Publishers

Hygiene[1]

Rationale for the Use of This Skill

Patients in healthcare facilities have at least as many needs for hygiene measures in their daily lives as you do in yours. Indeed, they may have considerably more because of perspiration from fever, drainage from wounds, odor from emesis, and other aspects of illness. Often, however, they cannot attend to those needs themselves without at least some help. It is the nurse's responsibility to provide patients with the opportunity for hygiene, assisting them as needed, taking into consideration their personal preferences, cultural differences, and physical disabilities, and delegating specific tasks as appropriate.[2]

▼ NURSING DIAGNOSIS

The principle nursing diagnosis for which the skills in this module are used is Bathing/Hygiene Self-Care Deficit: This may be related to a wide variety of health factors, among them fatigue and weakness associated with illness, specific neuromuscular deficits, painful conditions that inhibit activity, and lack of mental processes needed to plan and carry out activities.

GENERAL PROCEDURE FOR HYGIENE

There is a general approach you can use to help patients with the various aspects of hygiene. This can be modified according to the particular aspect of hygiene involved and the degree to which the patient is able to participate.

Assessment

1. Check the chart and nursing care plan for any information related to the patient's ability to participate in the procedure being planned—for example, diagnoses, activity orders, or any orders specific to hygiene.
2. Assess the patient to determine if there are other concerns of a higher priority than hygiene. For example, there may be a need for toileting. Assess for current symptoms related to the medical diagnosis, for fatigue or pain, and for level of se-

---

[1]For infant bathing procedure, see Module 19, Basic Infant Care. For perineal care procedure, see Module 17, Assisting with Elimination and Perineal Care.

[2]You will note that rationale for action is emphasized throughout the module by the use of italics.

dation. Remember that hygiene may be of a lower priority than rest for the patient who is short of breath or experiencing pain. Assess also for hygiene preferences.
3. Check to see whether needed special supplies or equipment are already in the room.

Planning

4. Determine whether or not you will need any assistance.
5. Determine what supplies and equipment are needed.
6. Wash your hands *for infection control.*
7. Obtain the needed supplies.

Whenever you are doing a procedure that has the potential for bringing you into contact with body secretions, you should put on clean gloves *for infection control.* You may wish to carry a pair of clean gloves with you at all times. Gloves should be disposed of by turning them inside out as they are removed, leaving the soiled surface enclosed inside the glove, and then discarding them in the wastebasket. *This provides added protection for housekeeping personnel.*

Implementation

8. Identify the patient *to be sure you are carrying out the procedure for the correct patient.*
9. Explain to the patient what you plan to do and how he or she can participate.
10. Provide for the patient's privacy.
11. Raise the bed to the appropriate working level.
12. Carry out the hygiene procedure planned.
13. Watch the patient carefully for signs of fatigue or other adverse responses. While giving the bath, you will also have an opportunity to carry out other assessments such as examining the skin or evaluating the patient's cognitive ability and psychosocial concerns.
14. Care appropriately for all equipment and supplies used. These are usually cleaned and stored for the next hygiene activities.
15. Wash your hands *for infection control.*

Evaluation

16. Evaluate in terms of the following criteria:
    a. Fatigue
    b. Feelings about comfort and cleanliness
    c. Objective signs of cleanliness

Documentation

17. Document the hygiene measure as appropriate for your facility. In many facilities, hygiene measures are recorded on a flow sheet. Information about the patient's preferences and ability to participate is recorded on the nursing care plan. Any information about physical signs and

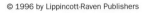© 1996 by Lippincott-Raven Publishers

symptoms identified during the procedure can be recorded either on a flow sheet or on the progress notes.

Figure 18–1 is an example of flow sheet entries. Table 18–1 provides some common abbreviations used for hygiene procedures.

SPECIFIC PROCEDURES FOR HYGIENE

For each procedure discussed, some steps of the General Procedure may be modified. We have included the modified steps as well as references to the steps of the General Procedure that remain the same.

SHIFT	23-07	07-15	15-23	23-07	07-15	15-23	23-07	07-15	15-23	23-07	07-15	15-23
PERSONAL HYGIENE: BATH: (Complete Bed Bath, Shower c̄/s̄ help, Sit Shower, Bath c̄ help)	A.M. care	CBB c̄ assist	P.M. care									
ORAL:	Self	Self	Self									
BACK CARE:		lotion rub	lotion rub									
PERI-CARE:		Self										
CATH CARE:		N/A										
ACTIVITY: (Bedrest, Amb c̄ help, Dangle, Chair c̄/s̄ help, Up Ad Lib, BR c̄ BRP)		Chair x 2 15"	Chair x 1 20"									
TURNED & POSITIONED	q 2 h	q 2 h when in bed	q 2 h when in bed									
DEEP BREATHE & COUGH	q 2 h	q 2 h	q 2 h									
ELIMINATION: BM (Number & Description)		1 formed										
SLEEP PATTERNS: (Naps, 1 hour intervals, etc)	Restless	Naps at intervals	Asleep @ 2200									
DIET:	Breakfast	Lunch	Dinner	Breakfast	Lunch	Dinner	Breakfast	Lunch	Dinner	Breakfast	Lunch	Dinner
Type	2 Gm Na											
Amount taken (All, none, fraction)	All	3/4	All									
Calorie Count												
SIGNATURES 23-07	M. Johnson RN											
07-15	B. Kucinski, R.N.											
15-23	D. Aquaro RN											
DATE	2-22-99			2-23			2-24			2-25		

ADDRESSOGRAPH:

THE SWEDISH HOSPITIAL MEDICAL CENTER
SEATTLE, WASHINGTON

N-1546 Nursing Rev. 6/80 FC/TSHMC
ACTIVITIES OF DAILY LIVING AND TREATMENT

Figure 18–1. Flow sheet entries for hygiene procedures and activities of daily living.

© 1996 by Lippincott-Raven Publishers

Table 18–1. Common Abbreviations Used for Charting Hygiene Procedures on Flow Sheets	
Abbreviation	**Meaning**
CBB	Complete bedbath
PBB	Partial bedbath
Self	Patient bathed self
N/A	Not applicable
X2	Done twice (times 2)
X3	Done three times (and so forth)

BATHING PROCEDURES

Apply the principles of infection control and body mechanics described in Module 14, Bedmaking, to giving various types of bedbaths. *Because a patient receiving a bedbath is very likely to stay in bed while the bed is being made,* you may need to refer again to the procedure for making an occupied bed.

Complete Bedbath

Assessment
1.–3. Follow the steps of the General Procedure for Hygiene.

Planning
4.–6. Follow the steps of the General Procedure.
7. Gather the necessary supplies:
  a. Basin for water
  b. Soap (some patients may have their own)
  c. Laundry hamper or bag
  d. Clean linen in the order of use (if you plan to make the bed as well)
  e. Bath blanket, towels, and washcloths as needed. (Remember, you will want to leave a fresh towel and washcloth at the bedside for use at other times during the day.)
  f. Clean gown or pajamas
  g. Necessary toiletries. (Some patients will bring their own toothbrush and paste or powder, deodorant, comb, and the like; others will not.)
  h. Clean gloves (two pairs)

Implementation
8.–11. Follow the steps of the General Procedure.
12. Carry out the bedbath as follows:
  a. Arrange for top covering. A bath blanket has traditionally been used to cover the patient during the bath. *This absorbent flannel blanket helps to prevent chilling and does not become "clammy" if it gets wet.* In the interest of cost containment, some facilities are no longer stocking bath blankets. Instead the top sheet is used for a cover during the bath. In such a case, be especially careful not to get the covering wet because it will feel clammy and uncomfortable. If a bath blanket is available, remove the top linen, placing a bath blanket over the patient before removing the top sheet. (See Module 14, Bedmaking, Occupied Beds, step 12, page 311.)
  b. Give oral care at this point if you have not done so already. (See Oral Care, pages 402–405.) Be sure to wear gloves.
  c. Obtain water for the bath. This may be done when you are rinsing the oral hygiene articles.
  d. Position the patient for the bath. Usually the supine position is used unless the patient cannot tolerate it. In some cases it may be necessary to use a semi-Fowler's or even Fowler's position *for the patient's comfort or safety.* Move the patient to your side of the bed *to decrease the need for reaching.*
  e. Bathe the patient in the following order:
    (1) Spread a towel across the patient's chest, tucking it under the chin.
    (2) Make a mitt out of the washcloth. Tucking one edge of the washcloth under your thumb, wrap it in thirds around your hand, tucking the final edge under your thumb as well (Fig. 18–2). Bring the far edge of the washcloth up and tuck it under the near edge. *Using a mitt prevents loose, cool ends of the cloth from dragging across the patient and causing discomfort.* As long as the mitt does not come apart, it may be left on the hand.
    (3) Wash the patient's face. This is generally done *without* soap, but be certain to ask patients for their preference. Many patients are able to do this portion of the bath themselves. Wash the eyes from the inner canthus to the outer canthus; rinse the cloth after washing each eye.
      Use gentle but firm strokes when you wash the face, *so that the patient feels clean.*
      Be sure to wash *behind* the ears as well as on the upper surfaces, using soap.
      You may want to use soap on the neck even if you did not on the face. Wash just the front and the sides of the neck. *The back part can be washed when the back is done.* Rinse and dry the neck after washing.

© 1996 by Lippincott-Raven Publishers

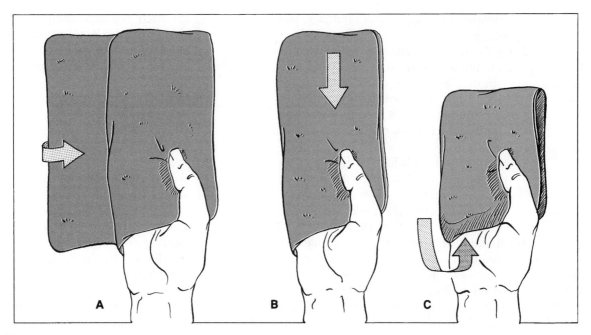

Figure 18–2. Folding a mitt for bathing. (**A**) Fold washcloth lengthwise in thirds around your hand. (**B and C**) Fold top end of cloth down under and tuck under bottom end.

(4) Remove the patient's gown.

(5) Place the towel lengthwise under the far arm. If you have moved the patient toward the side of the bed on which you are working, it should not be too far to reach, especially if you place a towel across the patient's chest and have patient place the arm on top of it (Fig. 18–3).

Do the far arm first *to avoid leaning over or dripping dirty water on the part that is already washed.* Using long, firm strokes toward the center of the body (*to increase venous return*), wash the far hand, arm, and axilla in that order. Cover the arm with half of the towel while rinsing out the washcloth *to prevent chilling from the evaporation of water from the skin.* Rinse and dry thoroughly.

Often the hands have been washed before the bath or are not very dirty. Some patients, however, enjoy the opportunity to soak their hands in a basin. In any case, wash the hands thoroughly, being certain to dry well between the fingers. Use an orangewood stick to clean under the nails if needed.

(6) Next, place the towel under the near arm and wash the near hand, arm, and axilla in the same way.

(7) Fold the bath blanket down to the waist. Place the towel over the chest

and fold it back as you wash. You can then leave it over the patient *to prevent chilling* as you rinse the cloth.

Wash the chest, being certain to wash, rinse, and dry thoroughly under the breasts of a female patient. Leave the chest covered with the towel while

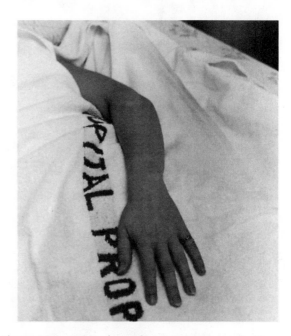

Figure 18–3. Draping for washing a patient's arm. Position patient's arm across body, with towel lengthwise underneath. (Courtesy Ivan Ellis)

© 1996 by Lippincott-Raven Publishers

rinsing the mitt. Rinse and dry the chest.

(8) Fold the bath blanket down to the pubic bone, leaving the towel over the chest. Wash, rinse, and dry the lower abdomen, paying particular attention to the umbilicus. Remove the towel and replace the bath blanket over the chest and arms.

(9) Remove the bath blanket from the far leg only, tucking it under the near leg and up around the hip *to avoid exposure and drafts.* Place the towel lengthwise under the far leg (Fig. 18–4).

(10) Bending the leg at the knee, slide the basin onto the bed and place the patient's foot in it. Place the foot carefully in the basin, *so as not to spill the water.* In some facilities the basins used for bathing may be too small to carry out this procedure for patients with large feet.

(11) Wash the leg, using long, firm strokes toward the center of the body. *You should not rub the muscle hard enough to potentially dislodge clots that may have formed in the large deep veins.* Dry the leg.

(12) Wash and rinse the foot, being careful to

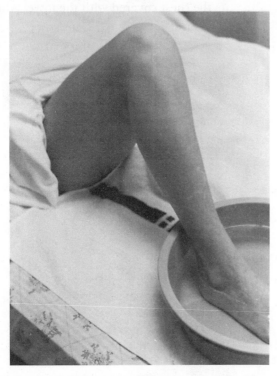

Figure 18–4. Draping for washing the patient's leg. Uncover only one leg at a time, keeping the rest of the patient's body covered. (Courtesy Ivan Ellis)

do each toe separately. Remove the basin from the bed. Dry the foot, giving special attention to the areas between the toes *to prevent irritation and injury to the skin.*

(13) Wash the near leg and foot in the same way (steps 9–12).

(14) Change the bath water and put on gloves.

(15) Wash the genital area. In many cases, patients will be able to wash themselves. In this case, your responsibility is to ensure that everything needed is within reach. You may want to stay within hearing distance or instruct the patient to call you with the call light. Be sure the patient understands what you expect to be done. You might say "Can you wash your own genital area?" or "I'll set things up and give you some privacy to wash your own genital area." If the patient does not understand that term, you might use the term "private area."

If patients are not able to wash their own genital area, you should do so. Put on clean gloves *for infection control. (There are always normal flora in the genital area and there may also be organisms from subclinical infections. These organisms may infect small breaks in your skin, or may be transmitted to other patients if handwashing is not thorough.)* Wash, moving gently from front to back (clean to dirty), making certain to wash and dry carefully between opposing skin surfaces (see Module 17, Assisting with Elimination and Perineal Care).

(16) Take off and dispose of gloves.

(17) Change the bath water.

(18) Turn the patient on the side, facing away from you. Very few patients will be comfortable lying on the abdomen, although this may be done. Drape the patient as shown in Fig. 18–5, with the bath blanket drawn down to the hips and a towel tucked lengthwise behind and beside the back.

(19) Wash, rinse, and dry the back of the neck and the back, using long, firm strokes.

(20) Put on your second pair of gloves.

(21) Wash, rinse, and dry the buttocks. If the patient is incapacitated, you will then wash the perianal area.

(22) Remove and discard gloves.

© 1996 by Lippincott-Raven Publishers

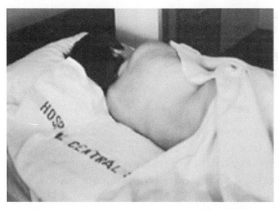

Figure 18–5. Draping for washing the patient's back. (Courtesy Ivan Ellis)

(23) Give a back rub at this point if the purpose is *to stimulate or invigorate the patient.* If, however, you wish to make the back rub a more relaxing experience for the patient, wait until after all care is completed. At this time lotion may also be applied to dry skin areas such as heels, elbows, feet, etc.

f. Help the patient put on a clean gown or pajamas.

g. Comb or brush and arrange the patient's hair (see Hair Care, pages 405–406).

h. File or cut the patient's fingernails and toenails. Because some facilities do not permit nail cutting, especially of diabetic patients or those with peripheral vascular disease, be sure you know the policy and follow it.

i. Assist the male patient with shaving at this point. You may have to assemble his shaving equipment, which will vary depending on the type of razor he prefers. If he is unable to shave himself, this task is also your responsibility. Some facilities have an electric razor you can use. Be sure to review the procedure for cleaning the razor after use. *This is essential to infection control.* If your facility requires you to use a safety razor and you do not know how, ask for assistance. If the patient is not able to indicate preferences regarding a mustache or beard, be sure to ask a family member before shaving the patient. Some elderly women develop facial hair. They may prefer to leave it in place or prefer to shave. Follow the patient's preferences.

j. Make the occupied bed (see Module 14, Bedmaking, Occupied Beds, pages 311–313). Be sure to return the bed to the low position at the completion of this procedure *for safety.*

k. Set the patient's room in order; wash, dry,

and return the bath basin to the patient's storage unit; and put away the patient's personal articles, leaving a washcloth and towel for use during the day. Clean off the overbed table. Be sure patients have within reach the call light and everything they will need throughout the day.

13.–15. Follow the steps of the General Procedure.

Evaluation

16. Follow the General Procedure.

Documentation

17. Follow the General Procedure.

Partial Bedbath

A partial bedbath is given for several reasons, *including a patient's inability to tolerate a full bath and a lack of need or desire for a full daily bath.* A partial bedbath usually includes the face, neck, hands, axillae, and perineum. The back may also be included if the patient can tolerate it. Provide a back rub for any patient on bed rest.

Self-Bedbath

This type of bath is given *when a patient is, for some reason, unable to take a shower or a tub bath but is able to move about freely in bed.* The self-bedbath is usually a complete bath. Your responsibility is to provide the basin of water, bath blanket, and other necessary articles and to be ready to assist at the call of the patient. Your assistance may be needed for the feet and legs, and is necessary for the back and buttocks. Do not omit the back rub simply because a patient is able to bathe unaided.

Sometimes a patient may be moved to a sink and allowed to bathe using running water. In this instance put all of the supplies close to the sink and arrange for the patient to have privacy to bathe. A bath blanket can be used to drape the leg or shoulders as needed to prevent chilling and provide for patient modesty.

Tub Bath

Tub baths are generally used *for hygiene, although at times therapeutic agents (such as bath oils for dry skin or anti-pruritic agents) can be added.* If your facility requires a physician's order for a tub bath, be sure you have the order before you offer the patient a bath. Check your facility's procedure manual for special instructions regarding tub baths and for the method of cleaning and disinfecting the tub between patient.

© 1996 by Lippincott-Raven Publishers

Assessment

1.–3. Follow the steps of the General Procedure for Hygiene.

Planning

4. Follow the General Procedure.

5. Determine what supplies and equipment are needed and prepare the tub area. *It is frustrating for everyone involved to arrive at the tub room only to find it already in use.* After checking to make sure the tub is clean, fill the tub about half full with warm water (100°–115°F; 37.7°–46.1°C).

6.–7. Follow the steps of the General Procedure.

Implementation

8.–9. Follow the steps of the General Procedure.

10. Assist the patient to the tub room. Be certain to check which method of ambulation is appropriate. Bring all needed items (towel, deodorant, pajamas, and the like) .

11. Hang a sign on the door indicating that the room is occupied *to protect the privacy of the patient.*

12. Carry out the tub bath as follows:

   a. Help the patient into the tub.

   b. Assist the patient as needed. If the patient is quite helpless, you may need a second person to assist while you wash. Some patients may be able to support themselves but will need your help with the bath. If the patient is quite independent, you may leave for a few minutes while the bath is being taken. The bed may be made at this time. Be certain, however, to tell the patient how to use the emergency call signal before you leave. If the patient seems weak, do *not* leave. Be sure to wash the patient's back.

   c. Drain the water and assist the patient out of the tub. Draining the water first decreases the chance of a fall. *The warm water may cause pooling of blood in the lower part of the body. Blood pressure may then drop when the patient stands, causing dizziness and instability.* Get help if you think you might need it. *Both you and the patient are too valuable to injure.*

   d. Assist the patient with drying.

   e. Help the patient to put on a clean gown or pajamas.

   f. Assist the patient back to the room.

13. Follow the General Procedure.

14. Return to the tub room.

   a. Clean the tub as directed in the facility procedure manual.

   b. Discard the used linen.

   c. Put the "unoccupied" sign on the door or notify the staff person next in line that the tub is ready for use.

15. Follow the General Procedure.

Evaluation

16. Follow the General Procedure.

Documentation

17. Follow the General Procedure.

Shower

A patient may take a standing shower independently, or a shower may be given in a shower chair. In any case, patients usually prefer showers to bedbaths. If your facility requires a physician's order for a patient to have a shower, be sure you have the order before offering the patient a shower.

Assessment

1.–3. Follow the steps of the General Procedure for Hygiene.

Planning

4.–6. Follow the steps of the General Procedure.

7. Obtain needed supplied and prepare the shower area. This may be in the patient's room or there may be a shower located elsewhere on the unit.

Implementation

8.–9. Follow the steps of the General Procedure.

10. Assist the patient to the shower room or stall. If the patient will walk, be sure you have provided slip-proof slippers or shoes. If a chair shower is to be given, you can transport the patient in the shower chair. The safest way to do this is to pull the chair backward down the hall, with at least one hand grasping the patient's shoulder.

11. If the shower is located outside the patient's room, hang a sign on the door indicating that the room is occupied *to protect the privacy of the patient.*

12. Carry out the shower as follows.

   a. Assist the patient as necessary. Run the shower until the water is warm (100°–115°F; 37. 7°–46. 1°C); then adjust it to the patient's preference. Place a paper shower mat or bath towel on the floor *to prevent slipping.*

   At this point, a patient who can take a shower independently may be left alone (with a call bell within reach), but for no more than 10 minutes. A patient having a chair shower may need assistance throughout or only at the end of the shower, depending on the reason the patient needs to sit during the shower. If the patient is able to be independent, check frequently to be certain that the patient is all right. *Some shower chairs are less stable than others,* and you may determine that no patient should be left alone in the shower chair.

© 1996 by Lippincott-Raven Publishers

b. Assist the patient with drying if necessary. Help the patient put on a clean gown or pajamas.

c. Assist the patient back to the room.

13. Follow the General Procedure.

14. Return to the shower room.

a. Clean the stall and shower chair in the manner prescribed by your facility.

b. Discard used linen.

c. Put the "unoccupied" sign on the door.

15. Follow the General Procedure.

Evaluation

16. Follow the General Procedure.

Documentation

17. Follow the General Procedure.

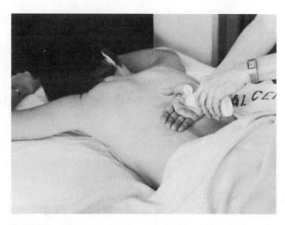

Figure 18–6. Retaining touch during back rub. At least one hand should remain in contact with the patient's back at all times, even when you are pouring lotion. (Let the back of your hand rest on the patient's back.) (Courtesy Ivan Ellis)

PROCEDURE FOR GIVING A BACK RUB

Research indicates that the back rub may decrease anxiety, help alleviate pain perception, decrease muscle tension and fatigue, stimulate circulation, and enhance immune system function. Unfortunately, the back rub has often been considered superfluous because it is not related to specific "high-tech" medical care. This has resulted in its being discarded as unneeded when time pressures are great. Nurses who understand the value of a well-done back massage use it as a planned part of nursing care.

Tradition dictates a back rub during or after the bath and at bedtime. These are often convenient times, but other times may fit into the plan of care better. For the person confined to bed, massage over pressure areas may be needed every 2 hours when turning is done. For the person experiencing pain, the back rub may be scheduled with the pain medication to enhance its effectiveness.

Use lotion to decrease friction on the skin and counteract the potential for dry skin in the institutional setting. In the past, alcohol was used for back rubs, but that has been found to dry skin. It is a nice touch to warm the lotion slightly before use by placing it under warm running water for a few moments. Once you begin a back rub, *it is more pleasant and relaxing for the patient* if at least one hand remains in contact with the patient's back until you have finished (Fig. 18–6). This is not difficult to do if the lotion is within easy reach.

Be aware of the patient's response to your touch and question the patient about areas that are especially tight or tense. Ask which areas the patient would like special attention to be given to. Also give special attention to any reddened areas, rubbing gently around them (never on them) to stimulate circulation. *When reddened areas do not subside quickly,*

the tissue beneath may be in the beginning stages of breaking down. Vigorous massage to the reddened area may actually be damaging to this tissue.

There are many acceptable ways to perform a back rub. Long smooth flowing movements over the length of the back tend to be relaxing. Kneading motions will often relax specific tight muscle groups. Circular motions will stimulate circulation in a specific area. The following is a suggested procedure for general use.

Assessment

1.–3. Follow the steps of the General Procedure for Hygiene.

Planning

4.–6. Follow the steps of the General Procedure.

5. Secure lotion.

Implementation

8.–11. Follow the steps of the General Procedure.

12. Carry out the back rub:

a. Move the patient close to your side of the bed *to decrease the distance you need to reach.* Position the patient on the abdomen if possible. If this is not possible because of the patient's condition or the presence of tubes, a side-lying position with the patient facing away from you is adequate, also. Pull the top covers down below the buttocks.

b. Pour a small amount of lotion into your hand and rub your palms together, *to get the lotion on both hands and warm it slightly.*

c. With your feet apart (the outside one ahead of the inside one *so that you can rock back and forth while maintaining good posture and body mechanics*), place your hands at the sacral area, one on either side of the spinal column.

© 1996 by Lippincott-Raven Publishers

d. Rub toward the neckline, using long, firm, smooth strokes.

e. Pause at the neckline and, using your thumbs, rub up into the hairline, while using your fingers to massage the sides of the neck.

f. With a kneading motion, rub out along the shoulders. Continue the kneading motion and move down one side of the trunk with both hands until you are again at the sacral area.

g. Then, placing your hands side by side with the palms down, rub in a figure 8 pattern over the buttocks and sacral area (Fig. 18–7). Move the figure 8 back and forth to include the entire buttocks area, *which is subjected to ongoing pressure in the bedridden patient.*

h. Next, again using the kneading motion, move up the opposite side of the back toward the shoulder.

i. Ask the patient if there are any areas that he or she would especially like rubbed.

j. Complete the back rub using long, firm strokes up and down the back (shoulders to sacrum and back to shoulders).

k. Replace the top covers, reposition the patient, and lower the bed.

13. Follow the General Procedure.
14. Return the lotion to the bedside stand.
15. Follow the General Procedure.

Evaluation
16. Follow the General Procedure.

Documentation
17. Follow the General Procedure.

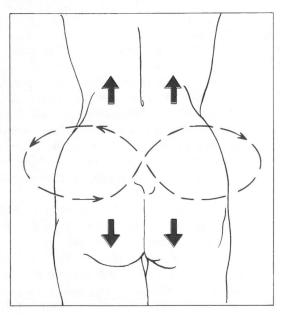

Figure 18–7. Figure-8 technique in the back rub.

ORAL CARE

Ideally the patient should be offered the opportunity for oral care before breakfast, after all meals, and at bedtime. Not all patients will want oral care this frequently, but it should still be offered. Oral care is especially important for patients who are receiving oxygen and for patients who have nasogastric tubes in place, as well as for those on NPO (nothing by mouth). Many will be able to take care of this aspect of their hygiene independently, provided the equipment is conveniently placed. For the patient who is not able to request oral care, the nurse should add oral care to the nursing care plan so that it is not overlooked.

Patients who can sit in Fowler's or even semi-Fowler's position can often do most of their oral care independently. If patients can do their own oral care but are confined to bed, you should provide the necessary articles.

PROCEDURE FOR TOOTHBRUSHING

Brushing is correctly done using a small, soft brush. Many dentists recommend a four-row, level, straight-handled brush. It is wise to rinse after eating if brushing cannot be done. Mouthwashes can be used if desired, but remember that their antiseptic value is questionable.

Assessment
1.–3. Follow the steps of the General Procedure for Hygiene.

Planning
4.–6. Follow the steps of the General Procedure.
7. Obtain the necessary supplies: toothbrush, toothpaste or powder (usually brought to the facility by the patient), cup of water, emesis basin, and face towel; some patients also use dental floss.

Implementation
8.–11. Follow the steps of the General Procedure.
12. Provide oral care.
    a. Place a towel under the patient's chin, tucking it behind the shoulders.
    b. Put on clean gloves *for infection control.*
    c. Moisten the toothbrush with water from a glass and spread a small amount of toothpaste on it. If no cleansing agent is available, plain water is adequate. Baking soda and mouthwash are substitutes that also freshen the breath.
    d. Brush the teeth, allowing the patient to expectorate into the emesis basin.

(1) Holding the brush at a 45° angle, use a small, vibrating, circular motion with the bristles at the junction of the teeth and gums. *This removes plaque that forms at the base of the tooth.* Use the same action on the front and the back of the teeth.

(2) Use a back-and-forth brushing motion over the biting surfaces of the teeth *to remove food particles and plaque from tooth crevices.*

(3) Brush the tongue *to decrease sordes on the tongue and the resident bacterial count*, then rinse the mouth.

    e. Allow the patient to rinse the mouth with water, followed by a mouthwash if desired.

    f. Wipe the patient's mouth.

13. Follow the General Procedure.

14. Care for equipment.

    a. Rinse equipment and return it to its appropriate place.

    b. Remove and dispose of gloves.

    c. Return bed to low position.

15. Follow the General Procedure.

Evaluation

16. Follow the General Procedure.

Documentation

17. Follow the General Procedure.

Flossing

Flossing should be done once daily *to remove plaque (microorganisms trapped in a mucous base) that is not reached by brushing and which, if not removed, causes tooth and gum disease.* Plaque forms in 24 hours and eventually becomes impossible to remove without dental instruments. Floss is correctly held as demonstrated in Fig. 18–8. Remember, however, that control of the floss is more important than how it is held.

Carry out flossing both between the teeth and between the gums and each individual tooth, taking care not to injure the delicate mucous membranes. The mouth should be rinsed after flossing *to remove debris.*

PROCEDURE FOR ORAL CARE FOR UNCONSCIOUS PATIENTS

Unconscious patients are completely dependent on you for their oral care. *Because these persons may be "mouth breathers" and are not taking food or fluids by mouth,* sordes (a collection of bacteria and residue of mucous and other mouth secretions that collects on the tongue, teeth, and lips) accumulates rapidly. A suitable procedure for the oral care of unconscious patients is as follows:

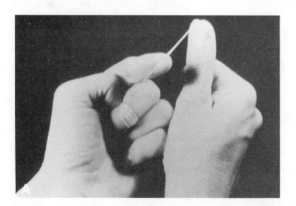

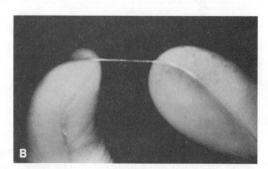

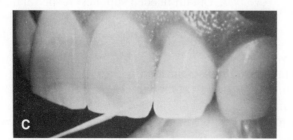

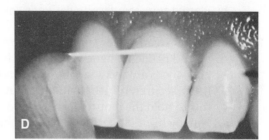

Figure 18–8. Patient flossing the teeth.

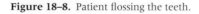

© 1996 by Lippincott-Raven Publishers

Assessment

1.–3. Follow the steps of the General Procedure for Hygiene.

Planning

4.–6. Follow the steps of the General Procedure.

7. Assemble the supplies and equipment. You will need a tongue blade wrapped in gauze to hold the mouth open, applicators, a toothbrush, cleansing agent, a lip lubricant, towel, and clean gloves. Suction or an asepto syringe and an emesis basin are needed to remove cleansing agents from the mouth. Many facilities have prepared mouth care kits that include needed items.

Additional tongue blades wrapped in gauze, sponge mouth swabs, or a light-weight wash-cloth may be substituted for applicators. A variety of cleansing agents can be used. A mixture of hydrogen peroxide and water (half and half) *has good cleansing properties and is not cariogenic.* However, this may cause mouth discomfort in some individuals. Further dilution to one part hydrogen peroxide to three parts water may prevent this. If discomfort continues, it should not be used. (Both buttermilk and milk of magnesia have been used traditionally, but they are cariogenic.) *Commercial agents often contain lemon juice, which can etch the teeth if used frequently, and glycerin, which actually absorbs moisture from the tissue.* Therefore, the use of such agents is not recommended, particularly for unconscious patients or patients who are receiving nothing by mouth. Avoid highly foaming products such as toothpaste because they are harder to remove and may be aspirated by the patient. A dilute mouthwash solution is often a good option. A water-soluble lubricant or lip salve may be used to lubricate lips.

Implementation

8.–11. Follow the steps of the General Procedure.

12. Give oral care.

   a. Raise the bed to a comfortable working height and place the patient in semi-Fowler's position with the head turned toward you. If the patient's head cannot be raised, leave patient flat and turn the head toward you.

   b. Place a towel under the patient's chin, tucking it in beneath the shoulders.

   c. Put on clean gloves *for infection control.*

   d. Place a padded tongue blade (made by wrapping 4 ×4s around a tongue blade and taping them securely) in the patient's mouth. Use this to hold the mouth open and prevent the patient from biting down on your hands or utensils.

   e. Moisten toothbrush very lightly with cleansing agent.

   f. Brush all tooth surfaces, tongue, and mouth surfaces as previously discussed.

   g. Using oversized cotton-tipped applicators or other substitute, clean all surfaces of the mouth, including the palate, inner cheeks, and tongue. If a large accumulation of sordes is present, it may be necessary to remove the sordes in stages, so as not to damage the tissue.

   h. Rinse the patient's mouth with small amounts of water, either allowing it to drain into the emesis basin by gravity or using an asepto syringe or suction to aspirate it.

   i. Wipe the patient's mouth.

   j. Lubricate the lips as needed.

   k. Return the bed to the low position.

13.–15. Follow the steps of the General Procedure.

Evaluation

16. Follow the General Procedure.

Documentation

17. Follow the General Procedure.

PROCEDURE FOR CARE OF DENTURES

Patients often want to care for their dentures themselves. If so, your responsibility, once again, will be to provide them with the necessary articles. A patient may have brought a denture brush and cleansing agent to the hospital, but if not, a regular toothbrush and paste or powder will suffice. Provide the patient with a partially filled bath basin over which to wash the dentures, *so that if they fall they will not break.* The patient will also need a glass of water *for rinsing.*

If you care for the dentures yourself, keep the following procedures in mind:

Assessment

1.–3. Follow the steps of the General Procedure for Hygiene.

Planning

4.–6. Follow the steps of the General Procedure.

7. Obtain needed supplies. A special denture brush and denture cleaner may be available. If not, use a regular toothbrush and cleansing agent. Obtain clean gloves.

Implementation

8.–11. Follow the steps of the General Procedure.

12. Clean the dentures.

   a. Put on clean gloves *for infection control.*

   b. Assist the patient with removal by applying downward pressure with the index fingers from above the upper denture. It may help if

© 1996 by Lippincott-Raven Publishers

the patient inflates the cheeks *to break the suction.* Lower dentures lift out easily. If no assistance is needed, it works well to have the patient remove the dentures and place them in a denture cup for you.

c. Handle dentures with care. *If dropped, they often break.* For this reason they are usually cleaned over a sink that is partially filled with water, *to break the fall in case they are dropped.* Some people like to pad the basin with a towel instead of putting water in it. Hold the teeth close to the bottom of the sink so if dropped they do not fall far.

d. Take the dentures to the sink in the denture cup. Use a denture brush if the patient has one. Note that the longer side of the brush is used for the tooth surface and the smaller part for brushing the inner surface. Hold the dentures close to the bottom of the sink so if dropped they do not fall far. Rinse them thoroughly.

e. Have the patient rinse out the mouth before reinserting the dentures. Some like to use a soft toothbrush to brush the gums and tongue.

f. Return dentures to the patient, fitting the upper dentures in first. If dentures are to be stored (for an unconscious patient or at night if necessary), they should be stored in a covered container, carefully labeled, and preferably placed in a drawer or other area *where they are not likely to be brushed off onto the floor.* Whether they should be stored in water depends on the material of which they are made. Check with the patient or the patient's family. Cool water is used for storage. *A few drops of white vinegar or mouthwash in the storage water may help to prevent odor from clinging to the dentures.*

g. Dry the patient's mouth.

13.–15. Follow the steps of the General Procedure.

Evaluation
16. Follow the General Procedure.

Documentation
17. Follow the General Procedure.

PROCEDURES FOR HAIR CARE

Brushing and Combing

A patient's hair should be combed and brushed daily. Generally this is done along with other hygiene activities and at other times throughout the day as necessary. Hair care is especially important to the patient, *because morale is often directly related to appearance.*

Hair care is usually done after the bath. Whenever it is done, these are some important points to remember.

Assessment
1.–3. Follow the steps of the General Procedure for Hygiene.

Planning
4.–6. Follow the steps of the General Procedure.

7. Assemble the equipment. Patients will probably have brought their own comb, brush, and other hair care items to the facility. A mirror may be available as a part of the overbed table.

Implementation
12. Provide hair care.

a. Place a face or bath towel over the pillow *to keep it clean.*

b. Place patients who are able to comb and brush their own hair in Fowler's position with the hair care items on the overbed table. Assist as necessary.

   The helpless or unconscious patient may be flat or in a semi-Fowler's position.

c. Turn the patient's head away from you and bring the hair back toward you. Brush hair with few tangles in two or three large sections. Matted hair may have to be separated into small sections and treated with a cream rinse or alcohol *to remove the snarls.*

d. Hold a section of hair 2 to 3 inches from the end. Comb the end until it is free of tangles. Gradually move toward the scalp, combing 2 to 3 inches at a time until the hair is tangle-free. You should be very gentle *to avoid causing pain.*

e. Turn the patient's head in the opposite direction and repeat step d.

f. Arrange the hair as neatly and simply as possible. Braiding may be the most appropriate style for long hair. (The family can bring in barrettes and ribbons to make your job easier.) Use cream or spray if it is needed or if the patient wants it.

g. Remove towel.

13. Follow the General Procedure.

14. Place towel in a laundry hamper or bag. Clean the comb and brush and return them, along with the other toilet articles, to the bedside stand.

15. Follow the steps of the General Procedure.

Evaluation
16. Follow the General Procedure.

Documentation
17. Follow the General Procedure.

© 1996 by Lippincott-Raven Publishers

Shampooing

Many patients whose illnesses keep them in the hospital for only a few days do not want or need shampoos during that time. Other patients, however, may *need* shampoos, not only *to remove oil and dirt and to increase circulation to the scalp but to improve appearance and morale as well. A shampoo may be important for the patient who has had an electroencephalogram in which an electrode gel is used on the scalp or for the patient who has been in an accident.* Before giving a shampoo, check to see whether a physician's order is needed.

Generally, a shampoo is not given at the same time as the bath *because it is a tiring procedure.* The obvious exception is when a patient can shower. The equipment and general procedure you will use for those patients who need a shampoo and cannot shower will vary with the facility. In some places, the patient is taken on a stretcher to an area away from the room where there is a sink at the right height with room for the stretcher, too. In most facilities, however, the patient remains in bed and the shampoo is given using pitchers of warm water and a trough arrangement *to guide the water into a receptacle on the floor or chair beside the bed.*

Use this general procedure for giving a shampoo:

Assessment

1.–3. Follow the steps of the General Procedure for Hygiene.

Planning

4.–6. Follow the steps of the General Procedure.

7. Assemble the equipment, including bath blanket, two towels, shampoo, commercial rinse or vinegar, plastic square to protect the bed, pitcher, trough (if not available in the facility, you can make one from a plastic or rubber sheet with rolled towels under the edges), and basin to collect water (Fig. 18–9).

You will need gloves only if the patient has

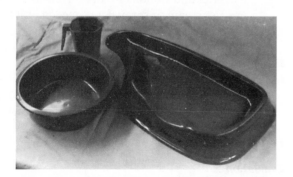

Figure 18–9. Shampooing the patient's hair in bed. Water is poured from the pitcher over the patient's hair, drains down through the trough beneath the patient's head, falls into the basin below. (Courtesy Ivan Ellis)

© 1996 by Lippincott-Raven Publishers

abrasions on the scalp (such as after an accident), or if the patient has other open areas, such as from a scalp condition, that might put you in contact with body substances.

Implementation

8.–11. Follow the steps of the General Procedure.

12. Shampoo hair.

   a. Fan fold the top linens to the foot and position a bath blanket over the patient (see Module 14, Bedmaking, Occupied Beds, step 12, page 311).

   b. Place the plastic square under the patient's head and shoulders.

   c. Place a towel around the patient's shoulders and neck, with the ends of the towel coming together in front.

   d. Place or arrange a trough under the patient's head with one end extending to the receptacle for water.

   e. Wet the hair, taking care to keep water out of the patient's eyes. Some patients like to hold a folded washcloth over their eyes *to protect them.*

   f. Shampoo and rinse twice, using only a small amount of shampoo and rinsing thoroughly. Use cream rinse or half-and-half vinegar and water rinse as desired by the patient. Rinse again.

   g. Dry the patient's hair, ears, and neck with a towel. If an electric hair dryer is available, you may find it helpful, particularly if a patient has long hair.

   h. Comb or brush and arrange the hair, allowing the patient to assist if able. If hair-setting materials are available, a female patient may wish to set, or have a family member or friend set, her hair, in which case you would comb it at a later time.

   i. Remove the plastic square, towels, trough, pitcher, and basin.

   j. Replace the top bed linen, removing the bath blanket after the top sheet is in place.

   k. Allow the patient to rest.

13.–15. Follow the steps of the General Procedure.

Evaluation

16. Follow the General Procedure.

Documentation

17. Follow the General Procedure.

PROCEDURES FOR EYE CARE

The eyes of the healthy individual need no special care other than that given during the usual bathing procedure. However, if there is a neurologic deficit that prevents the blink reflex from operating or if the person is comatose, the eyes need special care to prevent drying of the surface, which can lead to ulceration and permanent vision impairment.

The physician may order a product known as "artificial tears" to keep the eye surface moist or may order that the eyes be patched for protection.

Assessment

1. Check the chart to determine whether there is a physician's order for eye care.
2. Assess the patient's ability to blink.
3. Check to see whether there are eye care supplies in the patient's room. You will need a clean eye pad and tape. Commercially prepared eye pads are oval and *do not have lint that could get in the eye.* If these are not available, clean gauze squares can be substituted. Many hospitals use sterile pads *for extra safety from microorganisms. However, the eye will be closed, and the pad will contact only the exterior of the eyelid; therefore, sterile pads are not essential.* Follow the policy of your facility.

Planning

4. Wash your hands *for infection control.* Gloves are not usually used for this procedure because it is designed for well eyes, which do not have any secretions that are of danger to the nurse. Because the nurse will be touching only the skin surface of the face, clean, washed hands will prevent introducing microbes to the patient. Therefore, based on CDC Guidelines, gloves are not required but may be used as an option by the nurse.
5. Obtain the needed supplies.

Implementation

6. If the eyelids are not clean, clean them at this time. Use a clean washcloth and clear warm water. Wipe the exterior of each eye from the medial aspect to the lateral aspect. Dry the eyes in the same way.
7. If artificial tears are ordered, instill them into the eyes at this time. (See Module 46 for directions on administering eye drops.)
8. Observe the surface of the eyes closely *to detect any irritation or inflammation.*
9. Gently close each eyelid and hold it closed while the eyepad is placed over it.
10. Secure the eyepad with tape so that it holds the eye closed. *The eyelid will protect the surface of the eye from foreign bodies and allow tears to keep the surface moist.*
11. Repeat steps 9 and 10 for the second eye.
12. Put away or dispose of equipment.
13. Wash your hands *for infection control.*

Evaluation

14. Evaluate whether the pad is holding the eye closed.
15. Check skin around eye for irritation resulting from tape.

Documentation

16. Record routine care for eyes on a flow sheet or on the narrative progress notes. If eye medication was instilled, follow directions for recording medications (see Module 46, Irrigations).

Contact Lens Care, Removal, and Insertion

When a patient wears contact lenses, self-care is the best way to ensure that the care is done properly. However, an individual who enters a hospital in an emergency may have contact lenses in place that must be removed *to prevent complications associated with excessive wear.* During a stay, an incapacitated patient may need assistance with routine care and placement of contact lenses.

Assessment

1. Check to see if the patient has contact lenses in place.
2. Determine what type of lenses are being worn (ie, soft lenses or hard lenses).

Planning

3. Wash your hands *for infection control.*
4. Obtain a clean container in which to store the contact lenses. If a regular contact lens container is not available, use sterile specimen jars that have been carefully marked with the patient's name and the information that these are contact lenses. The left and right lenses should be separated and marked as left or right. Hard lenses may be stored dry; however, both hard and soft lenses may be stored in sterile saline or special soaking solution.

Implementation

5. Use a flashlight to examine the eye and determine where the contact lens is resting. *The lens will reflect light and be visible.* Without this, it is often difficult to see the lens.
6. Always wash your hands thoroughly before caring for contact lenses. Gloves are worn based on Standard Precautions. Unless you use fitted sterile gloves it is very difficult to handle contact lenses effectively with gloves on.
7. Care for the lenses in the following way:
   a. Hard lenses
      (1) *Remove each lens*

© 1996 by Lippincott-Raven Publishers

(a) Place a drop of saline or lens solution in the eye *to moisten the surface and facilitate removal.*

(b) Place one forefinger on the upper lid and one on the lower lid.

(c) Raise the upper lid and gently push in on the lower lid at the lower margin of the lens. *This should raise the lower edge of the lens and allow it to pop out.* A small contact lens suction device may also be used to remove the lens.

(2) *Clean each lens* Most facilities do not stock cleaning solutions; therefore, you may need to ask the family or other support person to bring in supplies. If none are available, use saline as a temporary measure.

(a) Be sure to hold the lens over a basin or sink with water in it in case you drop the lens.

(b) Clean the lens with lens cleaning solution by moistening the lens and rubbing it gently between your fingers.

(c) Rinse the cleaning solution off with sterile saline or wetting solution.

(3) *Replace each lens*

(a) Place the lens on the tip of the index finger with the concave surface up.

(b) Wet with wetting solution or sterile saline *to avoid drying the eye surface.*

(c) Hold the eye open with the thumb and index finger of the other hand.

(d) Tip the lens onto the surface of the eye.

(e) Have the patient blink *to position the lens.*

b. Soft lenses

(1) *Remove each lens*

(a) Place a drop of saline or lens wetting solution in the eye *to moisten the surface and facilitate removal.*

(b) Place the forefinger on the upper lid and the thumb on the lower lid and open the eye wide.

(c) Using the other forefinger and thumb, gently pinch up on the lens. *It is flexible and will fold and lift out.* The contact lens suction device can also be used to remove soft lenses.

(2) *Clean each lens*

(a) Place the lens in the palm of one hand.

(b) Apply a few drops of cleaning solution and rub both surfaces of the lens thoroughly *to remove accumulated sediment.*

(c) Rinse with rinsing solution or sterile saline *to remove cleansing agent.* Store in saline or replace in eye.

(3) *Insert each lens*

(a) Hold the lens carefully balanced, concave side up, on the end of a dry finger.

(b) Open eye with other thumb and forefinger.

(c) Place lens onto eye surface and hold for a second as it adheres.

(d) Have patient blink *to position the lens.*

Evaluation

7. Evaluate in terms of patient comfort and whether the patient can see adequately.

Documentation

8. Document that the patient wears contact lenses on the nursing care plan.

9. Note in the chart:

a. That contact lenses were removed

b. The disposition of contact lenses (whether they were sent home with a relative or stored in the bedside stand) *to prevent concern over their possible loss and to prevent liability of the hospital for loss of the lenses.*

Care of Glasses

It is probable that most nursing students have worn some type of eyeglasses, either regular glasses or sunglasses. Therefore, it seems somewhat unnecessary to describe the care of glasses. However, in the busy care environment, it is easy to forget certain essentials.

DATE/TIME	
4/10/99	Interim note: Contact lenses
1600	Contact lenses removed from both eyes, placed in labeled sterile specimen bottles, and sent home with Mrs. Evans (mother of patient). ———— J. Johnson, NS

Example of Nursing Progress Notes Using POR Format.

© 1996 by Lippincott-Raven Publishers

Cleaning Glasses

1. Wash glasses at the beginning of the day. *A soiled surface that is tolerable when it accumulates gradually during the day is very disturbing when the glasses are put on at the beginning of the day.*
2. Use water and soap to clean the glasses before polishing them dry. *This prevents the fine scratches on the surface of glasses that dust particles can cause.* Many glasses are now made of plastic, *which is much more susceptible to scratching than traditional glass;* therefore, extra care is needed.

Protecting Glasses

1. After glasses have been removed, place them in a labeled glasses case *for protection* if at all possible.
2. If a case is not available, place the glasses in a bedside drawer, *where they are more protected.*
3. Always place them with the glass surface up *to avoid scratches on the glass.* Be careful where glasses are placed *so that they do not get accidentally pushed onto the floor.*

PROCEDURES FOR CARE OF HEARING AIDS

Currently available hearing aids are finely adjusted electronic devices. They can be damaged by rough handling. The ear piece can be lifted out of the ear. A notation should be made on the nursing care plan or patient record of the need for a hearing aid and the ear in which it should be placed *to facilitate appropriate care by other caregivers.* Some individuals may wear hearing aids in both ears. In this case they need to be carefully marked "left" and "right" because *each ear piece is individually molded to fit that ear only.*

Cleaning the Hearing Aid

1. Gently wipe off the hearing aid with a dry tissue.
2. If ear wax has become embedded in the small opening in the ear piece, clean it out with a special cleaning instrument that comes with the hearing aid. The patient may have this at home. If this is not available, use a thin needle as a substitute.

Protecting the Hearing Aid

1. If the hearing aid is not going to be used for a period of days, remove the battery for storage. *This prolongs the life of the battery and protects the hearing aid.* Some individuals remove the battery each evening when the hearing aid is removed. *This also prolongs battery life* and may be particularly important for the long-term care resident.
2. Keep the hearing aid dry *because any moisture can interfere with its functioning.* Place the hearing aid in a bedside drawer or other safe place *to prevent its being accidentally pushed onto the floor.*

AM and PM Care

In many facilities, a regular routine exists for morning and evening hygiene procedures. These are usually designated as AM (morning) and PM (evening) care. *The purpose of these procedures is to provide an opportunity for patients to complete those activities that would be done independently if they were at home.*

AM care is designed to help the patient be ready to eat breakfast when it is served. Most people would like to use the toilet, commode, or bedpan, wash their face and hands, and brush their teeth before eating breakfast. At this time it is appropriate to check the bed of an incontinent patient and make sure it is clean and dry. *Attention to hygiene before meals can greatly enhance the patient's appetite and food intake.*

PM care is designed to help patients relax and prepare to sleep for the night. An opportunity to use the toilet, bedpan, or commode, wash their hands and faces, and brush their teeth is important. The bed may need straightening, and, if the patient has perspired excessively, a clean pillowcase and patient gown may be needed. This is the time when a back rub is especially appropriate *to help an individual relax.* Careful attention to PM care may eliminate the need for sleeping medication to enable an individual to sleep. The hospital is a strange environment, and many individuals who have no difficulty sleeping at home find themselves having difficulty sleeping in the hospital.

DATE/TIME	
4/10/99 4:00 PM	*Sensory: Wears hearing aid in left ear. Pt able to insert aid and adjust volume independently.* ——— K. Robertson, NS

Example of Nursing Progress Notes Using Narrative Format.

© 1996 by Lippincott-Raven Publishers

LONG-TERM CARE

In long-term care facilities, baths are rarely given every day. A bathing schedule is established that provides for complete baths once or twice a week or as necessary. *Because the residents are not physically active and do not perspire as much as younger adults, this kind of schedule usually meets the needs for personal comfort and odor control. Elderly individuals in long-term care may experience excessive drying of the skin, itching, and actual skin breakdown from too frequent bathing.*

Chair showers have traditionally been the most common method of bathing in long-term care. Many institutions are now adopting a variety of tub systems that allow residents to be placed in a whirlpool-type tub either by means of an attached mechanically lifted chair or by a door that opens down the side of the tub. Moisturizing skin cleansers are used in these tubs, and the whirlpool action cleans the skin and stimulates circulation while moistening the skin.

Bathing in long-term care is delegated to nursing assistants. However, the professional nursing personnel should plan for the hygiene needs of the individual resident.

When individuals enter long-term care, dentures are usually marked with the resident's name by an engraving process. This is especially important in settings where ambulatory, cognitively impaired individuals reside.

Each day residents who are not scheduled for a bath are assisted with AM care. AM care in these situations may include washing under the arms and perineal area as well as face and hands. The resident is then helped with whatever grooming tasks are desired, such as combing hair, shaving, putting on makeup, and so forth, and helped to dress for the day. In long-term care facilities, all residents for whom it is possible are urged to dress for the day. Dress may be adapted for special needs such as being wheelchair bound or incontinent.

PM care in the long-term care facility involves helping the person change from day wear into night wear. In addition, the individual is helped to complete the regular bedtime hygiene procedures such as oral care and washing the face and hands.

HOME CARE

When a patient is being discharged or if nursing care is provided in the home, the nurse assesses the person's ability to manage hygiene needs and whether adaptations in hygiene procedures are necessary.

Typically, individuals may be able to manage their own hygiene needs if special safety modifications are made. Safety bars and handles in the bathroom are often needed. A non-skid surface may be applied to the bottom of the tub. A bath stool in the tub and a hand-held shower may enable an individual who could not climb in and out of a tub or stand in a shower to be independent. Sometimes doorways need to be modified to allow a wheelchair to enter.

If the person will need assistance with hygiene after discharge, you may teach a family member how to provide it. If no one in the family is able to provide assistance, you may help the patient to arrange for a home health aide.

Home health aides provide personal care and assistance with simple tasks associated with daily living for those whose families or home care providers are not able to manage these tasks. The registered nurse visits the home and does the initial assessment to determine what level of care is needed and to develop the plan for nursing care. The actual care is then delegated to the home health aide with follow-up evaluation by the registered nurse. Home health aides may also do light housekeeping tasks such as making a meal, washing dishes, or running a vacuum cleaner. They do not do heavy house cleaning.

© 1996 by Lippincott-Raven Publishers

CRITICAL THINKING EXERCISES

• Mrs. Wilson is a newly admitted resident to the nursing home. She tells you that she just hates having to bathe in the morning. She is 85 years old and says she has bathed every night of her life! She walks with a walker and sits in the shower for baths. You know that she needs help with bathing although she is able to do much of it herself. As a nursing student, how can you serve as her advocate? Determine what further information you need before making any decisions. Whom should you consult? Recommend some options that might be available.

• James Wilson, age 74, was admitted 2 days ago with pneumonia associated with his chronic obstructive pulmonary disease. His record indicates that he has not been bathed since admission. You note that he has severe body odor and looks disheveled and unshaven. When you approach him to arrange a bath time, he states "I told that other nurse that I don't want a bath. It'll just make me short of breath again!" Analyze this situation to determine what concerns are present for both the patient and the staff. Develop a specific approach to Mr. Wilson's situation that you believe will result in his accepting a bath.

© 1996 by Lippincott-Raven Publishers

PERFORMANCE CHECKLIST

General Procedure for Hygiene	Needs More Practice	Satisfactory	Comments
Assessment			
1. Check chart for information related to patient's ability to participate in the procedure being planned.			
2. Assess patient for specific symptoms.			
3. Check to see what supplies are in room.			
Planning			
4. Determine assistance needed.			
5. Determine what supplies and equipment are needed.			
6. Wash your hands.			
7. Obtain needed supplies, including clean gloves if you may come into contact with body secretions.			
Implementation			
8. Identify patient.			
9. Explain procedure to patient.			
10. Provide for patient's privacy.			
11. Raise bed to appropriate working level.			
12. Carry out hygiene procedure planned.			
13. Watch patient for adverse responses.			
14. Care for equipment and supplies.			
15. Wash your hands.			
Evaluation			
16. Evaluate in terms of the following criteria: 　a. Fatigue			
b. Feelings about comfort and cleanliness			
c. Objective signs of cleanliness			
Documentation			
17. Document as appropriate for your facility.			

(continued)

© 1996 by Lippincott-Raven Publishers

Complete Bedbath	Needs More Practice	Satisfactory	Comments
Assessment			
1.–3. Follow Checklist steps 1–3 of the General Procedure for Hygiene (check chart, assess patient, check supplies).			
Planning			
4.–6. Follow Checklist steps 4–6 of the General Procedure (determine assistance, determine needed supplies, wash hands).			
7. Obtain supplies: basin, soap, hamper, clean linen, bath blanket, clean garment, toilet articles, gloves.			
Implementation			
8.–11. Follow Checklist steps 8, 9, 10, and 11 of the General Procedure (identify patient, explain procedure, provide privacy, and raise bed).			
12. Carry out the bedbath. **a.** Remove top linen and place bath blanket.			
b. Give oral care if not already done.			
c. Obtain water.			
d. Position patient (see Complete Bedbath, step 12d, page 396).			
e. Bathe the patient in the following order: (1) Spread towel across patient's chest.			
(2) Make mitt out of washcloth.			
(3) Wash patient's face.			
(4) Remove patient's gown.			
(5) Place towel under far arm and bathe, rinse, and dry far hand, arm, and axilla.			
(6) Place towel under near arm and bathe, rinse, and dry near hand, arm, and axilla.			
(7) Spread across patient's chest and wash, rinse, and dry chest to waist.			
(8) Wash, rinse, and dry abdomen.			
(9) Place towel under far leg.			

(continued)

© 1996 by Lippincott-Raven Publishers

Complete Bedbath *(Continued)*

	Needs More Practice	Satisfactory	Comments
(10) Place patient's foot in bath basin.			
(11) Wash, rinse, and dry far leg.			
(12) Wash, rinse, and dry far foot.			
(13) Wash near leg and foot.			
(14) Change the bath water and put on gloves.			
(15) Wash genital area or give patient an opportunity to do so.			
(16) Remove and dispose of gloves.			
(17) Change water.			
(18) Assist patient to turn and drape.			
(19) Wash, rinse, and dry neck and back.			
(20) Put on gloves.			
(21) Wash, rinse, and dry buttocks.			
(22) Remove and discard gloves.			
(23) Give back rub if desired.			
f. Help patient put on clean garment.			
g. Assist patient with hair care.			
h. Assist patient with nail care.			
i. Assist male patient with shaving.			
j. Make occupied bed and return to low position.			
k. Tidy up area.			
13.–15. Follow Checklist steps 13–15 of the General Procedure (watch patient response, care for equipment, wash your hands).			
Evaluation			
16. Evaluate as in step 16 of the General Procedure (fatigue, subjective comfort, and cleanliness).			
Documentation			
17. Document as in step 17 of the General Procedure.			

(continued)

© 1996 by Lippincott-Raven Publishers

Tub Bath	Needs More Practice	Satisfactory	Comments
Assessment			
1.–3. Follow Checklist steps 1–3 of the General Procedure for Hygiene (check patient record, assess patient, check for supplies in room).			
Planning			
4. Determine assistance needed as in step 4 of the General Procedure.			
5. Determine needed supplies and prepare tub area; fill tub with water.			
6.–7. Follow checklist steps 6 and 7 of the General Procedure (wash your hands, obtain supplies).			
Implementation			
8.–9. Follow Checklist steps 8 and 9 of the General Procedure (identify patient and explain procedure).			
10. Assist patient to tub room.			
11. Hang "occupied" sign.			
12. Carry out the tub bath a. Help patient into tub.			
b. Assist with bathing as needed.			
c. Drain water and assist patient out of tub.			
d. Assist with drying.			
e. Help with donning garments.			
f. Assist patient to return to room.			
13. Watch for adverse response as in step 13 of the General Procedure.			
14. Return to tub room and clean area.			
15. Wash hands			
Evaluation			
16. Evaluate as in step 16 of the General Procedure (fatigue, subjective comfort, cleanliness).			
Documentation			
17. Document as in step 17 of the General Procedure.			

© 1996 by Lippincott-Raven Publishers

(*continued*)

Shower	Needs More Practice	Satisfactory	Comments
Assessment			
1.–3. Follow Checklist steps 1–3 of the General Procedure for Hygiene (check patient record, assess patient, check for supplies in room).			
Planning			
4.–6. Follow Checklist steps 4–6 of the General Procedure (determine assistance, determine needed supplies, wash your hands.			
7. Obtain supplies and prepare shower room.			
Implementation			
8.–9. Follow Checklist steps 8 and 9 of the General Procedure (identify patient and explain procedure).			
10. Assist the patient to the shower room.			
11. Hang privacy sign on door.			
12. Carry out the shower. 　**a.** Assist patient as necessary.			
b. Assist patient with drying themselves and putting on a clean garment.			
c. Assist patient to return to room.			
13. Watch patient for adverse responses as in step 13 of the General Procedure.			
14. Return to the shower room and clean area.			
15. Wash your hands.			
Evaluation			
16. Evaluate as in step 16 of the General Procedure (fatigue, subjective comfort, cleanliness).			
Documentation			
17. Document as in step 17 of the General Procedure.			

(continued)

© 1996 by Lippincott-Raven Publishers

Back Rub	Needs More Practice	Satisfactory	Comments
Assessment			
1.–3. Follow Checklist steps 1–3 of the General Procedure for Hygiene (check patient record, assess patient, check for supplies in room).			
Planning			
4.–6. Follow Checklist steps 4–6 of the General Procedure (determine assistance, determine needed supplies, wash your hands).			
7. Obtain lotion.			
Implementation			
8.–11. Follow Checklist steps 8–11 of the General Procedure (identify patient, explain procedure, provide privacy, and raise bed).			
12. Carry out the back rub. **a.** Move patient to your side of bed and position.			
b. Pour small amount of lotion into hand and rub hands together.			
c. Place hands on sacral area, one on either side.			
d. Rub toward neckline.			
e. Massage into hairline.			
f. Knead along shoulders and down one side of trunk.			
g. Rub in figure-8 pattern over buttocks and sacral area.			
h. Knead up opposite side toward shoulders.			
i. Seek response from patient.			
j. Complete back rub by moving from shoulders to sacrum and back to shoulders.			
k. Replace covers, reposition patient, and lower bed.			
13. Watch for adverse responses as in step 13 of the General Procedure.			

(continued)

© 1996 by Lippincott-Raven Publishers

Back Rub *(Continued)*	Needs More Practice	Satisfactory	Comments
14. Return lotion to storage.			
15. Wash your hands.			
Evaluation			
16. Evaluate as in step 16 of the General Procedure (fatigue, subjective feelings, objective appearance of comfort).			
Documentation			
17. Document as in step 17 of the General Procedure.			
Oral Care Procedure			
(The student serving as patient should provide own toothbrush and cleansing agent.)			
Assessment			
1.–3. Follow Checklist steps 1–3 of the General Procedure for Hygiene (check patient record, assess patient, check for supplies in room).			
Planning			
4.–6. Follow Checklist steps 4–6 of the General Procedure (determine assistance, determine needed supplies, wash hands).			
7. Obtain supplies: toothbrush, toothpaste or powder, cup of water, emesis basin, face towel, dental floss, clean gloves			
Implementation			
8.–11. Follow Checklist steps 8–11 of the General Procedure (identify patient, explain procedure, provide privacy, and raise bed).			
12. Provide oral care. **a.** Place towel under patient's chin.			
b. Put on clean gloves.			
c. Moisten toothbrush and apply cleansing agent.			
d. Brush teeth (see Toothbrushing, page 402).			
e. Allow patient to rinse with water.			

(continued)

© 1996 by Lippincott-Raven Publishers

Oral Care Procedure *(Continued)*	Needs More Practice	Satisfactory	Comments
f. Wipe patient's mouth.			
13.–15. Follow Checklist steps 13–15 of the General Procedure (watch patient for adverse response, care for equipment and supplies, and wash hands).			
Evaluation			
16. Evaluate as in step 16 of the General Procedure (fatigue, subjective feelings, objective appearance of cleanliness).			
Documentation			
17. Document as in step 17 of the General Procedure.			
Oral Care for Unconscious Patients			
Assessment			
1.–3. Follow Checklist steps 1–3 of the General Procedure for Hygiene (check patient record, assess patient, check for supplies in room).			
Planning			
4.–6. Follow Checklist steps 4–6 of the General Procedure (determine assistance, determine needed supplies, wash hands).			
7. Obtain supplies: tongue blade wrapped in gauze, applicators, toothbrush, cleansing agent, lip lubricant, clean gloves, towel, suction or asepto syringe, emesis basin			
Implementation			
8.–11. Follow Checklist steps 8–11 of the General Procedure (identify patient, explain procedure, provide privacy, and raise bed).			
12. Provide oral care. **a.** Position patient.			
b. Place towel under patient's chin.			
c. Put on clean gloves.			
d. Place padded tongue blade in patient's mouth.			
e. Moisten toothbrush.			

(continued)

© 1996 by Lippincott-Raven Publishers

Oral Care for Unconscious Patients *(Continued)*	Needs More Practice	Satisfactory	Comments
f. Brush teeth (see Toothbrushing, page 402).			
g. Use swabs or gauze to cleanse all surfaces of the mouth.			
h. Rinse patient's mouth.			
i. Wipe patient's mouth.			
j. Lubricate lips as needed.			
k. Return bed to low position.			
13.–15. Follow Checklist steps 13–15 of the General Procedure (watch patient for adverse response, care for equipment and supplies, and wash hands).			
Evaluation			
16. Evaluate as in step 16 of the General Procedure (fatigue, subjective feelings, objective cleanliness of mouth).			
Documentation			
17. Document as in step 17 of the General Procedure.			
Care of Dentures			
Assessment			
1.–3. Follow Checklist steps 1–3 of the General Procedure for Hygiene (check patient record, assess patient, check for supplies in room).			
Planning			
4.–6. Follow Checklist steps 4–6 of the General Procedure (determine assistance, determine needed supplies, wash hands).			
7. Obtain supplies: denture brush and denture cleaner, if available, or toothbrush and cleansing agent, clean gloves.			
Implementation			
8.–11. Follow Checklist steps 8–11 of the General Procedure (identify patient, explain procedure, provide privacy, and raise bed).			

(continued)

© 1996 by Lippincott-Raven Publishers

Care of Dentures *(Continued)*	Needs More Practice	Satisfactory	Comments
12. Clean dentures. **a.** Put on clean gloves.			
b. Assist patient with removal of dentures.			
c. Handle dentures with care.			
d. Take to sink in denture cup and clean.			
e. Have patient rinse mouth and clean gums if desired.			
f. Replace moist dentures, upper first, or store dentures in denture cup.			
g. Dry the patient's mouth.			
13.–15. Follow Checklist steps 13–15 of the General Procedure (watch patient for adverse response, care for equipment and supplies, and wash hands).			
Evaluation			
16. Evaluate as in step 16 of the General Procedure (fatigue, subjective feelings, objective cleanliness of mouth).			
Documentation			
17. Document as in step 17 of the General Procedure.			
Hair Care			
Assessment			
1.–3. Follow Checklist steps 1–3 of the General Procedure for Hygiene (check patient record, assess patient, check for supplies in room).			
Planning			
4.–6. Follow Checklist steps 4–6 of the General Procedure (determine assistance, determine needed supplies, wash hands).			
7. Assemble the equipment: comb, brush, mirror, other hair care items, towel			
Implementation			
8.–11. Follow Checklist steps 8–11 of the General Procedure (identify patient, explain procedure, provide privacy, and raise bed).			

(continued)

© 1996 by Lippincott-Raven Publishers

Hair Care *(Continued)*	Needs More Practice	Satisfactory	Comments
12. Provide hair care. **a.** Place a towel over the pillow.			
b. Position patient.			
c. Turn head away and arrange hair toward you.			
d. Brush gently in two or three sections.			
e. Turn head toward you, rearrange hair, and repeat step d on the other side of the head.			
f. Arrange hair neatly and simply.			
g. Remove towel.			
13. Watch for adverse response as in step 13 of the General Procedure.			
14. Place towel in laundry hamper, clean comb and brush, and return to bedside stand.			
15. Wash hands.			
Evaluation			
16. Evaluate as in step 16 of the General Procedure (fatigue, subjective feelings, objective cleanliness).			
Documentation			
17. Document as in step 17 of the General Procedure.			
Shampooing			
Assessment			
1.–3. Follow Checklist steps 1–3 of the General Procedure for Hygiene (check patient record, assess patient, check for supplies in room).			
Planning			
4.–6. Follow Checklist steps 4–6 of the General Procedure (determine assistance, determine needed supplies, wash hands.			
7. Obtain supplies: trough, pitcher, basin, plastic sheet, shampoo, rinse agent, and towels.			

(continued)

© 1996 by Lippincott-Raven Publishers

Shampooing *(Continued)*	Needs More Practice	Satisfactory	Comments
Implementation			
8.–11. Follow Checklist steps 8–11 of the General Procedure (identify patient, explain procedure, provide privacy, and raise bed).			
12. Shampoo hair. **a.** Remove top linens and place bath blanket.			
b. Place plastic square under patient's head and shoulders.			
c. Place towel around patient's shoulders and neck.			
d. Arrange trough under patient's head.			
e. Wet the hair.			
f. Shampoo and rinse twice, rinsing thoroughly.			
g. Dry hair, ears, and neck.			
h. Assist the patient to comb and arrange hair.			
i. Remove equipment.			
j. Replace top linen and remove bath blanket.			
k. Allow patient to rest.			
13.–15. Follow Checklist steps 13–15 of the General Procedure (watch patient for adverse response, care for equipment and supplies, and wash hands).			
Evaluation			
16. Evaluate as in step 16 of the General Procedure (fatigue, subjective feelings, objective cleanliness).			
Documentation			
17. Document as in step 17 of the General Procedure.			
Eye Care			
Assessment			
1. Check for physician's orders.			

(continued)

© 1996 by Lippincott-Raven Publishers

Eye Care *(Continued)*	Needs More Practice	Satisfactory	Comments
2. Assess patient's ability to blink.			
3. Check to see whether supplies are in room.			
Planning			
4. Wash your hands.			
5. Obtain needed supplies.			
Implementation			
6. Clean eyelids if necessary.			
7. Instill artificial tears if necessary.			
8. Observe surface of eyes for irritation or inflammation.			
9. Close eyelid and place eyepad over it.			
10. Tape eyepad in place.			
11. Repeat steps 9 and 10 for second eye.			
12. Care for equipment.			
13. Wash your hands.			
Evaluation			
14. Evaluate whether eyepad is holding eye closed.			
15. Check skin around eye for tape irritation.			
Documentation			
16. Document eye care on flow sheet or progress notes.			
Contact Lens Care, Removal, and Insertion			
Assessment			
1. Ascertain presence of contact lenses.			
2. Determine type of lenses being worn.			
Planning			
3. Wash your hands.			
4. Obtain container for contact storage.			
implementation			
5. Use flashlight to check for lens position.			
6. Wash your hands and put on gloves.			

(continued)

© 1996 by Lippincott-Raven Publishers

Contact Lens Care, Removal, and Insertion *(Continued)*	Needs More Practice	Satisfactory	Comments
7a. Care for hard lenses:			
(1) Remove the lenses.			
(a) Place drop of saline or lens solution in the eye.			
(b) Place forefingers on upper and lower lid.			
(c) Raise upper lid and push in on lower lid at lens margin.			
(2) Clean the lenses.			
(a) Work over a basin or sink with water in it.			
(b) Use cleaning solution and rub lens gently between fingers.			
(c) Rinse off cleaning solution.			
(3) Replace the lenses.			
(a) Place lens on tip of finger, concave surface up.			
(b) Wet with wetting solution or sterile saline.			
(c) Hold eye open with thumb and forefinger of opposite hand.			
(d) Tip lens onto surface of eye.			
(e) Have patient blink.			
7b. Care for soft lenses:			
(1) Remove the lenses.			
(a) Place a drop of saline or lens wetting solution in the eye.			
(b) Place forefinger on upper lid and thumb on lower lid.			
(c) Gently pinch lens up with opposite thumb and forefinger.			
(2) Clean the soft lenses.			
(a) Place lens in palm of one hand.			
(b) Apply cleaning solution and rub both surfaces.			
(c) Rinse lens.			

(continued)

© 1996 by Lippincott-Raven Publishers

Contact Lens Care, Removal, and Insertion *(Continued)*	Needs More Practice	Satisfactory	Comments
(3) Insert the soft lenses. (a) Hold lens pinched between thumb and forefinger.			
(b) Open eye with other thumb and forefinger.			
(c) Place lens onto eye surface and release.			
(d) Have patient blink.			
Evaluation			
8. Evaluate in terms of patient comfort and patient vision.			
Documentation			
9. Document on the nursing care plan that patient wears contact lenses.			
10. Note on the chart the disposition of contact lenses that were removed.			
Care of Glasses			
1. Clean the glasses. **a.** Clean at the beginning of the day.			
b. Use soap and water, then polish dry.			
2. Protect the glasses. **a.** Place in glasses case.			
b. Place in bedside drawer or where they won't get knocked to the floor.			
c. Place with glass surface up.			
Care of Hearing Aids			
1. Clean the hearing aid. **a.** Use a dry tissue.			
b. Use special instrument to remove ear wax from opening.			
2. Protect the hearing aid. **a.** Remove battery if hearing aid will be out for several days.			
b. Keep dry.			

© 1996 by Lippincott-Raven Publishers

? **Q U I Z**

Multiple-Choice Questions

_____ 1. The temperature of the water for bathing and shampooing has been described as "warm." This means

   a. 75°–90°F.
   b. 90°–105°F.
   c. 100°–115°F.
   d. 110°–125°F.

_____ 2. The preferred position for bathing the patient in bed is

   a. prone.
   b. supine.
   c. semi-Fowler's.
   d. Fowler's.

_____ 3. The partial bedbath usually includes which of the following areas of the body? (1) face and neck; (2) hands; (3) axillae; (4) perineum

   a. 1 and 2
   b. 3 and 4
   c. 2, 3, and 4
   d. All of these

Short-Answer Questions

4. How are soft contact lenses stored? _____

_____

5. How are hard contact lenses removed? _____

_____

6. Why are glasses cleaned with soap and water instead of simply being polished while dry?

_____

_____

7. What should be done to store a hearing aid for several days?_____

_____

8. What is usually done for AM care? _____

_____

9. What is usually done for PM care? _____

_____

True-False Questions

_____ 10. A patient's face should be washed with soap and water.

_____ 11. When washing the arms, long, firm strokes toward the center of the body are used to decrease venous return.

_____ 12. The back of the neck is washed separately from the front of the neck.

© 1996 by Lippincott-Raven Publishers

_____   **13.** You should always cut and file the patient's toenails and fingernails.

_____   **14.** A patient should be offered the opportunity for oral care before breakfast, after all meals, and at bedtime.

_____   **15.** The unconscious patient does not need oral care.

_____   **16.** Toothbrushing is correctly done using a small, soft brush.

_____   **17.** Dentures should be brushed over a basin of water.

_____   **18.** The hair of the hospitalized patient should be washed and combed or brushed daily.

© 1996 by Lippincott-Raven Publishers

BASIC INFANT CARE

MODULE CONTENTS

RATIONALE FOR THE USE OF THIS SKILL
DIAPERING
Types of Diapers
Folding Cloth Diapers
Cleansing at Diaper Changes
Fastening Diapers
Skin Problems
DIAPERING PROCEDURE
Assessment
Planning
Implementation
Evaluation
Documentation
BATHING
General Information
Safety
Holding the Infant
Shampooing
Eye Care
Folds
Perineal Care
Cord Care
BATHING PROCEDURE
Assessment
Planning
Implementation
Evaluation
Documentation
FEEDING
BOTTLE-FEEDING PROCEDURE

Assessment
Planning
Implementation
Evaluation
Documentation
PROCEDURE FOR FEEDING SOLIDS
Assessment
Planning
Implementation
Evaluation
Documentation
RESTRAINTS AND SAFETY DEVICES
PROCEDURE FOR APPLYING
    RESTRAINTS AND SAFETY DEVICES
Assessment
Planning
Implementation
Evaluation
Documentation
SPECIFIC SAFETY PRECAUTIONS
Mummying
MUMMYING PROCEDURE
Assessment
Planning
Implementation
Evaluation
Documentation
HOME CARE
CRITICAL THINKING EXERCISES

PREREQUISITES

Successful completion of the following modules:

VOLUME 1
Module 1 An Approach to Nursing Skills
Module 2 Basic Infection Control
Module 3 Safety
Module 4 Basic Body Mechanics

Module 5   Documentation
Module 6   Introduction to Assessment
           Skills
Module 18 Hygiene

431

© 1996 by Lippincott-Raven Publishers

OVERALL OBJECTIVE

To provide basic daily care for infants and to implement safety measures in all aspects of care.

SPECIFIC LEARNING OBJECTIVES

Know Facts and Principles	Apply Facts and Principles	Demonstrate Ability	Evaluate Performance
1. Diapering			
a. Types			
Identify types of diapers in common use.			
b. Folding cloth diapers			
Know methods of folding cloth diapers and advantages of each method.	Determine appropriate way to fold diaper for particular situation.	Fold diaper in triangle-fold and rectangle-fold shapes.	
c. Cleaning			
State rationale for frequent diaper changes. Know purpose of cleaning perineal area and buttocks with each diaper change.	Decide when to change infant's diaper based on rationale. Given a situation, select appropriate materials for cleaning infant during diapering.		
d. Fastening diapers			
List two ways diapers are fastened.	Given a situation, determine appropriate way to fasten diaper.	Fasten diaper, handling safety pins correctly.	
e. Skin problems			
Describe symptoms of diaper rash and scald.	Given a description of infant, identify whether diaper rash or scald is present.	In the clinical setting, identify diaper rash and scald.	
f. Diapering procedure			
List steps of procedure.		Change infant's diaper correctly and safely, using appropriate materials and methods for cleaning.	Evaluate diapering by checking for fit and comfort. Evaluate own performance using Performance Checklist.
2. Bathing			
Discuss special considerations for bathing infant.	Given a situation, describe correct procedure for bathing infant.	Bathe infant correctly and safely.	Evaluate own performance with instructor.

(continued)

© 1996 by Lippincott-Raven Publishers

SPECIFIC LEARNING OBJECTIVES (Continued)

Know Facts and Principles	Apply Facts and Principles	Demonstrate Ability	Evaluate Performance
3. Bottle-feeding Describe two positions for bottle-feeding.	Plan appropriate feeding position for infant.	Bottle-feed infant.	Evaluate by measuring infant's intake.
a. Temperature State usual temperature for bottle. State method for testing temperature.	Given a situation, decide whether to warm formula.	Correctly distinguish safe temperature for bottle-feeding.	Evaluate own performance with instructor.
b. Burping Describe two positions for burping.		Burp infant after feeding.	Evaluate by checking whether infant has burped.
4. Feeding solids Describe two positions for feeding solids to infants.	Plan appropriate position for particular infant.	Feed solids to infant correctly.	Evaluate by recording infant intake.
a. Temperature State proper temperature for solid foods.	Identify safe method for warming infant's food.	Demonstrate method to determine temperature of food.	Evaluate own performance with instructor.
5. Safety measures *a. Tying a clove hitch* State purpose of clove-hitch restraint.	Identify situation in which clove-hitch restraint is needed.	Correctly and safely tie clove-hitch restraint.	Evaluate own performance using Performance Checklist.
b. Using crib restraints State purpose of crib restraint.	Identify situations in which crib restraints are needed.	Correctly and safely apply crib restraints.	Evaluate own performance using Performance Checklist.
c. Elbow restraints State purpose of elbow restraints.	Identify situations in which elbow restraints are needed.	Correctly and safely apply elbow restraints.	Evaluate own performance using Performance Checklist.
d. Mummying State purpose of mummying.	Identify situations in which mummying is needed. Given a situation, identify correct type of restraint to be used.	Correctly and safely apply mummy restraint to infant.	Evaluate own performance using Performance Checklist. Evaluate choice with instructor.

© 1996 by Lippincott-Raven Publishers

LEARNING ACTIVITIES

1. Review the Specific Learning Objectives.
2. Look up the module vocabulary terms in the glossary.
3. Read through the module as though you were preparing to teach the procedures to another person.
4. In the practice setting, do the following:
   a. Diapering
      (1) Inspect cloth and disposable diapers.
      (2) Practice folding cloth diapers using the rectangle-folded method. Fold them to provide extra thickness in the front (used for boys and for girls lying on the abdomen). Then refold to provide extra thickness in the back (used for girls lying on the back).
      (3) Diaper an infant manikin, using the Performance Checklist as a guide. Practice opening and closing safety pins with one hand while keeping the other hand on the "infant."
      (4) Arrange for your instructor to check you when you feel competent.
   b. Bathing
      (1) Bathe an infant manikin using the procedure described.
   c. Bottle-feeding
      (1) Practice holding an infant manikin for bottle-feeding.
      (2) Practice both methods of holding an infant manikin for burping.
      (3) Have your instructor check your performance.
   d. Feeding solids
      (1) Practice feeding solids to an infant manikin while holding it on your lap.
   e. Safety measures
      (1) Practice tying a clove-hitch knot. Have your instructor check the knot.
      (2) Improvise an arm or use a manikin's arm, and tie it to a stationary object (the bed frame or an armboard) using a clove-hitch knot.
      (3) Inspect elbow restraints if they are available.
      (4) Practice mummying an infant manikin using the two methods outlined in the module.
      (5) Have your instructor check your performance.

VOCABULARY

adhesions	colic	foreskin	smegma
burp	cradle cap	gastrocolic reflex	venipuncture
cardiac sphincter	expectorates	macerate	
clove hitch	fontanelle	macular	

© 1996 by Lippincott-Raven Publishers

Basic Infant Care

Rationale for the Use of This Skill

Hospitalized infants, whether healthy or ill, need basic infant care and expert nursing care. Nurses are typically responsible for teaching infant care to new parents and supporting parents who are caring for ill infants in the hospital. Although the current practice is to encourage parents and other family caregivers to provide as much direct care as possible to maintain family bonds, nurses must often become primary caregivers to very ill infants. Included in the care of hospitalized infants are diapering, bathing, and feeding. In addition, nurses must have the skills necessary to keep the infant safe in the healthcare environment. Special efforts are needed to maintain safety for infants, both in general care and throughout all procedures. To provide this safety, the nurse must carry out special measures and use equipment, such as restraints, correctly.[1]

DIAPERING

Types of Diapers

Some hospitals use disposable diapers, which have the advantage of decreasing laundry and ensuring that no cross-contamination occurs. These have a waterproof layer that protects the linen from urine and stool. Disposable diapers come in a variety of sizes (such as newborn, infant, and toddler), making proper fit possible. Disposable diapers also provide a way to assess the child's fluid status. The synthetic material used in the diaper "traps" a significant amount of urine, which can be extracted with a needle and syringe after the diaper has been removed. The urine can then be tested for specific gravity (see Module 12, Assisting With Diagnostic and Therapeutic Procedures). Disposable diapers may irritate infants who develop a skin sensitivity to paper and plastic products. Also, they may pose an environmental concern because of disposal problems.

Cloth diapers can be softer and less irritating for most infants. Omit plastic diaper coverings for infants whose skin is sensitive to urine accumulation *because these coverings hinder moisture evaporation.* Cloth diapers are usually prefolded when used in the healthcare setting and are available in three sizes. You can fold several diapers together *to provide an absorbent diaper for overnight use on older infants or toddlers.*

Folding Cloth Diapers

No one folding method is ideal, and you may devise your own adaptations for specific situations. If diapers are not prefolded or you need to revise the size, follow the directions described below for folding. *The purpose of any type of fold is to provide the following type of diaper:*

1. Is the correct size for the infant
2. Fastens safely and securely
3. Is thickest where greatest absorbency is needed
4. Is comfortable for the infant to wear
5. Retains urine and stool adequately

Rectangular folding provides the maximum width between the legs and is effective for containing loose stools. The size can be changed simply. For example, you can alter the width by changing the width of the initial fold, or alter the length by folding over the front or the back until the diaper is the desired length.

To fold, follow the diagrams in Figure 19–1.

1. Use a square diaper and fold the two outer edges in to form a long rectangle (A).
2. Divide the rectangle into thirds by either (B) folding the top third down to put the added thickness in the back or (C) folding the bottom third up to put the added thickness in the front.

Cleansing at Diaper Changes

Cleansing is needed any time a diaper is changed *because stool and urine left on the skin will cause skin irritation.* Facilities usually establish a routine for this procedure. Two methods are presented here.

1. Wash with a mild soap and water, then rinse thoroughly. Keep a washcloth and towel at the side of the crib for this purpose.
2. Use commercial disposable wipes that contain a nonallergenic agent baby oil or lotion for cleansing. Rinsing is usually not needed because no irritating substance is present, although some babies may be sensitive to components of any cleaning solution.

Fastening Diapers

Disposable diapers come with attached tapes for fastening; these are convenient and safe. Safety pins are used to fasten cloth diapers. Remember that open safety pins are *always* a hazard. Close pins as soon as they are removed, and place them out of reach. *Even if you have misjudged the infant's reach, the child will pick up a closed pin.*

---

[1]Note that rationales for action are emphasized throughout the module by the use of italics.

© 1996 by Lippincott-Raven Publishers

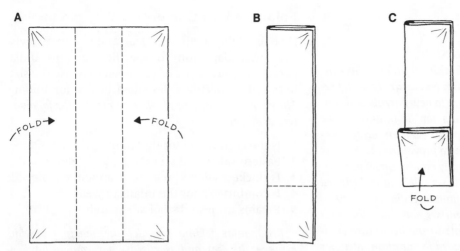

Figure 19–1. Folding a multilayer cloth diaper for a small infant. Place the thickly padded portion in front for boys and in back for girls.

When you are ready to fasten a diaper, place the pin horizontally, with the point toward the infant's side. *If the pin later opens, it will be less likely to cause injury* because it is pointed away from sensitive tissue. Also, always place your hand between the infant and the diaper you are pinning. *Then, if you push the pin completely through the diaper, you will stick your hand and not the infant.* If a safety pin does not slide easily into the diaper, stick the point into a bar of soap to lubricate it *so that it enters easily.*

After a cloth diaper has been put on the infant, place a leak-proof pad under the buttocks to protect linen. Diaper covers are not recommended for some infants because they can prevent evaporation and promote skin problems.

Velcro-fastening diaper covers are available. The diaper is folded as in Figure 19–1 and placed on the diaper cover. The cover and diaper are placed on the infant, and Velcro tabs on the corners of the diaper cover fasten the diaper securely. Diaper covers are used primarily in the home. They are constructed to allow a degree of evaporation, but you should check the infant's skin frequently when they are used.

Skin Problems

Diaper rash is a skin reaction that appears as a macular to solid redness in the perineal area. It may be caused by the following:

1. Prolonged contact with urine or feces
2. Irritation from ammonia formed as the urine decomposes
3. Maceration from wetness
4. Irritation from residual detergents or cleansing agents in a diaper
5. Irritation from the harsh surface of a diaper

Scald occurs rapidly and appears as a totally reddened area much like a burn. It happens when the stool or urine contains harsh ingredients that cause a chemical-type burn of the skin.

The best way to prevent diaper rash or scald is *to change diapers frequently and to clean the skin with each change to remove residual urine or feces. Allowing the infant to go without wearing a diaper for several hours each day and to be placed only on a water-proof pad allows the skin to dry and decreases rash. If the infant is wearing disposable diapers, a change to cloth diapers or inserting holes in the disposable ones may also help control diaper rash. If diaper rash persists, consult a physician. Infants also are prone to* Candida *(a fungal infection), which looks similar to diaper rash.*

If an infant is having frequent, loose, or diarrheal stools, apply a heavy, non–water-soluble ointment (petroleum jelly or another water-barrier ointment) at the time of the diaper change *to protect the skin from contact with the stool.* You must check your facility's policy regarding the use of ointments.

You can also use powders to help the skin remain dry. Do not let powder get into the air, where the infant might inhale it, because *it is an irritant to the respiratory tract.* Place a small amount on your hand and smooth it over the infant's skin. Use only a thin coating; *large amounts tend to gather in clumps that can irritate the skin. Some infants are sensitive to the perfume in baby powder, and this can cause skin irritation also.* Because of the problems associated with its use, some facilities do not use baby powder. Cornstarch is an

© 1996 by Lippincott-Raven Publishers

inexpensive substitute that does not tend to cause irritation; however, it may contribute to the growth of *Candida*.

DIAPERING PROCEDURE

Most healthcare facilities have a policy requiring nurses to wear clean gloves for all diaper changes (see Body Substance Precautions in Module 2, Basic Infection Control). The gloves are changed between infants. Because many newborns are not bathed until their temperature stabilizes, the mother's blood may be present on the infant, and the nurse may come in contact with it. Also, the infant has an immature immune system that prevents vigorous response to pathogens causing infection. *Gloves prevent contact with and transmission of pathogens.* In addition, practice conscientious handwashing before and after changing diapers.

Assessment

1. Assess the infant's diaper for soiling.
2. Determine the infant's physical development, with emphasis on its ability to roll over and grasp.

Planning

3. Wash your hands *so that you do not introduce microorganisms to the infant.*
4. Select the type and size of diaper, pins if needed for closure, and cleansing equipment.
5. If appropriate, obtain toys (such as a mobile) to divert the infant's attention.

Implementation

6. Fold the diaper if necessary.
7. Place the infant on his or her back in the crib or on a clean, padded surface. Make sure the infant is safe from falling. *Never* leave an infant with the crib side rails down or out of the crib.
8. Put on clean gloves, and unfasten the soiled diaper. If using a cloth diaper, close the safety pins as you remove them, and set them out of the infant's reach.
9. Remove the soiled diaper, using the clean portion of the diaper to wipe away any stool. Clean from the anterior region to the posterior region *so that you do not contaminate the urinary meatus with bacteria from the rectal area.*
10. Using the equipment for cleansing, clean the entire diaper area thoroughly. If there is a large amount of stool or urine, the infant may need more extensive bathing. Change all wet or soiled clothing. Place a clean diaper over the penis of a male infant to protect yourself against sudden voiding.
11. Lift the infant's buttocks by grasping both ankles with one hand, and place a clean diaper under the infant (Fig. 19–2).
12. Pull the front of the diaper up between the infant's legs, *so that it fits snugly around the abdomen.* Fasten with pins or tapes (Fig. 19–3). Always put the pins into the diaper so that the point is toward the outside. That way, if the pin comes open, it will be less likely to scratch the infant.
13. Be sure that the infant is secure and protected from falling.
14. Dispose of the soiled diaper and your gloves.
15. Wash your hands.

Evaluation

16. Check the diaper for secure fit and comfort.

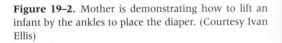

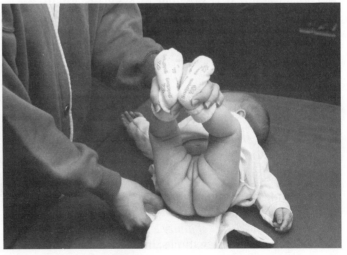

Figure 19–2. Mother is demonstrating how to lift an infant by the ankles to place the diaper. (Courtesy Ivan Ellis)

© 1996 by Lippincott-Raven Publishers

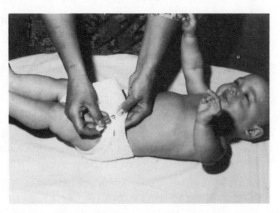

Figure 19–3. The diaper is in place and the pin inserted horizontally with the point toward the side, away from the infant. (Courtesy Ivan Ellis)

Documentation

17. Document any unusual appearance or odor of the urine and stool. When the amount of output is critical, you may be required to document the number of diaper changes, weigh diapers before and after use, or measure specific gravity of the urine (see Module 12, Performing Common Laboratory Tests.) This information is usually noted on a flow sheet.

BATHING

General Information

An infant is given a bedbath in much the same manner as an adult. It is essential to keep the infant warm and safe. Special considerations for bathing an infant include the following.

Safety

Everything must be within reach before beginning; one hand must remain in contact with the infant at all times *to prevent falls.*

Holding the Infant

Any method of holding an infant must *provide support for the head and neck and keep the infant close to your body to lessen the chance of injury or dropping.* The *football hold* does all of these things. In the football hold, the infant is held with the head in the palm of the

hand, the back on the forearm, and the feet between the arm and your side (Fig. 19–4).

If the infant can sit in a basin with support, keep one of your arms behind the infant, holding onto the infant's far arm. *This leaves your other arm free yet keeps the infant secure.* Even with an older infant who can sit unaided, you should still keep one hand on the infant at all times. Remember, a tub is slippery, and infants move very quickly. Do not immerse an infant whose umbilicus is not completely healed *because an infection might result.*

Shampooing

This is usually done each time an infant is bathed to *prevent a scale accumulation called cradle cap.* Hold the infant football-style, with the head over the basin so that the scalp can be gently scrubbed and thoroughly rinsed with strokes going away from the infant's face.

Eye Care

Without soap, clean each eye from inner to outer canthus, using a clean area of the washcloth for each eye *so that microorganisms are not transferred from one eye to the other.*

Folds

Infants have many creases and folds. Wash and dry carefully in all of them. *Moisture left in creases causes skin breakdown.*

Perineal Care

For the female infant, be sure to clean between the labia and in all folds from front to back. For the uncircumcised male infant, *gently* retract the foreskin

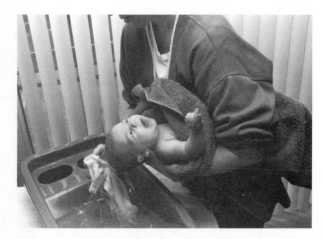

Figure 19–4. The "football" hold supports the infant's head and leaves one hand of the care provider free. (Courtesy Ivan Ellis)

© 1996 by Lippincott-Raven Publishers

only as far as it will go easily, and return it to its normal position after cleansing the exposed surfaces. *Secretions left under the foreskin may cause irritation and infection, with resulting adhesions.*

Cord Care

When the newborn still has the cord stump in place, you must perform cord care. This includes carefully inspecting the base of the cord for signs of infection (such as redness, drainage, or odor) and cleaning it with alcohol. The area also is kept dry, and the infant is not bathed in a basin or sink until the cord detaches (in 1–4 weeks). The cord falls off in the same way a scab falls off a small wound.

BATHING PROCEDURE

Assessment
1. Determine the infant's physical development and size.
2. Check for clothing, linen, and supplies needed.

Planning
3. Wash your hands *for infection control.*
4. Gather the necessary equipment. You will need a basin, sterile cotton balls, mild soap, a washcloth, a towel, clean clothing for the infant, and possibly clean linen for the crib or bed.

Implementation
5. Identify the infant *to be sure you are carrying out the procedure for the correct infant.*
6. Fill the basin with warm water. Check the temperature by using a sensitive part of your arm, such as the elbow. It should be comfortably warm, never hot, *to prevent burns.*If a bath thermometer is available, use water at 100° to 105°F (37.7°–40.5°C).
7. Place the basin on a firm surface.
8. With sterile cotton balls, wash the infant's eyes from nose area to outer area. Wash and dry the infant's face. Soap on the face is not needed.
9. Hold the infant securely in the football hold previously described, with the head over the basin.
10. Shampoo the scalp. Use your fingertips, not your fingernails, and massage firmly. If any loose skin cells are present, remove them from the hair with a fine-tooth comb. Do not hesitate to wash over the fontanelles (soft spots). In some facilities, the scalp (including the area behind the ears) is wiped with a small amount of baby oil on a cotton ball *to help prevent scales.*
11. Rub the head dry with a towel.
12. Undress the infant. (You should keep the infant dressed during the shampoo *to prevent chilling.*)
13. Hold the infant securely as you place him or her in the water. Use a towel in the basin *to decrease slipping.*
14. Keep one hand securely on the infant while bathing with the other *to prevent injury* (Fig. 19–5).
15. Wash and rinse the shoulders, arms, and chest, and then move down the body.
16. Lift the infant out of the water, and lay him or her on the towel.
17. Wrap the infant while you dry *to prevent chilling.*
18. Diaper and redress the infant.
19. If the crib must be made, place the infant at one end while you make up the other.
20. Put side rails up before you leave the infant. Refasten the crib net if necessary *for safety.*
21. Empty and clean the basin.
22. Dispose of soiled linen.
23. Wash your hands *for infection control.*

Evaluation
24. Check the infant for comfort and safety.

Documentation
25. Document observations made during the bath.
26. Enter the bath on the checklist or flow sheet for daily care.

FEEDING

Many newborns are breast-fed after birth. Others receive a well-balanced formula administered by a bottle. Most bottles are now made of plastic, with a plastic liner bag used for a single feeding and then

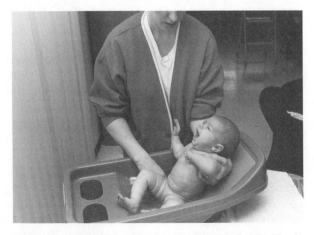

Figure 19–5. Bathing an infant in a basin while holding firmly to prevent slipping. (Courtesy Ivan Ellis)

© 1996 by Lippincott-Raven Publishers

discarded. A screw-on nipple and rim completes the bottle-feeding equipment.

BOTTLE-FEEDING PROCEDURE

Assessment

1. Determine the infant's physical development, and assess the record for feeding difficulties.
2. Check the order for formula. Most institutions use a standard, well-balanced commercial formula.
3. Check to determine if a specialized nipple or feeding device is needed.

Planning

4. Correctly identify the formula *for safety.*
5. Determine whether the formula is to be warmed. Although warming the formula is optional, *an infant with decreased energy levels will have to use energy to restore body heat if given cold formula.* Also, *chilled food takes longer to digest.* Therefore, the feeding should be at room temperature or slightly warmer. If the feeding is warmer than room temperature, use it as soon as it is warmed *so that it is not a source of bacterial growth.* Most hospitals routinely use formula at room temperature.
6. Wash your hands *for infection control.*
7. Obtain and warm formula if necessary.
8. Test for temperature. This is commonly done by shaking a few drops of formula onto the inner aspect of the wrist. The formula should feel only lukewarm, not hot.

Implementation

9. Check the infant's identification *to be sure you are carrying out the procedure for the correct infant.*
10. Try to sit in a comfortable position, in a pleasant area, while you feed an infant. *Feelings and attitudes are transmitted to infants and affect their feeding and digestion.*
11. Ideally, hold the infant in your arms while you bottle-feed. When an infant cannot be removed from the crib (because of equipment, traction, need for oxygen), substitute hand touch and support for whole body contact. Tuck a bib or clean cloth under the infant's chin *to protect garments or linen.* Hold the infant with the head slightly elevated *to facilitate swallowing.* Hold the bottle so that the nipple is filled with fluid, not air (Fig. 19–6).

    Although sucking infants usually swallow some air, try to keep the amount to a minimum. *Excessive swallowed air causes distention, discomfort, and sometimes regurgitation.*

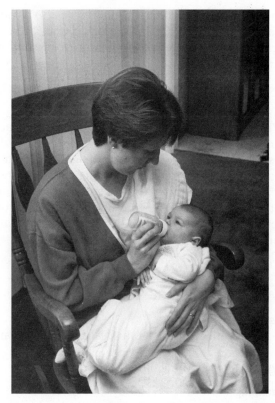

Figure 19–6. Bottle-feeding with an infant positioned so that he or she does not ingest air with the milk.m (Courtesy Ivan Ellis)

12. If the infant feeds quickly, remove the bottle for an occasional rest.
13. After the feeding is completed, burp the infant *to help expel swallowed air.* The two positions most commonly used are *on the lap* and the *over the shoulder* (Figs. 19–7 and 19–8).

    A small infant should be burped after each ounce and at the end of the feeding. Place the bottle on a clean, safe surface while you burp the infant; do not place it on the floor *because the floor is very contaminated.* By *gently* patting or rubbing the infant's back, you *encourage the relaxation of the cardiac sphincter and the release of retained air.* Place the bib or cloth where it will protect your clothing while you burp the baby.
14. Change the infant's diaper if necessary. *Small infants commonly defecate while eating because of the gastrocolic reflex.*
15. Return the infant to the crib. Position the infant on the side *so that if he or she expectorates, aspiration will not occur.* An infant positioned on the right side is more likely to burp air without bringing formula with it *because the sphincter is on the left side of the stomach.*
16. Wash your hands *for infection control.*

© 1996 by Lippincott-Raven Publishers

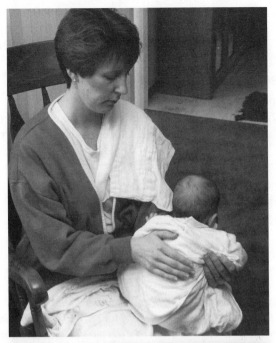

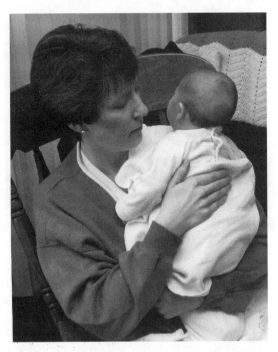

Figure 19–8. Holding an infant over the shoulder for burping. (Courtesy Ivan Ellis)

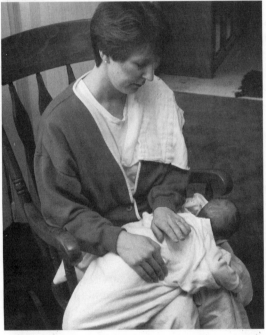

Figure 19–7. Holding an infant on the lap for burping—two positions. (Courtesy Ivan Ellis)

PROCEDURE FOR FEEDING SOLIDS TO AN INFANT

Assessment

1. Determine the infant's physical development. *Although it is not harmful to introduce solid foods to the young infant, the digestive tract is not physiologically ready for solid foods before 6 to 8 months.*
2. Identify the type of food ordered *to determine appropriateness for the infant's condition.*
3. Check to see whether any special feeding device is necessary.

Planning

4. Wash your hands *for infection control.*
5. Obtain the proper food and a small spoon.

Implementation

6. Identify the infant *to be sure you are carrying out the procedure for the correct infant.*
7. Position the infant comfortably, either on your lap (Fig. 19–9) or in a highchair (Fig. 19–10).
8. Use a bib *to protect the infant's clothing.*
9. Check the food *to be sure it is a comfortable temperature. Hot food can burn an infant's tender mouth, and chilled food takes longer to digest,* so slightly warm or room temperature food is usually used. Remember that infants have not established the strong likes and dislikes of adults and will usually eat what they are fed. They do, however, respond to nonverbal cues of aversion from the

Evaluation

17. Compare the infant's intake with usual intake and with the usual intake for an infant of this age and size.
18. Check the infant for comfort and safety.

Documentation

19. Record the kind and amount of formula taken.

© 1996 by Lippincott-Raven Publishers

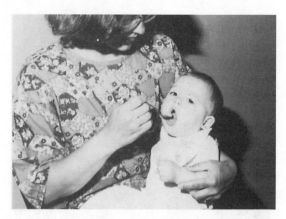

Figure 19–9. Feeding an infant on the lap. (Courtesy Ivan Ellis)

person who is feeding them. Also, feeding plain foods (cereals, vegetables) before feeding fruits usually results in better acceptance of the plain foods. *This is because once infants have tasted the naturally sweet fruit, they will prefer to continue eating it.*

10. Give small bites, and place them well into the infant's mouth.
11. Scrape the food that is pushed back out of the mouth into the spoon, and refeed. Hungry infants will often eat rapidly and complain loudly if food appears too slowly.

    Infants frequently put their hands into their mouths, smearing the food. You can minimize this by providing something for the infant to hold or by fending off the hands with your free hand, as shown in Figure 19–10.
12. When you have finished, clean any soiled areas.
13. If necessary, diaper the infant *because the stimulus of food often causes defecation.*
14. Wash your hands *for infection control.*

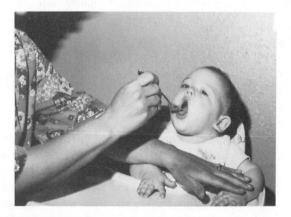

Figure 19–10. Feeding an infant in a high chair. (Courtesy Ivan Ellis)

© 1996 by Lippincott-Raven Publishers

Evaluation

15. Compare the infant's intake with usual intake and with the usual intake for an infant of this age and size.
16. Check the infant for comfort and safety.

Documentation

17. Document the amount of food taken. In some facilities or situations, you may also be required to record the kinds of foods taken.

RESTRAINTS AND SAFETY DEVICES

Maintaining safety for the infant is a major concern. Because it is impossible for an adult to be with the infant or young child at all times, special restraints and safety devices are used *to prevent falls, to prevent interruption of therapy,* and *to prevent the young child from behaving in ways that will cause harm* (such as scratching lesions or pulling off dressings). Many of these devices are nonrestraining so that the infant is not restricted in movement, although safety is provided. *For many procedures, the infant must be kept still and must be prevented from kicking or hitting at the person performing the procedure.* Restraints and safety devices are useful in many of these situations. It will be your responsibility to determine when they are needed and which type to use. (See Module 3, Safety.)

PROCEDURE FOR APPLYING RESTRAINTS AND SAFETY DEVICES

Assessment

1. Determine the infant's age and developmental level.
2. Identify hazards in the environment related to the infant's age and developmental level.
3. Identify the purpose for which the safety device is needed.

Planning

4. Plan the type of safety device to be used for the infant.
5. Plan for intervals at which to recheck the infant.
6. Wash your hands *for infection control.*
7. Obtain the appropriate safety device.

Implementation

8. Identify the infant *to be sure you are carrying out the procedure for the correct infant.*
9. Put the appropriate safety device in place, following either the instructions for use or the specific directions given below.

Evaluation

10. Check the circulation in the extremities distal to any restraint to determine whether the device is restricting circulation.

11. Check the skin under any restraint for moisture, redness, or skin damage.

12. Check the infant for safety and comfort.

13. Wash your hands *for infection control.*

Documentation

14. Note the type of safety device used, the reason for it, and the time applied.

15. Document all evaluative checks done.

SPECIFIC SAFETY PRECAUTIONS

Different kinds of safety devices, many of a nonrestraint type, are available for infants. *Crib nets* are used to keep an active infant or toddler in the crib while still allowing some freedom of movement. Clear plastic *domes* (Fig. 19–11) are also used for the same purpose.

Chest restraints can be used to secure an infant to a highchair. On occasion, these may be used to keep an infant from falling from a crib.

A soft *fabric tie* can be used to immobilize an extremity. Use a clove-hitch knot, *which ensures that the loop will not tighten and restrict circulation if the infant*

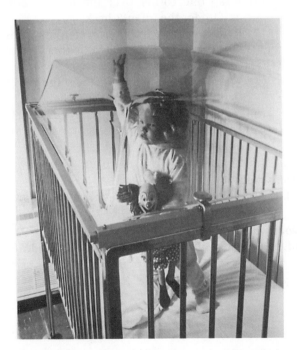

Figure 19–11. Plexiglas crib dome keeps a toddler safe from climbing or falling out.

© 1996 by Lippincott-Raven Publishers

struggles. Whenever you use a tie for a restraint, watch the infant closely to make sure that the child does not become entangled in it. Always attach the end of a tie to a stable part of the crib (bed), such as the frame, and not to a movable part, such as the side rail. *This prevents injury when the position of the movable part is changed.*

Elbow restraints are used to immobilize the elbow joint and *to prevent infants or young children from touching their own face and head.* To be effective, elbow restraints must be incorporated in a jacket or applied over a long-sleeved shirt and pinned at the wrist. *This prevents the infant from pulling the arms up and out of the restraint.* Commercial elbow restraints are widely available, but substitutes can be constructed from tongue blades, tape, and cardboard. Tying a clove hitch knot and applying elbow restraints are described in Module 3, Safety.

Mummying

One way to immobilize an infant safely during a procedure, such as venipuncture, is to wrap the infant tightly in a manner called *mummying* or *swaddling. A blanket or sheet can act as a safety device and allow a procedure to be done more quickly, protecting the infant from the harm that might occur if he or she moved during the procedure.* The entire body can be swaddled with the chest covered, exposing only the neck and head (Fig. 19–12). You can alter the swaddling to expose the chest or *to provide access to whatever part of the body is needed* (Fig. 19–13).

For the two mummying procedures discussed, step 9 of the General Procedure for Applying Restraints and Safety Devices has been modified. This modified step and references to the steps of the General Procedure that remain the same follow.

MUMMYING PROCEDURE

Assessment

1.–3. Follow the steps of the General Procedure.

Planning

4.–7. Follow the steps of the General Procedure.

Implementation

8. Follow the steps of the General Procedure.

9. Mummy the infant as follows:

    a. Head and neck exposed (Fig.19–12 A–C)

        (1) Obtain a clean, small sheet, and fold it into a triangle.

        (2) Place the sheet under the infant with the long, straight edge lying across and under

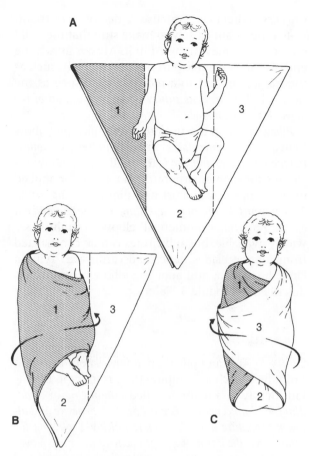

Figure 19–12. Mummy full-body restraint with the chest covered.

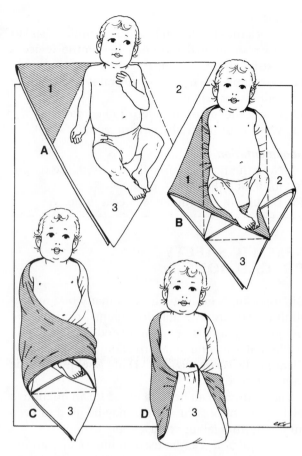

Figure 19–13. Mummy restraint with the chest exposed.

the shoulders and the opposite point under the feet (**A**).

(3) Fold one side corner over the infant's arm, across the chest, and around the other arm. Tuck this side under the infant's back (**B**). This securely anchors both arms.

(4) Fold the bottom point up over the feet.

(5) Wrap the other side corner over the top of and around the infant (**C**). Note that one person can then hold the infant, yet all extremities are restrained.

(6) Pin or simply hold in place. Adapt wrap for covering full body or exposing the chest.

b. Chest and abdomen exposed (Fig. 19–13 A–D)

(1) Start with a triangle-folded sheet.

(2) Place sheet under the infant as before (**A**).

(3) Wrap one corner over the infant's arm and under the infant's back.

(4) Repeat with the other arm (**B**). The ends of the sheet will emerge on either side of the infant's legs and hips.

(5) Wrap first one end and then the other tightly around the infant's legs (**C**).

(6) Fold the bottom point up over the feet.

(7) Pin or tuck the bottom edge over the infant's arms (**D**).

Evaluation
10.–13. Follow the steps of the General Procedure.

Documentation
14.–15. Follow the steps of the General Procedure.

© 1996 by Lippincott-Raven Publishers

HOME CARE

Most first-time parents receive instruction in carrying out basic infant care before leaving the healthcare facility. The most common procedures taught are diapering, bathing, and feeding. Because you may be involved in this activity, you should be familiar with the parents' knowledge level, what is to be taught, and the method to be used. Consult a text on health teaching techniques to plan an effective teaching activity.

When preparing an infant for discharge, whether it is a newborn or an older infant, the nurse should discuss infant care with the parent or other caregiver and determine whether the caregiver needs teaching regarding any aspect of infant care. Parents of first-born infants often participate in infant care classes before giving birth. Some hospitals provide regular classes for all new mothers on a variety of topics related to the mother's and the baby's care after discharge. You may be participating in these teaching programs as you become more experienced.

When the infant has been ill, the parents may have many questions and concerns about alterations or adjustments needed in the basic care they had been providing. As a beginning student, you may not be able to answer all of their questions, but you should be alert to their needs and obtain answers for them or seek another nurse to consult with them.

CRITICAL THINKING EXERCISES

• You are to teach five new parents (two couples and one single mother) how to diaper an infant. After consulting a text on health teaching, answer the following questions to prepare for this activity:

1. What physical environment would be conducive to learning?
2. What information should you assess regarding the parents' current level of knowledge?
3. What items would you need for the class? Make a list.
4. How would you describe the items and their use for the parents?
5. How could you involve the parents attending the class?

• After answering all of the questions, mentally go through the procedure as you would for the class.

© 1996 by Lippincott-Raven Publishers

✔ PERFORMANCE CHECKLIST

Diapering Procedure	Needs More Practice	Satisfactory	Comments
Assessment			
1. Assess the infant's diaper for soiling.			
2. Determine physical development of infant.			
Planning			
3. Wash your hands.			
4. Select type of diaper, pins if needed, and cleansing equipment.			
5. Obtain diversional toys if appropriate.			
Implementation			
6. Fold diaper if necessary.			
7. Place infant on back in safe, clean location.			
8. Put on clean gloves, unfasten diaper, close pins if used.			
9. Remove soiled diaper, wiping away any stool.			
10. Clean perineal area thoroughly.			
11. Lift infant, placing clean diaper underneath.			
12. Pull diaper upward between legs, and secure.			
13. Determine that infant is safe.			
14. Dispose of soiled diaper and gloves.			
15. Wash your hands.			
Evaluation			
16. Check diaper for fit and comfort.			
Documentation			
17. Document changes according to policy; Note any unusual characteristics.			
Bathing Procedure			
Assessment			
1. Determine infant's physical development.			
2. Check clothing, linen, and supplies needed.			

(continued)

© 1996 by Lippincott-Raven Publishers

Bathing Procedure *(Continued)*	Needs More Practice	Satisfactory	Comments
Planning			
3. Wash your hands.			
4. Gather the necessary equipment: basin, mild soap, sterile cotton balls, wash cloth, towel, clean clothing, and clean linen.			
Implementation			
5. Identify infant.			
6. Fill basin with warm water (100–105°F; 37.7°–40.5°C).			
7. Place basin on safe surface.			
8. Wash and dry infant's face.			
9. Hold infant over basin.			
10. Shampoo scalp.			
11. Rub head dry with towel.			
12. Undress infant.			
13. Hold infant securely, and place in basin.			
14. Keep one hand on infant while bathing.			
15. Wash and rinse shoulders, arms, chest, and so forth.			
16. Lift infant out of water, and place on towel.			
17. Wrap infant while you dry to prevent chilling.			
18. Diaper and redress infant.			
19. Place infant at one end of crib while making other end.			
20. Put up side rails and refasten crib net.			
21. Empty and clean basin.			
22. Dispose of soiled linen.			
23. Wash your hands.			
Evaluation			
24. Check infant for comfort and safety.			
Documentation			
25. Document observations made during bath.			
26. Enter bath on checklist or flow sheet.			

© 1996 by Lippincott-Raven Publishers

(continued)

Bottle-Feeding Procedure	Needs More Practice	Satisfactory	Comments
Assessment			
1. Determine infant's physical development.			
2. Check order for type of formula.			
3. Check need for specialized feeding device.			
Planning			
4. Identify formula.			
5. Determine whether formula is to be warmed.			
6. Wash your hands.			
7. Obtain formula and warm if necessary.			
8. Test formula for temperature on wrist.			
Implementation			
9. Check infant's identification.			
10. Pick up infant, and sit in a comfortable position.			
11. Hold infant in your arms. Tuck bib under infant's chin, and slightly elevate the head.			
12. Remove bottle for occasional rest.			
13. Burp infant.			
14. Change infant's diaper if needed.			
15. Return infant to crib. Position infant on right side or on abdomen with head to side.			
16. Wash your hands.			
Evaluation			
17. Compare infant's intake with usual intake for an infant of this age and size and with usual intake for this child.			
18. Check infant for comfort and safety.			
Documentation			
19. Record kind and amount of formula taken.			
Procedure for Feeding Solids			
Assessment			
1. Determine infant's physical development.			

(*continued*)

© 1996 by Lippincott-Raven Publishers

Procedure for Feeding Solids *(Continued)*	Needs More Practice	Satisfactory	Comments
2. Check order for type of food.			
3. Check need for specialized feeding device.			
Planning			
4. Wash your hands.			
5. Obtain correct food and spoon.			
Implementation			
6. Identify the infant.			
7. Position infant.			
8. Put bib on infant.			
9. Check temperature of food.			
10. Give small bites.			
11. Refeed as needed.			
12. Wash infant as needed.			
13. Diaper if necessary.			
14. Wash your hands.			
Evaluation			
15. Compare infant's intake with usual intake for an infant of this age and size and with usual intake for this child.			
16. Check infant for comfort and safety.			
Documentation			
17. Document amount of food taken and kinds of food if this is policy.			
General Procedure for Applying Restraints and Safety Devices			
Assessment			
1. Determine infant's age and development.			
2. Identify environmental hazards.			
3. Identify purpose.			
Planning			
4. Plan type of device to be used.			
5. Plan intervals for rechecking infant.			

(continued)

© 1996 by Lippincott-Raven Publishers

General Procedure for Applying Restraints and Safety Devices *(Continued)*	Needs More Practice	Satisfactory	Comments
6. Wash your hands.			
7. Obtain device.			
Implementation			
8. Identify infant.			
9. Put device in place.			
Evaluation			
10. Check circulation in extremities distal to restraint.			
11. Check skin under restraint.			
12. Check infant for comfort and safety.			
13. Wash your hands.			
Documentation			
14. Note type of device used and time applied.			
15. Document evaluative checks.			
Mummying			
Assessment			
1.–3. Follow steps 1–3 of the General Procedure for Applying Restraints and Safety Devices (check infant's age and development; identify environmental hazards; identify purpose for application).			
Planning			
4.–7. Follow steps 4–7 of the General Procedure (plan type of device to be used; plan intervals for checking the infant; wash hands; obtain device).			
Implementation			
8. Identify infant.			
9. Mummy infant as follows: **a.** Head and neck exposed: (1) Get and fold clean sheet.			
(2) Place sheet under infant.			
(3) Fold one corner over arm, across chest, around other arm, and under back.			
(4) Fold bottom up.			

(continued)

© 1996 by Lippincott-Raven Publishers

General Procedure for Applying Restraints and Safety Devices *(Continued)*	Needs More Practice	Satisfactory	Comments
(5) Fold second corner over top of infant and around body firmly.			
(6) Pin or hold in place.			
b. Chest and abdomen exposed: (1) Obtain triangle-folded clean sheet.			
(2) Place sheet under infant.			
(3) Wrap one corner over arm and under back.			
(4) Repeat for other side.			
(5) Wrap ends securely around legs.			
(6) Fold bottom point up over feet.			
(7) Pin or tuck bottom edge over arm.			
Evaluation			
10.–13. Follow Checklist steps 10–13 of the General Procedure (check circulation; check skin; check infant for comfort and safety; wash your hands).			
Documentation			
14.–15. Follow Checklist steps 14 and 15 of the General Procedure (note type of device used and time applied; record evaluative checks).			

© 1996 by Lippincott-Raven Publishers

? QUIZ

Short-Answer Questions

1. What is one reason it is advisable to use cloth rather than disposable diapers for the infant?
   _____

2. Why is the perineal area cleaned at the time of a diaper change? _____
   _____

3. What should be done with safety pins while changing a baby's diaper? _____
   _____

4. Differentiate between diaper rash and scald. _____
   _____

5. What precaution should be taken when using baby powder, and why? _____
   _____

6. How would you test a bottle-feeding for proper temperature? _____
   _____

7. What is one method of minimizing the amount of air swallowed during bottle-feeding?
   _____
   _____

8. Why should you feed an infant plain food (such as cereal) before fruits? _____
   _____

9. Why is a clove hitch used to tie an arm restraint? _____
   _____

10. List three safety measures that must be followed when bathing an infant.
    a. _____
    b. _____
    c. _____

11. What nursing measures could be used to protect the skin of an infant who has diarrhea?
    _____
    _____

12. In what position should the infant be placed after eating to decrease the chance of regurgitation
    and possible aspiration? _____
    _____

© 1996 by Lippincott-Raven Publishers

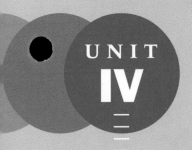

Assisting With Activity and Rest

MODULE 20
Transfer

MODULE 21
Ambulation: Simple Assisted and Using Cane, Walker, or Crutches

MODULE 22
Range-of-Motion Exercises

MODULE 23
Caring for Patients With Casts and Braces

MODULE 24
Applying and Maintaining Traction

MODULE 25
Special Mattresses and Therapeutic Frame and Beds

MODULE

20

TRANSFER

MODULE CONTENTS

RATIONALE FOR THE USE OF THIS
    SKILL
NURSING DIAGNOSES
SAFETY
GENERAL PROCEDURE FOR TRANSFER
  Assessment
  Planning
  Implementation
  Evaluation
  Documentation
SPECIFIC TRANSFER TECHNIQUES
Bed to Chair: One-Person Maximal Assist
Bed to Chair: One-Person Minimal Assist
Bed to Chair: Two-Person Maximal Assist
Chair to Chair: Two-Person Lift
Bed to Chair: Two-Person Lift
Six-Point Seated Transfer: Two-Person Lift
Bed to Chair: Mechanical Lift
Horizontal Slide: Using a Transfer Slider
    Board
Horizontal Lift: Two- or Three-Person
    Assist
LONG-TERM CARE
HOME CARE
CRITICAL THINKING EXERCISES

PREREQUISITES

Successful completion of the following modules:

VOLUME 1

Module 1 An Approach to Nursing Skills
Module 2 Basic Infection Control
Module 3 Safety
Module 4 Basic Body Mechanics
Module 5 Documentation
Module 6 Introduction to Assessment
          Skills
Module 15 Moving the Patient in Bed
          and Positioning

© 1996 by Lippincott-Raven Publishers

OVERALL OBJECTIVE

To transfer a patient from a bed to a chair, wheelchair, commode, or stretcher with maximum comfort and safety for the patient and nurse.

SPECIFIC LEARNING OBJECTIVES

Know Facts and Principles	Apply Facts and Principles	Demonstrate Ability	Evaluate Performance
1. Reasons for transfer List four reasons for patient's activity.	Given a patient situation, state purpose of activity.	In clinical setting, state reasons for patient's activity.	Evaluate own rationale with instructor.
2. Safety List common hazards encountered when doing transfers.	Recognize hazards in a particular situation.	Provide safe setting for transfer.	Determine that patient was not injured in transfer.
3. Assessment of patient State reasons for knowing patient's diagnosis and capabilities.	Give examples of how different diagnoses and capabilities would affect plans for transfer.	Gather data on patient's abilities and diagnoses before moving patient.	After transfer, review procedure to find whether more data would have helped. Validate with instructor.

4. Transfer of patient
    a. Bed to chair
    b. Bed to stretcher
    c. Chair to chair
List steps of usual transfer procedures.
	Plan modification of procedures for particular patient situation.
	Identify best procedure to use in specific situation.
		Successfully transfer patient:
		    a. From bed to chair or commode
		    b. From bed to stretcher
		    c. From chair to chair or commode
			Evaluate own performance using Performance Checklist.

© 1996 by Lippincott-Raven Publishers

LEARNING ACTIVITIES

1. Review the Specific Learning Objectives.
2. Read the section on posture and body mechanics and ambulation (in the chapter on activity and rest) in Ellis and Nowlis, *Nursing: A Human Needs Approach,* or comparable material in another textbook.
3. Look up the module vocabulary terms in the glossary.
4. Study the module as though you were preparing to teach the content to another person. Mentally practice the skills.
5. In the practice setting, do each of the following, being sure to communicate effectively with the "patient" as you proceed:
   a. Place a colored tie or scarf around your partner's left arm and another on the left leg (or right arm and right leg). This will be the non-functional side.
   b. Transfer your partner from a supine position in bed to an upright position sitting on the side of the bed. This is called dangling and is often preparatory to any type of transfer.
   c. Transfer your partner from the bed to a chair using a one-person, maximal-assist transfer.
   d. Transfer your partner from the bed to a chair using a one-person, minimal-assist transfer.
   e. With a third person, transfer your partner from a bed to a chair using a two-person, maximal-assist transfer.
   f. Transfer your partner from chair to chair and from bed to chair using each of the two-person lift transfer techniques.
   g. Transfer your partner from bed to chair using a mechanical lift device if one is available.
      (1) Obtain the lift.
      (2) Review the specific directions for its use.
      (3) Practice raising and lowering the device without a person in it.
      (4) Using the directions in this module, transfer another student from a bed to a chair and back to the bed using the lift.
      (5) Ask the student who was transferred to describe how it felt.
   h. Transfer your partner from a bed to a stretcher using a horizontal slide and then using a two- or three-person horizontal lift.
   i. Change roles as patient and nurse, and repeat all of the transfers until each person participating has had an opportunity to be in each role.

VOCABULARY

contact guard assistance	hydraulic	stand-by assistance
dangling	orthostatic hypotension	supine
horizontal	out of bed	weight-bearing

© 1996 by Lippincott-Raven Publishers

Transfer

Rationale for the Use of This Skill

Moving patients out of bed is beneficial for them. The movement maintains and restores muscle tone, stimulates the respiratory and circulatory systems, and improves elimination. Patients need only dangle their legs over the side of the bed or sit in a chair at the bedside for a few minutes to improve their physical and psychological well-being. Many patients are unable to move at all or need some assistance in moving. It is the nurse's responsibility to help by moving patients, directing them in the best techniques for self-movement, and seeing that enough people are on hand to ensure the safety of the patient and staff during transfer.

Properly helping a patient from the bed to a chair is an important nursing function, in which you play a vital role by giving the patient physical support and encouragement. Pay special attention to safety precautions and to the basics of body mechanics to ensure the safety of all involved.

The level of activity is usually determined by a physician's orders, but nursing assessment and judgment are necessary to determine the best method for carrying out the order.[1]

▼ NURSING DIAGNOSES

A nursing diagnosis related to moving patients is Impaired Physical Mobility. Patients may be completely unable to move themselves or need assistance in doing so. Reasons for Impaired Physical Mobility include decreased strength, pain or discomfort, and neuromuscular or musculoskeletal impairment. Another nursing diagnosis to keep in mind when moving patients is Activity Intolerance. The person with Activity Intolerance may need assistance to move with safety.

SAFETY

Falls are the most common hazard to a patient being transferred. The patient may become dizzy or have less strength than expected, or the nurse may not be strong enough to accomplish the task. Consider these possibilities carefully before beginning the transfer so that you can plan the specific measures you will take to maintain safety for the patient. For

[1]Note that rationales for action are emphasized throughout the module by the use of italics.

example, if the patient is very large or hard to handle, consider having other nurses assist you or using a mechanical lift.

If a patient begins to fall, lower the patient to the bed, the chair, or the floor in a way that *prevents injury.* Especially protect the head from a blow. If a patient does fall, complete a thorough assessment before you move the patient to determine if there are any injuries. *Moving may increase the severity of a fall-related injury.* This assessment may be done by an experienced registered nurse, but in some instances, should be done by a physician. Consult the policy in your facility.

Another hazard in moving patients is the pull on indwelling tubings (such as catheters or IV tubing). Take care to move tubings as necessary without dislodging them.

Bruising from striking side rails or furniture is another hazard of transferring the patient. Position the patient carefully *to prevent him or her from striking against side rails or furniture.* Be sure the patient is wearing shoes or slippers (with firm soles) when stepping onto the floor. *Floors tend to be slick, creating the potential for slipping. Small objects may be on the floor that could injure the foot. Additionally, floors in healthcare settings are considered contaminated with microorganisms.*

GENERAL PROCEDURE FOR TRANSFER

Assessment

1. Review the patient's records for medical diagnosis, current problems, and physician's orders indicating any restrictions to be observed. For example, a patient with a recently repaired fractured hip may be allowed to rest only 25% of body weight on the affected side, whereas a postoperative patient who has had an appendectomy may not be restricted in any way. Check with other nurses, and consult the patient record and Kardex to obtain information regarding any transfer plans.

2. Assess the patient. Is the patient capable of moving all extremities? Does the patient have any specific disabilities that would affect movement? Is one side stronger? Does the patient have the endurance to sustain activity? How was the patient transferred before? Has the patient received any medication that will affect balance, ability to follow directions, or judgment? You may need to take vital signs before transfer to evaluate the patient's response effectively. Assess the patient for pain. Some patients may need to be medicated

© 1996 by Lippincott-Raven Publishers

for pain before they are able to move effectively. Does the patient know how to participate, or can the patient follow instructions? Asking the patient appropriate questions will often provide this information. Some patients may not be able to provide accurate information. If the patient wears glasses or a hearing aid, be sure they are in place *to ensure maximum cooperation.*

3. Identify what equipment is available for moving patients and who is available to assist you.

Planning

4. With the data in hand, devise a plan to transfer the patient in the safest and most convenient manner, taking into account proper body mechanics for you and the patient. Be realistic. You may need more than one person to transfer a heavy or severely disabled patient.
5. Wash your hands *for infection control.*
6. Obtain any equipment that you or the patient will need.

Implementation

7. Identify the patient *to be sure you are carrying out the procedure for the correct patient.*
8. Put shoes or slippers on the patient. *Firm-soled shoes give the patient a sense of security and prevent slipping.* If shoes are not available, leather-soled slippers can be used. Always put ordered braces and appliances on a patient before he or she is transferred.
9. Put transfer belt on patient if indicated. Transfer belts, sometimes called gait belts, are useful assistive devices. The belt is made of heavy twill with a buckle that stays fastened when pressure or force is applied. It is placed around the patient's waist *to give those assisting with the activity a way to hold onto the patient firmly.* The belt must be applied snugly enough *to hold the patient in a secure fashion* but not so snugly *as to be uncomfortable.* Be careful that a female patient's breasts do not become caught under the belt.

   In the past, these belts were available only in physical therapy departments, so many nurses were not familiar with their use. Now, however, they are commonly found on the clinical unit, sometimes in every patient room. In many nursing homes, the nursing assistants wear a transfer belt around their own waists so that it is immediately available for use. Once you have used one, you will be convinced of its value.

   Use a transfer belt for all transfers except those for which the procedure specifically states the belt is not needed. When a belt is not available, devise a substitute from items on hand. A drawsheet can be folded and wrapped around the patient's waist. If the sheet is thin enough to permit tying it, do so. If it is too bulky to tie, cross it in back and grasp the ends along with the side when you use it for lifting. A patient's gown can be another substitute. Tie it around the patient's waist and use it as you would a transfer belt. A patient may even have a regular leather belt that can be used, but be careful that a narrow belt does not cut into the patient.

10. Lower the entire bed and the head of the bed. Some beds are lowered by an electrical control at the side or foot of the bed, and some are lowered manually by crank. Make these mechanical devices work for you.
11. As simply as possible, explain to the patient what you intend to do or how you intend to help and how he or she is expected to participate. Ask if there are any questions. It is essential that you appear confident. It also is important not to rush the patient.
12. Carry out the specific procedure as outlined.
13. Retake vital signs as appropriate for evaluation of response.
14. Wash your hands.

Evaluation

15. Evaluate using the following criteria:
    a. Patient's body alignment is correct.
    b. Patient does not experience pain and is comfortable.
    c. Patient remains safe without injury.
    d. Patient did not experience excess fatigue, and vital signs remain stable.
    e. The nurse(s) involved used correct body mechanics and maintained personal safety.

Documentation

16. Document on the Kardex or nursing care plan the following:
    a. Best means of transfer and any aids or devices needed
    b. Number of people needed to help
    c. Patient's ability to cooperate
17. Each time a transfer is carried out, document the following. This is commonly done using a flow sheet. In some facilities, it is done on the nursing progress notes in either a narrative or a SOAP format:
    a. The exact nature of the activity
    b. The time it was carried out
    c. The patient's response to the activity; consider pain, fatigue, pulse and respiration rate, blood pressure changes, and dizziness.

© 1996 by Lippincott-Raven Publishers

SPECIFIC TRANSFER TECHNIQUES

Review Module 4, Basic Body Mechanics, *to under-stand the rationale for the way you move patients.* For each transfer procedure discussed, some steps of the General Procedure may be modified. The modified steps and references to the steps of the General Procedure that remain the same follow.

Bed to Chair: One-Person Maximal Assist

Assessment

1.–3. Follow the steps of the General Procedure for Transfer.

Planning

4.–6. Follow the steps of the General Procedure.

Implementation

7.–11. Follow the steps of the General Procedure.

12. Transfer the patient from bed to wheelchair or armchair.

   a. Angle the wheelchair or armchair at a 45-degree angle to the bed so that the chair is on the patient's stronger side. If the footrests are removable, remove them at this time; otherwise, fold them out of the way. *This arrangement will allow the patient to pivot on the stronger leg.*

   b. Lock the bed and wheelchair *to prevent them from moving during transfer.* Be sure the patient sees the chair and its position. If the patient is visually impaired, explain the location of the wheelchair, and if possible, place the patient's hand on it *to promote a feeling of security.*

   c. Begin with the patient in a supine position, with the hips placed where the bed will bend as the head of the bed is raised, and close to the edge of the bed.

   d. Raise the head of the bed so that the patient is in a sitting position. (*This decreases the effort for you and the patient.*) Raise the bed slowly *so that the patient does not get dizzy.*

   e. Slide one arm under the patient's legs and place the other arm behind the patient's back. Swing the patient's legs over the side of the bed while pivoting the patient's body, so that the patient ends up sitting on the edge of the bed with the feet hanging down.

   f. Allow the patient to sit for a few minutes *to prevent light-headedness or orthostatic hypotension,* which can occur with any sudden change in circulation caused by lowering the legs and raising the head. Support the patient if he or she feels dizzy.

   g. Position the patient's feet firmly on the floor and slightly apart, with the patient's hands on the bed. *To protect yourself from injury,* do not let the patient hold on to you. *If the patient is holding on to you and begins to fall, you may receive a back injury from the twisting weight applied to your spine.*

   h. Take a wide stance, bend your knees, and grasp the patient at the sides of the belt. You may want to straddle the patient's weaker leg with your own legs, or you may want to stabilize the patient's knees by supporting them with your own knees (Fig. 20–1).

   i. Inform the patient that you will assist him or her to a standing position on a count of "one, two, three, *stand*" and that he or she should lean slightly forward and push up with the hands on the bed.

   j. On the count, straighten your knees, assisting the patient to a standing position.

   k. Stand close to the patient, and pivot to the chair.

   l. Instruct the patient to place both hands on the arms of the chair.

   m. Lower the patient to the seat.

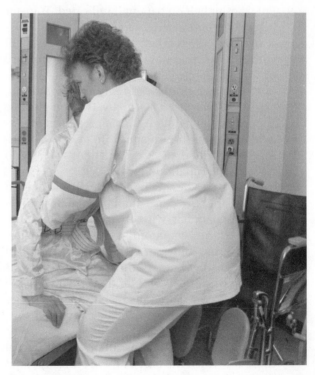

Figure 20–1. Bed to wheelchair: One-person maximal assist. Supporting the patient's knees between your knees adds stability.

© 1996 by Lippincott-Raven Publishers

n. Be sure the patient's body is positioned firmly back in the seat *for good posture.*

13.–14. Follow the steps of the General Procedure.

Evaluation

15. Follow the steps of the General Procedure.

Documentation

16.–17. Follow the steps of the General Procedure.

This same technique can be used to transfer a patient from one chair to another or from a wheelchair to the toilet.

Bed to Chair: One-Person Minimal Assist

Proceed as you would for the one-person maximal-assist transfer described previously, with two exceptions. It is not necessary to brace the patient's knees, nor is a transfer belt usually necessary. *You will be primarily providing balance, not supporting the patient's weight* (Fig. 20–2).

Bed to Chair: Two-Person Maximal Assist

Assessment

1.–3. Follow the steps of the General Procedure for Transfer.

Planning

4.–6. Follow the steps of the General Procedure.

Implementation

7.–11. Follow the steps of the General Procedure.

12. Transfer the patient from bed to wheelchair or armchair.

    a. Put the bed in the flat position, and lock it.

    b. Position the wheelchair or armchair next to the bed, at a 45-degree angle, with the seat facing toward the bed. Secure the brakes.

    c. Help the patient to a sitting position on the edge of the bed as described in the one-person maximal assist, steps 12e and f.

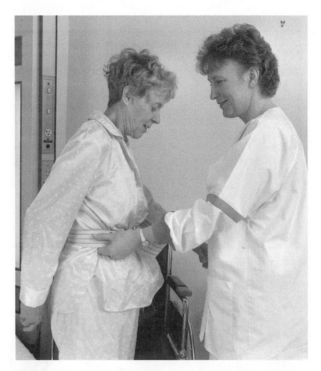

Figure 20–2. Bed to wheelchair: One-person minimal assist. Your function is primarily to provide balance.

    d. Have the patient place both hands on the bed.

    e. Nurse 1 stands in front of the patient (one-person maximal assist, steps 12g and h), grasping the belt at the sides.

    f. Nurse 2 stands between the wheelchair and the bed with one knee on the bed and grasps the transfer belt at the patient's back (Fig. 20–3).

    g. Nurse 1 informs the patient that the move will occur on a count of "one, two, three, *lift.*"

    h. Nurse 1 signals "one, two, three, *lift.*" Both assistants lift and pivot the patient at the same time, and then lower the patient into the wheelchair.

    i. Be sure the patient's body is positioned

DATE/TIME	
9/6/98 8:30 AM	Transferred from bed to chair and back with two-person maximal assistance. Up in chair for 15 min. Stated felt dizzy and weak after transfer. Vital signs remained stable.
	C. Jensen N.S.

Example of Narrative Charting.

© 1996 by Lippincott-Raven Publishers

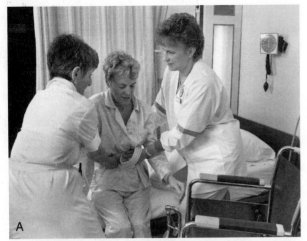

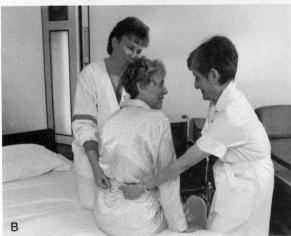

Figure 20–3. Bed to wheelchair: Two-person maximal assist. **(A)** the bed is flat so that nurse 2 can place one knee on the bed. **(B)** Both nurses grasp the transfer belt.

straight and firmly back in the wheelchair *for good posture.*

13.–14. Follow the steps of the General Procedure.

Evaluation

15. Follow the steps of the General Procedure.

Documentation

16.–17. Follow the steps of the General Procedure.

Chair to Chair: Two-Person Lift

This lift, often referred to as a "bucket lift," has a high potential for back injury for nurses *because one nurse must lift from a bent position.* Another concern with this technique is that *the nurses' arms may place pressure on the brachial plexus under the patient's arms, causing injury.* For these reasons, many facilities encourage staff to use the six-point seated transfer (described below) instead of this lift. This lift can be done safely if nurse 1 is tall, quite strong, and uses good body mechanics; nurse 2 is careful to be in a position to support the patient's body weight; and the patient can keep the arms and shoulders in a rigid position so that weight is not placed on the brachial plexus. Therefore, it is presented for your information.

Assessment

1.–3. Follow the steps of the General Procedure for Transfer.

Planning

4.–6. Follow the steps of the General Procedure.

Implementation

7.–11. Follow the steps of the General Procedure.

12. Transfer the patient from chair to chair or commode. The transfer belt is not used for this transfer technique.
 a. Place the chairs (or commode and chair) side by side, facing in the same direction.
 b. Remove the footrests from the wheelchair, or fold them out of the way, and lock or brace the chair (or commode).
 c. The taller nurse (1) stands behind the chair.
 d. The shorter nurse (2) stands facing the patient.
 e. Nurse 1 folds the patient's arms across the patient's chest. The nurse then reaches under the patient's arms from behind the patient and grasps the opposite wrists.
 f. Nurse 2 bends knees and hips, adopting a squatting position, and grasps the patient

DATE/TIME	
9/7/98 10:30 AM	S "I felt dizzy and weak while I was moving. It was a good thing you both were there; I'd have landed on the floor if I tried it myself."
	O Before transfer, P-86, R-22, BP 130/76; after transfer, P-90, R-24, BP 134/82
	A Physically stable in response to activity.
	P Continue transfers with two-person assist until feels more stable. M. Wyatt R.N.

Example of Nursing Progress Notes Using SOAP Format.

© 1996 by Lippincott-Raven Publishers

under the knees to support the legs (Fig. 20–4).

  g. Nurse 1 informs the patient that the move will occur on the count of "one, two, three, *lift*."

  h. Nurse 1 counts ("one, two, three, *lift*"), and both lift at the same time. Nurse 1 controls the timing because that nurse bears the greatest weight.

  i. When the word "lift" is said, both nurses lift the patient and move over to the second chair (or commode), lowering the patient immediately, slowly, and smoothly.

13.–14. Follow the steps of the General Procedure.

Evaluation

15. Follow the steps of the General Procedure.

Documentation

16.–17. Follow the steps of the General Procedure.

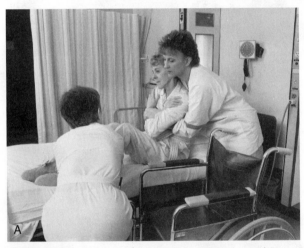

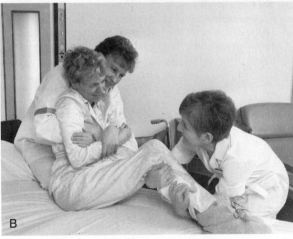

Figure 20–4. Bed to chair: Two person "bucket" lift. One person lifts from behind the person, grasping the arms for a firm hold. The second person lifts under the person's legs.

© 1996 by Lippincott-Raven Publishers

Bed to Chair: Two-Person Lift

This transfer has the same problems identified for the chair to chair: two-person lift. The same factors are needed to maintain safety.

Assessment

1.–3. Follow the steps of the General Procedure for Transfer.

Planning

4.–6. Follow the steps of the General Procedure.

Implementation

 7.–11. Follow the steps of the General Procedure.

12. Transfer the patient from bed to chair, wheelchair, or commode. The transfer belt is not used for this transfer technique.

  a. Put the bed flat, and lock it.

  b. Set the wheelchair parallel to the bed, and secure its brakes. If the armrests are removable, remove the one next to the bed.

  c. Slide the patient to the edge of the bed.

  d. Nurse 1 slides one arm under the patient's arms and begins lifting the shoulders. The nurse places one knee on the bed and slides his or her arms around the patient until both arms are under the patient's arms and the patient is sitting, leaning on the nurse's chest.

  e. Nurse 1 crosses the patient's arms on the chest, grasping the opposite wrists in front of the patient.

  f. Nurse 2 squats beside the bed and slides both arms under the patient's thighs from the same side.

  g. Nurse 1 informs the patient that he or she will be moved on a count of "one, two, three, *lift*."

  h. Nurse 1 counts ("one, two, three, *lift*"), and both nurses lift the patient onto the wheelchair (or commode). A third person can help in this lift, sliding arms under the patient's buttocks *so that all three people can lift at one time.*

13.–14. Follow the steps of the General Procedure.

Evaluation

15. Follow the steps of the General Procedure.

Documentation

16.–17. Follow the steps of the General Procedure.

Six-Point Seated Transfer: Two-Person Lift

This transfer may be used to move the patient from bed to chair, wheelchair, or commode or from chair to bed and back. This procedure can easily be adapt-

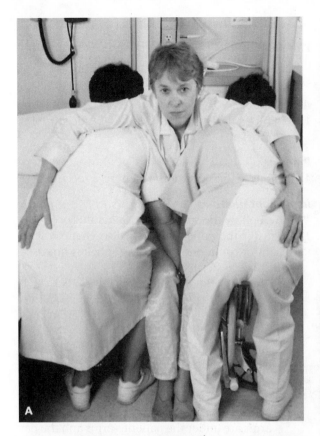

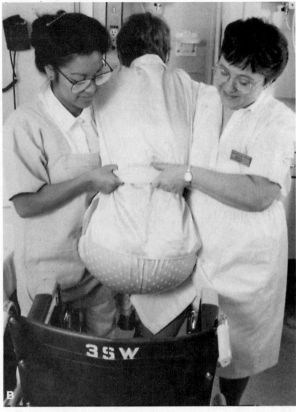

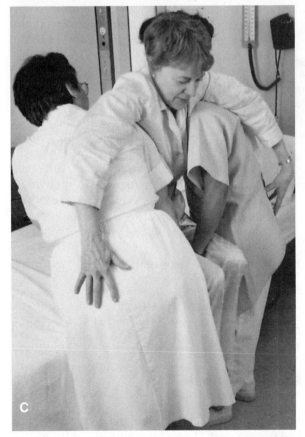

Figure 20–5. Six-point seated transfer: Two-person lift (**A**) The patient leans forward with her arms resting over the backs of the nurses. (**B**) The nurses lift the patient by coming to a complete standing position with their shoulders back. (**C**) The patient is lowered to the stretcher or bed.

© 1996 by Lippincott-Raven Publishers

ed to transfer between any two surfaces on which the patient can sit. *Physical therapists state that this transfer provides greater protection from back injury for personnel and eliminates the potential for brachial plexus injury that the traditional two-person lift creates.* It is called a six-point transfer because the patient uses both arms for support and each of two nurses using both arms for support.

Assessment

1.–3. Follow the steps of the General Procedure for Transfer.

Planning

4.–6. Follow the steps of the General Procedure.

Implementation

7.–11. Follow the steps of the General Procedure.
12. Transfer the patient.
- **a.** Place the two seats (chairs, commode and chair, or wheelchair and bed) so that the sitting surfaces are at right angles to one another, and lock both.
- **b.** If the armrests on the chair(s) are removable, remove both.
- **c.** Both nurses stand facing the patient, one on each side. This lift is easier to accomplish if the nurses are approximately the same height.
- **d.** Secure a transfer belt around the waist of the patient. If trousers with a belt are worn, the belt can be used instead of a transfer belt in this lift because the weight of the patient is not pulling on the groin due to the seated position.
- **e.** Both nurses lean forward with knees flexed and feet in a wide stance; place the forearm nearest to the patient around and under the closest thigh of the patient from the inner side. (An alternative is to secure a transfer belt around both thighs of the patient and grasp the transfer belt).
- **f.** Instruct and assist the patient to lean forward and rest arms over the backs of the nurses (Fig. 20–5A). If the patient is unable to do this because of arthritic or contracted shoulder joints, the patient's arms are placed along the tops of his or her thighs and slid toward the knees as the patient leans forward.
- **g.** Both nurses grasp the patient's waistband or the transfer belt with their outside hands.
- **h.** Inform the patient that the move will begin on the count of "one, two, three, *lift*." To be sure that only one nurse is giving directions, determine who will be spokesperson before starting.
- **i.** One nurse counts (one, two, three, *lift*"), and

both nurses lift the patient straight up by coming to a complete standing position with shoulders back. The patient will be in a flexed forward sitting position (Fig. 20–5B).
- **j.** Turn and place the patient onto the next chair or bed in a sitting position (Fig. 20–5C).
13.–14. Follow the steps of the General Procedure.

Evaluation

15. Follow the steps of the General Procedure.

Documentation

16.–17. Follow the steps of the General Procedure.

Bed to Chair: Mechanical Lift

The mechanical lift enables nurses to lift heavy patients or those who are badly incapacitated without relying on physical strength. All lifts have a sturdy frame that supports the patient's weight; a sling or seat of some type, which is positioned under the patient; and a mechanical lifting mechanism. One such lift was devised specifically to assist in providing hygiene to the patient (Fig. 20–6).

Consult the direction for specifics about the particular brand and model used in your facility. The following is a general outline of the procedure when using a device with a sling. Two people are usually needed *to ensure the patient's safety.* Two people are essential for incapacitated patients who cannot support their own heads. The transfer belt is not used for this transfer technique.

Assessment

1.–3. Follow the steps of the General Procedure for Transfer.

Planning

4.–6. Follow the steps of the General Procedure.

Implementation

7.–9. Follow the steps of the General Procedure.
10. Raise the bed to a comfortable working position.
11. Explain to the patient what the lift is for and how it works. Emphasize the safety of the procedure *because the patient may be frightened by the large mechanical device.*
12. Using the mechanical lift, transfer the patient.
- **a.** Place the patient in the supine position.
- **b.** Place the sling by rolling the patient side to side and slipping it under the body in the same way you would place a sheet under a patient in bed. If the patient is not clothed (as in a transfer to a tub, for example), cover the patient with a bath blanket.

  For the patient's safety, position the sling

© 1996 by Lippincott-Raven Publishers

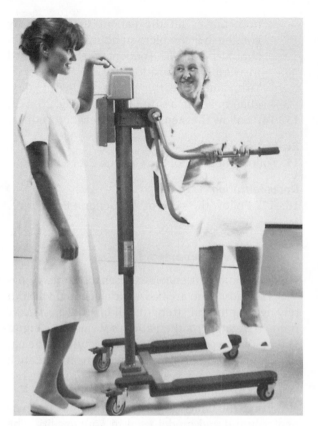

Figure 20–6. Electric mechanical lift chair. The patient can be transferred, transported, and showered using this lift chair.

correctly. If the lower edge of the sling is too high, the patient could slip feet first out of the sling. If the lower edge is too low (on a two-piece sling), the patient could "fold up" and slip out of the sling.

(1) *One-piece sling:* Place the bottom edge just above the knees. The top edge can extend behind the shoulders or to the head.

(2) *Two-piece sling:* Place one of the canvas strips behind the patient's thighs *so that it forms a seat for the sling.* Position the second canvas strip under the patient's shoulder blades so that it supports the patient's trunk in a semireclining position.

c. Lower the bed. *This allows you to keep the lift in a lower, more stable position.*

d. Position the lift by the bed, *so that the lifting arm extends above the patient.* If the support legs are adjustable, put them in their widest, *most stable position.*

e. Place the patient's arms across the chest, *keeping them out of the way during the lift.*

f. Fasten the chains of the lift to the sling. The chains to the seat section should be slightly

longer than the chains to the trunk section *to create a semireclining position when the sling is lifted.* When you fasten the chains, make sure that the hooks are pointed away from the patient *to prevent them from jabbing the patient.* Be careful not to catch skin folds in the metal edges and chains *to prevent skin damage.*

g. Nurse 1 stands at the patient's head *to support the head and guide the patient during the lift.*

h. Nurse 2 operates the device to raise the patient. Most newer devices are electrical and may be operated through a switch that raises and lowers the device. Older devices often operate by means of a hydraulic pump. If a hydraulic pump is used, nurse 2 makes sure the valve is closed and begins pumping, gradually lifting the patient off the bed.

With either type of device, lift until the patient just clears the bed and no higher. *The higher the lift, the less stable its balance* (Fig. 20–7).

i. Nurse 1 guides the patient, and nurse 2 guides the lift as it is maneuvered away from the bed.

j. Double-check the position of the bath blanket if you are transporting the patient to a tub. You may want to place additional coverings around the patient's buttocks and shoulders *to keep the patient warm and to provide for modesty.*

k. Slowly, keeping careful balance, move the lift to the chair, tub, or other bed. *If you move*

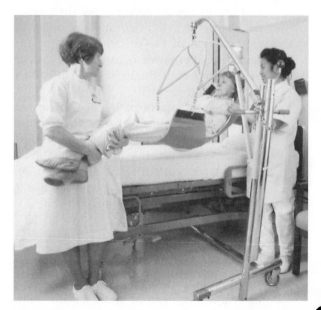

Figure 20–7. Hydraulic mechanical lift sling. Pump until the patient just clears the bed.

© 1996 by Lippincott-Raven Publishers

rapidly, the sling will begin to sway, lessening stability.

l. Position the patient above the next resting place, with special attention to the correct positioning of the hips.

m. Lower the patient slowly. If using an electrical device, turn the switch to the position to lower the patient, correcting the positioning as the patient moves downward. Turn it off when the patient is on the bed.

If using a hydraulic lift, release the hydraulic valve carefully, and lower the patient very slowly. Do not open the valve too far, *which would cause the patient to move down too abruptly.*

n. Turn off the switch or close the valve as soon as the patient's weight is on the chair. Otherwise *the support arm will lower onto the patient.*

o. Detach the chains from the sling, and remove the lift. The sling usually remains under the patient in the new position, so that the reverse procedure, back to the bed, is easy. If you have transferred the patient to another bed, remove the sling by turning the patient from side to side.

13.–14. Follow the steps of the General Procedure.

Evaluation

15. Follow the steps of the General Procedure.

Documentation

16.–17. Follow the steps of the General Procedure.

Horizontal Slide: Using a Transfer Slider Board

A slick plastic board is used in many facilities to enable the patient to be moved between a stretcher and a bed. *The board facilitates moving the patient because its slick surface reduces friction.*

Assessment

1.–3. Follow the steps of the General Procedure for Transfer.

Planning

4.–6. Follow the steps of the General Procedure.

Implementation

7. Follow the steps of the General Procedure.

8.–11. Omit steps 8 through 11 of the General Procedure.

12. Transfer the patient horizontally in the following manner:

a. Nurse 1 stands on the side of the bed where the stretcher is placed (usually closest to the door), and nurse 2 stands on the opposite side of the bed.

b. Nurse 1 lowers the side rail nearest the door and places the stretcher with the slider board, covered with a sheet, alongside the bed.

c. Nurse 2 rolls the patient away from the stretcher while nurse 1 slides the board across the dividing space between the stretcher and the bed and partially under the patient. *This provides a firm, smooth surface on which to slide the patient to the stretcher* (Fig. 20–8).

d. Nurse 2 rolls the patient back over partially onto the slider board and pulls the cover sheet out on the far side of the bed, rolling the patient as necessary to accomplish this.

e. Nurse 1 reaches across the stretcher and grasps the sheet firmly at the level of the patient's shoulders and hips.

f. Nurse 2 lifts the edge of the sheet transferring the patient's weight toward the slider board as nurse 1 firmly pulls the sheet and the patient across the slider board onto the stretcher. If the patient is incapacitated or very heavy, additional assistance may be needed on the stretcher side to support the head and pull the patient.

DATE/TIME	
8/1/98	S *"I feel a little tired, but otherwise okay."*
0930	O *Transported to bath tub via mechanical lift. Bathed and returned to bed at 0815. No complaint of pain or dizziness. P = 84, R = 18, BP stable at 144/80.*
	A *Tolerates transport and bathing procedures as outlined on care plan.*
	P *Continue bathing twice weekly (Monday and Thursday) as indicated on care plan.*
	J. Van Dyke, RN

Example of Nursing Progress Notes Using SOAP Format.

© 1996 by Lippincott-Raven Publishers

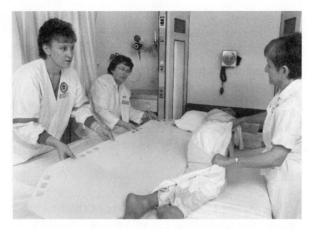

Figure 20–8. Plastic slider board to facilitate transfer from the bed to the stretcher.

> **g.** If the patient is being returned to bed, re-move the transfer sheet by turning the pa-tient side to side. The transfer sheet remains under the patient if the patient will soon be transferred again (such as from the stretcher to the x-ray table).

13.–14. Follow the steps of the General Procedure.

Evaluation

15. Follow the steps of the General Procedure.

Documentation

16.–17. Follow the steps of the General Procedure.

Horizontal Lift: Two- or Three-Person Assist

You might be more likely to use this transfer in a long-term care setting, where patients usually have fewer tubes and attachments than in acute care set-tings. In acute care settings, this transfer technique is most commonly used to move a patient from a bed to an ambulance stretcher or from the ambulance stretcher to the bed *because the ambulance stretcher is at a different height than the bed.*

Assessment

1.–3. Follow the steps of the General Procedure for Transfer.

Planning

4.–6. Follow the steps of the General Procedure.

Implementation

7. Follow the steps of the General Procedure.

8.–11. Omit steps 8 through 11 of the General Pro-cedure.

12. Transfer the patient as outlined below. The transfer belt is not used for this transfer tech-nique.

> **a.** Place the stretcher at the foot of the bed, at a right angle to it, with the brakes secured.
> **b.** Move the patient to one side of the bed.
> **c.** Nurse 1, the tallest, stands at the patient's head and slides arms under the patient's neck and shoulders.
> **d.** Nurse 2, the next tallest, stands at the pa-tient's waist and hips and slides both arms under the patient.
> **e.** Nurse 3, the shortest, stands at the patient's knees and slides both arms under the lower legs and thighs. If only two nurses are used, nurse 1 is at the head and chest, and nurse 2 is at the hips and legs.
> **f.** Nurse 2 instructs the patient that the lift will occur on the count of "one, two, three, *lift.*"
> **g.** Using the elbows as levers, all nurses roll the patient toward themselves in a hugging mo-tion. Then the patient is lifted on the count "one, two, three, *lift.*"
> **h.** Holding the patient against their bodies, the nurses walk together, with synchronized steps, to the side and backward, until they are parallel to the stretcher (Fig. 20–9).

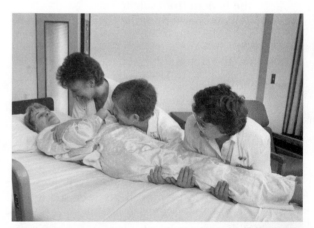

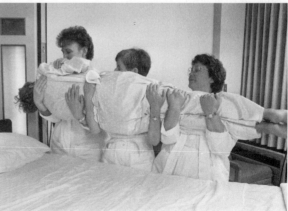

Figure 20–9. Horizontal lift: Three-person assist. Nurse 1 (the tallest) slides his arms under the patient's neck and shoulders.

© 1996 by Lippincott-Raven Publishers

ACTIVITIES OF DAILY LIVING--FLOW SHEET

DATE	10/12/99			10/13/99			10/14/99			10/15/99		
SHIFT	23-07	07-15	15-23	23-07	07-15	15-23	23-07	07-15	15-23	23-07	07-15	15-23
Personal Hygiene	Ø	Bed bath	PM care	Ø	Self bed bath	PM care	Ø	Self bed bath	PM care	Ø	Chair shwr	PM care
ACTIVITY	Ø	Bed rest	Bed rest	Ø	Chair max asst.	Chair max asst.	Ø	Chair max asst.	Chair max asst.	Ø	Chair min asst.	Chair min asst.
Elimination	Ø	1/1	Ø	Ø	Ø	1/1	Ø	1/1	Ø	Ø	Ø	1/1
Sleep/Rest	Slept all noc	×2 1h	@ 2200	Slept all noc	×2 1h	@ 2200	All noc	Ad lib	→	All noc	Ad lib	→
DIET:	Bkfst	Lun.	Din.	Bkfst	Lun.	Din.	Bkfst	Lun.	Din.	Bkfst	Lun.	Din.
Type	Low Na	→	→	Low Na	→	→	Low Na	→	→	Low Na	→	→
Amount	1/2	1/2	3/4	1/2	1/2	1/2	3/4	1/2	3/4	3/4	3/4	3/4
Initials	MR	GW	RT	MR	GW	RT	MR	GW	RT	MR	GW	RT

Figure 20–10. Example of nursing progress note using flow sheet.

i. At the count ("one, two, three, *down*."), the patient is placed on the stretcher.

13.–14. Follow the steps of the General Procedure.

Evaluation

15. Follow the steps of the General Procedure.

Documentation

16.–17. Follow the steps of the General Procedure (Fig. 20-10).

© 1996 by Lippincott-Raven Publishers

LONG-TERM CARE

During a shift, care providers in long-term care settings have the potential to be involved in more transfers where maximum assistance is needed than those in most acute care settings. A serious concern is the potential for repetitive strain injury to the back. The Occupational Safety and Health Administration is studying the problem and considering ways that workers can be protected from injury. It is critical that these care providers use tech- niques and mechanical devices designed to reduce the need for their physical exertion. Thus, you may see mechanical lifts used more frequently in long-term care. Many new types of lifting devices are being developed as their value is demonstrated through fewer on-the-job injuries. When a two-person lift is needed, the authors recommend the six-point seated transfer.

HOME CARE

Those caring for patients at home also need to know how to carry out safe and effective transfers. You may be asked to teach family members appropriate procedures for their situation. It may also be useful for you to assess the home environment so that it can be adapted to accommodate the client's needs, including adequate space and special equipment necessary for maximum safety.

CRITICAL THINKING EXERCISES

• Martha Evans fractured her hip in a fall at home. The surgeon repaired the fracture 2 days ago and has just ordered that Ms. Evans be up in a chair with no weight-bearing on the affected leg. Ms. Evans is alert and oriented and states that she fell when she got dizzy, although she has no idea why that might have happened. She is a thin, slightly frail woman who looks her 77 years. Based on this information, choose a method of transfer. Explain what additional information you would like to have before transferring the patient into a chair. Describe the specific criteria you will use to evaluate Ms. Evans' transfer.

• Maude Jefferson is an 84-year-old nursing home resident. She goes to the dining room in a wheelchair for her meals. Although she can walk a few steps to a chair with assistance, she is unsteady and states that she is afraid of falling. You are to plan her care for the day. Evaluate the various types of transfers possible in relation to the abilities and deficits Ms. Jefferson appears to have. Identify the reasons each particular transfer technique would be appropriate or inappropriate for use with this individual. Plan an appropriate transfer technique.

© 1996 by Lippincott-Raven Publishers

✔ **PERFORMANCE CHECKLIST**

General Procedure for Transfer	Needs More Practice	Satisfactory	Comments
Assessment			
1. Check patient's diagnosis and restrictions.			
2. Assess patient.			
3. Identify equipment and help available.			
Planning			
4. Devise plan for transfer.			
5. Wash your hands.			
6. Obtain equipment needed.			
Implementation			
7. Identify patient.			
8. Place shoes or slippers on patient.			
9. Put transfer belt on patient if needed for the transfer technique being used.			
10. Lower the entire bed.			
11. Explain method of transfer to patient.			
12. Carry out specific procedure.			
13. Retake vital signs.			
14. Wash your hands.			
Evaluation			
15. Evaluate using the following criteria: a. Patient's body alignments correct.			
b. Patient is comfortable.			
c. Patient remains safe.			
d. Patient's vital signs remain stable.			
e. Nurse(s) involved maintained safety and used proper body mechanics.			
Documentation			
16. Record on Kardex or nursing care plan: a. Best method and aids to use			
b. Number of people needed to help			
c. Patient's ability to participate			

(continued)

© 1996 by Lippincott-Raven Publishers

General Procedure for Transfer *(Continued)*	Needs More Practice	Satisfactory	Comments
17. Record on patient's chart: **a.** Activity carried out			
b. Time of activity			
c. Patient's response			
Bed to Chair: One-Person Maximal Assist			
Assessment			
1–3. Follow checklist steps 1–3 of the General Procedure for Transfer (check patient's diagnosis and restrictions; assess patient; identify equipment and help available).			
Planning			
4.–6. Follow checklist steps 4–6 of the General Procedure (devise plan for transfer; wash your hands; obtain equipment needed).			
Implementation			
4–11. Follow checklist steps 7–11 of the General Procedure (identify patient; place shoes or slippers on patient; put transfer belt on patient if indicated; lower the entire bed; explain method of transfer to patient).			
12. Transfer the patient from bed to wheelchair or armchair as outlined below: **a.** Angle chair to bed on patient's stronger side.			
b. Lock or brace bed and chair.			
c. Have patient in supine position.			
d. Raise head of bed slowly.			
e. Swing patient's legs over side of bed while pivoting patient's body to achieve sitting position.			
f. Allow patient to sit for a few moments.			
g. Place patient's feet slightly apart, and position patient's hands on the bed.			
h. Straddle patient's knees with your own, keeping wide stance and knees bent, and grasp belt.			
i. Inform patient of signal.			

(continued)

© 1996 by Lippincott-Raven Publishers

Bed to Chair: One-Person Maximal Assist *(Continued)*	Needs More Practice	Satisfactory	Comments
j. On the count, straighten your knees, lifting patient to a standing position.			
k. Stand close to patient, and pivot to chair.			
l. Instruct patient to place hands on armrests.			
m. Lower patient to seat.			
n. Be sure patient's buttocks are positioned in back of seat.			
13.–14. Follow checklist steps 13 and 14 of the General Procedure (retake vital signs, and wash hands).			
Evaluation			
15. Evaluate using the criteria in checklist step 15 of the General Procedure (patient's body alignment is correct; patient is comfortable; patient remains safe; patient's vital signs remained stable; and Nurse(s) involved maintained safety and used proper body mechanics).			
Documentation			
16.–17. Record as in checklist steps 16 and 17 of the General Procedure (on the Kardex or nursing care plan, best method and aids to use, number of people needed to help, and patient's ability to participate; on the patient's chart, activity carried out, time of activity, and patient's response).			
Bed to Chair: Two-Person Maximal Assist			
Assessment			
1.–3. Follow checklist steps 1–3 of the General Procedure for Transfer (check patient's diagnosis and restrictions; assess patient; identify equipment; and help available).			
Planning			
4.–6. Follow checklist steps 4–6 of the General Procedure (devise plan for transfer; wash your hands; obtain equipment needed).			

(continued)

© 1996 by Lippincott-Raven Publishers

Bed to Chair: Two-Person Maximal Assist *(Continued)*	Needs More Practice	Satisfactory	Comments
Implementation			
7.–11. Follow checklist steps 7–11 of the General Procedure (identify patient; place shoes or slippers on patient; put transfer belt on patient if indicated; lower the entire bed; explain method of transfer to patient).			
12. Transfer the patient from bed to wheelchair or armchair as outlined below: **a.** Put bed in flat position, and lock it.			
b. Position wheelchair at 45-degree angle and lock.			
c. Assist patient to sit.			
d. Have patient place hands on bed.			
e. Nurse 1 stands in front of patient and grasps belt at sides.			
f. Nurse 2 stands between chair and bed, with one knee on bed, and grasps belt at back.			
g. Nurse 1 informs patient of signal.			
h. Nurse 1 signals, and both lift.			
i. Position patient crrectly in chair.			
13.–14. Follow checklist steps 13 and 14 of the General Procedure (retake vital signs, and wash hands).			
Evaluation			
15. Evaluate using the criteria in checklist step 15 of the General Procedure (patient's body alignment is correct; patient is comfortable; patient remains safe; patient's vital signs remain stable; and Nurses involved maintained safety and used proper body mechanics).			
Documentation			
16.–17. Record as in checklist steps 14 and 15 of the General Procedure (on the Kardex or nursing care plan, best method and aids to use, number of people needed to help, and patient's ability to participate; on the patient's chart, activity carried out, time of activity, and patient's response).			

(continued)

© 1996 by Lippincott-Raven Publishers

Chair to Chair: Two-Person Lift	Needs More Practice	Satisfactory	Comments
Assessment			
1.–3. Follow checklist steps 1–3 of the General Procedure for Transfer (check patient's diagnosis and restrictions; assess patient; identify equipment and help available).			
Planning			
4.–6. Follow checklist steps 4–6 of the General Procedure (devise plan for transfer; wash your hands; obtain equipment needed).			
Implementation			
7.–11. Follow Checklist steps 7–11 of the General Procedure (identify parent; place shoes or slippers on patient; lower the entire bed; and explain method of transfer to patient).			
12. Transfer the patient from chair to chair or commode as outlined below:			
a. Place chairs (chair and commode) side by side.			
b. Remove footrests from chair, and lock or brace chair (commode).			
c. Taller nurse (nurse 1) stands behind chair with patient.			
d. Shorter nurse (nurse 2) stands facing patient.			
e. Nurse 1 crosses patient's arms and grasps wrists from behind.			
f. Nurse 2 squats and grasps patient around knees.			
g. Nurse 1 informs patient of signal.			
h. Nurse 1 counts.			
i. On *"lift,"* both nurses lift patient and move to second chair (or commode).			
13.–14. Follow checklist steps 13 and 14 of the General Procedure (retake vital signs, and wash hands).			

(continued)

© 1996 by Lippincott-Raven Publishers

Chair to Chair: Two-Person Lift *(Continued)*	Needs More Practice	Satisfactory	Comments
Evaluation			
15. Evaluate using the criteria in checklist step 15 of the General Procedure (patient's body alignment is correct; patient is comfortable; patient remained safe; patient's vital signs remained stable; and Nurses involved maintained safety and used proper body mechanics).			
Documentation			
16.–17. Record as in checklist steps 16 and 17 of the General Procedure (on the Kardex or nursing care plan, best method and aids to use, number of people needed to help, and patient's ability to participate; on the patient's chart activity carried out, time of activity, and patient's response).			
Bed to Chair: Two-Person Lift			
Assessment			
1.–3. Follow checklist steps 1–3 of the General Procedure for Transfer (check patient's diagnosis and restrictions; assess patient; identify equipment and help available).			
Planning			
4.–6. Follow checklist steps 4–6 of the General Procedure (devise plan for transfer; wash your hands; obtain equipment needed).			
Implementation			
7.–11. Follow checklist steps 7–11 of the General Procedure (identify patient; place shoes or slippers on patient; explain method of transfer to patient; lower the entire bed).			
12. Transfer the patient from bed to chair, wheelchair, or commode as outlined below: **a.** Put bed flat, and lock it.			
b. Position chair parallel to bed and secure brakes.			
c. Slide patient to edge of bed.			

(continued)

© 1996 by Lippincott-Raven Publishers

Bed to Chair: Two-Person Lift *(Continued)*	Needs More Practice	Satisfactory	Comments
d. Nurse 1 slides arm under patient's shoulders and maneuvers patient to sitting position.			
e. Nurse 1 crosses patient's arms over chest and grasps opposite wrists.			
f. Nurse 2 squats beside bed and slides arms under patient's thighs.			
g. Nurse 1 informs patient of signal.			
h. Lift at nurse 1's signal.			
13.–14. Follow checklist steps 13 and 14 of the General Procedure (retake vital signs, and wash hands).			
Evaluation			
15. Evaluate using the criteria in checklist step 15 of the General Procedure (patient's body alignment is correct; patient is comfortable; patient remain safe; patient's vital signs remain stable; and Nurses involved maintained safety and used proper body mechanics).			
Documentation			
16.–17. Record as in checklist step 16 and 17 of the General Procedure (on the Kardex or nursing care plan, best method and aids to use, number of people needed to help, and patient's ability to participate; on the patient's chart, activity carried out, time of activity, and patient's response).			
Six-Point Seated Transfer: Two-Person Lift			
Assessment			
1.–3. Follow checklist steps 1–3 of the General Procedure for Transfer (check patient's diagnosis and restrictions; assess patient; identify equipment and help available).			
Planning			
4.–6. Follow checklist steps 4–6 of the General Procedure (devise plan for transfer; wash your hands; obtain equipment needed).			

(continued)

© 1996 by Lippincott-Raven Publishers

Six-Point Seated Transfer: Two-Person Lift *(Continued)*	Needs More Practice	Satisfactory	Comments
Implementation			
7.–11. Follow checklist steps 7–11 of the General Procedure (identify patient; place shoes or slippers on patient; put transfer belt on patient if indicated; lower the entire bed; explain method of transfer to patient).			
12. Transfer the patient as outlined below: **a.** Place the two seats at right angles and lock both.			
b. Remove both armrests from wheelchair.			
c. Both nurses stand facing patient.			
d. Secure transfer belt around patient's waist if patient is not wearing trousers.			
e. Both nurses place forearm nearest patient under thighs of patient from inner side (or secure transfer belt around both thighs of patient, and grasp transfer belt).			
f. Instruct and assist patient to lean forward with arms resting over the backs of nurses.			
g. Both nurses grasp patient's waistband or transfer belt with outside hand.			
h. Inform patient of signal.			
i. Count. Both nurses lift patient straight up by coming to a complete standing position with shoulders back. Patient flexes forward.			
j. Turn and place patient onto chair or bed.			
13.–14. Follow checklist steps 13 and 14 of the General Procedure (retake vital signs, and wash hands).			
Evaluation			
15. Evaluate using the criteria in Checklist step 15 of the General Procedure (patient's body alignment is correct; patient is comfortable; patient remained safe; patient's vital signs remain stable; the nurses involved used safety and proper body mechanics).			

(continued)

© 1996 by Lippincott-Raven Publishers

Six-Point Seated Transfer: Two-Person Lift *(Continued)*	Needs More Practice	Satisfactory	Comments
Documentation			
16.–17. Record as in checklist steps 16 and 17 of the General Procedure (on the Kardex or nursing care plan, best method and aids to use, number of people needed to help, and patient's ability to participate; on the patient's chart, activity carried out, time of activity, and patient's response).			
Bed to Chair: Mechanical Lift			
Assessment			
1.–3. Follow checklist steps 1–3 of the General Procedure for Transfer (check patient's diagnosis and restrictions; assess patient; identify equipment and help available).			
Planning			
4.–6. Follow checklist steps 4–6 of the General Procedure (devise plan for transfer; wash your hands; obtain equipment needed).			
Implementation			
7.–9. Follow checklist steps 7–9 of the General Procedure (identify patient and place shoes or slippers on patient).			
10. Raise bed to comfortable working position.			
11. Explain lift to patient.			
12. Using the mechanical lift, transfer the patient as indicated below: **a.** Place patient in supine position.			
b. Position sling correctly, and drape patient if necessary.			
c. Place bed in low position.			
d. Position lift over patient.			
e. Place patient's arms across chest.			
f. Fasten lift's chains.			
g. Nurse 1 stands at patient's head.			
h. Nurse 2 operates device.			

(continued)

© 1996 by Lippincott-Raven Publishers

Bed to Chair: Mechanical Lift *(Continued)*	Needs More Practice	Satisfactory	Comments
i. Nurse 1 guides and supports patient's head while nurse 2 moves lift away from bed.			
j. Double-check draping.			
k. Slowly move lift to new position.			
l. Position patient above next resting place.			
m. Lower patient slowly.			
n. Turnoff switch or close valve.			
o. Detach chains from sling.			
13.–14. Follow checklist steps 13 and 14 of the General Procedure (retake vital signs and wash your hands).			
Evaluation			
15. Evaluate using the criteria in checklist step 15 of the General Procedure (patient's body alignment is correct; patient is comfortable; patient remains safe; patient's vital signs remain stable; Nurses involved maintained safety and used proper body mechanics).			
Documentation			
16.–17. Record as in checklist steps 16 and 17 of the General Procedure (on the Kardex or nursing care plan, best method and aids to use, number of people needed to help, and patient's ability to participate; on the patient's chart, activity carried out, time of activity, and patient's response).			
Horizontal Slide: Using a Transfer Slider Board			
Assessment			
1.–3. Follow checklist steps 1–3 of the General Procedure for Transfer (Check patient's diagnosis and restrictions; assess patient; identify equipment and help available).			
Planning			
4.–6. Follow checklist steps 4–6 of the General Procedure (devise plan for transfer; wash your hands; obtain equipment needed).			

(continued)

© 1996 by Lippincott-Raven Publishers

Horizontal Slide: Using a Transfer Slider Board *(Continued)*	Needs More Practice	Satisfactory	Comments
Implementation			
7. Identify the patient as in checklist step 7 of the General Procedure.			
8.–11. Omit steps 8–11 of the General Procedure.			
12. Transfer patient from bed to stretcher using a slide: **a.** Nurse 1 stands on side of bed by stretcher and nurse 2 is on opposite side of the bed.			
b. Nurse 1 lowers side rail and places stretcher with slider board covered with sheet alongside the bed.			
c. Nurse 2 rolls patient toward him or her while nurse 1 slides the board across the dividing space and under patient.			
d. Nurse 2 rolls patient back over partially onto board, rolling the patient as necessary.			
e. Nurse 1 grasps sheet at shoulders and hips.			
f. Nurse 2 lifts sheet, transferring patient's weight as nurse 1 firmly pulls sheet and patient across slider board to stretcher.			
g. Remove sheet if patient is being returned to bed.			
13.–14. Follow checklist steps 13 and 14 of the General Procedure (retake vital signs, and wash your hands).			
Evaluation			
15. Evaluate using the criteria in checklist step 15 of the General Procedure (patient's body alignment is correct; patient is comfortable; patient remains safe; patient's vital signs remain stable; nurse(s) involved maintained safety and used proper body mechanics.)			

(continued)

© 1996 by Lippincott-Raven Publishers

Horizontal Slide: Using a Transfer Slider Board *(Continued)*	Needs More Practice	Satisfactory	Comments
Documentation			
16.–17. Record as in checklist steps 16 and 17 of the General Procedure (on the Kardex or nursing care plan, method of transfer and aids to use, number of people needed, and patient's ability to participate; on the patient's chart, activity carried out, time of activity, and patient's response.)			
Horizontal Lift: Two- or Three-Person Assist			
Assessment			
1.–3. Follow checklist steps 1–3 of the General Procedure for Transfer (check patient's diagnosis and restrictions; assess patient; and identify equipment and help available).			
Planning			
4.–6. Follow checklist steps 4–6 of the General Procedure (devise plan for transfer; wash your hands; obtain equipment needed).			
Implementation			
7. Identify patient as in checklist step 7 of the General Procedure.			
8.–11. Omit steps 8–11 of the General Procedure.			
12. Transfer the patient as outlined below: **a.** Place stretcher at right angle to bed.			
b. Move patient to edge of bed.			
c. Tallest nurse (1) stands at patient's head and shoulders.			
d. Second tallest nurse (2) stands at patient's waist and hips.			
e. Shortest nurse (3) stands at patient's legs.			
f. Nurse 2 informs patient of signal.			
g. Using elbows as levers, roll and lift at signal.			

(continued)

© 1996 by Lippincott-Raven Publishers

Horizontal Lift: Two- or Three-Person Assist *(Continued)*	Needs More Practice	Satisfactory	Comments
h. Nurses hold patient and walk to stretcher.			
i. At signal, nurses place patient on stretcher.			
13. and 14. Follow checklist steps 13 and 14 of the General Procedure (retake vital signs, and wash your hands).			
Evaluation			
15. Evaluate using the criteria in checklist step 15 of the General Procedure (patient's body alignment is correct; patient is comfortable; patient remains safe; patient's vital signs remain stable; and Nurses involved maintained safety and used proper body mechanics).			
Documentation			
16.–17. Record as in checklist steps 16 and 17 of the General Procedure (on the Kardex or nursing care plan, best method and aids to use, number of people needed to help, and patient's ability to participate; on the patient's chart, activity carried out, time of activity, and patient's response).			

© 1996 by Lippincott-Raven Publishers

? **Q U I Z**

Short-Answer Questions

1. List four reasons for patient activity.

   a. _____

   b. _____

   c. _____

   d. _____

2. State two reasons for having the patient wear shoes or slippers with firm soles when being transferred.

   a. _____

   b. _____

3. What should you do if a patient begins to fall during a transfer?

   _____

4. How would right-sided paralysis affect a patient's transfer?

   _____

5. What is the purpose of a transfer belt?

   _____

6. Name two transfer techniques for which a transfer belt is used.

   a. _____

   b. _____

7. Why is a patient changed from a lying-down to a sitting position slowly?

   _____

8. State two criteria that may be used in evaluating the transfer of a patient.

   a. _____

   b. _____

9. The response of a patient to transfer might be documented by observing

   _____ , _____ , and _____ .

10. In what situation would you use a plastic transfer slider board? _____

   _____

11. What are the safety concerns related to doing a two-person lift to transfer a patient from a bed to a chair? _____

   _____

© 1996 by Lippincott-Raven Publishers

MODULE

21

AMBULATION: SIMPLE ASSISTED AND USING CANE, WALKER, OR CRUTCHES

MODULE CONTENTS

Rationale for the Use of This Skill
Nursing Diagnosis
General Procedure for Ambulation
  Assessment
  Planning
  Implementation
  Evaluation
  Documentation
PROCEDURES FOR SPECIFIC TYPES
  OF AMBULATION
Simple Assisted Ambulation
Using a Cane

Using a Walker
Crutchwalking
  Adjusting Crutches for Size
  Determining the Appropriate Gait
  Standing, Walking, and Sitting Using
    Crutches
  Crutchwalking Up Stairs With Railing
  Crutchwalking Up Stairs Without Railing
  Crutchwalking Down Stairs
LONG-TERM CARE
HOME CARE
CRITICAL THINKING EXERCISES

PREREQUISITES

Successful completion of the following modules:

VOLUME 1
Module 1 An Approach to Nursing Skills
Module 2 Basic Infection Control
Module 3 Safety
Module 4 Basic Body Mechanics
Module 5 Documentation

© 1996 by Lippincott-Raven Publishers

OVERALL OBJECTIVE

To assist patients to ambulate safely, taking into account their capabilities and when indicated, using the appropriate assistive device(s).

SPECIFIC LEARNING OBJECTIVES

Know Facts and Principles	Apply Facts and Principles	Demonstrate Ability	Evaluate Performance
1. Reasons for physical activity			
List four ways physical activity can improve patient status.	Given a patient situation, state purpose(s) for physical activity.	In clinical experiences, give rationale for patients' physical activities.	
2. Safety			
List common hazards of ambulation and of assistive devices.	Recognize hazards in a patient situation.	Provide safe setting for ambulation. Maintain correct body mechanics for self and patient.	Determine that patient was not injured in ambulation.
3. Assessment of patient			
State reasons for knowing patient's diagnosis and capabilities.	Give examples of how different diagnoses and capabilities would affect plans for ambulation.	Gather data on patient's abilities and diagnoses before ambulating patient.	After ambulation, review procedure to find whether more data would have helped. Validate with instructor.
4. Ambulation of patient			
State ways of supporting patient while ambulating. Describe various gait patterns used for cane, walker, or crutches.	Plan specific means of support for a particular patient. Given a patient situation, describe gait pattern that would be used for each assistive device.	Ambulate patient safely with supervision. Correctly assist patient with use of assistive devices.	Evaluate own performance using Performance Checklist.
5. Documentation			
List data to be recorded on nursing care plan. List data to be recorded on patient's chart.	Given a patient situation, determine what should be recorded on nursing care plan and on patient's chart.	In the clinical setting, update nursing care plan on patient's ambulation status. In the clinical setting, chart activity and patient's response.	Evaluate own performance using Performance Checklist.

© 1996 by Lippincott-Raven Publishers

LEARNING ACTIVITIES

1. Review the Specific Learning Objectives.
2. Read the chapter on activity and rest in Ellis and Nowlis, *Nursing: A Human Needs Approach*, or a comparable chapter in another textbook.
3. Look up the module vocabulary terms in the glossary.
4. Read through the module as though you were preparing to teach the module content to another person. Mentally practice the techniques.
5. In the practice setting, do the following:
   a. Practice ambulation with a partner. Take turns being the patient and being the nurse. Use a colored tie or scarf to mark one of the patient's legs as the affected leg.
   b. Using the procedures in the module, practice each ambulation technique. Review the teaching and explanations for the patient each time. When you are the patient, evaluate your partner's performance using the Performance Checklist. Practice each of the following techniques:
      (1) Simple assisted ambulation
      (2) Using a cane
      (3) Using a walker
      (4) Using crutches (including three-point gait, three-point-plus-one gait, four-point gait, sitting down with crutches, and crutches on stairs)
   c. When you believe that you have mastered these skills, ask your instructor to evaluate your performance.
6. In the clinical setting, do the following:
   a. Observe a physical therapist's technique for ambulating patients.
   b. Seek opportunities to ambulate patients.
   c. Ask your instructor to approve your plan and supervise you.

VOCABULARY

gait
gait belt
FBW full weight-bearing
LOB loss of balance
PWB partial weight-bearing
SBA stand-by assist

© 1996 by Lippincott-Raven Publishers

Ambulation: Simple Assisted and Using Cane, Walker, or Crutches

Rationale for the Use of This Skill

Ambulation maintains and restores muscle tone, muscle strength, and joint flexibility. In addition, it helps individuals improve balance. Mobility also improves appetite and stimulates the respiratory and circulatory systems, increasing the effective functioning of each system. It stimulates bowel action, thus facilitating bowel elimination. It also enhances the patient's psychological well-being, which is a move toward optimal health.[1]

▼ NURSING DIAGNOSIS

The ambulation techniques in this module are valuable for patients who have the nursing diagnosis of Impaired Physical Mobility. The specific etiology and defining characteristics will help to determine which assistive devices or methods of assistance are appropriate.

GENERAL PROCEDURE FOR AMBULATION

The following is a general approach to help patients walk and can be modified as needed for each patient.

Assessment

1. Identify the patient's capabilities.
2. Identify the activity ordered.
3. Check the patient's previous level of activity.
4. Determine whether assistive devices were previously used.
5. Take pulse, respirations, and blood pressure *to provide a baseline.*

Planning

6. Plan for pain relief, if indicated, before ambulation. Be sure to allow enough time for the medication to take effect before the patient begins to ambulate.
7. With the patient, set a tentative goal for how far the patient will ambulate.
8. Decide how much support the patient will need.
9. Plan to use a specific technique.
10. Wash your hands *for infection control.*

[1]Note that rationales for action are emphasized throughout the module by the use of italics.

Implementation

11. Identify the patient *to be sure that you are carrying out the procedure for the correct patient.*
12. Explain to the patient what you are planning to do, and encourage questions *so that he or she can participate fully in the activity.*
13. Obtain the patient's robe and shoes. The patient must be covered *for warmth and modesty.* Firm-soled, supportive shoes are best for ambulation *because they give the patient additional stability.* If shoes are not available, use slippers. If at all possible, avoid "scuffs," which can easily slip off, and cloth slippers, which tend to slide on smooth floors. The area should be litter-free and spill-free *so that the patient does not fall or slip.*
14. Adjust the bed to low position, and help the patient to stand, using the techniques and devices discussed in Module 20, Transfer, and later in this module.
15. Using the directions given for the specific type of ambulation, assist the patient to ambulate.
16. Watch the patient carefully for signs of fatigue or faintness or for other adverse responses. If the patient feels faint, move him or her to the nearest chair to sit with the head down *to enhance blood flow to the brain.* Ask someone else to get a wheelchair *so you can return the patient to bed.*

    It is wise to be familiar with the environment when you are ambulating a patient *so that you know where the patient can sit and rest if he or she becomes weak or unsteady.*

    If the patient loses balance slightly, help him or her regain balance. If the knees buckle and the patient makes no attempt to straighten up, control the descent to the floor. Do not try to hold the patient up: *this is likely to cause you injury and is often unsuccessful anyway.* Simply steady and support the patient, making sure that the patient's head does not strike anything, as you allow him or her to slide slowly to the floor. You will need help to return the patient to bed.
17. After completing the desired ambulation, return the patient to bed or to a chair, and position for comfort.
18. Recheck pulse, respirations, and blood pressure.
19. Wash your hands *for infection control.*

Evaluation

20. Compare preambulation and postambulation vital signs, and note major changes, such as a drop or rise in blood pressure of more than 10 mm Hg, a rise in respirations to tachypnea, or a change in pulse of more than 20 beats/min.
21. Check the patient's fatigue or pain level.

© 1996 by Lippincott-Raven Publishers

22. Ask whether the patient feels better as a result of the exercise.
23. Evaluate effects on overall strength, balance, and ability to ambulate.
24. Evaluate use of special techniques or assistive devices.

Documentation

25. Document the activity as appropriate for your facility. In most instances, any new information about times planned for activity, the best method, assistive aids or number of people needed, and the patient's ability to participate is recorded on the nursing care plan. The specific activity carried out, the time, the distance ambulated, and the patient's response and abilities are usually noted on the patient's chart, either on a flow sheet or in the nurse's progress notes.

PROCEDURES FOR SPECIFIC TYPES OF AMBULATION

For each procedure discussed, some steps of the General Procedure may be modified. The modified steps and references to the steps of the General Procedure that remain the same follow.

Simple Assisted Ambulation

Assessment

1.–5. Follow the steps of the General Procedure for Ambulation.

Planning

6.–10. Follow the steps of the General Procedure.

Implementation

11.–14. Follow the steps of the General Procedure.
15. Assist the patient to ambulate.
    a. In most cases, walk on the patient's weaker or affected side *so that if the patient falters, you can give assistance and support.* However, if the patient has poor balance and tends to lean toward the person assisting, walk on the patient's strong side, *so that the patient's weight is shifted to the strong leg, rather than the weak leg, when he or she leans.*
    b. Support the patient as you walk, but do not allow the patient to put an arm around your shoulders. *If the patient starts to fall, the weight could place a twisting strain on your back and cause severe injury.* Instead, offer support by extending an arm bent at the elbow with the palm up. The patient can then rest a hand on your arm. *You can maintain firm support, and*

the patient can determine how much support is needed.

Another way to provide safety with minimal support is to use a gait belt (sometimes called a transfer and ambulation belt) around the patient's waist. This is a strong webbing belt with a safety release buckle. In this instance, you walk on the patient's weaker side and slightly behind, with one hand grasping the belt in the center back. The other arm may be extended at the patient's side for the patient to grasp (Fig. 21–1).

If you do not know the patient, you may wish to begin with a gait belt and then evaluate whether it is needed.
    c. Walk slowly and with an even gait. *It is very difficult for a patient if your gait is uneven;* therefore, avoid speeding up and slowing down. Synchronize your steps with the patient's. Also, try to make your steps the same size as the patient's, *which will make your supportive arm feel more stable to the patient. By using smooth, coordinated movements, you give the patient confidence in you and diminish fear of falling.*

16.–19. Follow the steps of the General Procedure.

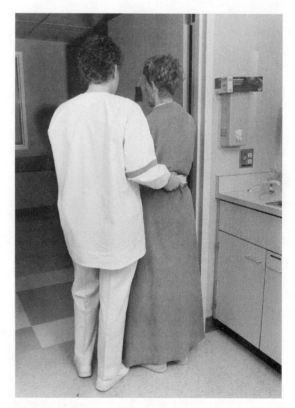

Figure 21–1. Ambulation. The nurse stands on the patient's weaker side and grasps the ambulation belt. The patient also may hold a cane on the stronger side. (Courtesy Ivan Ellis.)

© 1996 by Lippincott-Raven Publishers

Evaluation
20.–24. Follow the steps of the General Procedure.

Documentation
25. Follow the General Procedure.

Using a Cane

A cane is used by those who need help with balance or who are able to bear weight on both legs but have one leg weaker than the other. All canes should have a rubber tip *to prevent slipping.* The height of the cane should be that of the wrist, allowing for 25% to 30% bend at the elbow when the patient places weight on the cane. If the cane is used to help in balance, encourage the patient to use a normal gait and to go slowly *so that the cane is easy to use.* This does take time to perfect. A quad cane is used *when maximum support is needed* (Fig. 21–2).

When a cane is used to augment a weak leg, a special gait is often useful. The gait usually is taught by a physical therapist, who also is responsible for securing and measuring the cane. You support the therapist's instructions and help the patient practice.

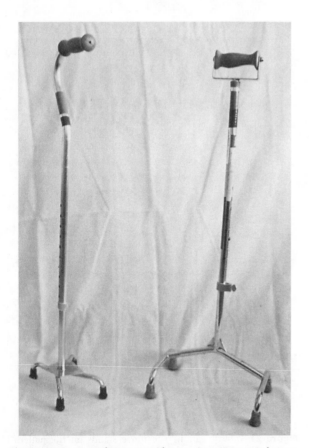

Figure 21–2. A quad cane provides maximum support for ambulation. (Courtesy Ivan Ellis.)

Assessment
1.–5. Follow the steps of the General Procedure for Ambulation.

Planning
6.–10. Follow the steps of the General Procedure.

Implementation
11.–13. Follow the steps of the General Procedure.
14. Omit step 14 of the General Procedure.
15. Assist the patient to ambulate using a cane.
  a. Teach the patient to stand up from a sitting position, as follows:
    (1) Grasp the cane in the hand *opposite* the affected leg *for support.*
    (2) Slide the hips forward in the chair *to make standing easier.*
    (3) Grasp one arm of the chair with the free hand. With the other hand, grasp the cane and the chair arm, if possible. If the patient cannot grasp both, only the cane is grasped.
    (4) Push to a standing position, using the arms of the chair *for support.* Encourage this type of independence. If the patient needs help to stand, give only the help that is needed, and allow maximum independence. *This will help to develop muscle strength and balance and promote psychological well-being.*
    (5) After standing, pause in place, *to gain balance and to place the cane initially. This keeps the patient from tripping on the cane.* Balance is best maintained if the cane is placed close to the foot *so that the patient remains erect, not bent over* (Fig. 21–3).
  b. Walk to the side and slightly behind the patient *to provide support if needed.* You may want to use a gait belt until you have determined that the patient is strong enough to walk without the added support.
  c. Teach the patient to carry out the gait pattern, as follows:
    (1) Move the cane ahead approximately 4 to 6 inches.
    (2) Move the affected leg ahead opposite the cane.
    (3) Place the weight on the affected leg and the cane.
    (4) Move the unaffected leg forward. The steps of both legs should remain equal *to promote a normal walking pattern* (Fig. 21–4).
    (5) Repeat the sequence.
  d. Teach the patient to sit, as follows:

© 1996 by Lippincott-Raven Publishers

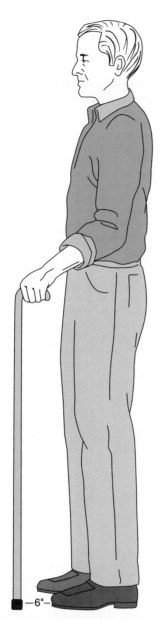

Figure 21–3. Proper cane stance. Cane on strong side; elbow slightly flexed. Cane is to the side and 6 inches in front of the foot.

(1) Using the cane, approach the chair, turn around, and back up to the chair.
(2) Reach behind to grasp one arm of the chair with the free hand. With the other hand, grasp the cane and the other arm of the chair, if possible. If the patient cannot grasp both, only the cane is grasped.
(3) The patient lowers himself or herself into the chair, placing the cane beneath the chair so that someone else does not fall over it. If the cane is a quad cane, it is

placed to the side of the chair, within easy reach of the patient.
16.–19. Follow the steps of the General Procedure.

Evaluation
20.–24. Follow the steps of the General Procedure.

Documentation
25. Follow the General Procedure.

Using a Walker

Walkers are assistive devices used by patients who have at least one weight-bearing leg and arms strong enough to bear partial weight. They also may be used by patients with generalized weakness and those with balance problems. *A walker gives greater support and stability than a cane.* Walkers are of two types, pick-up and rolling. The pick-up walker is more stable; *it does not slip when the patient leans on it* (Fig. 21–5). The *rolling walker* allows a smooth, normal gait but is less steady. Usually, the physical therapist determines which style of walker will be used. When there is a question, the more stable pick-up walker is generally recommended. Walkers can be adjusted in height. Ideally, they should reach slightly below waist level *so that the handgrips can be grasped with comfort and so that the arms are slightly flexed to give strength to the support.*

Assessment
1.–5. Follow the steps of the General Procedure for Ambulation.

Planning
6.–10. Follow the steps of the General Procedure.

Implementation
11.–13. Follow the steps of the General Procedure.
14. Omit step 14 of the General Procedure.
15. Assist the patient to ambulate using a walker.
   a. Teach the patient to stand up from a sitting position, as follows:
   (1) Place the walker in front of the seat. (You may wish to place a gait belt on the patient's waist until you are certain the patient is stable.)
   (2) Place both hands on the arms of the chair and push up to a standing position. You can grasp the gait belt for safety if needed. The patient uses the chair instead of the walker when getting up *because the lower chair allows him or her to push with more force. Furthermore, the walker is less stable, and the patient could pull it over when trying to use it to stand.*
   (3) Move the hands to the handgrips of the walker one at a time *to maintain balance during the transfer.*

© 1996 by Lippincott-Raven Publishers

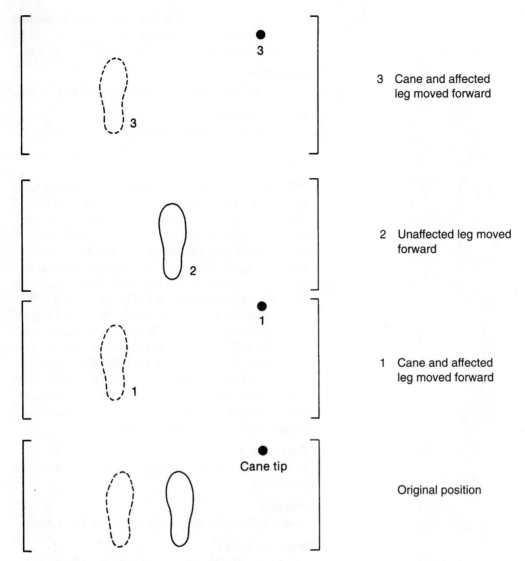

3 Cane and affected
leg moved forward

2 Unaffected leg moved
forward

1 Cane and affected
leg moved forward

Cane tip

Original position

Figure 21–4. Walking with a cane. Dashed lines indicate partial weight-bearing by the affected leg. A normal alternating stride is used, in the order shown.

b. Walk closely behind and slightly to the side of the patient.
c. Teach the patient to carry out the gait pattern, as follows:
  (1) Move the walker and the affected leg simultaneously ahead 4 to 6 inches.
  (2) Place weight on the arms *for support.* Place partial weight on the affected leg, if permitted. If no weight-bearing is allowed on the affected leg, the arms must support all the weight.
  (3) Move the unaffected leg forward.
  (4) Repeat the pattern.
d. Teach the patient to sit, as follows:
  (1) Turn around in front of the chair and back up until the legs touch the chair. *This places the patient in the correct position to sit directly onto the chair.* The walker is used for support during this maneuver.

  (2) Reach behind with one hand and then the other to grasp the arms of the chair.
  (3) Using the arms of the chair *to provide support and balance,* lower into the chair.
16.–19. Follow the steps of the General Procedure.

Evaluation
20.–24. Follow the steps of the General Procedure.

Documentation
25. Follow the General Procedure.

Crutchwalking

The physical therapist is usually responsible for initiating the crutchwalking process. This includes correctly adjusting the length of the crutches, determining the gait appropriate for the patient's condition, and initiating patient teaching.

  You must be aware of the basis for the therapist's

© 1996 by Lippincott-Raven Publishers

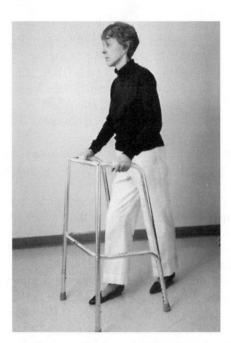

Figure 21–5. Using a walker for ambulation. Note that the arms are slightly bent, and the walker is placed squarely in front of the person.

The top of the crutch rests against the chest wall, with approximately 2 inches between the crutch top and the axilla (Fig. 21–7). The patient should not rest on the crutches in a way that puts pressure on the axillae. Doing so *causes pressure on the nerves that control the hand and can lead to numbness, tingling, muscle weakness, and even paralysis from nerve damage (crutch palsy).*

The handgrip should be placed so that the elbows are slightly flexed (approximately 30 degrees) when the hands grasp the grip. *The arm is stronger and more*

decisions *so that you can reinforce the teaching.* In addition, in some settings, you may be expected to carry out some of these functions when a physical therapist is not available.

Adjusting Crutches for Size
Crutches are adjusted so that when a patient stands upright, the tip of the crutch rests approximately 6 inches in front of the foot and 2 inches to the side of the foot (Fig. 21–6).

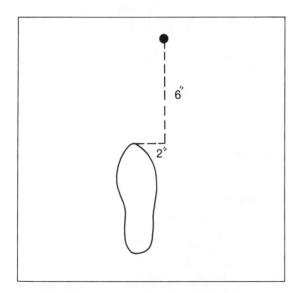

Figure 21–6. Measuring crutch position. Position the crutch tip 2 inches to the side of the foot and 6 inches ahead.

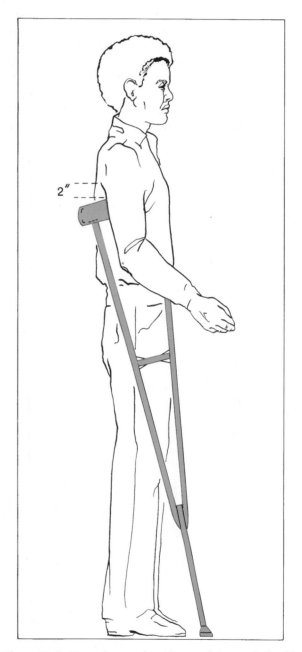

Figure 21–7. Measuring crutches. The top of the crutch should fall 2 inches below the axilla.

© 1996 by Lippincott-Raven Publishers

stable in this position than when fully extended. Also, if the arm is fully extended, the *patient may experience discomfort from strain on the elbow joint.*

Determining the Appropriate Gait

The gait is chosen according to the patient's weight-bearing ability. As you read the directions for the various gaits, you will note that some allow for no weight-bearing, some allow for partial weight-bearing, and one allows for full weight-bearing on both legs (using the crutches for balance and stability). The patient's physician will indicate whether full or partial weight-bearing is allowed. The physical therapist usually plans the specific gait pattern. The following are common gait patterns:

1. *Three-point gait.* This gait is used for patients able to bear weight on only the unaffected leg. The other leg is held off the floor (Fig. 21–8) and may be balanced straight ahead of the patient or bent at the knee and held behind the patient. Teach the patient to do the following:

   a. Support the weight on the unaffected leg.
   b. Lift crutches and affected leg simultaneously, and place forward 4 to 6 inches.
   c. Shift the weight to the crutches.
   d. Step forward on the unaffected leg so that the foot is slightly behind the crutches.
   e. Shift the weight to the unaffected leg.
   f. Repeat the pattern.

2. *Variations of the three-point gait:* Weaker patients may have to move one crutch forward at a time *to maintain better balance and support.* Very strong patients may swing the unaffected leg up past the crutches on each step. This is called the *swing-through gait* (Fig. 21–9).

3. *Three-point-plus-one gait*: This gait is used for patients who have one unaffected leg and one leg that can bear partial weight. This also is called the *three-point-with-partial-weight-bearing gait* (Fig. 21–10). Teach the patient to do the following:

   a. Stand in the crutch stance with full weight on the unaffected leg and the affected side bearing only partial weight.

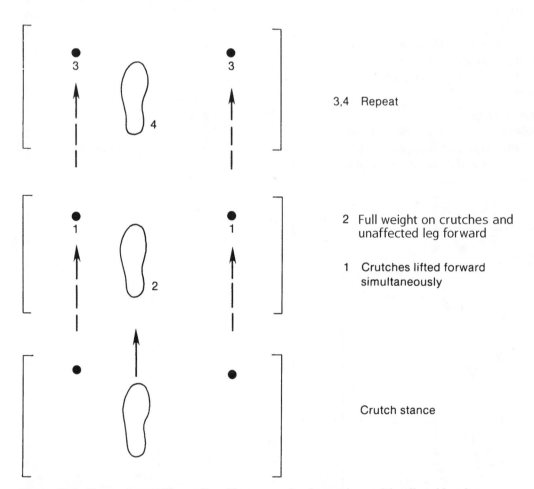

3,4 Repeat

2 Full weight on crutches and
    unaffected leg forward

1 Crutches lifted forward
    simultaneously

Crutch stance

Figure 21–8. Three-point gait. The unaffected foot moves after the crutches, and the affected foot does not touch the floor.

© 1996 by Lippincott-Raven Publishers

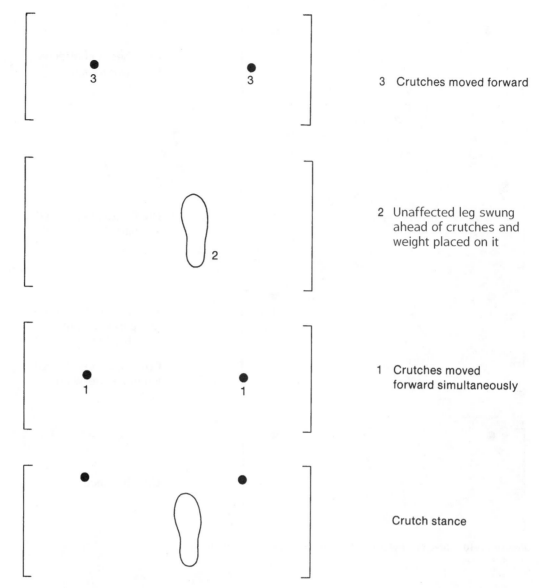

3 Crutches moved forward

2 Unaffected leg swung ahead of crutches and weight placed on it

1 Crutches moved forward simultaneously

Crutch stance

Figure 21–9. Swing-through gait. The unaffected foot comes down in front of the crutches with each step, and the affected foot does not touch the floor.

b. Shift all the weight to the unaffected leg.

c. Move the crutches and the affected leg forward 6 to 12 inches.

d. Shift the weight to the hands on the crutches, with partial weight on the affected leg.

e. Step ahead on the unaffected leg in front of the crutches. The length of the steps for both legs should be similar *to encourage a normal, even stride*.

f. Shift the weight back to the unaffected leg.

g. Repeat the pattern.

4. *Four-point gait*: This gait is used for patients with muscular weakness, lack of balance, or lack of coordination (Fig. 21–11). Teach the patient to do the following:

a. Start with the weight on both legs and both crutches. Move each leg and each crutch independently.

b. Move left crutch forward.

c. Move right leg forward.

d. Move right crutch forward.

e. Move left leg forward.

f. Repeat the pattern.

Standing, Walking, and Sitting Using Crutches

Ideally, a person using crutches should be able to ambulate safely and independently. For this to happen, the patient must understand how to use the crutches and must practice using them. Teach and

© 1996 by Lippincott-Raven Publishers

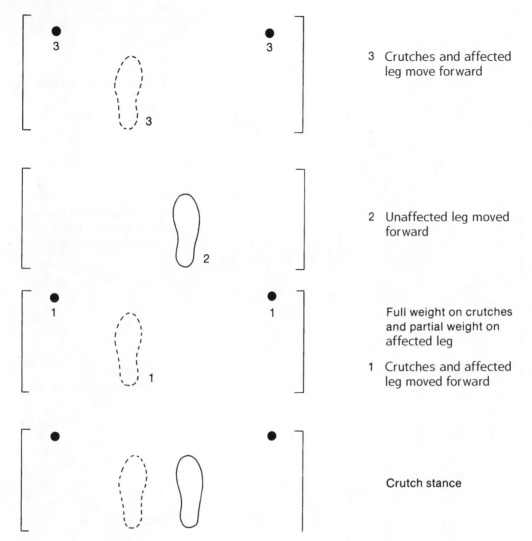

3 Crutches and affected leg move forward

2 Unaffected leg moved forward

Full weight on crutches and partial weight on affected leg

1 Crutches and affected leg moved forward

Crutch stance

Figure 21–10. Three-point-plus-one gait. The crutches move with the affected leg as it bears partial weight.

reinforce methods, encouraging the patient to ask questions about anything that is not clear.

To encourage independence, stand beside and slightly behind the patient. Be prepared to catch the patient if needed, but allow him or her to proceed unaided. A gait belt may be used.

Assessment
1.–5. Follow the steps of the General Procedure for Ambulation.

Planning
6.–10. Follow the steps of the General Procedure.

Implementation
11.–13. Follow the steps of the General Procedure.
14. Omit step 14 of the General Procedure.
15. Assist the patient to ambulate using crutches.

a. Teach the patient to stand up from a sitting position, as follows:
   (1) Stand up as a smooth movement.
   (2) Place the feet securely on the floor if possible.
   (3) To make standing easier, slide the hips forward on the chair.
   (4) Hold both crutches in the hand of the unaffected side.
   (5) Grasp the arm of the chair with the hand on the side opposite the crutches. Alternatively, push up on the bed or the seat of the chair.
   (6) Push up from the chair, using the arms of the chair or the chair or bed surface.
   (7) Stabilize the body by standing on the unaffected leg.

© 1996 by Lippincott-Raven Publishers

(8) Place the crutches under both arms.

b. Have the patient take the crutch stance. The patient balances on the unaffected leg or on both legs if weight-bearing is allowed. Carefully position the crutches under each arm, keeping the tips approximately 2 inches to the side and 6 inches in front of the feet. *This stance provides good balance.*

c. With the patient maintaining balance, implement ambulation using any of the various crutch gaits:

(1) Three-point gait

(2) Three-point-plus-one gait

(3) Four-point gait. (See "Determining the Appropriate Gait," p. 498, for a detailed description of each gait.)

d. No matter which gait has been used for walking, teach the patient to sit, as follows:

(1) Walk up to the chair, using the appropriate gait.

(2) Turn around, so that the back is to the chair and the backs of the legs touch the seat of the chair. Use the crutches *for support while turning.* Do not step on the non–weight-bearing leg.

(3) Grasp both crutches with one hand.

(4) Reach back with the other hand to grasp the arm of the chair.

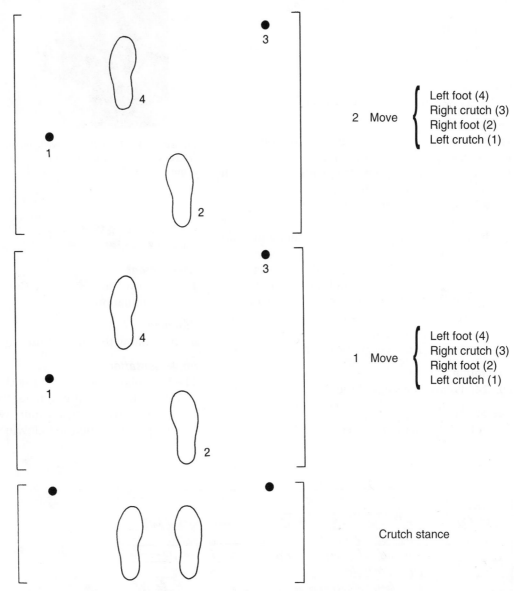

2 Move {
Left foot (4)
Right crutch (3)
Right foot (2)
Left crutch (1)
}

1 Move {
Left foot (4)
Right crutch (3)
Right foot (2)
Left crutch (1)
}

Crutch stance

Figure 21–11. Four-point gait. Each foot and each crutch is moved independently to achieve a smooth alternating gait.

© 1996 by Lippincott-Raven Publishers

(5) Lower into the chair, using the support of the crutches and the chair.

(6) Sit back in the chair, using proper body mechanics. Legs may be elevated depending on the physician's order.

(7) If legs are elevated, do not hyperextend the knees *because doing so can lead to poor circulation.*

16.–9. Follow the steps of the General Procedure.

Evaluation

20.–24. Follow the steps of the General Procedure.

Documentation

25. Follow the General Procedure.

Crutchwalking Up Stairs With Railing

Assessment

1.–5. Follow the steps of the General Procedure for Ambulation.

Planning

6.–10. Follow the steps of the General Procedure.

Implementation

11.–13. Follow the steps of the General Procedure.

14. Omit step 14 of the General Procedure.

15. For crutchwalking up stairs with railing, teach the patient to do the following:

a. Hold both crutches under one arm as if to walk (Fig. 21–12).

b. Place the other hand on the railing in front of the body.

c. Raise the unaffected leg to the first step, and pull up with hand on rail (Fig. 21–13A).

d. Pull up the affected leg, and advance crutches.

e. Again, raise the unaffected leg, pulling up the affected leg and advancing crutches.

16.–19. Follow the steps of the General Procedure.

Evaluation

20.–24. Follow the steps of the General Procedure.

Documentation

25. Follow the General Procedure.

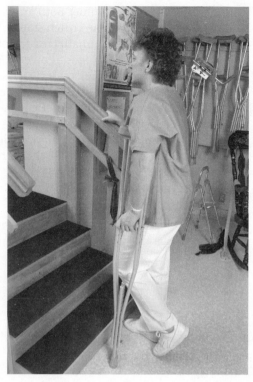

Figure 21–12. Preparing to walk up stairs with railing using crutches. Both crutches are held under one arm as if to walk. (Courtesy Ivan Ellis.)

Crutchwalking Up Stairs Without Railing

Assessment

1.–5. Follow the steps of the General Procedure for Ambulation.

Planning

6.–10. Follow the steps of the General Procedure.

Implementation

11.–13. Follow the steps of the General Procedure.

14. Omit step 14 of the General Procedure.

15. For crutchwalking up stairs with railing, teach the patient to do the following:

DATE/TIME	
11/7/99	TPR—98⁴—76—18 BP 116/72. Amb. length of hall
7:30 AM	using crutches with three-point swing-through gait.
	Remained stable and steady. Postambulation: PR 84-22
	BP 120/82. Uses gait correctly. States understands
	procedures for getting up and sitting down. — R. Riska, NS

Example of Nursing Progress Notes Using Narrative Format.

© 1996 by Lippincott-Raven Publishers

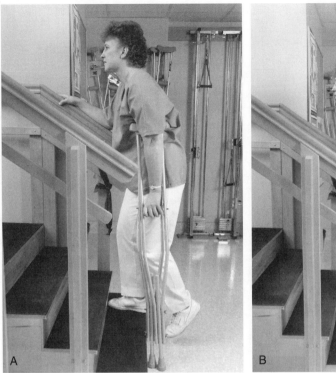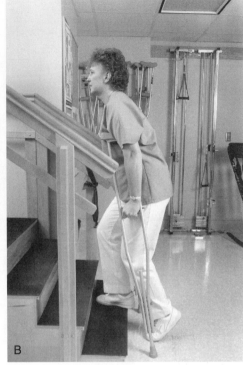

Figure 21–13(A). Walking up stairs with railing. With one hand on the railing, the unaffected leg is raised to the next step, followed by the affected leg and crutches. (Courtesy Ivan Ellis.) **(B).** Walking up stairs without railing. The unaffected leg is raised to the next step, the affected leg is pulled up, and the crutches are advanced to the same step. (Courtesy Ivan Ellis.)

a. Position the crutches under the arms as if walking.

b. Put weight on hands.

c. Raise the unaffected leg to the first step, and pull up the affected leg (Fig. 21–13B).

d. Advance the crutches to the step on which you are standing.

e. Again, raise the unaffected leg to the next

higher step, and pull up the affected leg, advancing the crutches as before.

16.–19. Follow the steps of the General Procedure.

Evaluation

20.–24. Follow the steps of the General Procedure.

Documentation

25. Follow the General Procedure.

DATE/TIME	
11/7/99 8:30 AM	Limited mobility rel. to long leg cast. TPR 98⁴ — 76 — 18 BP 116/72.
	S "I really have the hang of these crutches, and getting up and down is easy."
	O Amb. length of hall using crutches with three-point swing-through gait. Remained stable and steady. Postambulation PR 84–22 BP 120/82. Used gait correctly.
	A Making satisfactory progress in crutch walking.
	P Encourage patient to increase ambulation distance gradually. R. Riska, NS

Example of Nursing Progress Notes Using SOAP Format.

© 1996 by Lippincott-Raven Publishers

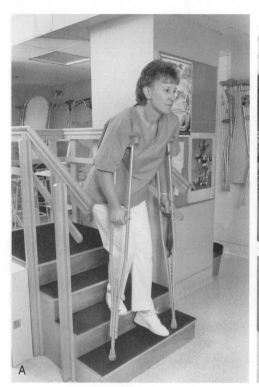
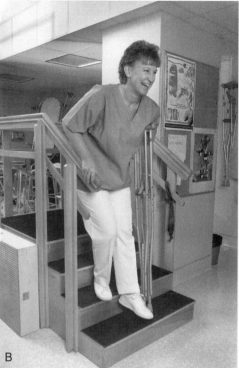

Figure 21–14. (A) Walking down stairs without railing. With weight on the unaffected leg, the crutches are placed on the next lower step, partial weight is placed on the hands and crutches, and the affected leg is moved to the lower step. **(B)** Walking down stairs with railing. With both crutches held under one arm and the other hand grasping the railing, the crutches are placed on the next lower step; partial weight is placed on the hand, crutches, and railing; and the affected leg is moved to the lower step. (Courtesy Ivan Ellis.)

Crutchwalking Down Stairs

For descending steps, reverse the procedures outlined above, taking into account the presence or absence of a railing. Until the patient is confident and performs well with crutchwalking, particularly when maneuvering on stairs, special precautions should be taken *to prevent falls.* If a second person grasps the belt on the robe or a gait belt from behind, *additional stability is ensured.*

Assessment
1.–5. Follow the steps of the General Procedure for Ambulation.

Planning
6.–10. Follow the steps of the General Procedure.

Implementation
11.–13. Follow the steps of the General Procedure.
14. Omit step 14 of the General Procedure.
15. For crutchwalking down stairs, teach the patient to do the following:

a. Position crutches under arms as if walking.
b. Place weight on unaffected leg.
c. Place crutches on next lower step.
d. Put partial weight on hands and crutches.
e. Move affected leg to lower step.
f. Put total weight on crutches and affected leg (Fig. 21–14A).
g. Move unaffected leg to same step as crutches and affected leg.
h. If a railing is present, hold both crutches with one arm, and use the other to grasp the railing (Fig. 21–14B). *The railing provides more stability than the two crutches will provide.*

16.–19. Follow the steps of the General Procedure.

Evaluation
20.–24. Follow the steps of the General Procedure.

Documentation
25. Follow the General Procedure.

© 1996 by Lippincott-Raven Publishers

LONG-TERM CARE

A major focus in all long-term care facilities is assisting the residents to stay as independent as possible. Supporting residents in maintaining their activity is an important component of that independence. Contrary to what many think, residents in long-term care can increase their ability to engage in activity with regular exercise. Assistance when necessary and encouragement to continue efforts help to sustain motivation in this process. Safety is a major concern because those who reside in long-term care facilities are often fragile and susceptible to falls.

Regular exercise programs in long-term care facilities can contribute to a feeling of increased well-being for all residents. Recent research has shown that even people in their 80s can benefit from regular muscle-strengthening exercises.

HOME CARE

Typically, more barriers to maintaining activity exist for those receiving care at home. Stairs, narrow doors, rugs, furniture placement, and inadequate lighting may all pose problems for the person trying to ambulate. You can assist clients and families to identify safety concerns and barriers to ambulation. When these problems have been identified, you can often be a resource for planning modifications. Handrails and grab bars may be installed in bathrooms and hallways. Area rugs that slip may be removed. Night lights, brighter light bulbs, and white lines painted on the edges of steps make it easier for individuals with disabilities to ambulate safely. The goal is to prevent injury and maintain or increase the present level of activity.

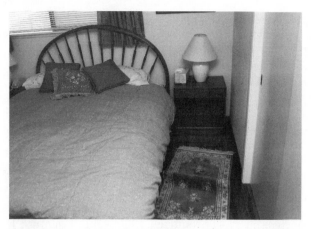

Figure 21–15. The grandmother's room. What changes will help increase safety? (Courtesy Ivan Ellis.)

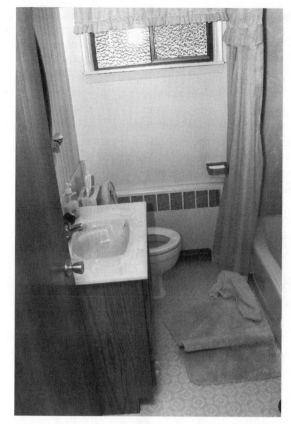

Figure 21–16. The bathroom that the grandmother uses. What changes will help increase safety? (Courtesy Ivan Ellis.)

CRITICAL THINKING EXERCISES

A frail 84-year-old woman living with her family has balance problems occasionally, but she does not require assistive devices. You are making a home visit and find the situations described below. Analyze each situation, and suggest appropriate interventions or possible alternatives.

1. The living room, dining room, kitchen, two bedrooms (one used as an office), one bathroom, and a powder room are located on the first floor. Three bedrooms, one bathroom, and a sewing room are located on the second floor. The grandmother's room is on the second floor. Two teenagers occupy the other two upstairs bedrooms. The daughter and her husband sleep in the bedroom on the first floor. Suggest alternatives to these arrangements and implications for the family.

2. Above is a photograph of the grandmother's room. Identify four changes that should be made to increase her safety (Fig. 21–15).

3. Above is a photograph of the bathroom that the grandmother uses. Determine what changes should be made to increase her safety (Fig. 21–16).

© 1996 by Lippincott-Raven Publishers

General Procedure for Ambulation	Needs More Practice	Satisfactory	Comments
Assessment			
1. Identify patient's capabilities.			
2. Identify activity ordered.			
3. Check previous level of activity.			
4. Determine whether assistive devices were used previously.			
5. Take pulse, respirations, and blood pressure.			
Planning			
6. Plan for pain relief, if indicated, before ambulation.			
7. Set tentative goal.			
8. Decide on support needed.			
9. Plan specific technique needed.			
10. Wash your hands.			
Implementation			
11. Identify patient.			
12. Explain procedure to patient.			
13. Obtain robe and shoes, and clear floor of litter or spills.			
14. Adjust bed to low position, and help patient stand.			
15. Assist the patient to ambulate according to the specific procedure below.			
16. Provide safety.			
17. Return patient to bed, and position for comfort.			
18. Recheck pulse, respirations, and blood pressure.			
19. Wash your hands.			
Evaluation			
20. Compare preambulation and postambulation vital signs.			
21. Check fatigue or pain level.			

(*continued*)

© 1996 by Lippincott-Raven Publishers

General Procedure for Ambulation *(Continued)*	Needs More Practice	Satisfactory	Comments
22. Ask how patient feels.			
23. Evaluate overall strength, balance, and ability to ambulate.			
24. Evaluate use of special techniques or assistive devices.			
Documentation			
25. Document according to facility policy.			
Simple Assisted Ambulation			
Assessment			
1.–5. Complete checklist steps 1–5 of the General Procedure for Ambulation (identify patient's capabilities, activity ordered, previous level of activity; assistive devices; take vital signs).			
Planning			
6.–10. Complete checklist steps 6–10 of the General Procedure (plan for pain relief; goal; support needed, technique; wash your hands).			
Implementation			
11.–14. Complete checklist steps 11–14 of the General Procedure (identify patient; explain procedure; obtain robe and shoes; clear floor of litter or spills; adjust position of bed, and help patient stand).			
15. Assist the patient to ambulate. **a.** Walk on appropriate side for patient's condition and ability.			
b. Offer support to the patient.			
c. Walk slowly and with an even gait.			
16.–19. Complete checklist steps 16–19 of the General Procedure (provide safety; return patient to bed; position for comfort; recheck vital signs; wash your hands).			

(continued)

© 1996 by Lippincott-Raven Publishers

Simple Assisted Ambulation *(Continued)*	Needs More Practice	Satisfactory	Comments
Evaluation			
20.–24. Complete steps 20–24 of the General Procedure (compare vital signs; check for fatigue and pain; ask how the patient feels; evaluate overall strength, balance, and ability to ambulate; evaluate use of special techniques or assistive devices).			
Documentation			
25. Document according to facility policy.			
Using a Cane			
Assessment			
1.–5. Complete checklist steps 1–5 of the General Procedure for Ambulation (identify patient's capabilities, activity ordered, previous level of activity, assistive devices; take vital signs).			
Planning			
6.–10. Complete checklist steps 6–10 of the General Procedure (plan for pain relief; goal, support needed, technique; wash your hands).			
Implementation			
11.–13. Complete checklist steps 11–13 of the General Procedure (identify patient; explain procedure; obtain robe and shoes; clear floor of litter and spills).			
Implementation			
14. Omit Step 14 of the General Procedure.			
15. Assist the patient to ambulate using a cane. **a.** *Standing:* Teach patient to do the following: (1) Hold cane in hand opposite affected side.			
(2) Move hips forward in chair.			
(3) Grasp arms of chair.			
(4) Push to standing position.			
(5) Gain balance.			
b. Nurse stands to side of and behind patient.			

(continued)

© 1996 by Lippincott-Raven Publishers

Using a Cane *(Continued)*	Needs More Practice	Satisfactory	Comments
c. *Gait pattern:* Teach patient to do the following: (1) Hold cane ahead 4–6 ins.			
(2) Move affected leg ahead, opposite cane.			
(3) Put weight on affected leg and cane.			
(4) Move unaffected leg ahead.			
(5) Repeat sequence.			
d. *Sitting:* Teach patient to do the following: (1) Turn around and back to chair.			
(2) Grasp arm of chair.			
(3) Lower self into chair.			
16.–19. Complete checklist steps 16–19 of the General Procedure (provide safety; return patient to bed; position for comfort; recheck vital signs; wash your hands).			
Evaluation			
20.–24. Complete steps 20–24 of the General Procedure (compare vital signs; check for fatigue and pain; ask how the patient feels; evaluate overall strength, balance, and ability to ambulate; evaluate use of special techniques or assistive devices).			
Documentation			
25. Document according to facility policy.			
Using a Walker			
Assessment			
1.–5. Complete checklist steps 1–5 of the General Procedure for Ambulation (identify patient's capabilities, activity ordered, previous level of activity, assistive devices; take vital signs).			
Planning			
6.–10. Complete checklist steps 6–10 of the General Procedure (plan for pain relief, goal, support needed, technique; wash your hands).			

(continued)

Using a Walker *(Continued)*	Needs More Practice	Satisfactory	Comments
Implementation			
11.–13. Complete checklist steps 11–13 of the General Procedure (identify patient; explain procedure; and obtain robe and shoes).			
14. Omit step 14 of the General Procedure.			
15. Assist the patient to ambulate using a walker. **a.** *Standing:* Teach patient to do the following: (1) Place walker in front of seat.			
(2) Put both hands on arms of chair, and push up to a standing position.			
(3) Move hands to walker one at a time.			
b. Stand behind and slightly to side of patient.			
c. *Gait pattern for pick-up walker:* Teach patient to do the following: (1) Move walker and affected leg ahead 4–6 ins.			
(2) Place weight on arms with partial weight on affected leg if permitted.			
(3) Move unaffected leg forward.			
(4) Repeat pattern.			
d. *Sitting:* Teach patient to do the following: (1) Turn around, and back up to chair.			
(2) Reach behind to grasp arms of chair, one hand and then the other.			
(3) Lower self into chair.			
16.–19. Complete Checklist steps 16–19 of the General Procedure (provide safety; return patient to bed; position for comfort; recheck vital signs; wash your hands).			
Evaluation			
20.–24. Complete steps 20–24 of the General Procedure (compare vital signs; check for fatigue and pain; ask how the patient feels; evaluate overall strength, balance, and ability to ambulate; and evaluate use of special techniques assistive devices).			

(continued)

© 1996 by Lippincott-Raven Publishers

Using a Walker *(Continued)*	Needs More Practice	Satisfactory	Comments
Documentation			
25. Document according to facility policy.			
Crutchwalking			
Assessment			
1.–5. Complete checklist steps 1–5 of the General Procedure for Ambulation (identify patient's capabilities; activity ordered, previous level of activity, assistive devices; take vital signs).			
Planning			
6.–10. Complete checklist 6–10 of the General Procedure (plan for pain relief, if indicated; set goal, support needed, technique; wash your hands).			
Implementation			
11.–13. Complete checklist steps 11–13 of the General Procedure (identify patient; explain procedure; obtain robe and shoes).			
14. Omit step 14 of the General Procedure.			
15. Assist the patient to ambulate using crutches. **a.** *Standing:* Teach patient to do the following: (1) Do the procedure as a smooth movement.			
(2) Place feet securely on the floor.			
(3) Slide hips forward on the chair.			
(4) Hold both crutches in the hand of the unaffected side.			
(5) Grasp arm of chair with hand opposite from crutches.			
(6) Push up from the chair.			
(7) Stabilize body by standing on the unaffected leg.			
(8) Place crutches under both arms.			
b. Have patient take crutch stance, with crutch tips approximately 2 in to side and 6 in ahead of feet.			

(continued)

1996 by Lippincott-Raven Publishers

Crutchwalking *(Continued)*	Needs More Practice	Satisfactory	Comments
c. Gait pattern (1) *Three-point gait:* Teach patient to do the following: (a) Support weight on unaffected leg.			
(b) Lift crutches and affected leg forward 4–6 in simultaneously.			
(c) Shift weight to crutches.			
(d) Step forward with unaffected leg.			
(e) Shift weight to unaffected leg.			
(f) Repeat pattern.			
(2) *Three-point-plus-one (partial weight-bearing):* Teach patient to do the following: (a) Take crutch stance, with full weight on unaffected leg and partial weight on affected leg.			
(b) Shift weight to unaffected leg.			
(c) Move crutches and affected leg forward 6–12 ins.			
(d) Shift weight to hands on crutches, with partial weight on affected leg.			
(e) Step unaffected leg ahead with same-sized steps.			
(f) Shift weight to unaffected leg.			
(g) Repeat pattern.			
(3) *Four-point gait:* Teach patient to do the following: (a) Take crutch stance with weight on both legs and both crutches.			
(b) Move left crutch forward.			
(c) Move right leg forward.			
(d) Move right crutch forward.			
(e) Move left leg forward.			
(f) Repeat pattern.			
d. *Sitting down with crutches:* Teach patient to do the following: (1) Walk to chair.			

(continued)

© 1996 by Lippincott-Raven Publishers

Crutchwalking *(Continued)*	Needs More Practice	Satisfactory	Comments
(2) Turn around so back is to chair and backs of legs touch chair.			
(3) Grasp both crutches in one hand.			
(4) Reach back with free hand and grasp arm of chair.			
(5) Lower self into chair using support of both crutches and chair.			
(6) Sit back in chair using proper body mechanics.			
(7) Do not hyperextend knees if legs are elevated.			
16.–19. Complete steps 16–19 of the General Procedure (provide safety; return patient to bed; position for comfort; recheck vital signs; wash your hands).			
Evaluation			
20.–24. Complete steps 20–24 of the General Procedure (compare vital signs; check for fatigue and pain; ask how the patient feels; evaluate overall strength, balance, and ability to ambulate; and evaluate use of special techniques or assistive devices).			
Documentation			
25. Document according to facility policy.			
Crutchwalking Up Stairs With Railing			
Assessment			
1.–5. Complete checklist steps 1–5 of the General Procedure for Ambulation (identify patient's capabilities, activity ordered, previous level of activity, assistive devices; take vital signs).			
Planning			
6.–10. Complete checklist steps 6–10 of the General Procedure (plan for pain relief, goal, support needed, technique; wash your hands).			

(continued)

© 1996 by Lippincott-Raven Publishers

Crutchwalking Up Stairs With Railing *(Continued)*	Needs More Practice	Satisfactory	Comments
Implementation			
11.–13. Complete checklist steps 11–13 of the General Procedure (identify patient; explain procedure; obtain robe and shoes; clear floor of litter and spills).			
14. Omit checklist step 14 of the General Procedure.			
15. Teach the patient to do the following: **a.** Hold both crutches under one arm as if to walk.			
b. Place other hand on railing in front of body.			
c. Raise unaffected leg to first step, and pull up with hand rail.			
d. Pull up affected leg, and advance crutches to next step.			
e. Again, raise unaffected leg, and pull up affected leg, advancing crutches.			
16.–19. Complete steps 16–19 of the General Procedure (provide safety; return patient to bed; position for comfort; recheck vital signs; wash your hands).			
Evaluation			
20.–24. Complete steps 20–24 of the General Procedure (compare vital signs; check for fatigue and pain; ask how the patient feels; evaluate overall strength, balance, and ability to ambulate; evaluate use of special techniques or assistive devices).			
Documentation			
25. Document according to facility policy.			
Crutchwalking Up Stairs Without Railing			
Assessment			
1.–5. Complete checklist steps 1–5 of the General Procedure for Ambulation (identify patient's capabilities; activity ordered, previous level of activity, assistive devices; take vital signs.)			

(continued)

© 1996 by Lippincott-Raven Publishers

Crutchwalking up Stairs Without Railing *(Continued)*	Needs More Practice	Satisfactory	Comments
Planning			
6.–10. Complete checklist steps 6–10 of the General Procedure (plan for pain relief, goal, support needed, technique; wash your hands).			
Implementation			
11.–13. Complete checklist steps 11–13 of the General Procedure (identify patient; explain procedure; obtain robe and shoes; clear floor of litter and spills).			
14. Omit checklist step 14 of the General Procedure.			
15. Teach the patient to do the following: **a.** Position crutches under arms as if walking.			
b. Put weight on hands.			
c. Raise unaffected leg to first step, and pull up affected leg.			
d. Advance crutches to step on which patient is standing.			
e. Again, raise unaffected leg to next higher step.			
16.–19. Complete steps 16–19 of the General Procedure (provide safety; return patient to bed; position for comfort; recheck vital signs; wash your hands).			
Evaluation			
20.–24. Complete steps 20–24 of the General Procedure (compare vital signs; check for fatigue and pain; ask how the patient feels evaluate overall strength, balance, and ability to ambulate; evaluate use of special techniques or assistive devices).			
Documentation			
25. Document according to facility policy.			
Crutchwalking Down Stairs			
Assessment			
1.–5. Complete checklist steps 1–5 of the General Procedure for Ambulation (identify patient's capabilities, activity ordered, previous level of activity, assistive devices; take vital signs.)			

(continued)

© 1996 by Lippincott-Raven Publishers

Crutchwalking Down Stairs *(Continued)*	Needs More Practice	Satisfactory	Comments
Planning			
6.–10. Complete checklist steps 6–10 of the General Procedure (plan for pain relief, goal, support needed, technique; wash your hands).			
Implementation			
11.–13. Complete checklist steps 11–13 of the General Procedure (identify patient; explain procedure; obtain robe and shoes; clear floor of litter and spills).			
14. Omit checklist step 14 of the General Procedure.			
15. Teach the patient to do the following: **a.** Position crutches under arm as if walking.			
b. Place weight on unaffected leg.			
c. Place crutches on next lower step.			
d. Put partial weight on hands and crutches.			
e. Move affected leg to lower step.			
f. Put total weight on crutches and affected leg.			
g. Move unaffected leg to same step as crutches and affected leg.			
h. If railing is present, hold crutches with one arm, and use other to grasp railing.			
16.–19. Complete steps 16–19 of the General Procedure (provide safety; return patient to bed; position for comfort; recheck vital signs; wash your hands).			
Evaluation			
20.–24. Complete steps 20–24 of the General Procedure (compare vital signs; check for fatigue and pain; ask how the patient feels; evaluate overall strength, balance, and ability to ambulate; and evaluate use of special techniques or assistive devices).			
Documentation			
25. Document according to facility policy.			

© 1996 by Lippincott-Raven Publishers

? QUIZ

Short-Answer Questions

1. Name four ways in which physical activity can improve patient status.

   a. _____

   b. _____

   c. _____

   d. _____

2. What is the major hazard of ambulation for patients? _____

3. Why are shoes better than most slippers for ambulation? _____

4. What types of assistive devices could be used for a person with one affected leg and one unaffected leg? _____

5. How is the crutch length determined? _____

6. Which gait patern is indicated for the patient with muscular weakness, lack of balance, or lack of coordination? _____

7. Describe the safest way to teach a patient to stand up from a chair to use a walker. _____

8. On which side does the patient hold a cane? _____

9. When a patient using crutches sits down, what should he or she do with the crutches? _____

10. Which gait is appropriate for a patient using crutches who cannot bear weight on one leg? _____

11. When crutchwalking down stairs without a railing, what is the order of crutches, affected leg, and unaffected leg? _____

12. Name three safety precautions related to ambulation you would discuss with a patient recovering at home. _____

MODULE

22

RANGE-OF-MOTION EXERCISES

MODULE CONTENTS

RATIONALE FOR THE USE OF THIS
   SKILL
NURSING DIAGNOSIS
RANGE-OF-MOTION EXERCISES
Goals of Range-of-Motion Exercises
Contraindications to Range-of-Motion
   Exercises
TYPES OF JOINTS
JOINTS NEEDING EXERCISE
TYPES OF RANGE OF MOTION
Active
Active-Assistive
Passive

Continuous Passive Motion
SEQUENCE OF EXERCISES
TIME OF EXERCISE
GENERAL PROCEDURE FOR RANGE-OF-
   MOTION EXERCISES
   Assessment
   Planning
   Implementation
   Evaluation
   Documentation
LONG-TERM CARE
HOME CARE
CRITICAL THINKING EXERCISES

PREREQUISITES

Successful completion of the following modules:

VOLUME 1
Module 1   An Approach to Nursing Skills
Module 2   Basic Infection Control
Module 3   Safety
Module 4   Basic Body Mechanics
Module 5   Documentation
Module 6   Introduction to Assessment Skills
Module 15 Moving the Patient in Bed and Positioning
Module 18 Hygiene

© 1996 by Lippincott-Raven Publishers

OVERALL OBJECTIVE

To perform range-of-motion (ROM) exercises on patients' joints, using proper sequence and joint positioning.

SPECIFIC LEARNING OBJECTIVES

Know Facts and Principles	Apply Facts and Principles	Demonstrate Ability	Evaluate Performance
1. Goals of ROM			
State two goals of ROM.	Given a patient situation, identify goal of ROM.	In the clinical setting, identify goal of ROM for a specific patient.	Evaluate with instructor.
2. Contraindications to ROM			
State two major contraindications to ROM.	Given a patient situation, identify whether a contraindication to ROM is present.	In the clinical setting, assess patient to determine presence of contraindications to ROM.	Evaluate with instructor.
3. Types of joints			
Name the six types of joints.	Describe the various joints and movements of the six types.	In the clinical area, note the various joint movements as you perform ROM.	Evaluate your observations with instructor.
4. Joints to be exercised			
State principles for deciding which joints need exercising.	Given a patient situation, describe side of body or joints requiring ROM.	In the clinical area, perform ROM on appropriate joints for particular patient.	Evaluate decision-making with instructor.
5. Types of ROM			
Know three types of ROM.	State reasons for selecting a specific kind of ROM for a specific patient.	In the clinical area, select correct kind of ROM for patient.	Check decision with instructor.
6. Sequence used for exercising various joints			
List order for exercising various joints.		Use prescribed sequence, making adaptations for particular patients.	Evaluate own performance using Performance Checklist.
7. Special attention to certain joints			
Explain rationale for exercise of particular functional joints.	Determine mobility or lack of mobility of key joints.	Emphasize functional joints when doing ROM.	
8. Performing ROM			
Give frequency of ROM for optimum benefit to patient.	Determine frequency of ROM for particular patient.	Do ROM at predetermined intervals.	Evaluate frequency by checking joint flexibility.

(continued)

© 1996 by Lippincott-Raven Publishers

SPECIFIC LEARNING OBJECTIVES (Continued)

Know Facts and Principles	Apply Facts and Principles	Demonstrate Ability	Evaluate Performance
9. Teaching ROM Explain why it is important for patients to participate in ROM.	Determine what information patient needs.	Teach patient about ROM procedures.	Evaluate patient's knowledge of ROM.
10. Documentation List data needed for chart.	Determine correct manner of recording data for facility.	Record procedure correctly, adding pertinent data.	Evaluate own performance with instructor.

© 1996 by Lippincott-Raven Publishers

LEARNING ACTIVITIES

1. Review the Specific Learning Objectives.
2. Read the section on ROM and active and passive exercises (in the chapter on activity and rest) in Ellis and Nowlis, *Nursing: A Human Needs Approach*, or comparable material in another textbook.
3. Review the anatomy of the skeletal and muscular systems.
4. Look up the module vocabulary terms in the glossary.
5. Read through the module, and study the figures. Mentally practice the procedure. Study the material as if you were preparing to teach these skills to another person.
6. In the practice setting, do the following, using the Performance Checklist as a guide:
   a. Standing, move the joints on one side of your body through ROM. Begin with your neck.
   b. Practice ROM with a partner for one side of the body.
   c. Change positions, and have your partner perform ROM on one side of your body.
   d. Together, evaluate your performances of steps b and c.
7. In the clinical setting, do the following:
   a. Perform ROM on a patient with your instructor's supervision.
   b. Evaluate your performance with the help of your instructor.

VOCABULARY

abduction	dorsiflexion	internal rotation	rotation
adduction	eversion	inversion	saddle joint
ball-and-socket joint	extension	opposition	supination
circumduction	external rotation	pivotal joint	synovial fluid
condyloid joint	flexion	plantar flexion	ulnar deviation
contracture	gliding joint	pronation	
contraindicate	hinge joint	proximal	
distal	hyperextension	radial deviation	

© 1996 by Lippincott-Raven Publishers

Saddle Joints

The two bones forming the joint rest together in convex and concave position. They have the ability to assume right angles allowing for flexion, extension, adduction, and abduction. The thumbs are saddle joints.

Gliding Joints

The bones involved in a gliding joint rest and glide on one another. These joints are not obvious as actual joints when performing ROM. The foot and vertebrae of the spine have gliding joints. The wrist and ankle also have a gliding component but are essentially condyloid (wrist) and hinge (ankle) joints.

JOINTS NEEDING EXERCISE

When an individual is weak and inactive, exercises of all joints may be needed because the ordinary activities of daily living may not provide sufficient exercise of the joints to maintain ROM. In particular, elderly individuals may need assistance in planning for ROM exercises when a sedentary lifestyle places them at risk for loss of joint function. Daily ROM exercises are usually adequate to maintain full mobility for these individuals.

When extremities or joints are just weak or partially affected, focus your assessment on abilities and disabilities. How far can the patient move the joint independently? This may be indicated in degrees of motion. How far can the joint be moved with assistance? Is there any stiffness or barrier to passive movement?

Any joint that is completely immobile as a result of paralysis is in particular need of ROM exercises. When a patient is completely paralyzed on one side of the body, the joints ideally should be exercised four to five times daily *for full maintenance of joint flexibility.* In reality, however, the staff's time restrictions may limit the exercise to only one or two times a day. Of course, limited ranging does not lead to optimum joint mobility.

When a patient receives ROM for the first time, exercise affected and unaffected joints bilaterally to establish a baseline of normal functioning for the patient. With each ROM procedure, move each joint through its range six to eight times. If you also are bathing or ambulating the patient, you will not have to range all the joints many times *because several of the bathing movements are ROM movements.* As a nurse performing ROM, never force a joint to the point of pain *because this may injure the joint.* However, restor-ative therapy by a physical therapist may sometimes push a joint to the point of pain.

TYPES OF RANGE OF MOTION

Active

In active ROM, instruct the patient to perform the movements on a nonfunctioning joint. When patients are taught a planned ROM program, they feel more independent *because they are participating actively.* They also can carry out additional ROM *by participating in their own care.* Combing the hair exercises joints of the upper extremity; lifting the foot for bathing exercises joints of the lower extremity. Encourage other appropriate activities as well.

Active-Assistive

Active-assistive ROM is carried out with patient and nurse participating. Encourage the patient to carry out as much of each movement as possible, within the limitations of strength and mobility. You support or complete the desired movement.

Passive

Passive ROM is performed by a nurse or other care provider on a patient's immobilized joints. Your assessment skills are needed *to determine which parts or joints must be exercised and with what frequency.*

Continuous Passive Motion

After certain types of major knee surgery (such as a knee replacement), restoring the patient's ROM is a significant concern. In such cases, a machine called a continuous passive motion (CPM) device may be used. The CPM device provides a sling support for the thigh and calf, with a hinged connection at the knee. A foot plate maintains the foot at a right angle to prevent foot drop. The CPM device is placed in the bed under the leg; the motor is placed under the bed and plugged into a convenient outlet. The leg is then positioned in correct alignment with the knee at the flex point and secured to the CPM device with Velcro straps. (Usually padding or an artificial sheepskin is placed under the leg for comfort.) A control allows you to set the degree of flexion ordered by the surgeon. When the machine is turned on, it automatically flexes and extends the knee joint at a slow, continuous rate.

When caring for a patient using a CPM device, determine how many hours the device is to be used

© 1996 by Lippincott-Raven Publishers

and what degree of flexion should be set on it. Remove the leg from the CPM device for such activities as bathing, skin care, ambulating, or going to the bathroom. Some CPM devices have an on-off switch that allows for patient control, enhancing self-care. The patient using a CPM device will continue to have physical therapy for concentrated exercise.

SEQUENCE OF EXERCISES

Joints are exercised sequentially, starting with the neck and moving downward. Joints move in different ways: The knee and elbow move in just one direction; the neck, wrist, and hip move in several directions. Several movements can be done together. For example, flexion of the knee and external rotation of the hip can be done simultaneously, as can abduction and external rotation of the shoulder. Never grasp joints directly. Instead, grasp the extremities gently but firmly either distal or proximal to the joint. *This is more comfortable for the patient and results in easier movement through the entire ROM.* Cup the heel in your hand when exercising the leg. When it is necessary to support the joint itself, gently cup your hand under the joint and allow the joint to rest on the palm of the hand. *This prevents pressure on the joint.* Do not grasp the fingernails or toenails; *this can be uncomfortable for the patient.* When exercising extremities, work from the proximal joints toward the distal joints.

Every joint should receive adequate exercise, but it is crucial that several particular joints remain functional *to provide independence.* For example, flexion of the thumb must be maintained *so that there is opposition of the thumb to the other fingers—otherwise the patient's hand will be useless. Hip and knee extension allows the patient to walk successfully when he or she is again mobile. Maintaining ankle flexion helps to prevent footdrop, which interferes with walking.*

TIME OF EXERCISE

Bath time is an appropriate time to administer ROM. *The warm bath water relaxes the muscles and decreases their potential to spasm. Additionally, during the bath, areas are exposed so that the joints can be moved and observed.* Other appropriate times might be when the patient is rested in the morning or before bedtime.

Evaluate the effectiveness of the ROM regimen by observing the flexibility and range of the joints. Adjust the regimen to the patient's individual needs.

GENERAL PROCEDURE FOR RANGE-OF-MOTION EXERCISES

Note: After each movement, return the part to its correct anatomic position. Each joint movement is described separately here. Remember that it is possible to move two joints, such as the shoulder and the elbow, at the same time. Many of the movements listed in Table 24–1 are integrated in the exercises outlined below.

Assessment

1. Assess the patient's joint mobility and activity status to determine the need for ROM exercises.
2. Assess the patient's general health status to determine whether any contraindications to ROM exercises are present.
3. Assess the patient's ability and willingness to cooperate in ROM exercises.

Planning

4. Plan when ROM exercises should be done.
5. Plan whether exercises will be active, active-assistive, or passive and which joints will be included.

Implementation

6. Wash your hands *for infection control.*
7. Identify the patient *to be sure you are carrying out the procedure for the correct patient.*
8. Provide privacy by closing the door or pulling curtains around the bed.
9. Explain to the patient what you are about to do, and ask for the patient's cooperation.
10. Position the bed for effective working. Lower the head of the bed *so that the patient is in the supine position.* Raise the entire bed to a comfortable working level for you. Maintain your own proper body mechanics as you carry out the exercises for the patient *to avoid strain.*
11. Follow the procedure below to administer ROM to one side of the body. Complete ROM on joints you have determined should be exercised. A plan for exercising all joints follows.
    a. Neck (Fig. 22–1)
       (1) *Flexion*: Position the head as if looking at the toes.
       (2) *Extension*: Position the head as if looking straight ahead.
       (3) *Hyperextension*: Position the head as if looking up at the ceiling. The elderly person should not perform this movement, which can lead to pain or cervical fractures.

© 1996 by Lippincott-Raven Publishers

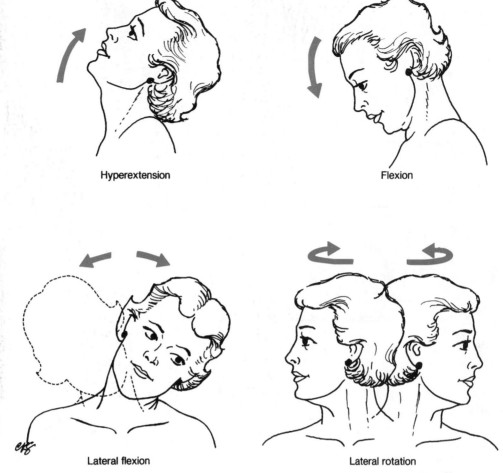

Hyperextension

Flexion

Lateral flexion

Lateral rotation

Figure 22–1. Exercising the neck. Hyperextension: Person lifts head straight backward with eyes toward ceiling. Flexion: Person lowers head to chest with eyes toward floor. Lateral flexion: Person moves head toward one shoulder and then the other. Lateral rotation: Person moves head in twisting motion from side to side.

(4) *Lateral flexion*: While the head is positioned looking straight ahead, tilt the head toward the shoulder, first to the left and then to the right.

(5) *Lateral rotation*: Position the head so that the head is looking first toward the right and then toward the left.

b. Shoulder (Fig. 22–2)

  (1) *Flexion*: Raise the arm forward and overhead. The elbow may be bent *to avoid the head of the bed*.

  (2) *Extension*: Return the arm to the side of the body.

  (3) *Vertical abduction*: Swing the arm out from the side of the body and up.

(4) *Vertical adduction*: Return the arm to the side of the body.

(5) *Internal rotation*: Swing the arm up and across the body.

(6) *External rotation*: Rotate the arm out and back, keeping the elbow at a right angle.

c. Elbow (Fig. 22–3). These movements can be performed in conjunction with the shoulder movements.

  (1) *Flexion*: Bend the elbow.

  (2) *Extension*: Straighten the elbow.

d. Wrist (Fig. 22–4)

  (1) *Flexion*: Grasping the palm with one hand and supporting the elbow with the other hand, bend the wrist forward.

© 1996 by Lippincott-Raven Publishers

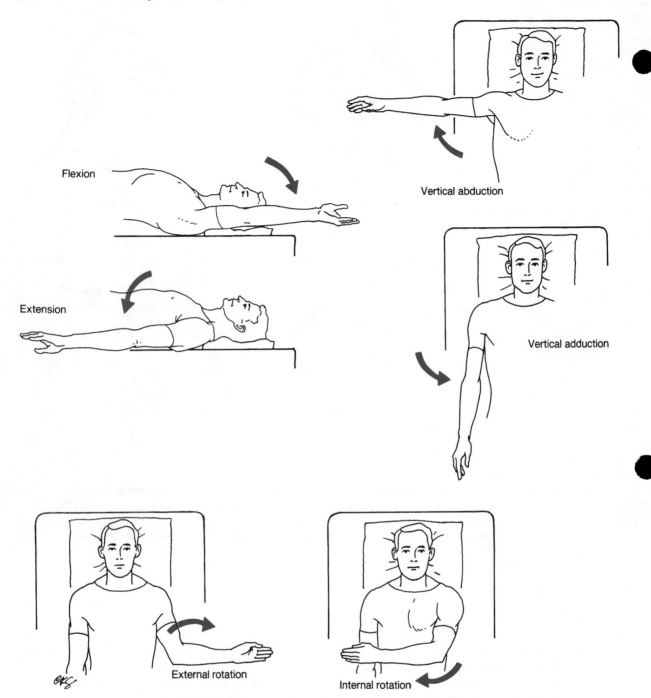

Figure 22–2. Exercising the shoulder. Flexion: Raise arm forward and overhead. Extension: Return arm to side of body. Vertical abduction: Swing arm out and up. Vertical adduction: Move arm downward to body. Internal rotation: Swing arm up and across body. External rotation: Rotate arm out and back.

© 1996 by Lippincott-Raven Publishers

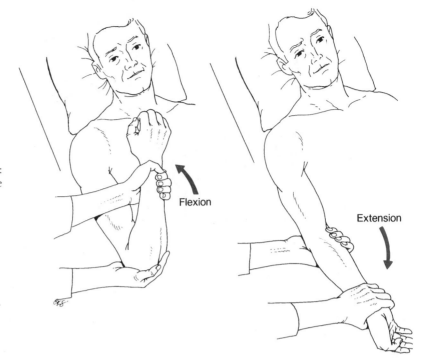

Figure 22–3. Exercising the elbow. Flexion: Cupping the elbow in the hand, bend the arm. Extension: Straighten the arm.

Flexion

Extension

(2) *Extension*: Straighten the wrist.
(3) *Radial deviation*: Bend the wrist toward the thumb.
(4) *Ulnar deviation*: Bend the wrist toward the little finger.
(5) *Circumduction*: Move the wrist in a circular motion.

e. Fingers and thumb (Fig. 22–5). *A hand can be partially functional* if a patient is able to place the thumb in opposition to the index finger or third finger. Therefore, take special care to exercise these joints as thoroughly as possible. You can move all three joints of each finger and the fingers and thumb through flexion and extension together.

(1) *Flexion*: Bend the fingers and thumb onto the palm.
(2) *Extension:* Return them to their original position.
(3) *Abduction*: Spread the fingers.
(4) *Adduction*: Return the fingers to the closed position.
(5) *Circumduction*: Move the thumb in a circular motion.
(6) *Opposition*: Touch the end of the thumb to each of the fingers in turn.

f. Hip and knee (Fig. 22–6). The hip and knee can be exercised together. Place one hand under the patient's knee, and with the other hand, support the heel.

(1) *Flexion*: Lift the leg, bending the knee as far as possible toward the patient's head.
(2) *Extension*: Return the leg to the surface of the bed and straighten.
(3) *Abduction*: With the leg flat on the bed, move the entire leg out toward the edge of the bed.
(4) *Adduction*: Bring the leg back toward the midline or center of the bed.

Note: Steps (3) and (4) can be performed with the knee bent. *This allows you to give better support to some patients and affords a greater range of movement.*

(5) *Internal rotation*: With the leg flat on the bed, roll the entire leg inward *so that the toes point in. This will rotate the hip joint internally.*
(6) *External rotation*: With the leg flat on the bed, roll the entire leg outward *so that the toes point out. This will rotate the hip externally.*

g. Ankle (Fig. 22–7)
(1) *Dorsiflexion*: Cup the patient's heel with

© 1996 by Lippincott-Raven Publishers

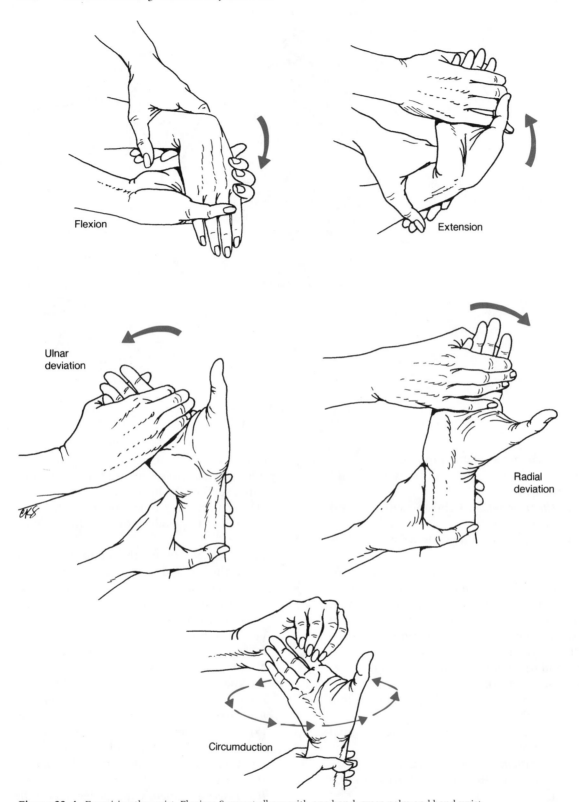

Figure 22–4. Exercising the wrist. Flexion: Support elbow with one hand; grasp palm and bend wrist forward. Extension: Straighten wrist. Lateral flexion for ulnar deviation: Bend the wrist toward the little finger. Lateral flexion for radial deviation: Bend the wrist toward the thumb. Circumduction: Move the wrist in a circular motion.

© 1996 by Lippincott-Raven Publishers

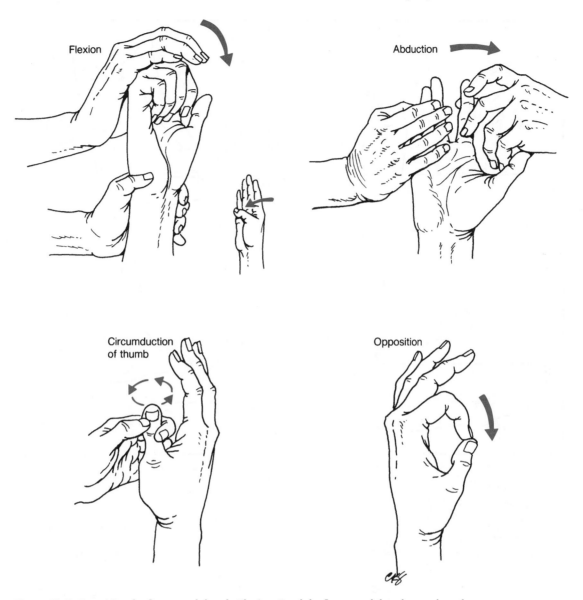

Figure 22–5. Exercising the fingers and thumb. Flexion: Bend the fingers and thumb onto the palm. Abduction: Spread the fingers. Circumduction of the thumb: Move thumb in circular motion. Opposition: Touch end of thumb to each of fingers in turn.

your hand, and rest the sole of the foot against your forearm. Steady the leg just above the ankle with your other hand. Put pressure against the patient's sole of the foot with your arm *to flex the ankle.*

(2) *Plantar flexion*: Change your hand from above the ankle to the ball of the foot. Move the other arm away from the toes, keeping the hand cupped around the heel, and push the foot downward *to point the toes.*

(3) *Circumduction*: Rotate the foot on the ankle, moving it first in one direction and then in the other.

h. Toes (Fig. 22–7)

(1) *Flexion*: Bend the toes down. Avoid grasping the nails *because this can be uncomfortable for the patient.*

(2) *Extension*: Bend the toes up.

i. Spine (Fig. 22–8). These exercises can be done only by an individual who is able to stand. Direct the elderly person to hold the back of a chair or a railing for balance while

(continued on page 536)

© 1996 by Lippincott-Raven Publishers

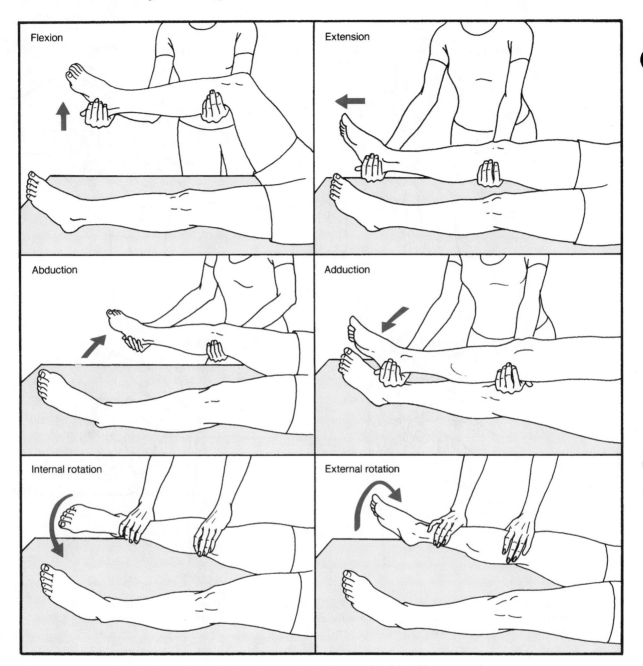

Figure 22–6. Exercising the hip and knee. Flexion: Cupping the heel in your hand, bend knee toward head. Extension: Return leg to bed. Abduction: Move leg outward to edge of bed. Adduction: Bring leg back to midline. Internal rotation: Roll entire leg inward. External rotation: Roll entire leg outward.

© 1996 by Lippincott-Raven Publishers

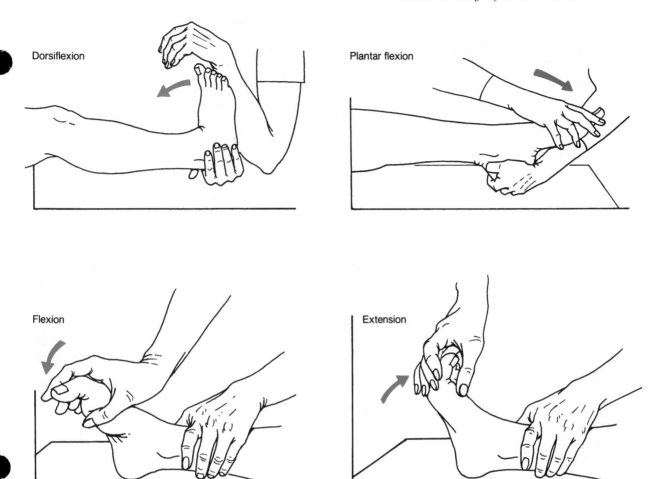

Figure 22–7. Exercising the ankle and toes. Ankle dorsiflexion: Cup heel, and using forearm, bend ankle toward upper body. Ankle plantar flexion: Cup heel and push ankle downward to point toes. Flexion of toes: Bend toes downward. Extension of toes: Bend toes upward.

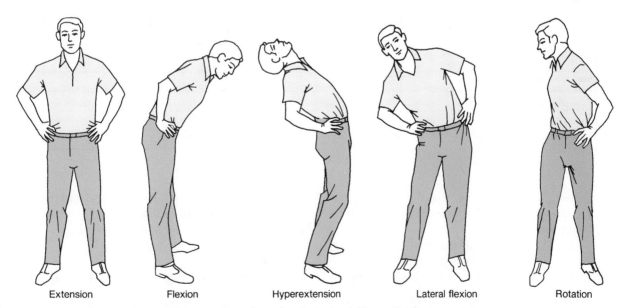

Figure 22–8. Exercising the spine. Extension: Stand straight. Flexion: Bend forward. Hyperextension: Bend backward. Lateral flexion: Bend toward the side. Rotation: Twist from the waist.

© 1996 by Lippincott-Raven Publishers

Fill in the parameters to be monitored. Refer to Standard & Individual Care Plans.
Parameter examples: Guaiac stools/emesis, urine fractionals, specific gravity, girth of limb/abd, bowel sounds, circulation of extremity, pedal pulses, frequent lab values.

CVA – L hemiplegia

Parameters Date	Time	L Upper Extremity					L Lower Extremity				Initial
		Shld. flex.	Shld. ext, ro	Elbow ext	Wrist ext	Finger ext	Hip abd	Hip ext	Knee ext	Ankle dorsiflexion	
Movement											
8/4	09	✓	✓	✓	✓	✓	✓	✓	✓	✓	JS
	21	✓	✓	✓	✓	✓	✓	✓	✓	✓	CB
8/5	09	✓	✓	✓	✓	✓	✓	✓	✓	✓	JS
	21	✓	✓	✓	✓	✓	✓	✓	✓	✓	CB
8/6	09	✓	✓	✓	✓	✓	✓	✓	✓	✓	SM
	21	✓	✓	✓	✓	✓	✓	✓	✓	✓	CB

Identify Initials with Signature:	4.	8.
1. *Joe Summers, RN*	5.	9.
2. *Carole Breen, RN*	6.	10.
3. *Sandra Matson, RN*	7.	11.

PARAMETER FLOW SHEET

Figure 22–9. Parameter flow sheet.

doing these exercises. If the person experiences back pain, the exercise should be stopped.

(1) *Extension*: Stand straight.

(2) *Flexion*: Bend forward from the waist.

(3) *Hyperextension*: Bend backward from the waist.

(4) *Lateral flexion*: Bend toward the side, first left, then right.

(5) *Rotation*: Twist from the waist to the side, first left, then right.

12. Wash your hands *for infection control.*

Evaluation

13. Evaluate the patient in terms of the following:

a. Fatigue

b. Joint discomfort

c. Joint mobility

© 1996 by Lippincott-Raven Publishers

Documentation

14. ROM is frequently documented on a flow sheet (Fig. 22–9) to facilitate record keeping. If no flow sheet is available, use a narrative nursing progress note. If there is any adverse response, you must make a narrative or SOAP note in addition to a flow sheet recording. Notations about the extent to which joints can be moved are usually made in degrees.

LONG-TERM CARE

Many long-term care facilities have an activities coordinator. These staff people frequently lead a daily exercise group for residents, during which active exercises are done. Even those confined to wheelchairs can join in the exercises. Bowling with special equipment and other types of activities may provide excellent ROM. As a staff nurse, you can encourage residents to participate in activities that provide this important movement.

Many elderly residents have the problem of fatigue. In these cases, it is useful to schedule ROM exercises for the morning hours *when fatigue may be less of a problem than it is later in the day.*

A large number of residents experience joint inflexibility due to arthritis. Move arthritic joints to maintain function, but avoid stress on the joints. Individuals with arthritis may benefit from a combination of active, active-assistive, and passive exercises. For the staff, scheduling ROM exercises at the same time each morning is most convenient because baths may be given only one to two times per week. If performing ROM *becomes routine and is done at the same time*, the patient or caregivers are more likely to remember it.

Many of the residents in long-term care facilities have suffered stroke or neuromuscular impairment. Receiving ROM exercise is essential for these people *to maintain joint mobility, strengthen muscles, and enhance the function of affected extremities.* An accurate assessment of these individuals is necessary before proceeding with ROM. Usually physical therapy assistants or activity aides carry out a physical therapy evaluation and a specific prescription for exercise. Restoration of function is an important goal in long-term care.

HOME CARE

As more incapacitated people are receiving care by family members in the home, maintaining the highest degree of mobility becomes a priority. Activities of daily living, such as eating, dressing, and ambulating, are enhanced when joint mobility is improved. If you are the nurse providing home care, you may perform ROM exercises for the patient and teach a family member to perform them on the person's joints. The nurse should encourage the disabled patient to participate as fully as possible *so that the person feels involved in the process.* If teaching the procedure, use a chart indicating the sequence of exercises. Use another chart showing progress to motivate the patient and the family member. Progress is usually slow, and improvements on a daily basis may be difficult to see.

CRITICAL THINKING EXERCISES

• Mildred Ogden was admitted to a long-term care facility from the hospital after suffering a stroke that left her right side paralyzed. She is receiving rehabilitative services that include physical therapy twice a week. Determine what factors you should consider when deciding whether she needs range-of-motion exercises provided by the nursing staff. Specify what joints might be most in need of ROM, and explain why. Who might be the best person to consult for assistance in making decisions regarding this aspect of care?

• Joseph French, age 75, was admitted with emphysema and pneumonia. His admission data state that he has been house bound due to shortness of breath for the last month. As he tries to turn over in bed, he says "This old body is pretty stiff!" Consider the problems associated with his medical diagnosis. Is this man a candidate for ROM exercises? If not, why not? If he is, determine what specific precautions are needed.

© 1996 by Lippincott-Raven Publishers

✔ PERFORMANCE CHECKLIST

General Procedure for Range-of-Motion Exercises	Needs More Practice	Satisfactory	Comments
Assessment			
1. Assess patient's joint mobility and activity status.			
2. Assess patient's general health status.			
3. Assess patient's ability and willingness to participate.			
Planning			
4. Plan time for exercises.			
5. Plan type of exercises.			
Implementation			
6. Wash your hands.			
7. Identify patient.			
8. Provide privacy.			
9. Explain to the patient what you are going to do, and elicit the patient's help.			
10. Position the bed for effective working.			
11. Follow the procedure below to administer ROM to one side of the body: a. Neck: (1) Flexion			
(2) Extension			
(3) Hyperextension			
(4) Lateral flexion			
(5) Lateral rotation			
b. Shoulder: (1) Flexion			
(2) Extension			
(3) Vertical abduction			
(4) Vertical adduction			
(5) Internal rotation			
(6) External rotation			

(*continued*)

© 1996 by Lippincott-Raven Publishers

General Procedure for Range-of-Motion Exercises *(Continued)*	Needs More Practice	Satisfactory	Comments
c. Elbow: (1) Flexion			
(2) Extension			
d. Wrist: (1) Flexion			
(2) Extension			
(3) Radial deviation			
(4) Ulnar deviation			
(5) Circumduction			
e. Fingers and thumb: (1) Flexion			
(2) Extension			
(3) Abduction			
(4) Adduction			
(5) Circumduction (thumb)			
(6) Opposition			
f. Hip and knee: (1) Flexion			
(2) Extension			
(3) Abduction			
(4) Adduction			
(5) Internal rotation			
(6) External rotation			
g. Ankle: (1) Dorsiflexion			
(2) Plantar flexion			
(3) Circumduction			
h. Toes: (1) Flexion			
(2) Extension			

(continued)

© 1996 by Lippincott-Raven Publishers

General Procedure for Range-of-Motion Exercises *(Continued)*	Needs More Practice	Satisfactory	Comments
i. Spine: (1) Extension			
(2) Flexion			
(3) Hyperextension			
(4) Lateral flexion			
(5) Rotation			
12. Wash your hands.			
Evaluation			
13. Evaluate: **a.** Fatigue			
b. Joint discomfort			
c. Joint mobility			
Documentation			
14. Document on flow sheet or narrative.			

© 1996 by Lippincott-Raven Publishers

? QUIZ

Short-Answer Questions

1. List two goals of ROM exercises.

   a. _____

   b. _____

2. Idendify two contraindications to ROM exercises.

   a. _____

   b. _____

3. Contractures occur when the stronger muscle group of an extremity shortens or pulls. These muscles are the _____

4. Examples of hinge joints are those of the

_____

5. One example of a saddle joint is the _____

6. The spine is an example of a _____ joint.

7. ROM that is performed by the patient is called _____

8. When the hand is held in an outward, upward position, it is called

_____

9. To comb the hair, the shoulder assumes a position of _____

Multiple-Choice Questions

_____ **10.** ROM should be performed

   a. every time a patient is repositioned.
   b. at bath time.
   c. when ordered by the physician.
   d. four to five times a day.

_____ **11.** Joints of the body should be exercised sequentially; that is,

   a. alternately, from one side to the other.
   b. from distal to proximal.
   c. from proximal to distal.

_____ **12.** "Scissoring" one leg over the other may bring about

   a. hip flexion.
   b. hip extension.
   c. adduction.
   d. circumduction.

© 1996 by Lippincott-Raven Publishers

MODULE

23

CARING FOR PATIENTS WITH CASTS AND BRACES

MODULE CONTENTS

RATIONALE FOR THE USE OF THIS
SKILL
NURSING DIAGNOSES
CASTS
CASTING MATERIALS
Plaster of Paris Casts
Fiberglass Casts
GENERAL PROCEDURE FOR ASSISTING
WITH THE APPLICATION OF A CAST
Assessment
Planning
Implementation
Evaluation
Documentation
SPECIFIC CASTING PROCEDURES
Assisting With the Application of a Plaster
of Paris Cast
Assisting With the Application of a
Fiberglass Cast
COMMON TYPES OF CASTS
CAST CHANGES AND ADAPTATION
Cast Changes
Bivalving
Windowing

IMMEDIATE CARE OF THE PATIENT IN A
CAST
CONTINUING CARE OF THE PATIENT IN
A CAST
BRACES
TYPES OF BRACES
Cervical Collar
Thoracic-Lumbosacral Spine Body Jacket
Boston Scoliosis Brace
Boston Brace
Anterior Spinal Hyperextension Brace
Cast/Brace Combinations
Knee and Leg Braces
GENERAL PROCEDURE FOR ASSISTING
WITH THE APPLICATION OF A BRACE
Assessment
Planning
Implementation
Evaluation
Documentation
EMOTIONAL SUPPORT
LONG-TERM CARE
HOME CARE
CRITICAL THINKING EXERCISES

PREREQUISITES

Successful completion of the following modules:

VOLUME 1
Module 1   An Approach to Nursing Skills
Module 2   Basic Infection Control
Module 3   Safety
Module 4   Basic Body Mechanics
Module 5   Documentation
Module 14   Bedmaking
Module 15   Moving the Patient in Bed
            and Positioning

Module 21   Ambulation: Simple Assisted
            and Using Cane, Crutches, or
            Walker
Module 22   Range-of-Motion Exercises

The following module may be needed for some situations:

Module 26   Applying Bandages and
            Binders

© 1996 by Lippincott-Raven Publishers

OVERALL OBJECTIVE

To assist efficiently with the application of a cast or brace, accurately assess the patient for complications, and prevent problems related to the presence of a cast or brace while providing psychological support.

SPECIFIC LEARNING OBJECTIVES

Know Facts and Principles	Apply Facts and Principles	Demonstrate Ability	Evaluate Performance
CAST APPLICATION			
1. Casting materials			
List common kinds of casting materials and describe characteristics of each.	Give advantages and disadvantages of each material for specific cases.	In the clinical setting, observe type of cast being used, and give reason patient is receiving particular type of cast.	Evaluate with instructor.
2. Procedure			
Explain steps of procedure for assisting with application of plaster of Paris and fiberglass casts.	Apply steps to specific casting situation.	If possible, assist with the application of a plaster of Paris or fiberglass cast in clinical setting.	Evaluate performance with instructor.
3. Types of casts			
Briefly discuss the four types of commonly used casts.	Given a patient situation, give rationale for type of cast applied.	In the clinical setting, observe presence of different types of casts, and know why each cast was used.	Evaluate with instructor.
4. Adaptations to casts			
Describe method and reason for bivalving or windowing a cast.	Given a patient situation, explain when and where bivalving or windowing might be appropriate.	In the clinical setting, observe a bivalved or windowed cast, and know why adaptation was done for specific patient.	Evaluate with instructor.
GIVING CARE			
1. Guidelines			
List steps to be taken when caring for the patient in a cast.	Given a patient situation, give rationale for specific steps taken for care of patient.	In the clinical setting, care for the patients in a cast.	Evaluate performance with instructor.
2. Problems			
State potential problems related to being in a cast.	Identify specific problems that may arise with a particular patient.	In the clinical setting, identify potential problems in nursing care plan.	Evaluate with instructor.

(*continued*)

© 1996 by Lippincott-Raven Publishers

SPECIFIC LEARNING OBJECTIVES (continued)

Know Facts and Principles	Apply Facts and Principles	Demonstrate Ability	Evaluate Performance
3. Preventive measures List measures that can be taken to avoid problems.	Identify preventive measures that could be taken with a particular patient.	In the clinical setting, incorporate preventive measures in nursing care plan.	Evaluate with instructor.
4. Emotional support State why emotional support is important for the patient in a cast.	Given a patient situation, show ways of offering emotional support.	In the clinical setting, include emotional support in nursing care plan.	Evaluate with instructor.
5. Documentation State information that should be recorded.	Given a patient situation, identify actions and observations to be documented.	In the clinical setting, document on patient's progress notes.	Review notes with instructor.
BRACE APPLICATION **1. Brace materials** List the materials commonly used to make braces.	Give specific purpose of materials.	In the clinical setting, observe what brace materials are used.	Report observations to instructor.
2. Procedure Explain steps of procedure for application of a brace.	Apply steps to a specific bracing situation.	If there is an opportunity, apply a brace in the clinical setting.	Evaluate performance with instructor.
3. Types of braces Briefly discuss four types of braces and the location of the body for which they are used.	Given a patient situation, give rationale for type of brace applied.	In the clinical setting, identify what types of braces are used and the rationale for use.	Evaluate with instructor.
4. Problems State potential problems that may occur for the patient who has a brace in place.	Identify specific problems that may arise for a particular patient.	In the clinical setting, record potential problems in the nursing care plan.	Evaluate with instructor.
5. Preventive measures List actions that can be taken to avoid problems.	Identify preventive actions that could be taken for a particular patient.	In the clinical setting, integrate preventive measures in your plan of care.	Evaluate with instructor.

(continued)

© 1996 by Lippincott-Raven Publishers

SPECIFIC LEARNING OBJECTIVES (continued)

Know Facts and Principles	Apply Facts and Principles	Demonstrate Ability	Evaluate Performance
6. Emotional support State rationale for importance of giving emotional support.	Given a patient situation, describe ways of offering emotional support.	In the clinical setting, include emotional support in your plan of care.	Evaluate your plan with your instructor.
7. Documentation State information that should be recorded.	Given a patient situation, identify actions and observations to be documented.	In the clinical setting, document on patient's progress notes.	Review documentation with your instructor.

© 1996 by Lippincott-Raven Publishers

LEARNING ACTIVITIES

1. Review the Specific Learning Objectives.
2. Read the section on immobilization (in the chapter on activity and rest) in Ellis and Nowlis, *Nursing: A Human Needs Approach,* or comparable material in another text.
3. Look up the module vocabulary terms in the glossary.
4. Read through the module as though you were preparing to teach these skills to another person. Mentally practice the specific procedure.
5. In the practice setting, observe any available casts, casting materials, or braces.
6. For casts, in the clinical setting, do the following:
   a. Read the material in your facility's procedure book on assisting with the application of a cast and the care of the patient in a cast.
   b. Review any written information designed for patient teaching regarding casts.
   c. Arrange with your instructor for an opportunity to observe or assist in the application of a cast.
   d. Review the care plan for a patient in a cast.
   e. Arrange with your instructor for an opportunity to care for a patient in a cast.
7. For braces, in the clinical setting, do the following:
   a. Read any material in your facility's procedure manual on the types and application of braces.
   b. Read any written material designed for teaching patients regarding their braces.
   c. Arrange with your instructor for an opportunity to apply a brace or assist a patient with a brace.
   d. Review the care plan for a patient wearing a brace.

VOCABULARY

bivalving	fiberglass cast	malleable	torso
cast padding	green cast	petaling	trapeze
cervical collar	isometric exercises	plaster of Paris cast	twist support
cure (a cast)	isotonic exercises	scoliosis	walking heel
epigastrium	kyphosis	stockinette	windowing
excoriation	logrolling	tepid	

© 1996 by Lippincott-Raven Publishers

Caring for Patients With Casts and Braces

Rationale for the Use of This Skill

The treatment of fractures by immobilizing a body part with a cast is very old, as is the treatment of sprains, skeletal abnormalities, and minor fractures with braces. To be effective and relatively problem free, casts and braces must be applied carefully. Highly trained technicians usually apply a specific cast or brace according to the physician's order. Some physicians, however, continue to apply casts for their patients.

Nurses seldom apply casts, but they do assist in their application and maintenance and should be competent and knowledgeable to recognize and prevent problems. Nurses should be able to gather the appropriate equipment and assist the person applying the cast. They also should be available to provide the patient with emotional support. Because the area or part being treated is covered by the cast, it is often difficult to discern problems unless the nurse carries out frequent and careful assessments. Nursing interventions also may prevent the occurrence of some problems.

Nurses commonly assist with the application of a brace. An understanding of the common types of braces used and how patients wear them is important for the nurse who must assist an individual to put on a brace correctly. Braces are often complicated devices and difficult for the patient and family to understand without proper instruction. The nurse provides teaching to support effective self-care and patient confidence in these situations.

Long-term immobilization of a body part caused by a cast or brace can lead to a variety of complications. These can, in large part, be prevented through conscientious nursing assessment and intervention. For problems that do arise, early intervention is essential. The nurse needs to be skillful in caring for the patient immediately after a cast or brace has been applied and in continuing care. Any cast or brace, regardless of type or size, forces the patient to make some immediate and long-term adaptations.[1]

▼ NURSING DIAGNOSES

Examples of some nursing diagnoses related to patients with casts and braces include:

Impaired Physical Mobility related to presence of long leg cast
Impaired Home Maintenance Management related to presence of body cast

Altered Tissue Perfusion related to peripheral compression caused by leg brace
Risk for Injury: Sensory or motor deficits related to pressure from casts, braces, crutches, or canes
Risk for Impaired Skin Integrity related to pressure from cast or brace

CASTS

Casts immobilize the trunk or a body part *so that a fracture of a bone, a dislocation, or an injury to soft tissue can heal.* The various casting materials are impregnated with a substance that hardens after being applied to the body part. To be effective, casts must be contoured or molded carefully to the surface being covered. Although padding is used on the skin, pressure from the hard casting material can produce complications in the covered area, including pain, decreased sensation, or skin breakdown.

CASTING MATERIALS

Many casting materials have been used over the years, and each has advantages and disadvantages for the patient. The physician orders the type of cast to be applied and the material to be used. The patient may be taken to a special casting room, where all the casting equipment is available. Or, instead, a "cast cart" with the materials may be brought to the location where the patient is being treated.

Two types of cast material are most often used today. The oldest, and still the most commonly used for casting is plaster of Paris. The second most frequently used material is fiberglass. These are described in greater detail below.

Padding or wrapping is used beneath both types of cast before the material is applied. Soft cotton material is the fabric of choice for the plaster of Paris cast *because it absorbs perspiration, thereby decreasing skin irritation.* Synthetic material is preferred for the fiberglass cast *because cotton can fray under the hardness of the fiberglass surface, causing skin-irritating particles to become embedded beneath the cast.*

Plaster of Paris Casts

When combined with water, Plaster of Paris, or calcium sulfate, forms gypsum, which is a hard but fairly light substance. Crinoline (a firmly woven cotton fabric) rolls impregnated with plaster of Paris are immersed in water and molded to a body part to

[1]Note that rationales for action are emphasized throughout the module by the use of italics.

© 1996 by Lippincott-Raven Publishers

form a cast. After drying, the resulting cast is hard and fits the body part exactly. Plaster of Paris is used *to immobilize fractures and damaged soft tissue parts and as a protective device for newly amputated limbs.*

The advantages of plaster of Paris casts are that they are hard, inexpensive, and relatively nonallergenic to most patients. Disadvantages are that the larger casts are quite heavy, and the material has a tendency to become crumbly if worn for long periods or if it becomes damp or wet. Casts made of plaster of Paris take 24 to 48 hours to dry completely. During this time, the extremity should be supported and not handled with the fingertips *because fingers may produce indentations that will create pressure points under the cast.*

Fiberglass Casts

The synthetic or fiberglass cast is sometimes referred to as a "light" cast because of its light weight. Rolls of synthetic cast material are in sealed moisture-proof packages that begin to harden as soon as the package is opened. These materials come in a wide variety of colors (such as purple, bright green, and yellow) and white. These are especially enjoyed by children.

Casts made from fiberglass, like those made from plaster of Paris, have advantages and disadvantages. Fiberglass is easier to apply, more rigid, and more durable than plaster of Paris. For these reasons, fiberglass is commonly used for children with minor fractures and injuries, because they are more active and may damage a softer cast. Another advantage is that the newer fiberglass casts dry in about 1 hour. Although these casts are more resistant to moisture and water than plaster of Paris casts, the manufacturer does not recommend that the patient shower or swim in such a cast, mainly *because the padding underneath will become wet and can macerate the skin.*

There are several disadvantages to fiberglass. It is more expensive than plaster of Paris. The substance is not as "forgiving" as plaster, so once the cast is molded to the part, *the rigidity may cause problems if even minimal swelling occurs.* When the cast is dry, *this rigidity may continue to cause problems for the underlying tissue.* For this reason, fiberglass is usually not used for elderly patients.

GENERAL PROCEDURE FOR ASSISTING WITH THE APPLICATION OF A CAST

Assessment

1. Review the patient's record to determine the kind of injury, and read the physician's notes about casting.

2. Inspect the skin over which the cast is to be applied for any abrasions or interruptions in skin integrity. Look for signs of edema that may intensify pressure caused by the cast. Surgical wounds are often exposed for inspection through a "window" (a small cut) after the cast has been applied.

3. Find out what the patient knows about the procedure *so that you can clarify, if necessary, any information that has been given.* Determine whether the physician has ordered a sedative to be given about 30 minutes before casting *to alleviate any anxiety or discomfort.*

Planning

4. Wash your hands *for infection control.*

5. Gather equipment appropriate to the type of cast on a cart if a special "cast cart" is not available.
   a. Stockinette. This soft, stretchy, ribbed tubular material comes in different circumferences. When pulled over a body part, it *provides a smooth surface and protection from the inner surface of the cast.* Choose an appropriate circumference and cut off a length 6 inches longer than the area to be casted.
   b. Large, heavy-duty scissors
   c. Cast padding
   d. A cast knife for trimming
   e. A cast saw in case windowing is needed (see "Windowing," page 556)
   f. Adhesive cloth tape
   g. A plastic apron and gloves; these are used by the physician or technician applying the cast *to protect the clothing and hands.*

Implementation

6. Identify the patient *to be sure you are performing the procedure for the correct patient.*

7. Drape the patient *so that there is no unnecessary exposure.* Place a plastic-covered sheet or pillow under the part to be casted *to protect the linen from moisture and casting materials.*

8. Offer the patient emotional support and reassurance.

9. Assist the person applying the cast.
   The person applying the cast may wish to incorporate twist supports and walking heels into the cast: Twist supports and walking heels can be incorporated during the wet or "green" stage or can be glued on later. Twists are made by twisting a roll, wrapping the ends around the two sites of attachment, then rolling another roll around the twist. When dry, this appears as a strong bar between two extremities or between an extremity and the patient's body (Fig. 23–1).
   The rough edges of the cast are trimmed with

© 1996 by Lippincott-Raven Publishers

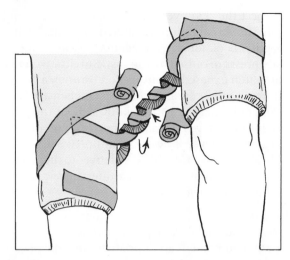

Figure 23–1. A "twist" support is made to act as a rigid bridge between the casts of two lower extremities. The wet casting bandage is twisted into a support and anchored into each leg cast.

a cast knife and may be covered with stockinette. The stockinette may simply be folded down over the outer surface of the cast and fastened with tape (Fig. 23–2). Edges also may be finished when the cast has dried using "petals" (see below).

10. When the casting is completed, clean excess material from the patient's skin *to prevent irritation.*

11. Position the patient so that the cast is supported and the patient is comfortable.
    a. Handle a cast carefully until it is completely dry. Use the flat palms of the hands *so that your fingers do not place indentations in the wet or damp cast because this weakens the surface and causes uneven pressure on the skin.*
    b. Place small plastic-covered pillows under and around the cast, leaving some air space at the sides until the cast is dry. Extending the pillows above and below the cast *allows the cast to dry more evenly and keeps the cast from pulling on muscle groups.*
    c. Elevate the extremity slightly higher than the heart. This will help prevent swelling of the tissues and excessive tightness of the cast *by improving venous return.*
    d. During the drying period, leave the cast uncovered. A fan or a hair dryer on a cool setting can be used to hasten the drying process. Never apply heat, *because it tends to dry the surface of the cast too quickly, causing cracking.*

12. Provide patient teaching, covering the following:
    a. Monitoring that will be done

b. Length of time cast takes to dry
c. How the cast feels as it dries
d. Importance of immediately reporting feelings of pain, pressure, or altered sensation
e. Need to keep the extremity immobile until the cast is dry

13. Care for equipment and supplies and clean area as needed.

14. Wash your hands.

Evaluation
15. Evaluate the following:
    a. Patient comfort
    b. Condition of the cast
    c. Neurovascular status, including circulation, motion, and sensation of the affected body part

Documentation
16. Document the following on the appropriate form:
    a. Type of cast applied
    b. Neurovascular status
    c. Patient comfort

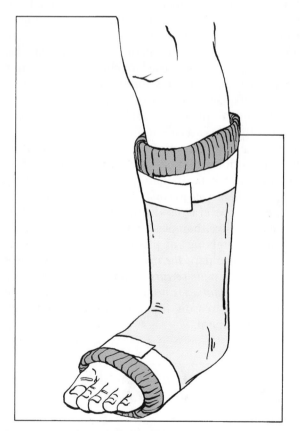

Figure 23–2. Folded stockinette protects the skin from the sharp edges of the cast.

© 1996 by Lippincott-Raven Publishers

DATE/TIME	
2/11/99 1520	Long leg cast applied to right leg by Dr. Stone. Toes warm to touch, pink, and easily moved. Returned to room. —————— S. Thayer, RN

(A) Example of Nursing Progress Notes Using Narrative Format.

DATE/TIME	
2/13/99 1420	Nursing Diagnosis: Alteration in comfort: Increasing pain in small area of thigh under long leg cast.
	S "It's just that one spot that keeps hurting."
	O Points to small area of cast and grimaces.
	A Pressure under cast causing tissue irritation.
	P Call physician, possible bivalving of cast. ———— S. Thayer, RN

(B) Example of Nursing Progress Notes Using SOAP Format.

SPECIFIC CASTING PROCEDURES

For each specific type of casting procedure discussed, some steps of the General Procedure may be modified. The modified steps and references to the steps of the General Procedure that remain the same follow.

Assisting With the Application of a Plaster of Paris Cast

Assessment

1.–3. Follow the steps of the General Procedure for Assisting With the Application of a Cast.

Planning

4. Follow the General Procedure.

5. Gather the equipment described in the General Procedure, plus the following:

    a. Rolls of plaster of Paris. Assemble more than you think might be needed, and include various widths. The physician will often want to reinforce certain areas or add more casting material than originally planned. It is frustrating not to have enough casting rolls on hand. Physicians usually elect to use the larger rolls *because they produce a smoother cast with less chance of undue constriction.*

    b. A bucket or deep container for immersing the rolls.

    c. Cotton cast padding. This padding consists of soft, thin cotton layers between two outer layers of more closely woven cotton material. It comes pressed into a "waffled" configuration to prevent wadding underneath the cast. Gather several rolls of various widths.

Implementation

6.–8. Follow the steps of the General Procedure.

9. Assist the person applying the cast.

    a. Fill the bucket with warm water. Put on gloves to protect your skin from the plaster. *Warm water facilitates the drying process.*

    b. Stand a plaster roll on its end in the water *so that absorption is more uniform.*

    c. As soon as the bubbling stops, remove the roll and gently squeeze (but do not twist) out the excessive water. "Free up" the end of the roll.

    d. Hand the roll to the person applying the cast. The casting rolls are wrapped around the body part in an overlapping fashion.

    e. Repeat steps b, c, and d until the cast has been completed.

10. Follow the General Procedure.

11. Plan for proper positioning and support for the cast, remembering that simple exposure to the air will dry a plaster cast in 10 to 20 hours, depending on the size and thickness of the cast. The patient may feel cold as a result of evaporation from the cast. Keep the rest of the body covered *to prevent chilling and discomfort.*

12. Provide patient teaching as in step 12 of the General Procedure. Also explain that the cast frequently feels cold as it dries.

13. Care for equipment and supplies, and clean the area as follows:

    a. Clean off any plaster on surfaces by wiping with a moist cloth immediately before the plaster dries.

    b. Return unused materials to the supply location, and discard opened packages.

© 1996 by Lippincott-Raven Publishers

c. Dispose of water from the plaster application in a special sink with a plaster trap. *Plaster will clog a regular sink.*

14. Follow the General Procedure.

Evaluation

15. Follow the General Procedure.

Documentation

16. Follow the General Procedure.

Assisting With the Application of a Fiberglass Cast

Assessment

1.–3. Follow the steps of the General Procedure for Assisting With the Application of a Cast.

Planning

4. Follow the General Procedure.
5. Gather the equipment described in the General Procedure, plus the following:
   a. Sealed rolls of fiberglass casting material
   b. Synthetic cast padding
   c. Can of fiberglass material for finishing cast

Implementation

6.–8. Follow the steps of the General Procedure.
9. Assist the person applying the cast.
   a. Cut open the packages of fiberglass materials one at time as they are needed.
   b. Hold the package so that the person applying the cast can lift the roll out of the package.
10.–11. Follow the steps of the General Procedure.
12. Provide patient teaching as in step 12 of the General Procedure. Also explain that the cast commonly feels hot as it dries.
13.–14. Follow the steps of the General Procedure.

Evaluation

15. Follow the General Procedure.

Documentation

16. Follow the General Procedure.

COMMON TYPES OF CASTS

There are many variations on the types of casts commonly used. Each type carries with it the complications specific to having a particular part of the body enclosed. Figure 23–3 illustrates the various casts.

Short arm or leg casts extend from below the elbow to the fingers or from below the knee to the toes. The elbow or knee can still be flexed.

Long arm or hanging arm casts extend from under the axilla to the fingers. The elbow is maintained in flexion so that the arm can be supported by a sling or strap. Module 26, Applying Bandages and Binders, gives directions for tying a sling. *Long leg casts* extend from above the knee to the toes.

Shoulder spica casts immobilize the upper torso and one shoulder and arm. A support bar is used *for stability,* and a window is cut over the epigastrium *to promote comfort after eating.*

Hip spica casts can extend over the torso from just under the axilla or from the lower rib cage downward, enclosing both hips. One, one and one-half, or both legs may be casted, depending on need. A support bar is used if both legs are enclosed, and a window is again placed at the epigastrium.

CAST CHANGES AND ADAPTATIONS

Casts may be changed or adapted for the needs of the patient.

Cast Changes

Casts are changed for a variety of reasons. The cast may become too tight as a result of swelling or weight gain. The cast may no longer immobilize effectively as a result of weight loss, a decrease in swelling, or a decrease in underlying muscle bulk related to disuse. In the infant or child requiring long-term casting, normal growth patterns can cause the original cast to become too snug, and a new one must be applied. Wrinkling of the padding under the cast can cause extreme discomfort and necessitate a change. The cast also can be changed because of the possibility of infection beneath it. The cast may soften, crumble, or become badly soiled or odoriferous. When this happens, a cast change may be needed.

Bivalving

A usable cast can be bivalved instead of being totally removed and discarded. An electric cast saw is used to cut the cast lengthwise in two pieces (Fig. 23–4).

This usually is done *because of swelling, infection, or discomfort* when a fracture is partially healed and although support is still needed, an enclosed cast is unnecessary. An elastic bandage wrap can be used when the patient is moving *to keep the two halves together.* The top half can be lifted off when the patient

© 1996 by Lippincott-Raven Publishers

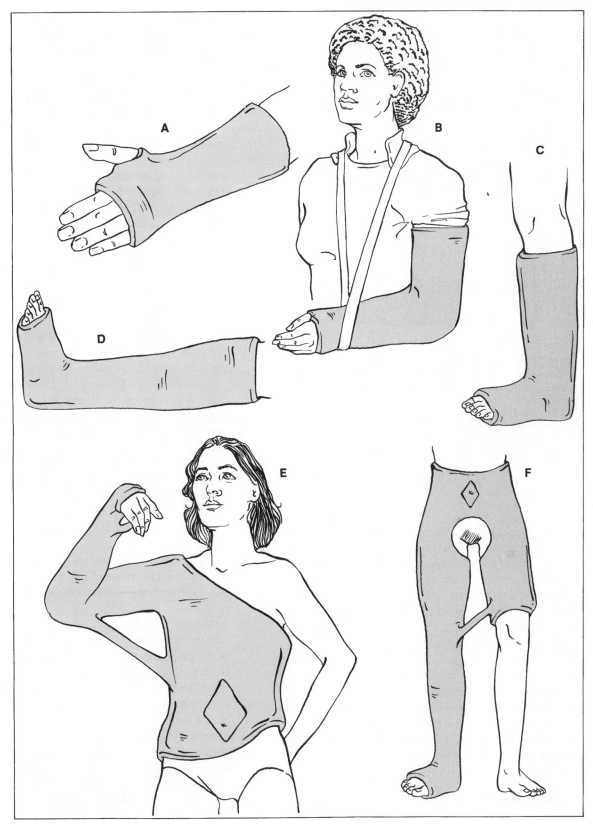

Figure 23–3. The various types of casts cover different parts of the body. The greater the surface of the body that is casted, the greater the chance for potential problems. **(A)** Short arm cast. **(B)** Hanging arm cast. **(C)** Short leg cast. **(D)** Long leg cast. **(E)** Shoulder spica cast. **(F)** Hip spica cast.

© 1996 by Lippincott-Raven Publishers

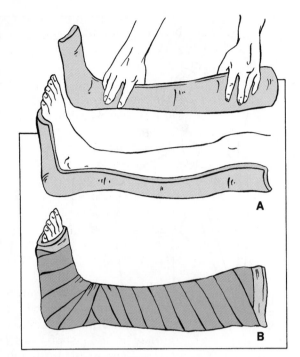

Figure 23–4. Bivalving. If the patient experiences swelling or infection, the cast may be bivalved (cut horizontally into two pieces). The top section can be removed to relieve pressure. The two halves are usually held together by elastic wrap to immobilize the casted area.

is resting *to relieve constant pressure from the cast* (see Fig. 23–4).

Windowing

Windowing involves cutting a square or diamond-shaped section from the cast *to allow for the observation and care of the skin underneath.* In some cases, this is done *to care for a surgical incision under the cast.* In others, pins that have been used to hold bones together must be removed through a window in the cast. Windows also are cut *to relieve pressure* when the tissue below includes a bony prominence or an area that will expand or swell. The swelling might be due to injury or, more commonly, to gastric enlargement caused by eating. Edges of windows should be "petaled" *to prevent skin irritation* (see step 2 of Continuing Care, p. 557). Handle the windowed part of a cast carefully, *because it is the weakest point, and cracking can occur.*

IMMEDIATE CARE OF THE PATIENT IN A CAST

The patient in a cast is at risk for specific problems. These problems are more likely to occur and to be more severe if a large proportion of the body or ex-

tremity is casted. Many important nursing actions can be taken to ensure the patient's comfort and safety. Consider the following guidelines carefully, and incorporate them into the plan of care for the patient immediately after casting. This plan of care may be carried out by the patient and family at home because many orthopedic procedures are done as day surgery. In such cases, the nurse must teach the patient and family.

1. Conduct circulation, motion, and sensation checks every hour while the cast is green, or in the drying stage. These are often referred to as CMS checks.
   a. *Circulation checks:* Check first for warmth of the toes or fingers of the extremity. Do not rely on the patient's report that the fingers or toes do not feel cool; *when the circulation is restricted, the patient's sensitivity is reduced.* Feel the surface of the skin with your own hand. Also, check for adequate circulation by observing the color of the nails (nail beds should be pink). Compare the pulse rates and quality of pulses of the two extremities. *Any differences could indicate that circulation is compromised.* Check for capillary filling by pressing on tissues. This causes blanching (loss of color) by emptying the capillary bed. Release the pressure and observe for the return of pink. It should return immediately. *Delayed capillary filling indicates that arterial circulation is impaired. When capillary filling is delayed, you should time how long it takes to occur. Swelling and darkening indicate impaired venous return.*
   b. Motion checks: Ask the patient to wiggle the fingers or toes. *Decreased ability to do this may indicate pressure on nerves from swelling or decreased circulation.*
   c. Sensation checks: Ask whether the patient can feel pressure when you press on the nails of the fingers or toes. Ask also about pain. Pain from the injury is expected, but *severe pain may result from decreased circulation or tissue swelling. Numbness or tingling may indicate pressure on nerves from the cast or from swelling.*
2. Ensure that the mattress is firmly supported if the patient is to remain in bed for any length of time. A firm surface *allows proper body alignment and supports a heavy cast.* In the hospital, beds usually have a flat metal surface supporting the mattress. In long-term care facilities, beds may have a flat spring. In this case, a special bed board is usually available to support the mattress. Placing a board between the mattress and box spring will provide the necessary support in the home.

© 1996 by Lippincott-Raven Publishers

3. Obtain a trapeze or side rails for the patient with a large, heavy cast or one who will remain in bed. *Such devices can help the patient move more easily in bed.* When this is not possible in the home, a rope tied to the foot of the bed and with a large knot where the patient can grasp it will help the patient move about in bed.

4. Use two care providers if you will be moving a patient with a large cast. One person can support the cast while the other assists the patient. Supporting the cast well *prevents undue strain on muscle groups adjacent to it.*

5. Encourage the patient to turn *after the cast is completely dry because turning prevents respiratory complications and helps elimination, as does other exercise.* Teach the patient to move in one plane *so that muscle groups are not stretched.*

6. Give instructions in performing isometric exercises if the patient is on continuous bed rest. These exercises *can help prevent loss of muscle tone and strength.*

7. Ensure that a nurse or physical therapist has given the ambulatory patient in a leg cast instructions in safe walking. *The weight of the cast can affect body balance,* leading to unsteadiness and possible falls. Assistive aids, such as a cane, crutches, or a walker, may be necessary (see Module 21, Ambulation: Simple Assisted and Using Cane, Walker, or Crutches) for such patients.

8. Document carefully on patients in casts. Whether your entry refers to a patient who has just been casted or to one who has been in a cast for some time, include specific findings relating to circulation, motion, and sensation as outlined previously. These observations are most often entered on a flow sheet. Also record any relevant psychological data.

CONTINUING CARE OF THE PATIENT IN A CAST

In 24 to 48 hours after the initial casting, the acute danger of swelling under the cast is gone; however, problems may still occur. The following should be part of the plan of care, whether the person is hospitalized or at home.

1. Conduct ongoing assessment of the following:
   a. Circulation, motion, and sensation. These checks (as described previously) are continued to identify any problems. After the initial period, the checks are gradually spaced out to longer and longer intervals until they are done just once a day by the patient.

   b. *Tightness or looseness. Either of these conditions can cause complications.* You should be able to slip one finger easily between the cast and the patient's skin.

   c. *Drainage.* Observe for signs of drainage coming through the cast. Report, record, and describe the size of any area stained with drainage. Most facilities have a policy of outlining the area of drainage with a felt-tipped pen, noting date and time. *This allows increases in drainage to be seen quickly. Because some patients can become anxious over this procedure,* reassure the patient that this is a method of assessment so that he or she does not become unduly alarmed.

   d. *Odor.* Check the odor of the cast. *A musty, foul odor can signal infection and should be reported immediately.*

2. Edge the cast. The edge of a cast must be finished in a way that protects the skin from the cast material and the cast material from perspiration, urine, or feces. This may be done when the cast is applied by folding padding material over the edges and fastening it on the outside of the cast; it also may be done after the cast is dry.
   a. Make adhesive petals by cutting small strips of adhesive tape into pointed or rounded ends. Place these strips perpendicular to the cast edge and then smooth over the edge and tuck inside the cast. Pointed petals wrinkle more readily than rounded ones. Moleskin cut into round sections *provides a smoother and softer surface and has less tendency to wrinkle up than tape* (Fig. 23–5). Commercially made cast-edging petals also are available.
   b. Protect casts that surround the perineal or anal area from soiling by edging or covering them with plastic secured by tape (Fig. 23–6).

3. Try to keep water or moisture away from a plaster of Paris cast when the patient is bathing or being bathed *so that the cast will not be damaged.*

4. Protect the exposed toes of a patient in a leg cast against cold with a heavy sock. Also prevent contact with sharp or dangerous objects; *because of the cast, the extremity cannot be flexed and withdrawn from danger.*

5. Discourage the patient from attempting to scratch beneath the cast with sharp objects. Sharp objects can *damage or even puncture the underlying skin surfaces.* These abrasions or injuries may remain undetected and become infected. Itching is usually present to some degree and is especially likely when the cast is in place for a long time. Physically, little can be done about this problem except changing the cast. The best intervention for itching is distraction. Keeping the mind focused on

© 1996 by Lippincott-Raven Publishers

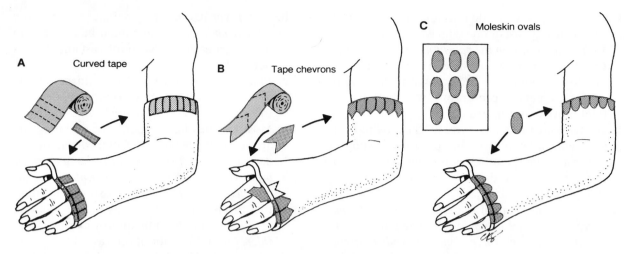

Figure 23–5. You can make "petals" by **(A)** cutting adhesive into small strips or **(B)** chevrons. You can also make petals from moleskin cut ovals **(C)**. Tuck petals smoothly over the edge of the cast to protect the skin from crumbling plaster and rough edges.

something interesting will make other sensations recede. A cool environment also helps, *because perspiration under the cast increases itching.* Sometimes the physician may recommend an over-the-counter analgesic, such as acetaminophen, to relieve itching at bedtime when it is hard to maintain distraction.

6. Assess for unpleasant odors caused by perspiration and bacteria, especially if the cast is extensive. These odors are different from the odor of infection. Commercial cast deodorants, which are sometimes mixed with the casting materials, are largely ineffective. A cast change is sometimes necessary if the odor becomes too unpleasant.

Never ignore the patient's complaints. *They could be the first indication of a problem that could develop into serious complications.* You should offer emotional support to all patients in casts. *Being encased within a cast of any size imposes restrictions on activities of daily living that concern and inconvenience the patient.*

BRACES

Braces are rigid devices that may be applied for several purposes:

1. *To provide protection and healing of minor fractures*
2. *To maintain therapeutic alignment for body parts*
3. *To protect soft-tissue injuries*
4. *To provide support after orthopedic surgery*
5. *To correct skeletal malformations*

Braces are made of cotton, soft or rigid plastic, metal, or a combination of these materials. Because of their many applications, braces are contoured to all parts of the body—cervical spine, lower spine, and extremities. Braces are available with movable joints when this feature is appropriate.

Some braces are named after the place they were developed. For example, the Boston, Milwaukee,

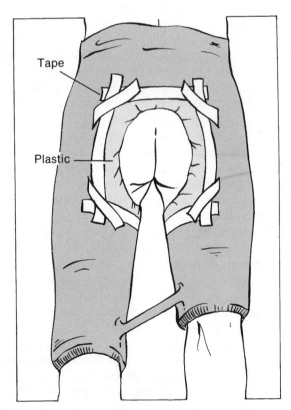

Figure 23–6. To protect casts surrounding the anal or perineal area from soiling, cut wide strips of plastic and tuck these smoothly over the soft padding around the cast edges. Tape the plastic in place on the cast. (Note the completed twist support.)

© 1996 by Lippincott-Raven Publishers

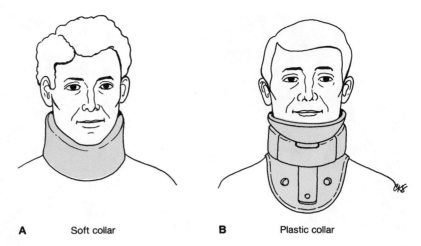

Figure 23–7. Cervical collar. The cervical collar is available in both padded cotton and rigid plastic materials. It is used for neck sprains and limits flexion and extension. Apply by encircling neck and fastening. **(A)** Soft collar. **(B)** Plastic collar.

A   Soft collar   **B**   Plastic collar

and Philadelphia braces were developed in the respective locations. Other braces are named after the designer, such as the Thomas brace. Many commercial companies produce the same brace under their own brand names.

Potential complications are associated with wearing braces. The patient may report initial discomfort and then develop skin problems. All braces should be applied over skin that is protected by clothing *so that excoriation does not occur.* Some braces have a protective soft inner lining sufficient for this purpose. The patient may have difficulty adjusting to changes in mobility if the brace is a body or leg brace.

Braces for patients in a healthcare facility are ordered from a commercial company that sends a representative to measure the patient *to ensure a correct fit.* Braces for children and adolescents may have to be refitted periodically *due to growth changes.* Older people also may need to have braces changed from time to time *due to shortening of the spine and structural changes in other bones.*

This module discusses only common types of braces and the appropriate parts of the body to which they are applied. The name "splint" is sometimes used for the term brace.

TYPES OF BRACES

Cervical Collar

The cervical collar is used for a neck strain. Trauma such as whiplash is treated by immobilizing the neck *so that neither flexion nor extension can occur.* It is difficult to rotate the head with a cervical collar in place.

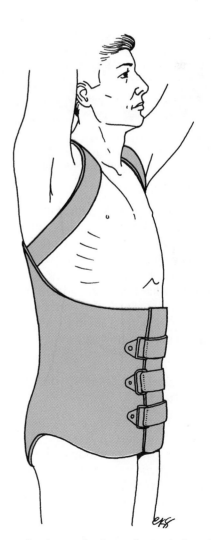

Figure 23–8. The thoracic-lumbosacral spine body jacket provides both anterior and posterior support. It is contoured to the body. Apply by wrapping around trunk and fastening with straps or Velcro. Adjust shoulder straps.

© 1996 by Lippincott-Raven Publishers

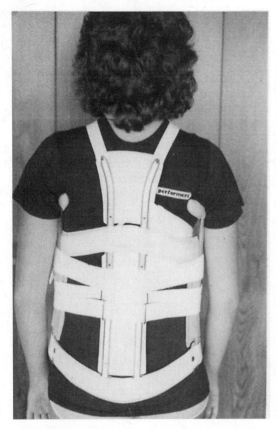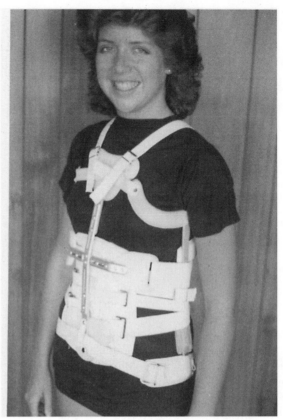

Figure 23–9. Boston scoliosis brace (Kosair). This brace has steel supports both anteriorly and posteriorly to correct lateral spinal curvature. It is fitted to the patient and is applied by holding the brace in place and adjusting with the straps provided.

In addition, the collar supports the weight of the head. Cervical collars are available in a soft version made from foam rubber with a cloth cover or a hard plastic collar with a padded cuff (Fig. 23–7).

To apply the cervical collar, encircle the neck as the patient looks straight ahead. Fasten firmly with the Velcro or straps provided with the specific collar being used. Check the patient for any impingement on breathing or swallowing.

Thoracic-Lumbosacral Spine Body Jacket

This is a multipurpose brace that provides anterior and posterior support. It is widely used for many types of orthopedic conditions. The brace may be worn *to prevent the progression of deformity in scoliosis.* It also may be worn after surgery *for scoliosis or other orthopedic surgery* (Fig. 23–8).

Boston Scoliosis Brace

The Boston Scoliosis Brace is effective as support for the thoracic-lumbar region. It can be used for a low-er back strain or for scoliosis if the curvature is primarily of the lower spine (Fig. 23–9). This brace has now replaced the heavier Milwaukee brace that was designed for the same purpose.

Boston Brace

The Boston brace supports the lumbosacral region. The brace is made of a rigid but flexible plastic material and is molded to the contours of the wearer. It is available with straps or Velcro fastenings (Fig. 23–10).

Anterior Spinal Hyperextension Brace

A brace that prevents anterior flexion of the thoracic spine is the anterior spinal hyperextension brace. It can be used *to prevent the progression of kyphosis in elderly patients.* The flexible soft plastic "plates" are comfortable for the patient and can be concealed under ordinary clothing (Fig. 23–11).

© 1996 by Lippincott-Raven Publishers

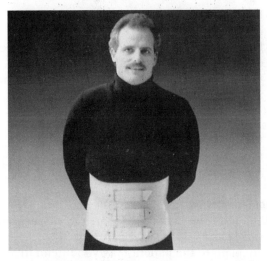

Figure 23–10. The Boston brace provides support to the lumbosacral region. Apply it by fitting it snugly around the body so that it is positioned around the lower spine and fasten with Velcro or straps.

Cast/Brace Combinations

Braces are applied in combination with casts in certain conditions. Patients undergoing amputation of the lower extremity may have a cast applied during the surgical procedure and a walking brace attached to the cast. These people begin ambulation earlier than they previously would have because of these assistive devices.

The cast/brace also is used with severe fractures, using the same rationale. The cast material protects the fracture, and the brace provides support for minimal weight-bearing earlier than would be possible without such devices (Fig. 23–12).

Knee and Leg Braces

Many kinds of knee and leg braces are available. Some are rigid so that the patient's knee is immobilized. Others are jointed *so that the patient can maintain knee joint mobility. Because these braces are complicated,* to be safe and effective, they require a person who has been instructed in the techniques for their

Figure 23–11. The anterior spinal hyperextension brace prevents anterior flexion of the thoracic spine. To apply, place in position and secure with straps that fasten at the back.

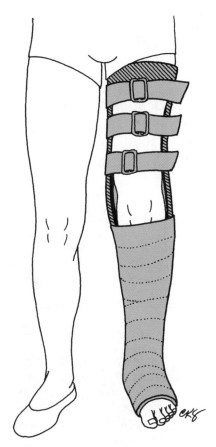

Figure 23–12. The combination of the cast and brace allows earlier ambulation for the person who has had a severe leg fracture. It is applied during the surgical procedure.

© 1996 by Lippincott-Raven Publishers

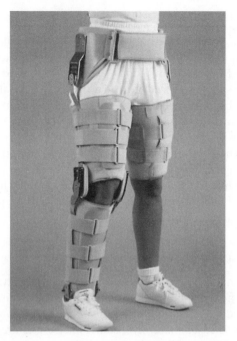

Figure 23–13. Knee and leg braces are available as rigid support or with the option of a flexible knee joint. This complex brace is designed for one leg but also has waist and opposite leg stabilizers. Most leg braces are designed to fit onto one leg only.

application. The study of sports medicine has greatly added to knowledge in this area (Fig. 23–13).

GENERAL PROCEDURE FOR ASSISTING WITH THE APPLICATION OF A BRACE

Assessment

1. Review the patient's record to determine the injury or condition and the type of brace ordered.

2. Read any instructions that accompany the brace.
3. Find out what information the patient has been given.
4. Determine the patient's understanding and how much assistance the patient can give.

Planning

5. Wash your hands *for infection control.*
6. Inspect the brace, and plan the method for application.

Implementation

7. Identify the patient *to be sure you are performing the procedure for the correct patient.*
8. Explain to the patient how you intend to apply the brace, and explain the various parts and fastening devices.
9. Have the patient put on clothing that will *provide protection from the pressure of the brace.*
10. Help the patient to a position that is the most convenient for application.
11. Apply the brace to the body part for which it is intended.

Evaluation

12. Evaluate the following:
    a. Effectiveness of the brace to fulfill its purpose
    b. Circulation, motion, and sensation of the part affected
    c. Patient comfort

Documentation

13. Document the type of brace applied and any observations.

DATE/TIME	
2/21/99 0930	*Instructed in application of jacket brace. Has difficulty getting out of bed to chair when wearing brace. Transferred to chair with assistance.* — B. Martin, NS

(A) Example of Nursing Progress Notes Using Narrative Format.

DATE/TIME	
4/1/99 8:00 AM	*Impairment of skin integrity related to pressure from brace* S *"It is a little sore over my upper back when the brace is on."* O *Nickel-sized reddened area over thoracic spine.* A *Pressure of brace causing tissue irritation.* P *Assess padding under brace and call physician if redness persists.* D. Dolan, RN

(B) Example of Nursing Progress Notes Using SOAP Format.

© 1996 by Lippincott-Raven Publishers

EMOTIONAL SUPPORT

Casts and braces are long-term treatments. Being in a cast or having to wear a brace places stress on the individual. People in casts realize that they are restricted physically and that they cannot easily perform some of their routine daily tasks. These tasks may be essential, such as bathing, eating, or moving around the setting rapidly. There also are minor inconveniences. In the healthcare facility, the patient may have difficulty finding a comfortable position in which to read in bed. As an outpatient, the person may have limited access to restaurants, theaters, and other social places. In the extreme, the person confined to bed in a body cast may understandably worry about safety *in the case of a fire or emergency.*

An adult of advanced age who is required to wear a spinal brace on a permanent basis may have feelings of lowered self-esteem *related to restrictions on activity. Body image is particularly important to teenagers, and some casts cannot be totally concealed under clothing.* To the teenager, this may be embarrassing and may lead to emotional distress. The teenager in a jacket brace cannot participate in sports with companions and may feel excluded.

Whatever the degree of stress, you can offer understanding and allow the person to talk about the temporary or permanent adjustments that must be made. If temporary, short-term planning can be done with the patient so that he or she feels some control over the situation. If the cast or brace is long term, you can emphasize activities the person can do and minimize attention to activities that must be postponed or eliminated. Planning realistically and positively *can greatly reduce stress.*

LONG-TERM CARE

Residents in long-term care facilities commonly are fitted with braces and sometimes admitted with a cast in place. In either situation, the nurse must understand the proper care and maintenance of patients with these devices. You should become familiar with the care of the specific cast that has been applied and how to assist with the application of a resident's brace. Following the general guidelines in this module will be useful in providing care.

Complications can arise *due to immobility and disuse of joints and muscles.* The resident may feel off-balance if ambulating *because of the weight of a cast if it is on one extremity.* The resident wearing a brace also may feel off-balance *due to the restriction on movement.* Until adjustments are made, safety and falls are a constant concern. You may have to assess for and obtain assistive devices and instruct the resident in their use.

Integrate into your plan of care regular range-of-motion exercises to keep the resident's other joints and muscles functional. Identifying measures for maintaining a good diet and adequate elimination also should be included in your plan.

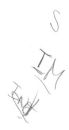

© 1996 by Lippincott-Raven Publishers

HOME CARE

People in the home may have casts or may be fitted with braces. Use the same principles of assessment and care as those used in the healthcare facility.

Casts and braces may interfere with the home maintenance role, *causing the person to feel more dependent on others than usual.* Some states have laws that prohibit a person with any cast or brace in place that inhibits full movement of the body from driving a motor vehicle. *This adds to the person's dependence and may affect the ability to fulfill important responsibilities.*

A home care nurse can instruct the client and family in ways to handle such situations and provide continuing assessment. An important part of this assessment includes the knowledge that even when a cast or brace has been in place for an extended time, *the potential for skin problems remains.* General concerns surrounding immobilization also must be taken into consideration for the client at home.

CRITICAL THINKING EXERCISES

• Jeff Whitman, age 22, was injured in a motorcycle accident. He has been admitted to your unit with a fractured hip, pelvis, and left femur that have been surgically fixated; a hip spica body cast has been applied. This is his first hospitalization. Synthesize information you know about psychosocial development, the process of bone healing, and cast care, and identify major priorities in nursing care for this young man.

• Amy Johnson, age 10, fell off her bike while riding and broke her left wrist. You have helped with applying a cast in the emergency room. She is to be discharged for care at home. Plan the teaching that will be necessary for Amy and her parents.

© 1996 by Lippincott-Raven Publishers

✔ PERFORMANCE CHECKLIST

General Procedure for Assisting With the Application of a Cast	Needs More Practice	Satisfactory	Comments
Assessment			
1. Review patient's record and doctor's notes.			
2. Inspect the skin over which the cast is to be placed for edema or interruptions in skin integrity.			
3. Find out what information has been given to patient and whether clarification is needed. Determine whether sedative has been ordered.			
Planning			
4. Wash your hands.			
5. Gather equipment appropriate to type of cast:			
a. Stockinette			
b. Scissors			
c. Cast padding			
d. Cast knife.			
e. Cast saw			
f. Cloth adhesive tape			
g. Plastic apron and gloves			
Implementation			
6. Identify patient.			
7. Drape patient.			
8. Offer emotional support and reassurance.			
9. Assist the person applying the cast.			
10. Clean excess material from patient's skin.			
11. Position the patient comfortably, and support the cast:			
a. Handle cast only with palms of hands until completely dry.			
b. Place small plastic-covered pillows under and around cast as appropriate.			
c. Elevate the extremity.			
d. Leave cast uncovered during drying process.			

(continued)

© 1996 by Lippincott-Raven Publishers

General Procedure for Assisting With the Application of a Cast *(Continued)*	Needs More Practice	Satisfactory	Comments
12. Provide patient teaching, covering the following: **a.** Monitoring			
b. Length of time cast takes to dry			
c. How a cast feels as it dries			
d. Importance of reporting feelings of pain, pressure, or altered sensation			
e. Need to keep the extremity immobile until cast is dry			
13. Care for equipment and supplies; clean area as needed.			
14. Wash your hands.			
Evaluation			
15. Evaluate the following: **a.** Patient comfort			
b. Condition of the cast			
c. Circulation, motion, and sensation of casted body parts			
Documentation			
16. Document the following: **a.** Type of cast applied			
b. Neurovascular assessment			
c. Patient comfort			
Assisting With the Application of a Plaster of Paris Cast			
Assessment			
1.–3. Follow checklist steps 1–3 of the General Procedure for Assisting With the Application of a Cast (review patient's record and doctor's notes; inspect the skin; find out what information patient has been given; determine whether sedative has been ordered).			
Planning			
4. Wash your hands as in checklist step 4 of the General Procedure.			

(continued)

© 1996 by Lippincott-Raven Publishers

Assisting With the Application of a Plaster of Paris Cast *(Continued)*	Needs More Practice	Satisfactory	Comments
5. Gather the equipment described in checklist step 5 of the General Procedure, plus the following: **a.** Rolls of plaster of Paris			
b. Bucket or deep container			
c. Cotton cast padding			
Implementation			
6.–8. Follow Checklist steps 6–8 of the General Procedure (identify patient; drape patient; offer emotional support).			
9. Assist the person applying the cast in the following way: (Wear gloves.) **a.** Fill bucket or container with warm water.			
b. Place first plaster of Paris roll in the water vertically.			
c. As soon as bubbles stop rising, remove roll and squeeze. "Free up" end of roll.			
d. Hand roll to person applying cast.			
e. Repeat steps b, c, and d until the cast has been completed.			
10. Clean excess material from patient's skin as in checklist step 10 of the General Procedure.			
11. Position the patient comfortably, and support the cast. Because the patient may feel cold as a result of evaporation from the cast, keep the rest of the body covered.			
12. Provide patient teaching as in checklist step 12 of the General Procedure. Also explain that the cast commonly feels cold as it dries.			
13. Care for equipment and supplies, and clean the area as follows: **a.** Clean plaster off surfaces by wiping with a moist cloth.			
b. Return unused materials and discard open packages.			
c. Dispose of water from the application in a special sink with a plaster trap.			
14. Wash your hands as in checklist step 14 of the General Procedure.			

(continued)

© 1996 by Lippincott-Raven Publishers

Assisting With the Application of a Plaster of Paris Cast *(Continued)*	Needs More Practice	Satisfactory	Comments
Evaluation			
15. Evaluate as in checklist step 15 of the General Procedure (patient comfort; condition of cast; circulation, motion, and sensation of casted body parts).			
Documentation			
16. Document as in checklist step 16 of the General Procedure (type of cast applied; neurovascular assessment; patient comfort).			
Assisting With the Application of a Fiberglass Cast			
Assessment			
1.–3. Follow checklist steps 1–3 of the General Procedure for Assisting With the Application of a Cast (review patient's record and doctor's notes; inspect the skin; find out what information patient has been given; determine whether sedative has been ordered).			
Planning			
4. Wash your hands as in checklist step 4 of the General Procedure.			
5. Gather the equipment described in checklist step 5 of the General Procedure, plus the following: **a.** Sealed rolls of fiberglass casting material			
b. Synthetic cast padding			
c. Can of fiberglass material			
Implementation			
6.–8. Follow checklist steps 6–8 of the General Procedure (identify patient; drape patient; offer emotional support).			
9. Assist the person applying the cast in the following way: **a.** Cut open packages of fiberglass materials as needed.			
b. Hold the package so the person applying the cast can lift out the roll.			

(continued)

© 1996 by Lippincott-Raven Publishers

Assisting With the Application of a Fiberglass Cast *(Continued)*	Needs More Practice	Satisfactory	Comments
10.–11. Follow checklist steps 10 and 11 of the General Procedure (clean excess material from patient's skin, and position patient comfortably and support cast).			
12. Provide patient teaching as in checklist step 12 of the General Procedure. Also explain that the cast commonly feels hot as it dries.			
13.–14. Follow checklist steps 13 and 14 of the General Procedure (care for equipment and supplies; clean area; wash your hands).			
Evaluation			
15. Evaluate as in checklist step 15 of the General Procedure (patient comfort; condition of cast; circulation, motion, and sensation of casted body parts).			
Documentation			
16. Document as in checklist step 16 of the General Procedure (type of cast applied, neurovascular assessment, patient comfort).			
Immediate Care of the Patient in a Cast			
1. Conduct circulation, motion, and sensation checks.			
2. Ensure that the mattress is firmly supported; use a bed board if needed.			
3. Obtain a trapeze or side rails as needed.			
4. Use two care providers when moving a patient with a large cast.			
5. Encourage the patient to turn when the cast is completely dry.			
6. Instruct the patient on bed rest in isometric exercises.			
7. Instruct the ambulatory patient with a leg cast in safe walking; use assistive devices as needed.			
8. Document carefully observations and patient's psychological response.			

(continued)

© 1996 by Lippincott-Raven Publishers

Continuing Care of the Patient in a Cast	Needs More Practice	Satisfactory	Comments
1. Conduct ongoing assessment of the following: a. Circulation, motion, and sensation			
b. Tightness or looseness			
c. Drainage			
d. Odor			
2. Edge the cast.			
3. Keep water or moisture away from plaster of Paris casts.			
4. Protect exposed toes from cold with a heavy sock.			
5. Discourage use of sharp objects for scratching underneath cast.			
6. Assess for unpleasant odors.			
General Procedure for the Application of a Brace			
Assessment			
1. Review patient's record to determine injury or condition and type of brace to be applied.			
2. Read any instructions accompanying the brace.			
3. Find out what information the patient has been given.			
4. Determine patient's understanding and degree of assistance.			
Planning			
5. Wash your hands.			
6. Inspect brace and plan application.			
Implementation			
7. Identify the patient.			
8. Explain to patient how you plan to apply brace.			
9. Have patient put on clothing *for protection*.			
10. Help patient to a convenient position.			
11. Apply brace to body part.			

(continued)

© 1996 by Lippincott-Raven Publishers

General Procedure for the Application of a Brace *(Continued)*	Needs More Practice	Satisfactory	Comments
Evaluation			
12. Evaluate the following: **a.** Effectiveness of brace			
b. Circulation, motion, and sensation of affected part			
c. Patient comfort			
Documentation			
13. Document type of brace applied and any observations.			

© 1996 by Lippincott-Raven Publishers

❓ QUIZ

Short-Answer Questions

1. The two kinds of casts are _____ and _____ .

2. Two advantages of a plaster of Paris cast are _____ and _____ .

3. Two advantages of a fiberglass cast are _____ and _____ .

4. The skin is inspected carefully before casting to prevent _____ .

5. The rough edges of a cast can be finished or covered by either of two methods, _____ and _____ .

6. When a person is in a cast or wearing a brace, the affected tissue is assessed for decreased circulation by checking _____ _____ .

7. Three kinds of materials used for constructing braces are _____ _____ .

8. Patients wearing braces may have difficulty ambulating because _____ .

Multiple-Choice Questions

_____ 9. Spica casts cover basically

   a. an arm or leg only.
   b. the body.
   c. the body and only one arm or leg.
   d. the body and one or more extremities.

_____ 10. Windowing is done to

   a. enlarge the cast.
   b. relieve pressure on underlying tissue.
   c. feel the fracture.
   d. do none of the above.

_____ 11. The toes or fingers of the patient in a green cast should be checked

   a. every 15 minutes.
   b. every hour.
   c. once per shift.
   d. once per day.

_____ 12. The brace on a child may have to be changed periodically due to

   a. increased activity.
   b. noncompliance.
   c. growth changes.
   d. wear and damage of the appliance.

_____ 13. Printed instructions for applying a brace will most likely come from

   a. the physician.
   b. the company supplying the brace.
   c. a nurse clinical specialist.
   d. the central supply department.

© 1996 by Lippincott-Raven Publishers

MODULE

24

APPLYING AND MAINTAINING TRACTION

MODULE CONTENTS

RATIONALE FOR THE USE OF THIS
  SKILL
NURSING DIAGNOSES
PURPOSES OF TRACTION
EQUIPMENT AND SETUP
The Traction Bed and Frame
Ropes
Pulleys
Weights
SPECIAL PROBLEMS FOR THE PATIENT
  IN TRACTION
SKIN TRACTION
TYPES OF SKIN TRACTION
Humerus (Side-Arm) Traction
Buck's Traction
Russell's Traction
Bryant's Traction
Pelvic Traction
Pelvic Sling Traction
Cervical Halter Traction
PROCEDURE FOR APPLYING SKIN
  TRACTION

Assessment
Planning
Implementation
Evaluation
Documentation
SKELETAL TRACTION
TYPES OF SKELETAL TRACTION
Balanced Suspension Traction
Skull Tongs Traction
Halo Traction
External Fixation Devices
PROCEDURE FOR MAINTAINING
  SKELETAL TRACTION
Assessment
Planning
Implementation
Evaluation
Documentation
CRITICAL THINKING EXERCISES

PREREQUISITES

Successful completion of the following modules:

VOLUME 1
Module 1   An Approach to Nursing Skills
Module 2   Basic Infection Control
Module 3   Safety
Module 4   Basic Body Mechanics
Module 5   Documentation
Module 6   Introduction to Assessment Skills
Module 15   Moving the Patient in Bed and Positioning
Module 22   Range-of-Motion Exercises
Module 26   Applying Bandages and Binders

© 1996 by Lippincott-Raven Publishers

OVERALL OBJECTIVE

To apply skin traction to the patient and maintain commonly used skin and skeletal traction devices effectively and safely.

SPECIFIC LEARNING OBJECTIVES

Know Facts and Principles	Apply Facts and Principles	Demonstrate Ability	Evaluate Performance
1. Purposes State two or more basic purposes of traction. Explain how pull or tension is applied to the tissue.	Apply principles when setting up traction appliances. Explain purpose of a particular type of traction for specific patient.	In the clinical setting, identify the type of traction used for a particular patient and the purpose of that traction.	Evaluate with insltructor.
2. Traction equipment Name various types of equipment used in setting up traction.	Given a patient situation, explain use of each piece of equipment.	In the clinical setting, locate equipment for traction.	Evaluate with instructor.
3. Special problems List, by body system, special problems that may arise from the immobilization imposed by traction.	Given a patient situation, assess patient, and suggest intervention for problems.	In the clinical setting, assess the patient for special problems using previously learned theory.	Evaluate with instructor.
4. Types of traction Explain the basic difference between skin and skeletal traction.	Given a patient situation, identify type of traction suitable for patient.	In the clinical setting, discuss the rationale for the type of traction being used to treat a particular patient.	Evaluate with instructor.

5. Procedures

   *a. Skin traction: Humerus (sidearm); Buck's; Russell's; Bryant's Pelvic; Pelvic
      sling; Cervical halter*

State position of bed and patient, equipment needed, direction needed, direction of pull, and special potential problems with each.	In the practice setting, correctly set up skin traction. With a patient in traction, determine purpose and effectiveness of treatment, and assess for potential problems.	In the clinical setting, care for the patient requiring skin traction, performing either application or maintenance.	Evaluate performance with instructor.

(continued)

© 1996 by Lippincott-Raven Publishers

Know Facts and Principles	Apply Facts and Principles	Demonstrate Ability	Evaluate Performance
b. Skeletal traction: Balanced suspension; Skull tongs; Halo traction; External fixation devices			
State position of bed and patient, equipment applied to the patient, direction of pull, and potential problems of each.	Given a patient in traction, determine purpose, and identify potential problems.	In the clinical setting, maintain skeletal traction under supervision.	Evaluate performance with instructor.
6. Documentation			
State what information should be recorded regarding the type of traction being used and the patient's response.	Given a patient situation, give an example of appropriate documentation.	In the clinical setting, document for a patient using either skin or skeletal traction.	Evaluate performance with instructor.

LEARNING ACTIVITIES

1. Review the Specific Learning Objectives.
2. Read the section on sensory disturbance in Ellis and Nowlis, *Nursing: A Human Needs Approach,* or comparable material in another textbook.
3. Look up the module vocabulary terms in the glossary.
4. Read through the module as though you were preparing to teach another person. Mentally practice the techniques described.
5. In the practice setting, do the following:
   a. Inspect the bed trapeze, pulleys, and weights available.
   b. Practice tying a traction knot.
   c. When you feel proficient doing this, have a partner check your knot, and you check your partner's knot.
   d. With a partner, practice applying one type of skin traction to experience the pulling sensation. Use both tape and a boot if possible.
   e. Together, evaluate the traction experience with attention to the feeling of immobility and psychosocial concerns.
   f. With a partner, practice applying Buck's traction and pelvic traction.
6. In the clinical setting, do the following:
   a. Arrange with your instructor for an opportunity to care for a patient in traction.
   b. Review the nursing care plan for this patient; pay particular attention to parts of the plan relating to traction or problems with immobilization.
   c. Administer care to the patient in traction, based on what you have learned.
   d. Evaluate your performance with your instructor.

VOCABULARY

anorexia	footdrop	occiput	thrombophlebitis
cervical traction	footrest	popliteal space	traction
countertraction	hairline fracture	prism glasses	trapeze
excoriate	humerus	pulley	whiplash
fixation	iliac crest	skull tongs	
foot board	integument	spreader bar	

© 1996 by Lippincott-Raven Publishers

Applying and Maintaining Traction

Rationale for the Use of This Skill

Traction devices are used to treat many injuries and conditions of the musculoskeletal system. Nurses on the unit can safely and effectively apply the simple, commonly used traction devices to keep an injured body part in proper alignment using the prescribed pull or tension. However, nurses or technicians with special training need to apply some of the more complicated traction devices. If reduction of a fracture requires surgery, the patient may return from the operating room to the unit with traction already in place. You are then responsible to maintain it properly. Traction and the immobility associated with it place the patient at risk for other complications, such as skin breakdown, muscle atrophy, urinary retention, hypoventilation, and pneumonia.[1]

▼ NURSING DIAGNOSES

Examples of some nursing diagnoses related to traction include the following:

Impaired Physical Mobility related to traction

Sleep Pattern Disturbance related to discomfort and confinement by traction device

Impaired Skin Integrity related to pin insertion sites

Risk for Infection related to presence of skeletal pin sites

Diversional Activity Deficit: Boredom related to confinement imposed by traction

PURPOSES OF TRACTION

Traction has several uses in the treatment of musculoskeletal conditions and injury. A pulling force on bones can be used to correct deformities. Immobilizing and aligning fractures with traction *encourages healing.* When traction is applied to muscles by a pull on the skin, *pressure on nerves can be decreased, providing relief from muscle spasm.* Through the use of pins and rods, which are inserted through the skin, traction can be exerted on bones (skeletal traction), *allowing more pull for the reduction of fractures or bony deformity.* Traction is most commonly applied to the

arms, legs, and spine, including the cervical spine, or neck.

Traction relies on the application of force or "pull" in two directions simultaneously to maintain the stability of a body part. Traction is commonly applied by using weights to pull in one direction and the body's own weight to provide pull or "countertraction" in the other direction. Traction also may be applied by arranging sets of weights that provide pull in opposing directions. Traction may be applied continuously or intermittently, depending on its purpose.

EQUIPMENT AND SETUP

The equipment and application methods for traction may vary somewhat from one healthcare setting to another. Essentially, the equipment consists of a traction bed, which provides correct body alignment for the patient. Traction pull is supplied by various ropes, pulleys, and weights. Discussions of each of these follow.

The Traction Bed and Frame

A regular hospital bed can be easily converted to a traction bed by installing a horizontal overhead bar attached to vertical bars at the head and foot. A trapeze device can be added to the overhead bar *to assist the patient to move* (Fig. 24–1).

All traction beds should have a firm, solid base under the mattress. Older beds with a spring base require the use of a bedboard *to provide a firm foundation, which helps maintain good body alignment.* Many

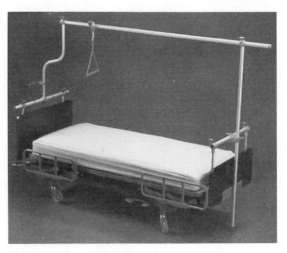

Figure 24–1. Bed prepared for traction application. The traction bars and overhead trapeze are in place. (Courtesy Zimmer, Inc., Warsaw, Indiana.)

---

[1]Note that rationales for action are emphasized throughout the module by the use of italics.

© 1996 by Lippincott-Raven Publishers

special mattresses and therapeutic beds and frames may be used for patients with special problems who also need traction (see Module 25, Special Mattresses and Therapeutic Frames and Beds).

Ropes

Inspect all ropes for kinking or fraying. Use only clean ropes in good condition. Ropes must hang freely without interference from bedding or bars. Wrap the ends of ropes near the patient's body with a pull tape *to prevent slipping and fraying*. You can do this by covering the end of the rope with adhesive tape and folding the two free ends of the tape over on themselves to form two pull tabs that can easily be removed (Fig. 24–2).

When tying ropes, use a traction knot, as shown in Figure 24–3. All knots are taped for safety *so that they do not separate*.

Pulleys

Be sure all pulleys move freely and function properly. Most pulleys are prelubricated. If they do not move easily, lubricate them with an oiled cotton sponge or silicone spray.

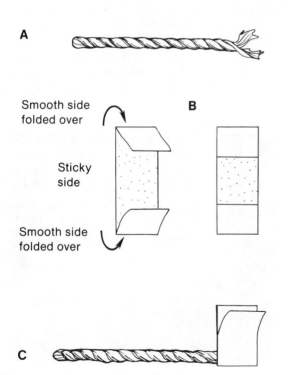

Figure 24–2. Pull-tape on end of rope. **(A)** Rope with frayed ends. **(B)** Prepared tape with folded-over ends to make removal easy. **(C)** Tape folded over end of rope to prevent further fraying.

© 1996 by Lippincott-Raven Publishers

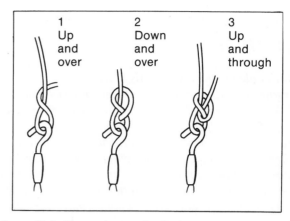

Figure 24–3. How to tie a traction knot.

Weights

The physician decides how much weight is to be applied. Metal blocks and sand bags, with hooks for attachment to the ropes, are used as weights. Weight is ordered by the physician in pounds. Each weight is marked with the number of pounds. Typically, a combination of weights is needed to achieve the desired traction. If weights are used intermittently, remove them slowly and gently while support is simultaneously given to the affected body part *to avoid jarring the patient*. You may need assistance to do this properly. Weights must hang freely from the pulleys at all times. When not in use, stack weights carefully out of the way *to avoid injuries*.

SPECIAL PROBLEMS FOR THE PATIENT IN TRACTION

Circulation, motor function, and sensation may be compromised by the pressure of a traction device on an extremity. Therefore, carry out routine circulation, motion, and sensation checks for patients in traction.

All patients in traction are immobilized to some degree, ranging from minimal restriction of activity to complete immobilization. Because of this immobilization, many body systems are at risk.

The *integument* (skin) is prone to breakdown in any area where there is pressure caused by the traction devices or from lying in bed. Frequent inspection, good hygiene, and massage are essential. You may need to adjust devices or place extra padding over bony prominences *to relieve pressure*.

The patient on bed rest in traction may have a slow *respiratory* rate and shallow breathing. Breathing exercises and frequent repositioning (within the confines of the traction requirements) may be needed *to prevent pulmonary complications*.

Active or passive range-of-motion exercises and other movements of the muscles and joints *can promote joint mobility, maintain muscle strength, and improve circulation in general.* This is especially important for extremities not in traction.

Gastrointestinal disorders may include anorexia (loss of appetite) and constipation. The diet should be as appealing as possible and have increased fiber content *to aid bowel function.* Stool softeners also may be prescribed. Taking at least 3,000 mL fluid per day also *helps to prevent constipation and maintain adequate urinary output.*

Pain can increase restlessness; therefore, adequate pain management is essential *for more effective traction and patient comfort.*

If the patient appears disoriented, you should give frequent explanations and reassurance. Avoid restraints if possible *because they often increase agitation and result in skin damage under the restraints.*

Boredom and sensory deprivation also can be problems for the immobilized traction patient. To lessen these, make the room as colorful and attractive as possible. Plan recreational activities for the patient. These might include music, television, crafts, or other activities suggested by the patient or family. These measures greatly *alleviate irritability, restlessness, and boredom.*

Patients may have secret fears of being trapped or abandoned in the event of a disaster. Discuss these fears openly with the patient and conscientiously deal with any concerns or complaints the patient may have *to avoid more serious problems.*

SKIN TRACTION

Skin traction applies traction to muscles or bones by pulling on the skin, using tapes or harnesses with protective padding. Skin traction has some limitations *because of the danger of skin irritation and breakdown.* It cannot be applied over skin that is broken or has poor blood supply *because of the danger of more serious tissue damage.* The weights are usually limited to less than 10 lb and are left on for less than 3 weeks.

Skin traction is generally used to treat fractures in children and minor fractures in adults and to temporarily immobilize fractures in adults before permanent fixation. It also is commonly used for muscle strains or spasms.

Although the physician decides the type of skin traction to be used, the nurse or a specially trained technician can apply it. Whether it can be removed intermittently to facilitate hygiene, elimination, or exercise depends on the physician's order or the facility's policy. The decision is usually guided by the purpose of the traction. For example, if the traction is being used to immobilize a fracture, it will generally not be removed. If the patient is being treated for muscle strain or spasm, the traction can usually be taken off for varying periods.

Be sure the skin is clean before traction is applied. Follow the policies of the physician or facility regarding skin preparation. Sometimes the area to be confined or taped is shaved. Tincture of benzoin is commonly applied to the skin *for protection.*

TYPES OF SKIN TRACTION

There are many variations of skin traction. This module discusses the following commonly used types: humerus (side-arm), Buck's, Russell's, Bryant's, traction, pelvic sling, and cervical halter traction.

Humerus (Side-Arm) Traction

Humerus skin traction is used for stabilizing fractures of the upper arm and for shoulder dislocations. The patient is in the supine position. The head may be elevated *for comfort* as long as the forearm is in flexion and is extended 90 degrees from and in the same plane as the body.

Traction is applied in two directions by producing one pull on the elbow and another on the hand. Procedures vary with the preference of the physician, but generally the following steps are used. Thoroughly cleanse the skin. Attach strips of a special commercial adhesive to the skin, with the ends of the tape protruding above the hand. Wrap the part with an elastic bandage. (Refer to Module 26, Applying Bandages and Binders, for complete directions.) Figure 24–4 shows the proper positioning of the ropes, pulleys, and weights. *To protect the skin over the bony prominence of the elbow,* use moleskin or lamb's wool padding.

Problems associated with this type of traction include skin breakdown, particularly over the elbow, and compromised circulation. Observe the patient's fingers closely for objective signs of coolness, pallor, or swelling, and ask about such subjective signs as numbness and tingling. *These are most often caused by wrappings that are too tight and interfere with circulation.* If any of these danger signs appear, rewrap the bandage *for comfort and safety.*

Buck's Traction

Buck's extension skin traction may be applied to one leg (unilateral) or both (bilateral). It is used primarily for immobilizing fractures of the femur, for low-

© 1996 by Lippincott-Raven Publishers

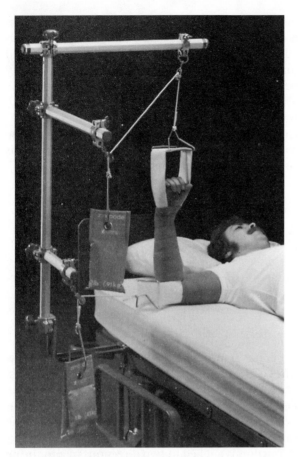

Figure 24–4. Humerus (side-arm) traction. The right angle of the elbow and the application of weights maintain alignment. (Courtesy Zimmer, Inc., Warsaw, Indiana.)

er spine "hairline" or simple fractures, and for temporary immobilization of a hip fracture. Muscle spasm of the lower back also can be treated with Buck's traction.

Place the patient in Buck's traction in the supine position with the bed flat. Position the head of the bed somewhat lower than the foot. Most electric beds are designed so that the foot end can be disengaged from the electric control, lowering the head to the desired level. This position allows the *weight of the patient's body to produce countertraction.*

Traction is applied in one direction on the leg or legs distally and with straight alignment. A foam and Velcro traction boot is commonly used to apply the traction and is the most convenient and comfortable means of doing so. An elastic bandage may be used instead of the boot to hold the footrest and side strips to the leg. If tape is used, apply wide strips lengthwise to the inner and outer aspects of the calf. Then pad and wrap the calf, and put in place a footrest and spreader bar. Position the ropes, pulleys, and weights at the foot of the bed (Figs. 24–5 and 24–6).

Problems include possible skin breakdown at the ankle and over the heel. Wrappings that are too tight

© 1996 by Lippincott-Raven Publishers

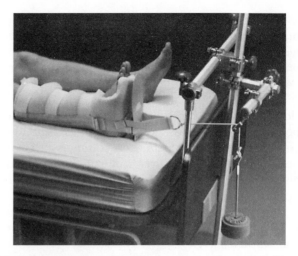

Figure 24–5. Unilateral Buck's extension traction using a foam boot with Velcro straps. Note the position of the leg and how the weight hangs freely. (Courtesy Zimmer, Inc., Warsaw, Indiana.)

may compromise the circulation. The foot should be in dorsiflexion on the footrest and should be covered only by light linen *to prevent footdrop (permanent plantar flexion of the foot).* If the diagnosis permits, remove the boot and wrappings *for observation and skin care,* and rewrap. When traction is held in place by elastic bandages only, rewrapping every 8 hours is usually essential.

Russell's Traction

Russell's traction combines, in principle, Buck's and balanced suspension traction (see pages 581 and 586). With children, Russell's traction is used to reduce or align fractures of the femur or treat knee injuries and is applied as skin traction. With adults,

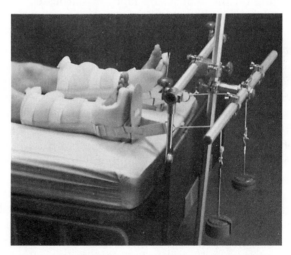

Figure 24–6. In bilateral Buck's extension traction, both legs are positioned in the same way with the same amount of weight attached. (Courtesy Zimmer, Inc., Warsaw, Indiana.)

Russell's traction is usually skeletal, with the pull being exerted on a pin or wire that has been surgically inserted through the proximal portion of the femur. Skeletal traction is used *because the skin in an adult could not tolerate the pull required for the reduction of the fracture.*

In general, with this type of traction, the patient is supine, and the bed is flat. If ordered, elevate the head to a more comfortable level. Russell's traction allows more mobility than Buck's or balanced suspension traction, and the patient can be in high Fowler's position and can move a little from side to side with care.

With this traction, two methods can be used to provide two-directional pull on the leg. In the first, two weights are used—one hung from an overhead bar lifting the knee and the second hung at the foot of the bed—exerting a proximal pull on the lower leg. In the second method, a single weight is added so that it exerts the two-directional pull used in the first method (Fig. 24–7).

Excessive pressure on the popliteal space behind the knee can impinge on nerves and constrict circulation. Pressure over the heel can irritate the skin and cause breakdown. Extra padding may have to be used. The foot must remain in flexion on the footrest *to prevent footdrop.* Put a sock on the foot *for warmth.* Continually assess the patient in Russell's traction.

Bryant's Traction

Bryant's traction is a variation of bilateral Buck's traction and is used for children younger than 2 years who have an unstable hip joint or a fracture of the femur. Traction boots are preferable to tape, particularly with children, *because the boots are less likely to cause skin breakdown.* Place the child supine with the bed flat. Apply traction boots to both lower legs. Thread ropes from the footrests of each boot through pulleys on the overhead bar and onto the foot of the bed, where a weight is hung. Suspend the legs so that the hips are flexed at 90 degrees to the bed surface. The buttocks should be a few inches off the mattress *to ensure proper traction on the legs* (Fig. 24–8). The traction must be applied to both legs *to maintain proper alignment of the affected leg.*

Children adjust surprisingly well and quickly to such an apparently uncomfortable position but are at risk for a variety of problems. Assess both feet frequently for decreased circulation, as evidenced by poor color, coolness, and decreased femoral, popliteal, or pedal pulses. Motion and sensation also may be decreased. Inspect the skin, including the back, for excoriation. When Bryant's traction is first applied, the child may need to have the upper body restrained for a short time until he or she no longer attempts to roll the body or pull on the traction ropes or boots.

Give the child in Bryant's traction additional support and comfort, and plan to spend extra time with the child. The family also can comfort and support the youngster and provide ideas for the amusement and diversion that are so important to the child's contentment.

Pelvic Traction

Pelvic traction is used to treat minor fractures of the lower spine, low back pain, and muscle spasm. A flannel or foam-lined canvas girdle or belt is placed

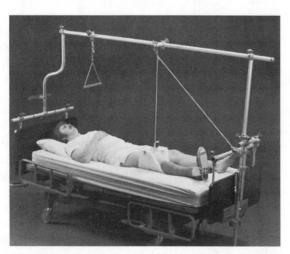

Figure 24–7. Russell's traction using a single weight. The sling supports the leg at the knee. (Courtesy Zimmer, Inc., Warsaw, Indiana.)

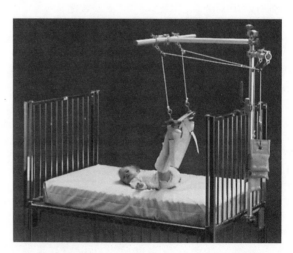

Figure 24–8. The small child in Bryant's traction. The buttocks are lifted slightly off the bed to enable the child's weight to serve as countertraction. (Side rails are lowered to show traction clearly. In the clinical setting, side rails would be in place unless someone is at the crib side.) (Courtesy Zimmer, Inc., Warsaw, Indiana.)

© 1996 by Lippincott-Raven Publishers

snugly around the patient's pelvic area, often over pajama bottoms. The belt is placed somewhat lower than an abdominal binder; the lower portion ends just below the greater trochanter. It is secured with buckles or Velcro closures, and traction is applied through straps sewn into it. Traction is applied in the direction of the foot of the bed, either with two weights—one weight pulling to each side of the bed—or with only one weight, which is attached to a connector bar (Fig. 24–9).

Orders on the position of the patient vary. The most common is William's position, in which the patient is supine with the knees elevated. The patient's head is usually not elevated higher than the knees except for meals. *For greater countertraction,* elevate the foot of the bed. In certain cases, the traction is ordered as intermittent, meaning that it may be removed for elimination or hygiene. These cases usually involve patients with muscle spasm or minor pathology. For more serious conditions, such as minor aligned vertebral fractures, the traction is usually ordered as continuous so that the pull will remain constant. A fracture pan is used for elimination in these cases.

If the pelvic belt becomes soiled, replace it. Inspect skin frequently *for irritation from the belt,* particularly over the iliac crests, and provide any special skin care or padding needed. You also may need to institute measures to prevent or relieve constipation. A correctly used footboard will keep the feet at right angles, *thereby preventing footdrop.* Foot and leg exercises and position changes *help to relieve cramping, maintain muscle tone, and prevent venous congestion, which could lead to thrombophlebitis.*

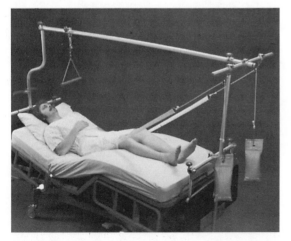

Figure 24–9. Pelvic traction. The knees and lower legs are elevated to flatten the lumbosacral curve of the spine, and the head is kept low to provide countertraction in the correct direction. (Courtesy Zimmer, Inc., Warsaw, Indiana.)

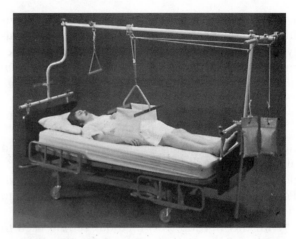

Figure 24–10. Pelvic sling traction. The sling supports the body and allows the pelvis to move as a unit without pull on the fracture site. (Courtesy Zimmer, Inc., Warsaw, Indiana.)

Pelvic Sling Traction

Pelvic sling traction is used to treat a fracture of the pelvis that has resulted in a separation of the pelvic bones. A flannel-lined sling provides compression on the pelvic region by suspending it slightly. Ropes are threaded through pulleys to a free-swinging weight at the foot of the bed. The patient is supine with the bed flat. Continuous traction is usually ordered, so problems of hygiene and elimination may arise. A footboard is needed, as in pelvic traction. Breathing exercises and exercises of the lower legs can help *prevent the complications of immobility* (Fig. 24–10).

Cervical Halter Traction

Cervical halter traction is used to treat a variety of conditions of the cervical spine (neck), including arthritis, "whiplash" injuries, spasms, and minor fractures.

A flannel-lined chin–head halter exerts pull on the cervical spine from the chin and occiput through a series of ropes and pulleys leading to a weight hanging freely over the head of the bed. Countertraction, if ordered, can be accomplished either by raising the head of the bed to a low Fowler's position or by placing the head of the bed on blocks. Place a rolled piece of flannel or a small, flat pillow under the neck *to increase extension and add to patient comfort. Use a footboard to help prevent footdrop* (Fig. 24–11).

The occipital area (back of the head) can develop a pressure ulcer; inspect it routinely. Be aware that the chin, cheeks, and ears also are susceptible to skin breakdown. The patient's diet may have to be modified if chewing becomes a problem. Obtain prism

© 1996 by Lippincott-Raven Publishers

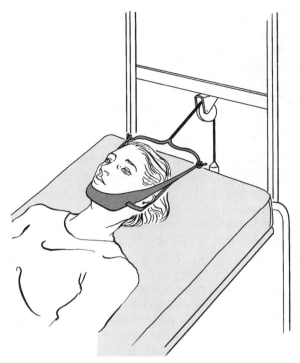

Figure 24–11. Cervical halter traction. To prevent skin breakdown, the ears must not be under the halter. The head of the bed is elevated for the body to provide countertraction.

glasses that direct vision upward and then horizontally *so that the patient can enjoy television and books while in the supine position and thus relieve boredom.*

PROCEDURE FOR APPLYING SKIN TRACTION

Assessment

1. Check the physician's order. The order will state the type of traction to be used, the weight to be applied, and allowances for or restrictions on the activity of the patient.
2. Assess the patient for possible complications of traction. *To prevent the complications of immobilization that have been discussed,* carefully assess the patient initially and at regular intervals thereafter. The assessment should include all systems with special emphasis on circulation, motor function, and sensation in any extremity affected by traction. If circulation, for example, is less than adequate, special padding over bony prominences may have to be added *to prevent skin breakdown.*

Planning

3. Wash your hands *for infection control.*
4. Ensure that any assistance you might need will be available.
5. Gather the equipment you need. Skin traction

may require several of the following: solutions, tapes, boots, bandages, harnesses, halters, ropes, pulleys, weights, padding, trapeze, spreader bars, footrests, footboard.

Implementation

6. Identify the patient *to be sure you are carrying out the procedure for the correct patient.*
7. Explain the procedure. Find out what the physician has told the patient and explain further if necessary. Explain the purpose of the traction, whether weights are to be used intermittently or continuously, and how much the patient will be allowed to turn or move. Some patients in traction, particularly those in continuous skeletal traction, cannot move as much as those in intermittent skin traction.
8. Provide for privacy, and drape the patient as appropriate.
9. Place the bed in proper position. *The degree of pull or tension required for effective traction often depends on the level of the bed and the relative position of the patient. With some types of skin traction, the patient's body weight serves as a counterbalance, necessitating elevation of the foot or the head of the bed.*
10. Cleanse and prepare the skin according to the procedure of the facility. If tape is to be applied, the skin is often shaved beforehand *so that pain and irritation when the tape is removed will be lessened.* Tincture of benzoin solution may be applied *to protect the skin* before any type of skin traction is initiated. (This is not done with cervical traction, *where the close proximity of the face makes it inadvisable.*)
11. Secure the traction by applying the tape, boots, slings, or halters appropriate to the specific procedure. Make sure all appliances are the right size for the patient.
12. Thread and knot ropes through lubricated pulleys. Check that both are aligned properly for the traction you are applying.
13. Using the hooks provided, attach ropes to the patient's appliance. Check for the security of the tapes, boot, or wrappings by gently tugging on the attached rope.
14. If more than one weight is to be applied, add one at a time with a gentle motion *to avoid jerking the body part.*
15. Tape the end of the rope *to prevent fraying.*
16. Carefully check that all appliances are functioning effectively.
17. Place the call signal, all personal possessions, and items needed for self-care within easy reach of the patient. *Having to reach for objects or call signals could not only misalign the traction, but also cause a fall.*

© 1996 by Lippincott-Raven Publishers

DATE/TIME	
5/12/99 1630	*Pelvic traction with 10 lb wt applied. C/o fatigue and discomfort in lower back after 2 h. Traction removed and off for 1 h, then reapplied. No skin redness.* ————————————— *A. Harford, RN*

Example of Nursing Progress Notes Using Narrative Style.

Evaluation

18. Evaluate using the following criteria:
   a. Patient is comfortable.
   b. Ropes, pulleys, and weights are correctly placed and unobstructed.
   c. Patient shows no signs of complications of immobility or impairment of skin integrity, circulation, motor function, or sensation.
19. Make any necessary adjustments. You may need to add padding to bony prominences. Take care not to exert any additional pressure when adding padding. Ropes and pulleys also may need some adjustments *to correct alignment.*
20. Wash your hands *for infection control.*

Documentation

21. Document the type of traction applied, any observations or concerns, and the patient's tolerance of the procedure.

SKELETAL TRACTION

Skeletal traction is accomplished by applying traction to wires, pins, or rods that have been surgically attached to or placed through bones. This type of traction, which exerts direct pull on the bones, allows up to 30 lb of weight to be applied for continuous periods of traction of up to 4 months. Although the skin is not covered or pulled, it is still at risk for breakdown, particularly in the elderly. Pulleys and ropes may abrade, and the traction may put shearing force on skin in contact with the bed.

Skeletal traction is used for more serious fractures of the bones and more often in adults than in children. *This is because with adults, more weight must be applied to align and reduce fractures effectively.*

Although the principles of care for the patient in skin and skeletal traction are similar, the nurse who cares for the skeletal traction patient has added responsibilities.

Skeletal traction is constant and must never be discontinued or interrupted without a specific order. The state of immobility is more complete, and frequent and conscientious assessment for potential problems is required. One important potential problem is that of infection, *because the skin barrier is bro-*

ken. Bone infections are very difficult to treat successfully. Circulation, motor function, and sensation may be impaired in an extremity being treated with traction.

Understandably, patients in skeletal traction may fear that they could not be moved or transferred quickly or easily in the event of a fire or natural disaster. It is sometimes advisable to explore these feelings and assure the patient that in such an event, they would be given special attention. Having the call bell constantly within reach of these patients *greatly allays fears.* Answer any questions the patient may have. *Because skeletal traction devices are usually applied in surgery,* the nurse's responsibilities center on maintenance and safety.

TYPES OF SKELETAL TRACTION

In this module, three of the more common types of skeletal traction are discussed: balanced suspension traction, skull tongs traction, and halo traction.

Balanced Suspension Traction

Balanced suspension traction is used to stabilize fractures of the femur. It can be the skin or skeletal type. If it is skeletal, a pin or wire is surgically placed through the distal end of the femur. If it is skin traction, tape and wrapping or a traction boot of the kind described under Buck's traction is used.

The patient is in the supine position, with the head of the bed elevated *for comfort.* As the name suggests, the affected leg is suspended by ropes, pulleys, and weights in such a way that traction remains constant, even when the patient moves the upper body.

Two important components of balanced suspension traction are the Thomas splint and the Pearson attachment. The Thomas splint consists of a ring, often lined with foam, that circles and supports the thigh. Two parallel rods are attached to the splint and extend beyond the foot. A Pearson attachment consists of a canvas sling that supports the calf. A footrest completes the setup (Fig. 24–12).

Parallel rods lead from the pin sites on the distal end of the femur to the attachment for the rope.

© 1996 by Lippincott-Raven Publishers

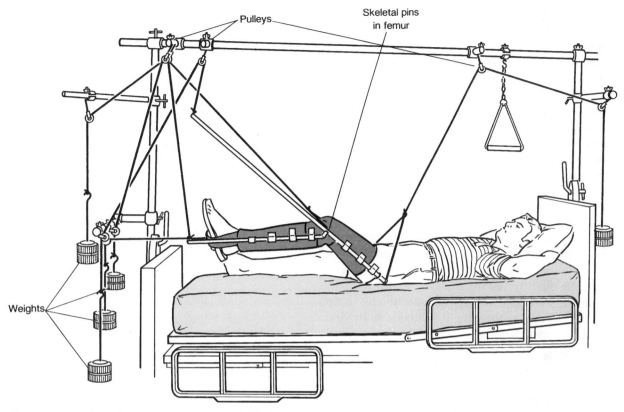

Figure 24–12. Balanced suspension traction. Pulleys provide directional pull to enable weights to support the extremity in correct alignment, while other weights exert traction on skeletal pins.

Traction to the femur is applied through a series of ropes, pulleys, and weights. These weights hang freely at the foot of the bed.

The skin should be inspected frequently *to identify problems early*. The ring of the Thomas splint can excoriate the skin of the groin. Special padding may have to be used. Again, the foot should always be at a right angle on the footrest *to prevent footdrop*. If pins are used for fixation, aseptic technique must be used around pin sites until they have healed. From then on, clean technique can be used. The pin sites are cleansed carefully with soap and water and rinsed thoroughly, unless this varies from policy. An antiseptic, such as povidone-iodine ointment, may then be applied. Dressings are usually not required. You should, however, constantly assess for infection at the pin sites. Indications include redness, heat, drainage, pain, or fever. Review your facility's policy on pin care.

Skull Tongs Traction

Skull tongs are used to immobilize the cervical spine in the treatment of unstable fractures or dislocation of the cervical spine. Although *Crutchfield tongs* were used almost exclusively in the past, *Gardner-Wells skull tongs* are in wide use. Some think these are less

likely to pull out than the Crutchfield tongs. The patient is prepared for either type with a local anesthetic to the scalp. The tongs are surgically inserted into the bony cranium, and a connector half-halo bar is attached to a hook from which traction can be applied (Fig. 24–13).

The patient is supine and is usually on a special frame instead of the regular hospital bed. If a hospital bed is used, two or more people are required to

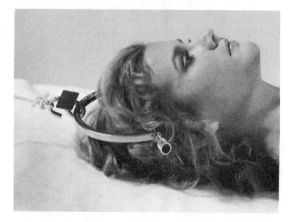

Figure 24–13. Skull tongs traction. Weights attached to the tongs provide traction to cervical vertebrae. The body weight provides countertraction. (Courtesy Zimmer, Inc., Warsaw, Indiana.)

© 1996 by Lippincott-Raven Publishers

assist the patient with any turning movements. The head of the bed may be elevated *to provide counter-traction.*

Because patients remain in this type of traction for an extended period, observe the precautions taken for the patient in other types of skeletal traction. Difficulties with the performance of activities of daily living, infection at the tong sites, and restlessness and boredom are common. It is useful to teach the patient range-of-motion exercises, provide good nutrition, and suggest recreational or occupational activities.

Halo Traction

Halo traction provides stabilization and support for fractured cervical vertebrae. The surgeon inserts pins into the skull. A half circle of metal frame connects the pins around the front of the head. Vertical frame pieces extend from the halo section to a frame brace that rests on the patient's shoulders. The halo traction allows the patient to be out of bed and mobile while stabilizing the cervical vertebrae until they heal. The frame cannot be removed because any movement of the vertebrae could injure the spinal cord (Fig. 24–14).

External Fixation Devices

An external fixation device is a frame of metal rods that connects skeletal pins. The rods extend and provide traction between the pin sites. Some external fixation devices are simple and have only two or

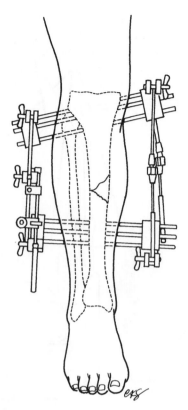

Figure 24–15. External fixation device. Metal rods exert traction between two sets of skeletal pins.

three connecting rods. Others are complex with rods arranged at different angles to maintain the position of fractured bone fragments.

An external fixation device has two major advantages. First, it is useful when skin wounds are present. A cast would cover these wounds, making infection a greater possibility. With an external fixation device the skin is uncovered, and wounds can be observed and treated as needed. In addition, the patient with an external fixation device is more mobile than one with a bed-based skeletal traction system. Therefore the complications of immobility are decreased (Fig. 24–15).

PROCEDURE FOR MAINTAINING SKELETAL TRACTION

Assessment

1. Check the physician's order. Because the patient has usually returned to the unit from the operating room, the order will be listed in the postoperative orders. It will state the weights to be used, any special restrictions on activity, and perhaps the position of the head or foot of the bed.

2. Carefully assess patients just returning to the unit

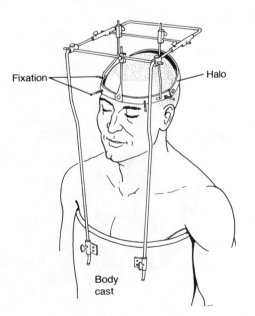

Figure 24–14. Halo traction. The external frame of the halo is attached to pins embedded in the skull.

© 1996 by Lippincott-Raven Publishers

from surgery for signs of general discomfort or pain. (See Module 45, Postoperative Care, for a more detailed discussion of this topic.) For other patients being maintained in skeletal traction, carry out a complete systems assessment, with particular attention to skin, respiratory, gastrointestinal, musculoskeletal, and psychosocial systems. Especially assess circulation, motion, and sensation in the extremities affected by the traction.

Planning

3. Wash your hands *for infection control.*
4. Ensure that any assistance you might need will be available.
5. Gather any equipment that assessment suggests you might need, such as pillows or padding.
6. If pain medication is ordered, be sure to give it long enough before the procedure for the patient to receive its full effect.

Implementation

7. Identify the patient *to be sure you are carrying out the procedure for the correct patient.*
8. Inspect the traction devices for effectiveness. Are all ropes and pulleys in proper alignment? Are ropes hanging freely? Are the correct weights attached?

9. Inspect all operative sites, such as pin or tong insertions. Is there any excessive bleeding? Are dressings clean and dry?
10. Carry out any nursing interventions appropriate to the problems identified in assessment. Give pain medication if needed (see Module 48, Administering Oral Medications).
11. Place the call signal and any personal items within reach of the patient.
12. Teach the patient methods for moving in bed and any appropriate exercises.

Evaluation

13. Evaluate using the following criteria:
    a. Patient is comfortable.
    b. Ropes, pulleys, and weights are correctly placed and unobstructed.
    c. Patient shows no signs of complications of immobility, infection around pin sites, or impairment of skin integrity, circulation, motor function, or sensation.
14. Make any necessary adjustments, such as correcting alignment or adding extra padding.
15. Wash your hands *for infection control.*

Documentation

16. Document any observations you have made and all nursing actions taken.

DATE/TIME	
3/16/99 12:30	Arrived on unit in balanced suspension traction for right leg. Right leg in good alignment. 10 lb wt hanging freely. All peripheral pulses on right leg strong. Leg pink and warm. Capillary refill immediate. Able to move toes. Pt senses touch and differentiates sharp and dull pressure. Moderate discomfort at fracture site. Medicated x1 with relief. Less restless, stated pain only mild and intermittent. ——— *S. Adams, RN*

Example of Nursing Progress Notes Using Narrative Style.

DATE/TIME		
5/19/99 1500	D:	Received from O.R. in Bryant's traction. Child anxious and crying. Toes and feet pink and warm to touch. Traction intact with 4 lb on each leg. Hips remain off bed.
	A:	Family member encouraged to stay at bedside. Proper positioning of traction taught to mother and father.
	R:	Patient more relaxed and drowsy; holding father's hand. Toes and feet warm to touch. ——— *S. Crowley, RN*

Example of Nursing Progress Notes Using Focus Format.

© 1996 by Lippincott-Raven Publishers

CRITICAL THINKING EXERCISES

Zachary, an active 19-month-old boy, has had an unstable left hip since birth. The physician has ordered him placed in Bryant's traction to correct this problem. How does his age affect his plan of care? Evaluate the physical and psychosocial concerns you should consider when developing his care plan. Describe how you will involve the parents in planning and providing care. Identify the outcomes that you anticipate.

© 1996 by Lippincott-Raven Publishers

PERFORMANCE CHECKLIST

Procedure for Applying Skin Traction	Needs More Practice	Satisfactory	Comments
Assessment			
1. Check the physician's order regarding type of traction and weights.			
2. Carry out systems assessment.			
Planning			
3. Wash your hands.			
4. Plan for any assistance you may need.			
5. Gather equipment appropriate to the type of traction ordered.			
Implementation			
6. Identify patient.			
7. Explain procedure. Clarify any questions.			
8. Provide privacy, and drape patient.			
9. Place bed in most effective position for type of traction being used.			
10. Cleanse and prepare skin according to facility policy.			
11. Apply appropriate tapes, boots, or halters.			
12. Thread and knot ropes, checking alignment.			
13. Attach ropes to patient's appliance, and check security.			
14. Gently add weights ordered one at a time.			
15. Tape loose ends of ropes.			
16. Check for functioning of all appliances.			
17. Place call signal and all personal items within reach of patient.			
Evaluation			
18. Evaluate using the following criteria: **a.** Patient comfortable.			
b. Ropes, pulleys, and weights correctly placed and unobstructed.			
c. No signs of complications of immobility or impairment of skin integrity, circulation, motor function, or sensation.			

(continued)

© 1996 by Lippincott-Raven Publishers

Procedure for Applying Skin Traction (Continued)	Needs More Practice	Satisfactory	Comments
19. Make any necessary adjustments, such as correcting alignment or adding padding.			
20. Wash your hands.			
Documentation			
21. Document type of traction applied, any observations you have made, all nursing actions taken, and patient's tolerance of procedure.			
Procedure for Maintaining Skeletal Traction			
Assessment			
1. Check the physician's order on the postoperative order sheet.			
2. Carry out systems assessment, including level of discomfort or pain.			
Planning			
3. Wash your hands.			
4. Plan for any assistance you may need.			
5. Gather any additional equipment you need based on assessment.			
6. Obtain any medication ordered.			
Implementation			
7. Identify patient.			
8. Inspect all traction devices, ropes, pulleys, and weights.			
9. Inspect pin or operative sites.			
10. Carry out nursing interventions for problems identified in assessment (including giving medication).			
11. Place call signal and personal items within reach of patient.			
12. Teach methods for moving in bed and any appropriate exercises.			

(continued)

© 1996 by Lippincott-Raven Publishers

Procedure for Maintaining Skeletal Traction *(Continued)*	Needs More Practice	Satisfactory	Comments
Evaluation			
13. Evaluate using the following criteria: a. Patient comfortable.			
b. Ropes, pulleys, and weights correctly placed and unobstructed.			
c. No signs of complications of immobility, infection around pin sites or impairment of skin integrity, circulation, motor function, or sensation.			
14. Make any necessary adjustments, such as correcting alignment or adding padding.			
15. Wash your hands.			
Documentation			
16. Document any observations you have made and all nursing actions taken.			

© 1996 by Lippincott-Raven Publishers

❓ Q U I Z

Short-Answer Questions

1. The primary difference between skin and skeletal traction is _____

_____

2. To prevent footdrop in patients in traction who must remain supine and immobile, a(n) _____ can be used to keep the feet in _____ .

3. List four common patient problems that may result from the immobilization associated with traction.

   a. _____

   b. _____

   c. _____

   d. _____

Matching Questions

4. Match the most likely area for potential skin breakdown with the type of traction listed below (more than one choice may be used):

   (1) _____ Humerus   **a.** elbow

   (2) _____ Buck's   **b.** groin

   (3) _____ Russell's   **c.** iliac crest

   (4) _____ Bryant's   **d.** heel

   (5) _____ Pelvic   **e.** occipital

   (6) _____ Cervical halter **f.** ankle

   (7) _____ Cervical tongs   **g.** chin

                              h. back

Multiple-Choice Questions

_____ **5.** A major advantage of a halo traction for a person with a cervical spine injury is that the

   a. vertebrae will heal more quickly.
   b. vertebrae are more stable than with any other type of fixation.
   c. person experiences less pain with a halo traction.
   d. person can be mobile.

_____ **6.** An external fixation device can be

   a. adjusted in tension by the nurse.
   b. removed for bathing and hygiene.
   c. applied when skin wounds are present.
   d. attached to a frame of weights and pulleys.

© 1996 by Lippincott-Raven Publishers

MODULE

25

SPECIAL MATTRESSES AND THERAPEUTIC FRAMES AND BEDS

MODULE CONTENTS

RATIONALE FOR THE USE OF THIS
   SKILL
SPECIAL MATTRESSES AND PADS
Sheepskin Pads
Foam Rubber Mattress Pads
Inflated Mattress
Alternating Pressure Mattress
THERAPEUTIC FRAMES AND BEDS
Turning Frame
Circle Bed
Obesity Bed
Static Steep Fowler's Position Bed

Static Low Air Loss Bed
Active Low Air Loss Bed
Air-Fluidized Bed (Static High Air Loss)
Rotation Bed
COMPARISON OF THERAPEUTIC
   FRAMES AND BEDS
PROCEDURE FOR USING SPECIAL
   MATTRESSES AND THERAPEUTIC
   FRAMES AND BEDS
LONG-TERM CARE
HOME CARE
CRITICAL THINKING EXERCISES

PREREQUISITES

Successful completion of the following modules:

VOLUME 1
Module 1   An Approach to Nursing Skills
Module 2   Basic Infection Control
Module 3   Safety
Module 4   Basic Body Mechanics
Module 5   Documentation
Module 6   Introduction to Assessment Skills
Module 14 Bedmaking
Module 15 Moving the Patient in Bed and Positioning

VOLUME 2
Module 24 Applying and Maintaining Traction (if the patient has traction in
          place)

© 1996 by Lippincott-Raven Publishers

OVERALL OBJECTIVE
To use special mattresses and therapeutic frames and beds effectively and safely, with emphasis on both physical and psychologic aspects of care.

SPECIFIC LEARNING OBJECTIVES

Know Facts and Principles	Apply Facts and Principles	Demonstrate Ability	Evaluate Performance
1. Rationale for use			
State two reasons for the use of special mattresses and therapeutic frames and beds.	Given a specific situation, identify reasons for use of specific device.	In the clinical setting, identify reason for use of special device with specific patient.	Evaluate with your instructor.
2. Special mattresses			
Name and describe three types of special mattresses.	Identify one precaution common to all three types of mattresses.	In the clinical setting, use special mattress correctly in specific situation.	Evaluate with your instructor.
3. Special frames and beds			
a. Specific types			
Name and describe eight therapeutic frames and beds. Name one unique feature of each device.	Identify two appropriate uses for each.	In the clinical setting, identify which special frame or bed is appropriate for a specific situation.	Evaluate with your instructor.
b. Manufacturer's instructions			
Locate and read manufacturer's instructions for any device used.	Given a patient situation and specific device, indicate how many people are needed to help.	In the clinical setting, read manufacturer's instructions and secure adequate number of people for specific procedure.	Evaluate using manufacturer's instructions.
c. Necessary equipment and accessories			
State equipment necessary and accessories available for each device.	Given a patient situation and a specific device, list equipment necessary for a specific procedure.	In the clinical setting, using manufacturer's instructions, gather necessary equipment for specific situation.	Evaluate using manufacturer's instructions.
d. Explanation to the patient			
State reasons for use of each device.	Given a patient situation and a specific device, describe what would appropriately be included in explanation to the patient.	In the clinical setting, prepare a patient appropriately for a procedure involving a specific bed or frame.	Evaluate with your instructor.

(*continued*)

© 1996 by Lippincott-Raven Publishers

SPECIFIC LEARNING OBJECTIVES (Continued)

Know Facts and Principles	Apply Facts and Principles	Demonstrate Ability	Evaluate Performance
e. Privacy			
State ways to provide for privacy.		In the clinical setting, provide for privacy of the patient about to undergo a procedure on a therapeutic frame or bed.	Evaluate with your instructor.
f. Operating the device			
List steps in operation of device used for specific procedure.	Given a specific device and procedure, describe how to proceed.	In the clinical setting, perform a procedure correctly for patient on a therapeutic bed or frame.	Evaluate with your instructor, using manufacturer's instructions.
List critical aspects of care of equipment as noted from manufacturer's instructions.	Given a specific situation, describe appropriate care of equipment.	In the clinical setting, care appropriately for equipment in use.	Evaluate with your instructor, using manufacturer's instruction.
g. Evaluating the procedure			
State two appropriate observations to make in evaluating procedure.	Given a specific situation, list observations and actions appropriate to procedure performed.	In the clinical setting, evaluate in relation to short- and long-term goals.	Evaluate with your instructor.
4. Documentation			
State at least two items of data to be included in record.	Given a patient situation, document appropriately using chart form provided.	In the clinical setting, document appropriately.	Evaluate with instructor.

© 1996 by Lippincott-Raven Publishers

LEARNING ACTIVITIES

1. Review the Specific Learning Objectives.
2. Read the section on special devices (in the chapters on Mobility and Activity and Rest and Sleep) in Ellis and Nowlis, *Nursing: A Human Needs Approach,* or comparable material in another textbook.
3. Look up the module vocabulary terms in the glossary.
4. Read through the module as though you were preparing to teach the contents to another person.
5. In the practice setting:
   a. Find out what special mattresses, frames, or beds are available in your setting.
   b. Read the instruction manual for each device.
   c. Working in groups of three (one patient and two nurses), practice using each device, with particular attention to safety measures and to explanations to the "patient" and the family or care giver.
6. In the clinical setting:
   a. Find out what special mattresses, frames, or beds are available in the facility. Observe them in use if possible.
   b. Read the instruction manual of those with which you are unfamiliar and the facility procedure for each device.
   c. Arrange with your clinical instructor for an opportunity to care for a patient using a special mattress, frame, or bed.

VOCABULARY

hypostatic pneumonia
pressure ulcer
pulmonary embolus

quadriplegia
radiolucent
renal calculi

© 1996 by Lippincott-Raven Publishers

Using Special Mattresses and Therapeutic Frames and Beds

Rationale for the Use of This Skill

Patients are placed on special mattresses, frames, and beds for a variety of reasons. One reason is to prevent and treat "pressure ulcers," or decubitus ulcers. Another is to keep the patient immobile to allow healing after disease, surgery, or fractures and to allow the patient to be turned without healing being disrupted. Patients who are immobile because of disease, injury, or other physical conditions may be placed on special devices. Frequent changes of position help to prevent the many complications of immobility (including hypostatic pneumonia, renal calculi, venous thrombosis, pulmonary emboli, and skin breakdown) and to promote physical and psychologic comfort.

Patients suffering from multiple fractures, extensive burns, quadriplegia, acute arthritis, or dermatitis may be placed on one of a number of special mattresses, frames, or beds. The device selected varies with the problems of the patient and the availability of the device, which is usually ordered by the physician after consultation with appropriate members of the healthcare team. Not only are special beds used in the long-term care setting, they may also be used in the home.

To use these devices effectively and safely, you must know which mattress, frame, or bed is appropriate in a specific situation, the principles on which it operates, and the details specific to its operation, such as the available attachments and the purpose of each attachment.[1]

SPECIAL MATTRESSES AND PADS

Several types of special mattresses have been designed *to assist in the prevention and treatment of pressure ulcers.* The primary goal of those that either inflate or operate on the principle of alternating pressure *is to reduce the pressure on capillaries to below 32 mm Hg either all of the time or for intermittent periods. Pressure above this level overcomes the internal blood pressure, and the capillaries collapse, increasing the risk of tissue damage and ulcer formation* (Thompson, Halloran, Strader, & McSweeney, 1993). This number is an average; persons with high blood pressure (hypertension) may be able to tolerate more pressure before capillary collapse occurs, whereas the capillaries of those with lower blood pressure may collapse with much less pressure.

[1]Rationale for action is emphasized throughout the module by the use of italics.

All special pads and mattresses are most effective when there is only one layer of untucked linen between the patient and the mattress. *This prevents the mattress from being confined by linen, so that it can inflate or provide the surface for which it was intended.* If dampness from excessive perspiration is a problem, a cotton blanket (or "sheet blanket") can be used *for extra absorption.*

With incontinent patients, using a single layer of linen may not be feasible. It may be necessary to use a moisture-proof pad under the patient's buttocks. If so, use as thin a layer of padding as possible and place it over the minimum area under the patient, *so that the mattress continues to benefit most of the skin that is at risk.* Check the patient frequently, and change the padding as needed *to keep the patient dry.*

Sheepskin Pads

Genuine or natural sheepskin pads have been used for a number of years for patients who are on bed rest and at risk for skin breakdown. These pads provide air to the surface of the skin, absorb moisture, and also contain natural lanolin, which further reduces the formation of pressure ulcers *by lubricating the skin and decreasing friction.* Rather than genuine sheepskin pads, commercial "sheepskin pads" are now available and used frequently. (These are made of an orlon pile, which does not absorb moisture or contain lanolin). Natural sheepskin pads are much more costly than those produced commercially. A recent study concluded that genuine sheepskin pads are much more effective with patients at risk for skin breakdown than are commercial pads (Marchand and Lidowski, 1993).

Foam Rubber Mattress Pads

The foam rubber mattress pad (often called an "egg-crate" or egg-carton mattress) is placed over the regular mattress on the bed. Its surface of rounded projections *allows air to circulate near the skin.* The result is twofold: *moisture is reduced, so that there is less danger of skin maceration, and pressure is distributed over a wider area, so that the pressure on any one spot is lower.* However, *the pressure remains above capillary pressure,* and therefore careful turning schedules are essential. These mattresses can be large enough to cover an entire bed or small enough to use with wheelchairs or other chairs. Again, only a single layer of linen should be used between the patient and the mattress *to allow for optimum air circulation and pressure distribution.*

© 1996 by Lippincott-Raven Publishers

Inflated Mattresses

A water-filled mattress is a special mattress that is placed on an ordinary bed; it is used *to distribute pressure evenly over the entire body*. It is similar in principle to the waterbed, which has become popular in recent years as a piece of bedroom furniture. The rubber mattress is filled with water so that the body floats. The feeling of weightlessness can induce nausea, and hip and knee contractures are common *because the pelvis tends to sink deeper than the trunk and lower extremities*. Although the outer covering is strong, take care with safety pins and other sharp articles *to avoid punctures and leaks*. Again, pressure may be above capillary pressure.

Air-inflated mattresses are used over the regular mattress and secured by corner straps. These "bed cushions" consist of interlocking layers of air compartments that are inflated using a special device. This mattress can be individualized to the body weight and needs of each patient by varying the amount of air infused. Capillary pressure is reduced to below 32 mm Hg. The mattress is for single patient use and can be cleaned easily with soap and water if soiled (Fig. 25–1).

One study stated that although various types of inflatable mattresses were effective in relieving pressure on the sacral area, they were ineffective in relieving pressure on the trochanter and heel (Stewart, Frieh, and McKay, 1992). This information has implications for nursing care; nurses should not be complacent by knowing that the sacral area is protected but should regularly inspect other skin areas for signs of irritation.

Alternating Pressure Mattress

The alternating pressure mattress is a plastic mattress that is placed on top of a standard mattress. *An attached motor alternately inflates and deflates tubular*

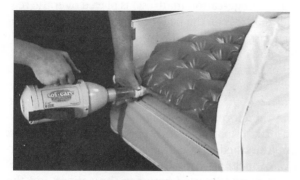

Figure 25–1. The air mattress is inflated with a special blower that should be kept with the mattress to reinflate it if necessary. (Courtesy Gaymar Industries, Inc., Orchard Park, New York.)

sections of the mattress every few minutes, so that the pressure against any section of the patient's body changes continuously. This constant motion can cause mild nausea, but the nausea usually disappears after the first few hours. You should warn the patient, family, and other staff to be careful with safety pins or other sharp objects *because punctures will cause the mattress to leak and be ineffective*. Use only a single layer of linen between the mattress and the patient *because multiple layers of linen tend to bunch up between the inflated tubes and minimize the pressure variation*. The covering used can be a regular sheet, or a cotton blanket can be used *for greater absorption*. Take care not to pinch or bend off the tubing that connects the mattress to the motor, *because this will interfere with the action of the mattress*.

THERAPEUTIC FRAMES AND BEDS

Recognizing that the use of therapeutic beds can greatly enhance the care of the immobilized patient, more physicians have been ordering these special beds over the past 5 years. Many of these are ordered for patients for whom the most careful nursing care cannot prevent skin complications. These patients may include those with extensive skin wounds (such as burn patients), those with multiple traumatic injuries, and those with very poor circulation. In this module, we present the major types of therapeutic beds. Although each brand may have some individual features, the major attributes are the same for each type. New beds are being developed, and new brand names of current types are constantly being developed. Therefore, you will need to examine the literature on a new type of bed to understand how it fits into patient care needs.

Because many of these beds are very expensive, they may be leased from the manufacturer. Their use must usually be ordered by the physician, who determines that the potential for complications is high. However, the nurses who care for the patient on an ongoing basis may be the first to identify the problem and suggest a physician's evaluation for use of one of these beds. In general, the more complex the bed, the greater the cost. Therefore, the bed that meets the patient's needs without providing unnecessary features is the best choice. Some of the manufacturers employ nurses as consultants to help with staff development and training. In large hospitals, the enterostomal therapist may be involved in this consultation.

Although a class may be provided to acquaint staff members with a brand that will be used in the insti-

© 1996 by Lippincott-Raven Publishers

tution, this class may not be available when a therapeutic bed is first ordered for a patient. Each bed comes with an instruction manual attached to it. Be sure to review that instruction manual *because each bed is somewhat different.*

Some general questions to consider for the use of each bed:

1. Are there special sheets, pads, or attachments to be used on the bed?
2. How is the bed operated?
3. How is the bed adjusted to allow cardiopulmonary resuscitation (CPR) to be performed?
4. Can the position of the bed be changed, and, if so, how?
5. How are elimination needs managed on this bed?
6. Are there any potential complications with the use of this bed? If so, what are they and how can they be prevented?
7. Are there alarms or signals? If so, what do they indicate and how should the nurse respond?

Of course, there is more information to learn, but the answers to these basic questions will allow you to begin care safely. You can then ask for additional instructions from a more experienced nurse and read the instruction manual more extensively.

Turning Frame

The turning frame (Stryker or Foster) is used *to maintain immobilization and, at the same time, provide for turning.* The frame, which may be used as a surgical table as well as a rehabilitation bed, has a bottom mattress or support attached to a frame on wheels. When the patient is to be turned, a second frame is fastened into place above the patient, and safety straps are applied. The patient is then turned laterally either from back to abdomen or from abdomen to back. Nursing care is planned around the turning schedule. The Stryker frame can be operated safely by one nurse if the wedge turning frame is used. *The wedge design prevents the patient from falling, because the opening is uppermost when the turn is made* (Fig. 25–2).

If the wedge turning frame is not used, two nurses must be present. Some facilities require two nurses to be present even when the wedge turning frame is used *to ensure safety and decrease patient anxiety.*

The frames have an opening in the bottom mattress to accommodate a bedpan. A face support is used when the patient is turned face down *to facilitate eating and reading.* Many patients have a fear of falling, however, and are not comfortable in that position, although some do adjust after some time on the frame.

Circle Bed

The circle bed is actually a frame designed for patients with severe injuries or other acute conditions in which the objective, again, is immobilization with provision for turning. The difference is that the circle bed turns vertically, and the bed and patient can be placed in several positions, including standing, sitting, and Trendelenburg positions (Fig. 25–3).

As in the turning frame, the patient is placed between two mattresses or supports if the turn is to be a complete one, and the bed is rotated using an electric or manual control. This bed will rotate a full 210° and can also be used as a tilt table *to help a patient regain gradually the ability to tolerate an upright position.* Also like the turning frame, there is an opening in the bottom mattress *to accommodate a bedpan,* and the patient can eat and read when in the face-down position. Turning can be a frightening experience for the patient, especially when going forward, and every effort should be made to make the turn as smooth as possible. Two nurses are usually required for maintaining safety during turns.

The patient can be transported to other areas of the facility on the circle bed, which makes transfer to a stretcher unnecessary. CircOlectric is one brand.

Obesity Bed

The use of a regular hospital bed may be inappropriate for the very obese patient; it may prove uncomfortable and unsafe. In addition, moving the very obese patient for weighing or into a chair may pose a problem for staff. The bed designed for the obese patient is somewhat wider than the conventional bed and designed to support 700 to 850 pounds (depending on the brand). The bed can be moved into a chair position and has hand supports for the patient to use when moving to a standing position. Some brands convert to a stretcher or an x-ray table, and one brand has a built-in scale.

Static Steep Fowler's Position Bed

This bed resembles a conventional bed but has a gel/foam mattress. In addition, the foot of the bed lowers to provide a chairlike position. This bed is most commonly used for patients with cardiac, respiratory, or neuromuscular disease who benefit from the reclining chair position to facilitate respirations and heart function.

© 1996 by Lippincott-Raven Publishers

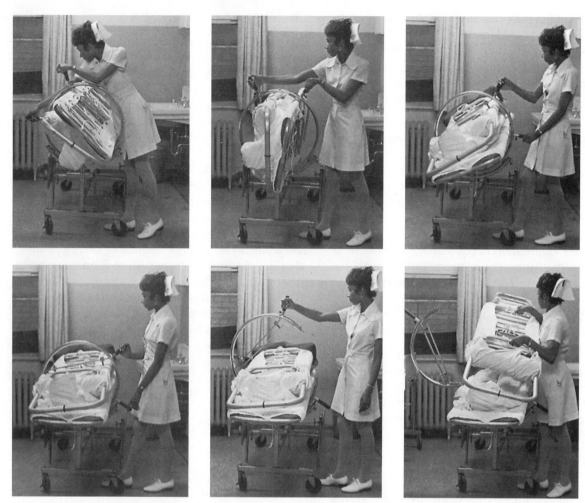

Figure 25–2. Turning a patient with the Stryker wedge turning frame. Note the top and bottom frame sections and the safety handles. (Courtesy Stryker Corporation, Kalamazoo, Michigan.)

Static Low Air Loss Bed

The static low air loss bed has many air-filled cushions. Each section of cushions may be filled to a different firmness, supporting the body evenly and decreasing pressure on bony prominences. Specially shaped cushions are available to facilitate positioning the patient on the abdomen. There are also special cushions to place under a cast or other appliance. Small cushions in the middle of the bed can be removed to make positioning and using a bedpan more convenient.

Some air is lost continually through the cushion surface and is replaced by a blower mechanism. The air loss can dry the skin. This may be a benefit for some patients and a problem for others. The temperature of the air can be controlled to warm or cool the patient as indicated. The cushions can be easily deflated to transfer the patient or to perform CPR.

The bed has side rails, and the head and knee sections move like a conventional hospital bed. The entire bed has high-low capability and can be moved

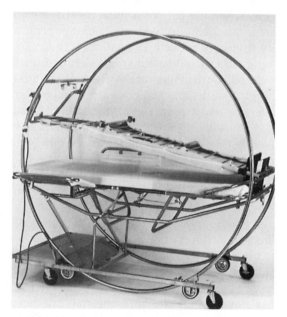

Figure 25–3. The circle bed has top and bottom frames and turns vertically. The bed can be stopped with the patient in a standing position. (Courtesy Stryker Corporation, Kalamazoo, Michigan.)

© 1996 by Lippincott-Raven Publishers

into the Trendelenburg position. The beds are firm enough to provide support for a patient with spinal cord injury. Fluids are not absorbed by the covering, and a fluid-repelling sheet is needed over the surface. Only specifically designed sheets and absorbent pads should be used on the surface; others may interfere with the effectiveness of the bed. Some brands are KinAir, Flexicair, Mediscus (Fig. 25–4), SMI 3000, and MegaAir (for obese patients).

Active Low Air Loss Bed

The active low air loss beds contain all of the features of the static beds, and in addition, rotate slightly (approximately 20°) from side to side or pulsate to stimulate circulation and to help mobilize respiratory secretions (Fig. 25–5).

Because of these added features, they are commonly used for patients who have cardiac or pulmonary problems in addition to skin and circulation problems. Brands include the Biodyne, TheraPulse, Restcue, and Pulmonair 40.

Air-Fluidized Bed (Static High Air Loss)

Tiny ceramic beads (finer than sand grains) are contained in a 12-inch thick "box" where the mattress would be. The "box" is covered with special fabric that fits loosely. Air is forced through the beads and out through the top covering. The air keeps the beads in constant motion, resulting in "fluidizing" of the surface. The surface yields to pressure, but supports the body's weight evenly. The person lying on such a bed has no body surface exposed to pressure greater than capillary pressure, so blood flow in the

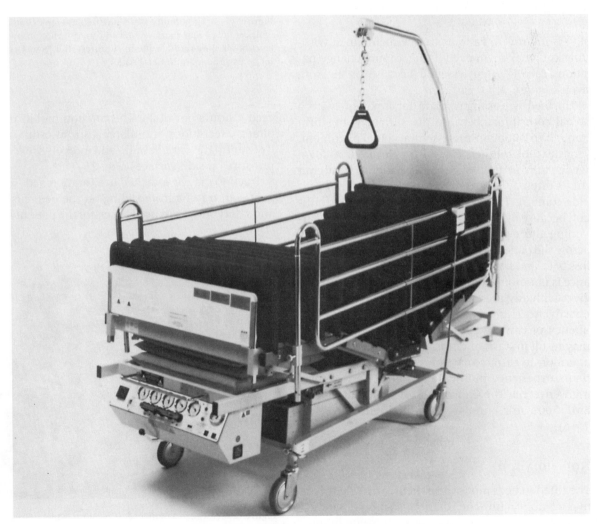

Figure 25–4. Static low air loss bed. The Mediscus Air Support System is a relief system designed for prevention and treatment of pressure ulcers. The system delivers measurable therapeutic support pressures below capillary closures with pressure gauges. (Courtesy Mediscus Products Inc., Signal Hill, California.)

© 1996 by Lippincott-Raven Publishers

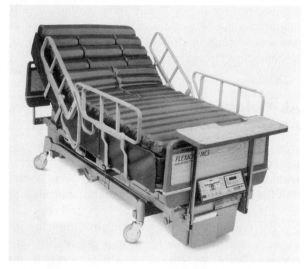

Figure 25–5. The Flexicare Low Airloss Therapy Unit provides the features of the static low air loss bed. (Courtesy Hill Rom Company, Inc., Charleston, South Carolina.)

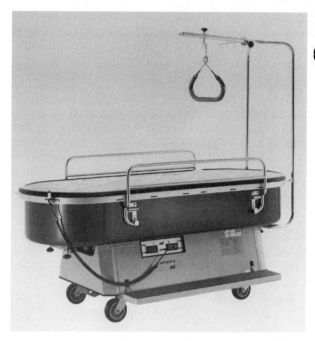

Figure 25–6. The Clinitron Air Fluidized Therapy Unit is filled with ceramic beads that are kept in constant motion by a high level of air flow through them. (Courtesy Hill Rom Company, Inc., Charleston, South Carolina.)

skin is improved. Patients can be maintained without skin breakdown even if they cannot change position. Pain is often lessened because of the soft, even support.

This bed is not appropriate for a patient with a spinal cord injury because the surface is not firm enough to maintain the essential spinal alignment. The head of the bed cannot be elevated. A foam wedge may be used to raise the patient's head, but this is often awkward to position and may not provide comfort. Transfer in and out of the bed is difficult because of the high, rigid sides of the "box" containing the ceramic beads. The constant air flow across the patient's skin is greater than in the low air loss beds and may dehydrate the patient if fluid balance is not monitored carefully. Because the surface gives with any pressure, the patient may not cough effectively. This, combined with a decreased frequency of turning because the skin is not at risk, may result in stasis of respiratory secretions. Careful attention to respiratory care is essential. Some patients experience disorientation due to the "floating" sensation. The Clinitron, Skytron, FluidAir, and SMI 5000 are brands of air-fluidized beds (Fig. 25–6).

Rotation Bed

The rotation beds move the patient from side to side to a 60° to 90° tilt. The rotation is approximately 7 minutes long but may be adjusted in some brands. Rotation is stopped for meals, care, and procedures, but the total time the rotation is off should not ex-

ceed 4 hours out of 24. The rotation mobilizes respiratory secretions, stimulates gastrointestinal activity, stimulates circulation, and prevents excessive pressure on skin surfaces (Fig. 25–7).

Traction may be attached to a rotation bed. To prevent skin trauma from sliding on the bed, cushions and safety straps are used to secure the patient in the

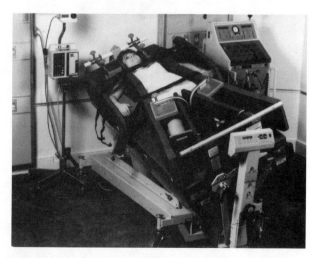

Figure 25–7. The rotation bed (Roto-Rest Kinetic Treatment Table) tilts from side to side to facilitate respiratory, gastrointestinal, and circulatory function. (Courtesy Kinetic Concepts, Inc., San Antonio, Texas.)

© 1996 by Lippincott-Raven Publishers

DATE/TIME	
1/30/98 1015	Patient placed on Clinitron Air - Fluidized unit per order. Health teaching in the following areas completed: _____
	1. Reason for bed _____
	2. Operation of bed _____
	3. Familiarize patient with bed _____
	4. Demonstration of control system _____
	5. Placement of the call signal _____
	6. Reassure patient and answer questions _____
	Patient to be assessed qh for first 8 h. ─── J. Buckwald, RN

Example of Nursing Progress Notes Using Narrative Format.

desired position. Some patients experience motion sickness from the movement. This is often temporary and subsides after some time. If it persists, the use of the bed may have to be discontinued. Brands include Keane Mobility, RotoRest, Tilt and Turn Paragon, and Mega Tilt and Turn (for obese patients).

COMPARISON OF THERAPEUTIC FRAMES AND BEDS

On the following pages, Table 25–1 provides a comparison of the special frames and beds just discussed. Appropriate points about each device are included.

PROCEDURE FOR USING SPECIAL MATTRESSES AND THERAPEUTIC FRAMES AND BEDS

Assessment

1. Assess the patient's need for a special mattress, therapeutic frame, or bed.
2. Check the order. Confer with the other members of the healthcare team and the physician if an order has not been written.
3. Check the patient unit for the supplies and equipment you will need to use the mattress, frame, or bed. This may include special sheets, cushions, safety belts, and other devices.

Planning

4. Review the manufacturer's instructions on setting up and using the particular device. Some beds must be started and the temperature established before the patient is transferred into the bed.
5. Wash your hands *for infection control.*

6. Gather needed equipment. Order items from the appropriate source if they are not in the patient's room or on the unit.

Implementation

7. Identify the patient *to be sure you are carrying out the procedure on the correct patient.*
8. Explain to the patient what you plan to do. Especially focus on the patient's participation and the sensations the patient will experience *to obtain maximum patient participation and decrease the patient's anxiety.*
9. Provide privacy.
10. Prepare the mattress, frame, or bed for the activity or procedure that will be done.
11. Carry out the procedure.
12. Make the patient comfortable.
13. Care for equipment.
14. Wash your hands.

Evaluation

15. Evaluate the patient's response to the procedure according to the following criteria:
    a. Safety and stability of the device
    b. Degree of physical comfort provided to the patient by the use of the mattress, frame, or bed; no skin irritation or impingement on patient's body parts
    c. Patient's psychologic response to the reason device is used or the device's effect on function
    d. Difficulties encountered

Documentation

16. Document either on the progress notes or on a flow sheet according to your facility's policy. Turning or other routine care is usually noted on a flow sheet. A progress note should be made if the patient's response was other than expected. The factors that require the ongoing use of a
(text continues on page 612)

© 1996 by Lippincott-Raven Publishers

Table 25–1. Comparison of the Most Common Therapeutic Frames and Beds

	Stryker Frame	Circle Bed	Rotation Bed	Air-Fluidized Bed	Static and Active Low Air Loss Beds
Indications for use	Used for cervical traction, spinal fusion, and laminectomy.	Used for patients with multiple fractures, extensive burns, quadriplegia, acute arthritis, dermatitis, spinal fusion.	Used for postural drainage of severely injured patients and for prevention of the complications of immobility (e.g., pressure sores, hypostatic pneumonia, deep vein thrombosis, pulmonary embolus).	Used for patients with limited movement, pain with movement or handling, and at risk for skin breakdown	Used for patients with limited movement, pain with movement or handling, and at risk for skin breakdown. Used for patients with orthopedic problems and spinal cord injury. Active bed provides increase in circulation.
Contraindications/ disadvantages	Should not be used if patient can be positioned on side, is broader than external frame, or is over 6 feet tall or 200 lb.	Should not be used if patient has unstable spine, because feet bear weight during turn, causing pressure on spine.	Constant motion may exacerbate diarrhea and nausea. Bed should be protected, because it is hard to clean. Movement increases risk of friction and shearing of skin. Warmth and sweating from waterproof cushions around body.	Not for patients with unstable spinal cord injury. Constant circulation of warm, dry air may affect temperature and hydration status. check patient closely. Difficult to elevate head. Difficult to transfer patient. May cause sagging at the hips. Coughing may be inhibited by lack of firm surface.	Bed does not absorb fluids.

© 1996 by Lippincott-Raven Publishers

Caring for equipment	Replace linen as necessary on anterior or posterior frame removed from bed. Store frame carefully where it will not get dirty or fall over and hurt someone.	Replace linen as necessary on anterior or posterior frame.	Special linen is needed for bed section.	Special sheets needed. The system should be cleaned every week and disinfected between patients.	Special sheets needed. The bed should be cleaned every week and disinfected between patients.
Special care techniques	Lock frame in place above patient. To turn the patient, you will need: (a) Anterior or posterior frame, correctly padded and covered (b) Two safety belts, one for chest, the other for thighs	To turn the patient, you will need: (a) Anterior or posterior frame, correctly padded and covered (b) Accessories include: safety/restraining straps traction bars IV bottle holders overbed table (c) Accessories include: footboard armrests tray table bedpan cervical traction	Bed is in constant motion. Posterior hatches open to allow care of cervical, thoracic, and rectal areas. Traction apparatus available. Be sure to close any posterior hatches opened while caring for patient.	(a) "Fluidized" temperature-controlled air flows constantly around patient. (b) Standard equipment foam wedge turn sheet IV holder side rails call signal	(a) Air cushions are inflated to meet individual needs of patient. (b) Standard equipment: turn sheet IV holder side rails call signal

(continued)

© 1996 by Lippincott-Raven Publishers

Table 25-1. Comparison of the Most Common Therapeutic Frames and Beds (Continued)

	Stryker Frame	Circle Bed	Rotation Bed	Air-Fluidized Bed	Static and Active Low Air Loss Beds
Special care techniques (continued)	Medicate patient if painful procedure is planned. When using wedge frame, turn patient toward yourself *to promote a greater feeling of security*—patients often have a fear of falling, especially when first on the frame. Narrowness of mattresse, as well as turning, contribute to fear. Attach anterior of posterior frame and fasten securely. Remove or adjust attachments as necessary. Secure safety belts (around both anterior and posterior frame and the patient)—	Medicate patient if painful procedure is planned. Stand facing patient and where patient can see you as you operate controls. Create calm quiet environment *to make patient less fearful— fear of falling is especially great when patients are turning face forward. Attach anterior or posterior frame and fasten securely. Remove or adjust attachments as necessary. Ask patient to hold onto frame if able. Otherwise restrain arms next to the body.	Medicate patient if painful procedure is planned. Bed can be placed in extreme lateral position. Care may be given and procedures performed through posterior hatches with bed in this position. Awake patient may benefit from presence of second person *for face-to-face contact and psychological comfort.* You may need to remove cushions or restraining straps or perform procedure through one of the posterior hatches. Be	Medicate patient if painful procedure is planned. Bed promotes relaxation, but the flotation sensation can have disorienting effect on patient. You may need to turn the unit off and on *several times to relieve patient's fear.* Rising airflow provides clean environment, and the special "filter sheet" is permeable to both rising flow of air and downward flow of fluids like plasma, blood, perspiration, and urine, thus removing them from contact with the patient.	Medicate patient if painful procedure is planned. Inflation may be altered in such a way as to accommodate a variety of positions for procedures. You may reassure patient during procedure by offering touch and comfort. Protect surface of bed with folded sheets. Adjust airflow pressure for patient comfort and convenience of carrying out procedure. Return to preset pressure readings.

Special care techniques *(continued)*

one around chest, the other around thighs. Be sure patient knows which way frame is to be turned. Arrange signal so that patient will know when you will turn frame (eg, on count of 3). Use smooth, uninterrupted motion and moderate speed. Remove frame that is now in uppermost position. If patient is now in prone position, use safety belts, because side rails cannot be used.

Be sure patient knows which frame is to be turned. Be sure patient is ready to be turned. Stand where you can see patient's face if verbal communication is not possible. Remove frame that is now in uppermost position. If patient is now in prone position, use safety belts, because side rails cannot be used.

certain to reposition patient and cushions carefully. Make sure all safety straps are carefully fastened.

Patient does not need to bel turned for skin care, but *should* be turned to maintain lung and kidney function. To turn, press down on bed beside patient while pulling patient toward you. Defluidize to provide firm surface for coughing. Instant "defluidization" can be accomplished if a firm surface is needed, as in cardiac arrest. If cardiac arrest occurs, be sure to unplug the bed at the wall socket *because if the bed is merely turned off, it will automatically restart after 30 minutes.*

Patient should be turned to check skin and maintain lung and kidney function. Patient is easily turned with a turn sheet. Change pressure settings to initiate changes in pressure on patient's tissues.

These units can be instantly deactivated *for purposes of administering resuscitation (CPR) in the event of a cardiac arrest.*

© 1996 by Lippincott-Raven Publishers

DATE/TIME	
9/2/99 1020	D: Patient stated, "My left hip is really sore when you turn me so that I am lying on it." Skin on left hip reddened and will not blanch. Warm to touch.
	A: Talked with family and physician regarding use of an alternative pressure mattress to prevent skin breakdown. Alternating pressure mattress placed on bed. Initiated 2 h. turning schedule.
	R: Patient states, "This mattress really helps." Turned without discomfort. N. Sanders, RN

Example of Nursing Progress Notes Using Focus Format.

therapeutic bed should be carefully documented. If the patient's condition has changed so that the bed is no longer essential, this should also be noted. *Reimbursement by third-party payers for the cost of therapeutic beds typically depends on adequate documentation of the patient's need.*

LONG-TERM CARE

Residents in long-term care now include greater numbers of persons with acute and chronic medical conditions in addition to the fragile elderly. Skin integrity is at risk with all of these residents. As a result, a special mattress or bed may be needed. To help the staff learn to operate these devices, in-service education classes can be conducted by representatives of the manufacturer or staff development department. Naturally, safety is an essential consideration in using any device.

Cost is also a factor. With a physician's order, most long-term care facilities provide these devices on a rental basis from the manufacturer. Depending on the resident's insurance, the service may be partially or totally reimbursed.

HOME CARE

The growing trend toward providing services to clients at home increases the need for the use of special mattresses and beds in the home. As a result, the home care nurse needs to be familiar with the equipment and be able to teach safe operation to caregivers.

The client's family may wish to purchase special pads or mattresses from commercial sources because these are less costly than special beds. With a physician's order documenting need, the insurer may reimburse the cost for these devices.

CRITICAL THINKING EXERCISES

Your patient, a 77-year-old woman, is thin and arthritic. She is out of bed for only a few hours each day. You notice that her sacrum and right hip are reddened and do not blanch with massage. If all special beds and mattresses were available, identify the bed or mattress that would be most effective and appropriate in preventing the formation of decubitus ulcers. Determine what additional nursing actions you could carry out to maintain this patient's skin integrity.

References

Marchand, A. C., & Lidowski, H. (1993). Reassessment of the use of genuine sheepskin for pressure ulcer prevention and treatment. *Decubitus, 6*(1), 44–47.

Stewart, T. P., Frieh, S. A., & McKay, M. G. (1992). The pressure relieving capabilities of seven replacement mattresses. Orchard Park, NY (A study funded by Gaymar Industries).

Thompson, J. H., Halloran, T., Strader, M. K., & McSweeney, M. (1993). Pressure-reduction products: Making appropriate choices. *Journal of Enterostomy Nursing, 20,* 239–244.

© 1996 by Lippincott-Raven Publishers

✔ PERFORMANCE CHECKLIST

Procedure for Using Special Mattresses and Therapeutic Frames and Beds	Needs More Practice	Satisfactory	Comments
Assessment			
1. Assess patient's need for special mattress, frame, or bed			
2. Check order.			
3. Check patient unit for supplies.			
Planning			
4. Review manufacturer's instructions.			
5. Wash your hands.			
6. Gather needed equipment.			
Implementation			
7. Identify patient.			
8. Explain procedure to patient.			
9. Provide privacy.			
10. Prepare mattress, frame, or bed for procedure.			
11. Carry out procedure.			
12. Make patient comfortable.			
13. Care for equipment.			
14. Wash your hands.			
Evaluation			
15. Evaluate using the following criteria: a. Safety and stability of the device			
b. Patient's physical comfort; no skin irritation or impingment on body parts			
c. Patient's psychological response to reason for use or effect on patient's function			
d. Difficulties encountered			
Documentation			
16. Document data on progress notes or flow sheet.			

© 1996 by Lippincott-Raven Publishers

QUIZ

Short-Answer Questions

1. Give two reasons for the use of special mattresses, frames, and beds.

a. _____

b. _____

2. Describe the principle by which the egg-crate mattress helps protect the skin.

_____

_____

3. Compare the construction of the Stryker frame with that of the circle bed.

_____

_____

4. List two precautions that the nurse should take when caring for the patient using an air-fluidized bed. _____

_____

5. What provision is made for administering resuscitation (CPR) measures to patients on the low air loss bed? _____

_____

Multiple-Choice Questions

_____   **6.** Which of the following is not an inflatable device?

  a. The low air loss bed
  b. An egg-crate mattress
  c. A waterbed
  d. The alternating positive pressure mattress

_____   **7.** Which of the following actions regarding x-rays is appropriate when caring for the patient on an air-fluidized bed?

  a. X-ray plates should be placed in pillow cases.
  b. The unit should be operating so that the x-ray plates stay in position.
  c. Always place a foam wedge beneath the patient's head.
  d. No x-rays should be taken.

_____   **8.** Capillary collapse occurs when surface pressure levels rise above

  a. 20 mm Hg.
  b. 32 mm Hg.
  c. 42 mm Hg.
  d. 50 mm Hg.

_____ 9. Bottom linen that covers a special mattress

    a. is tucked tightly so that the mechanism does not wrinkle it.

    b. is never tucked tightly because this interferes with the principle underlying the mattress.

    c. always consists of two sheets rather than one to protect the mattress.

    d. is always of special fabric and supplied by the manufacturer.

_____ 10. Which of the following special beds can be used for the patient with an unstable spinal cord injury?

    a. Air-fluidized bed

    b. Air mattress

    c. Low air loss mattress

    d. Water-inflated bed

© 1996 by Lippincott-Raven Publishers

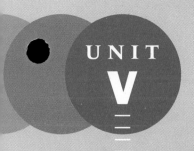

UNIT
V

Providing for Comfort, Elimination, and Nutrition

MODULE 26
Applying Bandages and Binders

MODULE 27
Applying Heat and Cold

MODULE 28
Administering Enemas

MODULE 29
Tube Feeding

MODULE

26

APPLYING BANDAGES
AND BINDERS

MODULE CONTENTS

RATIONALE FOR THE USE OF THIS SKILL

GENERAL INFORMATION

GENERAL PROCEDURE FOR APPLYING BANDAGES AND BINDERS

Assessment

Planning

Implementation

Evaluation

Documentation

APPLYING BANDAGES

Types of Bandages

Methods of Application

Circular

Spiral

Reverse-Spiral

Figure 8

Recurrent Fold

SPECIFIC PROCEDURES FOR APPLYING BANDAGES

Wrapping an Ankle and Lower Leg

Applying Elastic (Antiembolic) Stockings

Applying a Sequential Compression Device

Wrapping a Stump

Applying a Stump Stocking

APPLYING BINDERS

Types of Binders

SPECIFIC PROCEDURE FOR APPLYING BINDERS

Applying a Straight Abdominal Binder

Applying a Stretch Net Binder

Applying a T-Binder

Applying an Arm Sling

LONG-TERM CARE

HOME CARE

CRITICAL THINKING EXERCISES

PREREQUISITES

Successful completion of the following modules:

VOLUME 1

Module 1 An Approach to Nursing Skills

Module 2 Basic Infection Control

Module 3 Safety

Module 4 Basic Body Mechanics

Module 5 Documentation

Module 6 Introduction to Assessment Skills

© 1996 by Lippincott-Raven Publishers

OVERALL OBJECTIVE

To correctly apply commonly used bandages and binders.

SPECIFIC LEARNING OBJECTIVES

Know Facts and Principles	Apply Facts and Principles	Demonstrate Ability	Evaluate Performance
BANDAGES			
1. Types of methods used in application			
State common types of roll bandages and five methods of applying them.	Given a patient situation, determine appropriate type of bandage and method of application.	In the clinical setting, choose appropriate bandage and method of application.	Evaluate effectiveness of bandage.
2. Procedure			
Explain procedures for applying bandages.	Given a patient situation, explain rationale for selection of appropriate bandage and method chosen for application.	Replace existing bandage or apply new bandage correctly with supervision.	Evaluate own performance with instructor.
3. Documentation			
State information to be recorded.		Chart on patient's record.	Review progress notes with instructor.
BINDERS			
1. Types			
State types of binders most commonly used.	Given a patient situation, select appropriate binder.	In the clinical setting, select appropriate binder and method of application.	Evaluate own performance with instructor.
2. Procedure			
Explain selection of binder and method for applying.	Given a patient situation, state rationale for choice of binder and principles to be observed in application.	In the clinical setting, replace or apply binder correctly.	Evaluate appropriateness and effectiveness of binder.
3. Documentation			
State information to be recorded.		Chart on patient's record.	Review progress notes with instructor.
ARM SLING			
1. Type			
State size of adult sling and material used.			

(continued)

© 1996 by Lippincott-Raven Publishers

SPECIFIC LEARNING OBJECTIVES (continued)

Know Facts and Principles	Apply Facts and Principles	Demonstrate Ability	Evaluate Performance
2. Procedure Explain selection of sling and method for applying.	Given a patient situation, select appropriate sling.	Using Performance Checklist, correctly apply arm sling.	Evaluate own performance with instructor.
3. Documentation State information to be recorded.		Chart on patient's record.	Review progress notes with instructor.

© 1996 by Lippincott-Raven Publishers

LEARNING ACTIVITIES

1. Review the Specific Learning Objectives.
2. Look up the module vocabulary terms in the glossary.
3. Read through the module as though you were preparing to teach the contents to another person. Mentally practice the skills.
4. In the practice setting:
   a. Become familiar with the materials and available types of bandages and binders.
   b. Explain the purpose for the bandage or binder to the "patient" (partner) as it is applied.
   c. With a partner, practice bandaging, demonstrating each of the methods introduced, using the Performance Checklist.
   d. Reroll the bandages and have your partner apply the bandages to you, using the described methods.
   e. Together, evaluate one another's performance of steps b through d.
   f. Again with your partner, apply the straight abdominal binder, using the Performance Checklist.
   g. Have your partner apply this binder to you.
   h. Apply an arm sling to your partner.
   i. Have your partner apply an arm sling to you.
   j. Together, evaluate one another's performance of steps f through i.
5. In the clinical setting:
   a. Consult with your instructor about opportunities to apply bandages and binders to appropriate patients.
6. Evaluate your performance with your instructor.

VOCABULARY

circular bandage	girth	sequential compression device	straight abdominal binder
double T-binder	net binder	sling	stretch net binder
elastic bandage	recurrent bandage	spiral bandage	T-binder
figure 8 bandage	reverse-spiral		
gauze bandage	roller bandage		

© 1996 by Lippincott-Raven Publishers

Applying Bandages and Binders

Rationale for the Use of This Skill

There are a variety of reasons, and consequently a variety of methods, for applying bandages or binders. Some protect an underlying wound or dressing; others provide pressure, warmth, support, or immobilization.

It is important first to assess the needs of patients and then to select the device or material that best fulfills those needs. Physicians may order the specific type of bandage or binder to be used or may give only a general order.[1]

GENERAL INFORMATION

Most bandages are of a gauze material; binders are often made of muslin or elasticized fabric. Although dressings over open wounds are sterile, bandages or binders need not be sterile *when there are underlying sterile dressings to protect the wound.* To secure dressings, it is important to wrap in a manner that will be *tight enough to hold, yet loose enough to avoid constricting the body part in any way.* You will learn the proper tension with practice. *To keep a dressing clean,* adequately cover all edges and corners with the bandage or binder.

When you apply any bandage or binder, you must take certain precautions. Avoid bandaging over wrinkled dressings, *which can produce pressure on the wound or skin.* Also avoid applying a bandage or binder over a dressing that appears soiled, *which can indicate infection or provide a medium for the growth of infection-causing microbes.*

Approximately 30 minutes after you have applied a bandage or binder, check the patient for comfort. *A bandage or binder that is too tight can interfere with circulation, causing swelling, numbness, tingling, or color changes in the area distal to the binder.* Most bandages are applied on extremities from distal to proximal, *to facilitate venous return.*

GENERAL PROCEDURE FOR APPLYING BANDAGES AND BINDERS

Assessment

1. Identify the purpose of the particular bandage or binder for this patient *to plan appropriately.* You may also need to review the chart *to identify the patient's medical diagnosis.*

2. Identify the part of the body to be supported.
3. If the patient has had a bandage or binder in place, assess it for its effectiveness. Note the length of time the bandage has been in place as well as the color, temperature, sensation, and skin condition of the extremity or area of the body.

Planning

4. Plan the specific procedure to be used.
5. Wash your hands *for infection control.*
6. Obtain the appropriate bandage or binder and, if needed, the fastening devices.
7. Plan for intervals at which to recheck the bandage or binder. *Any bandage or binder that encircles an extremity must be checked more frequently because of the possibility that the device will compromise circulation. Binders around the trunk are less likely to cause circulatory problems but may become loose and wrinkle, causing discomfort. These bandages need less frequent checking. One check per shift is usually considered adequate. If the patient is conscious, the patient may be taught to check the bandage or binder and report discomfort, a decrease in circulation, or other symptoms of problems.*

Implementation

8. Identify the patient *to be sure you are carrying out the procedure for the correct patient.*
9. Explain to the patient the purpose of the bandage or binder, how long it is to be in place, and how it should feel. *This permits the patient to participate knowledgeably in his or her own healthcare by reporting discomfort or ineffective support.*
10. Provide for patient privacy and position the patient so that the appropriate part of the body is exposed.
11. Remove soiled or used bandage or binder, if present; wash hands.
12. Put the bandage or binder on the patient, using one of the specific techniques described. Teach the patient or caregiver how to apply the device if indicated and appropriate.
13. Examine the bandage or binder for neatness, lack of irritating wrinkles, and security *to determine whether it will stay comfortably in place.*
14. Assess the extremity distal to the bandage for circulation, motion, and sensation *to make sure the bandage or binder is not too tight or restricting. Tight bandages or binders that encircle an extremity can block venous return, leading to swelling. In addition, either the original bandage itself or the swelling may block arterial circulation to the distal extremity. This blocking of circulation may cause permanent nerve or other tissue damage. Judging the tightness of*

---

[1]Rationale for action is emphasized throughout the module by the use of italics.

© 1996 by Lippincott-Raven Publishers

any bandage, especially an elastic bandage, is difficult. Therefore, a planned program of assessing circulation, motion, and sensation of the extremity should be instituted whenever a bandage or binder is applied to an extremity. Teach the patient or caregiver to do this if the patient will go home with the bandage or binder in place.

15. Question the patient regarding comfort.
16. Wash your hands *for infection control.*

Evaluation

17. Evaluate using the following criteria:
    a. Patient comfort
    b. Effectiveness in holding dressings in place or providing support
    c. Safety regarding maintenance of tissue integrity, circulation, motion, and sensation

Documentation

18. Document on the progress notes or flow sheet:
    a. Time
    b. Type of bandage or binder applied
    c. Area to which bandage or binder was applied
    d. Assessment of circulation, motion, and sensation as appropriate
    e. Length of time the device was off and the condition of the skin underneath, if *reapplication* (Fig. 26–1 gives an example of a flow sheet entry.)

APPLYING BANDAGES

Types of Bandages

A variety of bandages can be used for wrapping limbs. *Roller gauze* is available in ½-inch, 1-inch, 2-inch, and 3-inch widths. This material does not stretch but is soft, strong, and comfortable. It can be easily molded to a part of the body with proper bandaging technique. Roller gauze is used to hold dressings in place. It is available in both sterile and non-sterile forms.

Another type of gauze bandage is a soft, meshlike flexible bandage that is stretchable. Kling is one brand of this type of bandage. Other brands of stretch gauze are also available. Commonly available in 2-inch, 3-inch, and 4-inch widths, it can be used on extremities, the head, and the torso. It can be part of the primary dressing or used to hold other dressings in place and can be either sterile or nonsterile. When applying a stretchable gauze bandage, keep the patient's extremities in a functional position while they are wrapped *to maintain correct alignment.*

Still another type of roller bandage is a heavier type of stretchable material commonly known as the elastic bandage. One brand that is used is Ace. Elastic bandages are used to provide constant pressure over an area or to support an injured joint. On a lower extremity, they also facilitate venous return. On an extremity, elastic hose, an elastic sleeve, or a sequential compression device can be used instead of an elastic bandage.

All bandages should be placed over clean, dry surfaces *to prevent the harboring and growth of microorganisms.* Change bandages frequently *to keep them clean.* Pad bony prominences *to prevent pressure.*

Methods of Application

There are five general methods of applying roll bandages: circular, spiral, reverse-spiral, figure 8, and recurrent fold. The circular-turn bandage is used *to secure a dressing or to cover a confined area of an extremity.* The spiral and reverse-spiral begin distally on an extremity and wind proximally, *to provide comfort to a wider area.* The figure 8 bandage is used over a joint *to provide easy flexion.* To bandage distal portions of extremities or a stump that has not been casted, the recurrent-fold technique *best provides the correct pressure.*

Before you begin to apply any type of roll bandage, firmly roll the bandage. Always unroll it with the rolled-up portion on top (Fig. 26–2) *to facilitate the process.* Secure the bandage with a strip of cloth or paper tape over the loose end, fastened to the bandage, not the skin. If the material is porous, use a metal clip with sharp small teeth on the undersurface. Metal clips are commonly used with Ace bandages, but a safety pin or tape also may be used.

Circular

With the roll on the inner aspect, unroll the bandage either toward you or laterally, holding the loose end until it is secured by the first circle of the bandage (Fig. 26–3). Two or three turns may be needed *to cover an area adequately.* Hold the bandage in place with tape or a clip.

Spiral

Begin with the circular method. After securing with one or two complete overlaps, place the bandage to overlap one-half or two-thirds of the width, and in this manner move up the extremity *to provide even support* (Fig. 26–4). Tape or clip the bandage in place.

© 1996 by Lippincott-Raven Publishers

Fill in the parameters to be monitored. Refer to Standard & Individual Care Plans.
Parameter examples: Guaiac stools/emesis, urine fractionals, specific gravity, girth of limb/abd, bowel sounds, circulation of extremity, pedal pulses, frequent lab values.

Parameters		EXTREMITY														Initial
						Circle Extremity Monitored LA (RA) LL RL										
Date	Time	COLOR 1.	CAPILLARY FILLING 2.	PULSE 3.	TEMPERATURE 4.	SENSATION 5.	MOTOR FUNCTION 6.	PAIN 7.	PAIN ON STRETCH 8.							
3/12	20	B	<3	W	Wm	Nb	N	Mod	O							EA
3/12	22	B	<3	W	Wm	Nb	N	M	O							EA
3/12	24	B	<3	W	Wm	Nb	N	M	O							JW
3/13	04	N	<3	S	Wm	Nb/T	N	M	O							JW
3/13	06	N	<3	S	Wm	Nb/T	N	M	O				*feeling all fingers*			JW
		1. N Normal B Blue P Pale														
		2. < 3 Sec. > 3 Sec.														
		3. S Strong W Weak A Absent														
		4. Wm Warm H Hot C Cool														
		5. N Normal T Tingle Nb Numb A Absent														
		6. N Normal W Weak A Absent														
		7. O None, M Mild, Mod Moderate, Sev Severe														
		8. O None, M Mild, Mod Moderate, Sev Severe														

PARAMETER FLOW SHEET

Identify Initials with Signature:		4.		8.	
1. *Ella Adams, RN*		5.		9.	
2. *Joy Williams, RN*		6.		10.	
3.		7.		11.	

ADDRESSOGRAPH:
McCarthy, Michael   M-76
338 - 19 - 3154

Dr. Costello

SWEDISH HOSPITAL MEDICAL CENTER
SEATTLE, WASHINGTON

Figure 26–1. A form for the nurse to use in recording color, motion, and sensation after a bandage or binder has been applied.

© 1996 by Lippincott-Raven Publishers

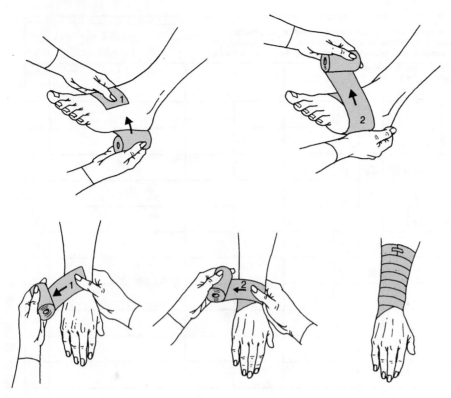

Figure 26–2. To facilitate unrolling the bandage, the nurse has the unrolled portion on the top.

Reverse-Spiral

Begin as you would for the spiral bandage. When the end is secured by the first turn, hold your thumb on the bandage as it approaches the side nearest you and fold over, reversing the direction downward (Fig. 26–5). Repeat this step with each turn, overlapping as before. When the desired area is covered,

end with a circular wrap and secure the bandage with tape or a clip.

Figure-8

This bandage is most often used on a joint. Make the first turns over the joint, securing with the overlap. Make the next turn higher than, or superior to, the

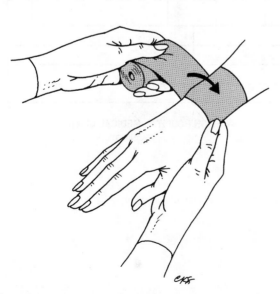

Figure 26–3. You may use a circular wrap for applying a bandage to a wrist.

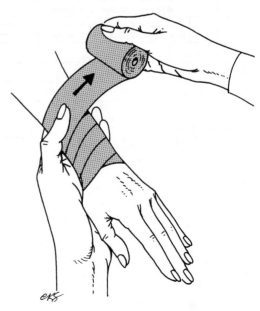

Figure 26–4. You may use a spiral wrap for applying a bandage to the wrist and forearm.

© 1996 by Lippincott-Raven Publishers

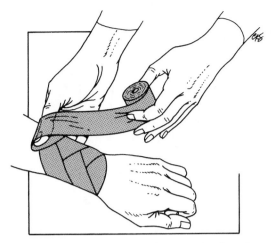

Figure 26–5. To use a reverse-spiral wrap to bandage the arm, hold the fold of the bandage in place with one hand as you reverse the spiral and wrap with your other hand.

joint. Make the following turn lower than, or inferior to, the joint (Fig. 26–6). Continue working in this manner, one turn above and one below. The figure 8 pattern *allows the joint to maintain its mobility without dislodging the bandage.* Secure the bandage with tape or a clip.

Recurrent Fold

The recurrent fold bandage can be adapted for use on many parts of the body. It is used for the finger, hand, toe, or foot. This type of bandage is also applicable for use as a head dressing (Fig. 26–7) or on the stump of an extremity.

To apply, hold the end of the bandage in place with one circular turn. Then, bring the roll down over the end of the body part (finger, hand, toe, foot, or stump) and back up behind. When used on the head, the circular turn is made, and then turns are made over and back across the top of the head. Subsequent turns are folded alternately to the right and

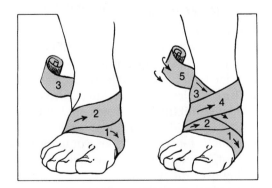

Figure 26–6. Following the numbers indicated above, you can use a finger wrap to bandage and give support to the ankle.

left of the initial center fold (Fig. 26–8). Keep your fingers in place at the top to secure the bandage until a circular turn or two can be made to complete the bandage (Fig. 26–9). Clip or tape in place.

SPECIFIC PROCEDURES FOR APPLYING BANDAGES

For each procedure discussed, some steps of the General Procedure may be modified. We have included completely the modified steps as well as references to the steps of the General Procedure that remain the same.

Wrapping an Ankle and Lower Leg

Assessment
1.–3. Follow the steps of the General Procedure for Applying Bandages and Binders.

Planning
4.–7. Follow the steps of the General Procedure.

Implementation
8.–11. Follow the steps of the General Procedure.
12. Wrap the ankle or leg.
   a. Keep the body part in a horizontal position for at least 15 minutes before bandaging *to ensure that veins have emptied.*
   b. Secure the bandage around the instep with a single circular wrap and form a figure 8 around the ankle itself.

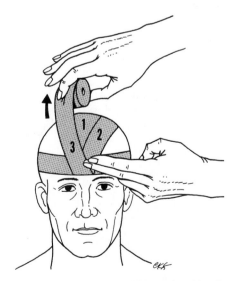

Figure 26–7. Using the recurrent fold on a head bandage. Hold the end of the bandage in place as you use your other hand to change directions and overlap. Continue overlapping to cover, making a final horizontal loop to secure the bandage.

© 1996 by Lippincott-Raven Publishers

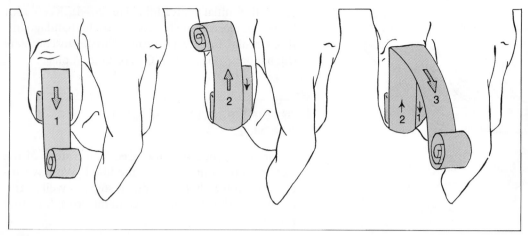

Figure 26–8. You can use the recurrent fold on the fingers and toes by following the same procedure as given for the head.

c. Wrap as far up the leg as desired, using a spiral wrap. To continue the wrap above the knee, use a reverse-spiral just below the knee *to secure the bandage firmly.* Always work from distal to proximal. This, as well as the elastic quality of the bandage, *promotes venous return.*

d. Clip or tape in place.

13.–16. Follow the steps of the General Procedure.

Evaluation

17. Follow the General Procedure.

Documentation

18. Follow the General Procedure.

Applying Elastic (Antiembolic) Stockings

Elastic stockings are used *to provide firm support to the soft tissue, preventing venous blood from pooling and blood clots from developing in the deep veins.* Elastic stockings are typically ordered for patients preoperatively (*to maintain venous return during the operative procedure*) and kept in place during the postoperative phase as well. They are also commonly used when a patient's mobility is limited and sometimes to prevent or treat orthostatic hypotension. Usually, elastic hose are applied before the patient gets out of bed. There are many different brands of elastic stockings. Some have openings *to allow the toes to be examined and circulation to be checked.* There are both knee-length and thigh-length types. Thigh-length stockings usually have a nonconstricting gusset set in at the inner aspect of the thigh. *To provide adequate pressure at the right place without impairing blood flow,* the correct size must be obtained. Check the directions on the brand you are using to determine the size. Because they are so firm, elastic stockings are often difficult to apply using the usual techniques for putting on hose. Most manufacturers recommend an "inside-out" technique (Fig. 26–10).

Assessment

1.–3. Follow the steps of the General Procedure for Applying Bandages and Binders.

Planning

4.–7. Follow the steps of the General Procedure.

Implementation

8.–11. Follow the steps of the General Procedure.

12. Apply the elastic stockings.

a. Slide your hand into the stocking to the foot.

b. Turn the leg of the stocking down over your hand until the leg is inside out but the foot is still right side out inside the leg.

c. Pull the foot of the stocking onto the patient's foot, carefully placing the heel of the stocking over the heel of the foot.

d. Gradually pull the stocking up over the leg by turning it right side out onto the leg.

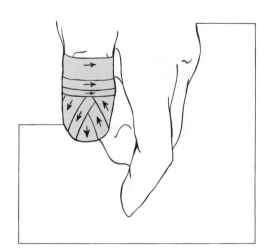

Figure 26–9. Recurrent bandages are secured with one or more horizontal loops.

© 1996 by Lippincott-Raven Publishers

DATE/TIME	
1/15/99 8:00 AM	*Elastic bandage applied to left ankle. Pt states it feels comfortable. Toes pink, warm, rapid capillary filling, no numbness or tingling. ———— A. Edge, SN*

Example of Nursing Progress Notes Using Narrative Format.

e. Make sure that the stocking fits smoothly without wrinkles and that the foot is correctly positioned. Do not turn down the top edge *to avoid restricting venous return.*

f. Repeat steps a through e for the other stocking.

Elastic hose should not be worn for longer than 8 hours at one time. At least every 8 hours the hose should be removed, the skin inspected, the legs elevated for 15 minutes *to promote venous return,* and the stockings reapplied. The skin of the feet and legs should be cleansed at least every 24 hours.

13.–16. Follow the steps of the General Procedure.

Evaluation

17. Follow the General Procedure.

Documentation

18. Follow the General Procedure.

Applying A Sequential Compression Device

A sequential compression device provides intermittent compression over the lower leg or thigh *to promote venous return and prevent deep vein thrombosis and pulmonary embolism.* Amounts of pressure exerted by the sleeve during the various phases of the cycle are adjustable and displayed on the control unit. It may be applied to one or both lower extremities. Such a device is contraindicated for patients with severe arterial disease of the lower extremities.

Various forms of sequential compression devices exist, but the typical device usually consists of a vinyl "sleeve" that fits over the ankle and calf (some versions include the thigh) and fastens with Velcro connectors. A control unit that is placed on the floor under the bed has a small pump that inflates and deflates channels in the sleeve to provide increasing and decreasing pressure.

The device must be ordered in the appropriate size for the individual patient. Instructions for how to measure calf and thigh circumference and length are included with the device. In some cases, elastic stockings are applied beneath the sequential compression device *for optimum clinical efficacy.*

Assessment

1.–3. Follow the steps of the General Procedure for Applying Bandages and Binders.

Planning

4.–7. Follow the steps of the General Procedure.

Implementation

8.–11. Follow the steps of the General Procedure.

12. Apply the sequential compression device.

    a. Place the vinyl sleeve over the ankle and calf. If it is a tubular sleeve, slide it on over the

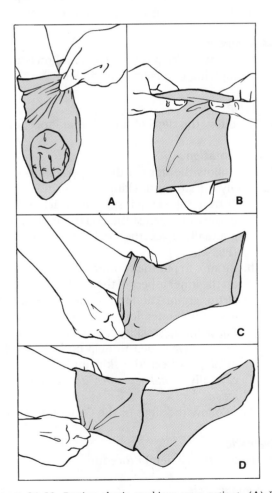

Figure 26–10. Putting elastic stockings on a patient. **(A)** Put hand inside the stocking and turn wrong side out. **(B)** Stretch the stocking at the heel to facilitate putting it on. **(C)** Pull the stocking over the heel. **(D)** Pull the stocking up over the leg.

© 1996 by Lippincott-Raven Publishers

foot, ankle, and calf. If it is a wrap style, align the leg on the open thigh-length sleeve according to the instructions included. Wrap the sleeve securely around the patient's leg and fasten the Velcro tabs, thigh section first (Fig. 26–11).

b. Attach the connector on the sleeve to the correct end of the connector tubing. Check carefully to be certain there are no kinks in the tubing.

c. Attach the other end of the connector tubing to the control unit.

d. Turn the power on and adjust or monitor pressure according to your facility's protocol.

e. Remove the device at least twice daily, for 20 to 30 minutes each time, to allow for ambulation and bathing. Replace immediately after ambulation or care.

13.–16. Follow the steps of the General Procedure.

Evaluation

17. Follow the General Procedure.

Documentation

18. Follow the General Procedure.

Wrapping a Stump

Assessment

1.–3. Follow the steps of the General Procedure for Applying Bandages and Binders.

Planning

4.–7. Follow the steps of the General Procedure.

Implementation

8.–11. Follow the steps of the General Procedure.

12. Wrap the stump according to the method preferred by the surgeon. Commonly, a recurrent bandage is placed on the stump first, and then a

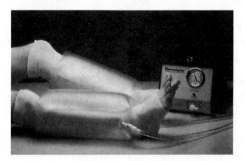

Figure 26–11. Sequential compression device and control unit.

spiral is started at the distal end of the stump and moved up to the thigh (Fig. 26–12). Pressure must be properly distributed, with slightly more pressure at the most distal portion of the stump, both *to enhance return circulation and to produce a smooth, even stump.* Alternatively, some surgeons prefer that a figure 8 bandage be wrapped from the stump up and around the hip and waist.

13.–16. Follow the steps of the General Procedure.

Evaluation

17. Follow the General Procedure.

Documentation

18. Follow the General Procedure.

Applying a Stump Stocking

An elastic support stump stocking may be used in place of an elastic wrap. This stocking is made of firmly woven stretch elastic in a rounded shape that is smooth and *provides even support to the tissue.*

Assessment

1.–3. Follow the steps of the General Procedure for Applying Bandages and Binders.

Planning

4.–7. Follow the steps of the General Procedure.

Implementation

8.–11. Follow the steps of the General Procedure.

12. Apply the stump stocking.

a. Turn the stocking inside out, placing the end of the tube against the end of the stump, and gradually invert the stocking over the stump (Fig. 26–13).

b. Be sure to put the shorter side of the stocking on the inner aspect of the thigh so that it stops at the groin. The longer side of the stocking fits on the outer, longer aspect of the thigh.

c. Some stump stockings have buckles that fasten to a waist belt to help hold the stocking in place. Check the skin under the buckles carefully *to make sure they are not causing irritation.*

13.–16. Follow the steps of the General Procedure.

Evaluation

17. Follow the General Procedure.

Documentation

18. Follow the General Procedure.

© 1996 by Lippincott-Raven Publishers

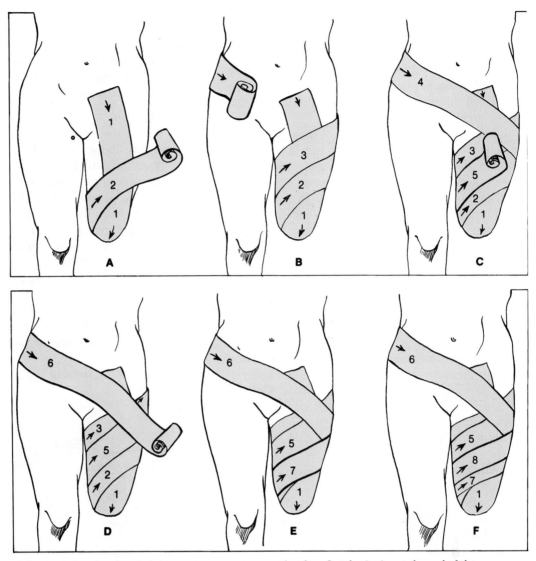

Figure 26–12. When bandaging a stump, use a recurrent bandage first, beginning at the end of the stump, and then wrap a spiral bandage up the thigh. (Courtesy University of Washington Department of Prosthetics-Orthotics, Seattle, Washington.)

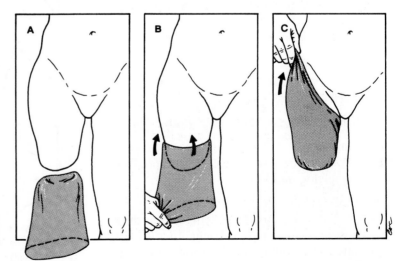

Figure 26–13. To apply the stump stocking, turn the stocking inside out, invert it over the end of the stump, and gently pull it to its right side over the stump.

© 1996 by Lippincott-Raven Publishers

APPLYING BINDERS

Types of Binders

Binders are generally used on the trunk of the body *to hold dressings in place or to support tissues.* They can be placed around the chest, the abdomen, or the pelvic area.

Binders are made of a variety of materials. They may be made of a wide strip of soft muslin, a strip of lightweight canvas material, an elastic fabric, or a stretch net fabric used to hold dressings in place.

Abdominal binders are usually straight and can be fashioned from any strong material—for example, a drawsheet or bath blanket. However, most are commercially made from a firm elastic fabric with Velcro fasteners across the front.

Stretch net binders are used to hold dressings in place, not for support. They are usually used around the abdomen or chest but can also be used on the extremities. They come in a variety of circumferences. Because these binders will stretch and are available in different widths and lengths, you do not have to measure the body part but should order a size you think is appropriate for the patient. The advantages of stretch net binders are that *they can be washed easily and dried quickly; they offer air circulation; and they stretch to conform to the shape of the part being bound.*

T-binders are designed to hold perineal dressings or packs in place. Single T-binders are used for female patients; double T-binders are used for male patients *so that the testicles are not unduly constricted.* Some T-binders are elastic with snap fasteners, some are muslin, and others are made of a disposable paper.

Slings (in effect, arm binders) are used to rest the arm in a right-angle position. They are often made from bright patterned material cut in a triangular shape.

SPECIFIC PROCEDURES FOR APPLYING BINDERS

Applying a Straight Abdominal Binder

Assessment

1.–3. Follow the steps of the General Procedure for Applying Bandages and Binders.

Planning

4.–5. Follow the steps of the General Procedure.

6. Measure the patient's girth and order the appropriate size abdominal binder, usually from the facility's central supply department. Abdominal binders for adult patients are available in sizes small, medium, large, and extra large. If you are unsure, call the central supply department with the measurements and the appropriate staff person will determine the correct size to send.

7. Follow the General Procedure.

Implementation

8.–11. Follow the steps of the General Procedure.

12. Apply the abdominal binder.

   a. Place the patient in the supine position. Ask the patient to lift upward, using the legs, or roll the patient onto the binder. Apply the binder smoothly and evenly *so that wrinkles do not cause pressure on the patient's skin.*

   b. Bring the ends of the binder upward around the patient's trunk.

   c. Overlap the edges of the binder snugly over the abdomen.

   d. Fasten using Velcro connectors or safety pins. Velcro fastenings are more comfortable for the patient than are the hard surfaces of pins (Figure 26–14).

13.–16. Follow the steps of the General Procedure.

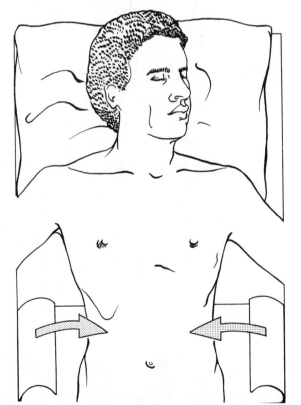

Figure 26–14. Straight abdominal binder. With patient lying in the supine position, overlap the edges of the straight abdominal binder snugly over the abdomen. Secure with Velcro or safety pins.

© 1996 by Lippincott-Raven Publishers

Evaluation

17. Follow the General Procedure.

Documentation

18. Follow the General Procedure.

Applying a Stretch Net Binder

Assessment

1.–3. Follow the steps of the General Procedure for Applying Bandages and Binders.

Planning

4.–7. Follow the steps of the General Procedure.

Implementation

8.–11. Follow the steps of the General Procedure.
12. Apply the stretch net binder.
   a. Gather the net in your hands.
   b. Stretch the net and slip it upward over the feet and legs to its position around the abdomen. Alternatively, slip it over the head and downward, surrounding the abdomen. Use the technique that is most comfortable for the patient. When stretch net binders are used around the chest, they are usually pulled over the head (Figure 26–15).
13.–16. Follow the steps of the General Procedure.

Evaluation

17. Follow the General Procedure.

Documentation

18. Follow the General Procedure.

Applying a T-Binder

Assessment

1.–3. Follow the steps of the General Procedure for Applying Bandages and Binders.

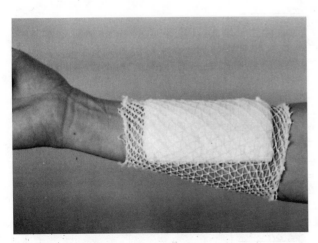

Figure 26–15. Stretch net binder. Gather and stretch net in your hands over extremity.

© 1996 by Lippincott-Raven Publishers

Planning

4.–5. Follow the steps of the General Procedure.
6. Select the appropriate binder according to the patient's sex (Fig. 26–16).
7. Follow the General Procedure.

Implementation

8.–11. Follow the steps of the General Procedure.
12. Apply the T-binder.
   a. Have the patient lift midsection or turn patient side to side and place the binder underneath the patient smoothly, with the waistband at waist level and the tails pointing down the midline of the back.
   b. Bring the waist tails around the patient and overlap.
   c. Bring the center tail (or tails) up between the patient's legs and over perineal dressings, taking care to touch only the outside of the dressings. Make sure the two tails of the double T-binder are on either side of the scrotum and penis.
   d. Join the center tail(s) to the waistband and secure the ends with safety pins.
13.–16. Follow the steps of the General Procedure.

Evaluation

17. Follow the General Procedure.

Documentation

18. Follow the General Procedure.

Applying an Arm Sling

Assessment

1.–3. Follow the steps of the General Procedure for Applying Bandages and Binders.

Planning

4.–5. Follow the steps of the General Procedure.
6. To make an arm sling from muslin, fold or cut (for less thickness) a 36-inch square of fabric diagonally.
7. Follow the General Procedure.

Implementation

8.–11. Follow the steps of the General Procedure.
12. Apply the arm sling, using one of the two following methods:
   a. Method A
      (1) With the patient facing you, place one end of the triangle over the unaffected shoulder.
      (2) Bring the long straight border under the hand on the affected side.
      (3) Loop upward, positioning the other end of the triangle over the affected shoulder.
      (4) Tie or pin the ends to one side of the

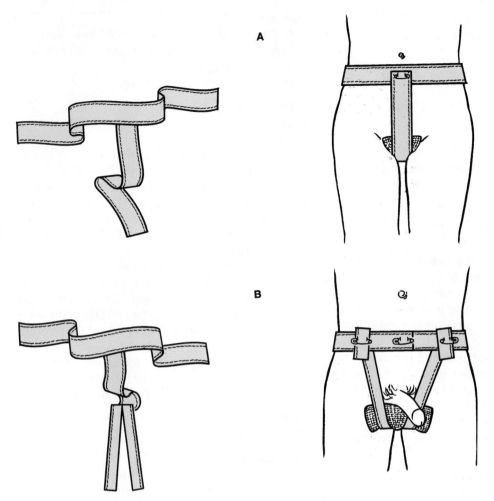

Figure 26–16. Disposable T-binders. To apply a T-binder, bring the waist tails around the patient's waist and the center tail or tails up between the patient's legs to hold the dressings in place. Secure the ends of the tails with safety pins.

DATE/TIME	
1/15/99 9:00 AM	*Right arm supported with sling. States no pain as long as arm not moved. Fingers pale, cool with slight swelling. Capillary filling rapid. No c/o numbness or tingling.* *A. Edge, SN*

Example of Nursing Progress Notes Using Narrative Format.

DATE/TIME	
1/15/99 0900	*High risk for altered peripheral circulation in left arm related to surgery on left elbow.* *S States no pain if arm not moved. No numbness or tingling reported.* *O Fingers pale, cool, slight swelling, capillary filling rapid.* *A Circulation stable at this time.* *P Assess circulation of left arm qh. Maintain sling on left arm.* *A. Edge, SN*

Example of Nursing Progress Notes Using SOAP Format.

© 1996 by Lippincott-Raven Publishers

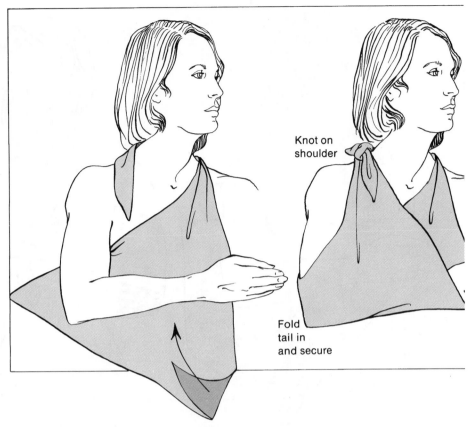

Figure 26–17. Arm sling—Method A. Place one end of triangle over unaffected shoulder. Bring other end of triangle over affected shoulder. Tie or pin ends to one side of the neck. Fold corner flat at elbow and secure with safety pins.

neck, using a square knot, or pin smoothly, using a safety pin. Never secure a sling at the back of the neck, *where pressure could be exerted.*

(5) Fold the corner flat and neatly at the elbow, and pin.

(6) Check the position—the hand should be supported in the sling (Fig. 26–17).

b. Method B

(1) With the patient facing you, place the sling across the body and underneath the arms, as shown in Figure 26–18.

(2) Bring the corner of the sling that is under the unaffected arm to the back.

(3) Bring the lower corner up over the affected shoulder to the back, and tie.

(4) Fold the sling neatly at the elbow, and pin.

(5) Check the position—the hand should be supported in the sling.

13.–16. Follow the steps of the General Procedure.

Evaluation

17. Follow the General Procedure.

Documentation

18. Follow the General Procedure.

Method B is preferred because the first kind of sling *can pull or strain the neck muscles, even when it is tied at the side* of the neck. In method B, the entire shoulder bears the weight of the immobilized arm.

Some commercially made slings are made of a canvaslike material. They have a support pocket for the forearm and straps that go over the shoulder (Fig. 26–19).

© 1996 by Lippincott-Raven Publishers

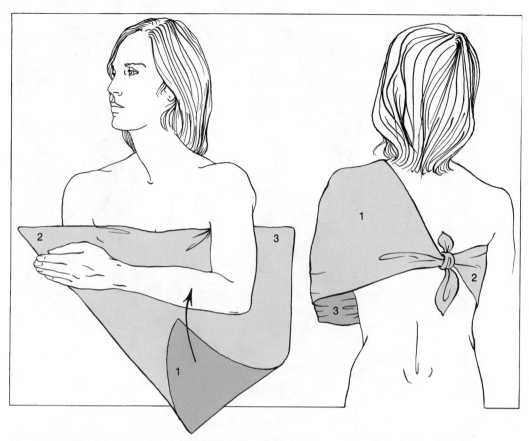

Figure 26–18. Arm sling—Method B. Place triangle under the arms. Bring the corner that is under the unaffected arm up over the shoulder to the back and the corner under the affected arm around the body to the back. Tie the ends. Fold corner flat at the elbows and secure with safety pins.

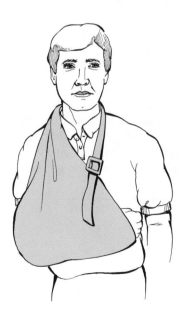
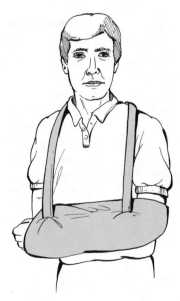

Figure 26–19. Commercial arm slings are made of a canvaslike material and have a pocket for the affected arm. They are supported by straps that go over the shoulder.

© 1996 by Lippincott-Raven Publishers

LONG-TERM CARE

The principles related to applying bandages and binders remain the same regardless of the setting in which they are used. However, *the circulation of some older adults residing in long-term care facilities may be more compromised than that of younger patients found in other settings. These residents may have decreased sensation as well, and hence they may be unaware of a bandage or binder that has become too snug. In addition, those who are unable to communicate their distress are at added risk.* Therefore, you may need to check circulation, sensation, and movement at more frequent intervals than in other settings.

Because of decreased mobility and poor venous return, many long-term care residents will wear elastic hose on a routine basis. These hose need to be laundered frequently, which will lead to diminished effectiveness over time. This means you will need to plan for sufficient pairs of hose so that some are always available. You also will need to engage in frequent evaluation of the effectiveness of the hose.

HOME CARE

Those who need to wear various types of bandages and binders at home need to know how to apply them safely and effectively and how often to check or change them. In some situations, the client will be able to do this without assistance. In other situations, a family member, friend, or neighbor may need to help.

Caution ambulatory clients who wear elastic hose that these stockings may roll down, creating a constricting band and compromising circulation. Your teaching will be specific to a given situation, but you might include teaching about how to change a sterile or clean dressing, how to assess circulation and skin condition, and principles of correct positioning. Encourage both clients and their families to telephone their care provider if questions or concerns arise.

CRITICAL THINKING EXERCISES

A 4-year-old girl has sustained an injury that will require her to have her left arm in a sling for 2 weeks. Describe and demonstrate to the child's mother an appropriate way to apply a sling. Write out instructions for the mother to take home.

© 1996 by Lippincott-Raven Publishers

✔ PERFORMANCE CHECKLIST

General Procedure for Applying Bandages and Binders	Needs More Practice	Satisfactory	Comments
Assessment			
1. Identify purpose.			
2. Identify part of body to be supported.			
3. Assess any previously placed bandage or binder for effectiveness and comfort. Note length of time in place and color, temperature, sensation, and skin condition of affected body part.			
Planning			
4. Plan the specific procedure to be used.			
5. Wash your hands.			
6. Obtain appropriate bandage or binder and fastening devices.			
7. Plan for times to recheck patient.			
Implementation			
8. Identify patient.			
9. Explain procedure to patient.			
10. Provide for privacy and position patient.			
11. Remove soiled or used bandage or binder, if present; wash your hands.			
12. Use specific technique planned.			
13. Examine for neatness, no wrinkles, security.			
14. Assess circulation, motion, and sensation distal to bandage.			
15. Question the patient regarding comfort.			
16. Wash your hands.			
Evaluation			
17. Evaluate using the following criteria: a. Patient comfort			
b. Effectiveness in holding dressings in place			
c. Safety regarding maintaining tissue integrity.			

(continued)

© 1996 by Lippincott-Raven Publishers

General Procedure for Applying Bandages and Binders (Continued)	Needs More Practice	Satisfactory	Comments
18. Document on progress notes or flow sheet: **a.** Time			
b. Type of bandage or binder applied			
c. Area to which applied			
d. Assessment of circulation, motion, and sensation			
e. Length of time device off and condition of skin underneath (if reapplication)			
Wrapping an Ankle and Lower Leg			
Assessment			
1.–3. Follow Checklist steps 1–3 of the General Procedure for Applying Bandages and Binders (identify purpose, identify part of body to be supported, assess any previously placed bandage or binder).			
Planning			
4.–7. Follow Checklist steps 4–7 of the General Procedure (plan procedure, wash hands, obtain bandage(s), plan times to recheck).			
Implementation			
8.–11. Follow Checklist steps 8–11 of the General Procedure (identify patient, explain procedure, provide for privacy and position, remove soiled or used bandage [if present], and wash hands).			
12. Wrap ankle or leg. **a.** Keep in horizontal position 15 minutes.			
b. Secure bandage around instep and form figure 8 around ankle.			
c. Wrap up leg, using spiral wrap. If wrapping above knee, use reverse-spiral just below knee. Move from distal to proximal.			
d. Clip or tape in place.			
13.–16. Follow Checklist steps 13–16 of the General Procedure (examine for neatness; check circulation, motion, and sensation; question patient regarding comfort; and wash hands).			

(continued)

© 1996 by Lippincott-Raven Publishers

Wrapping an Ankle and Lower Leg *(Continued)*	Needs More Practice	Satisfactory	Comments
Evaluation			
17. Evaluate as in Checklist step 17 (patient comfort, effectiveness, safety).			
Documentation			
18. Document as in Checklist step 18 (time; type of bandage; where applied; assessment of circulation, motion, and sensation; length of time off and condition of skin underneath [if reapplication]).			
Applying Elastic Stockings			
Assessment			
1.–3. Follow Checklist steps 1–3 of the General Procedure for Applying Bandages and Binders (identify purpose, identify part of body to be supported, assess any previously placed bandage or binder).			
Planning			
4.–7. Follow Checklist steps 4–7 of the General Procedure (plan procedure, wash hands, obtain stocking(s), plan times to recheck).			
Implementation			
8.–11. Follow Checklist 8–11 of the General Procedure (identify patient, explain procedure, provide for privacy and position, remove soiled or used bandage or binder [if present], and wash hands).			
12. Apply stockings. **a.** Slide hand into stocking to the foot.			
b. Turn leg of stocking down over hand.			
c. Pull foot of stocking onto patient's foot with heel of stocking over heel of foot.			
d. Turn stocking right side out onto leg.			
e. Ensure stocking fit smoothly and foot is positioned correctly.			
f. Repeat steps a–e for other stocking.			
13.–16. Follow Checklist steps 13–16 of the General Procedure (examine for neatness; check circulation, motion, and sensation; question patient regarding comfort, and wash hands).			

(continued)

© 1996 by Lippincott-Raven Publishers

Applying Elastic Stockings *(Continued)*	Needs More Practice	Satisfactory	Comments
Evaluation			
17. Evaluate as in Checklist step 17 (patient comfort, effectiveness, safety).			
Documentation			
18. Document as in Checklist step 18 (time; type of bandage or binder; where applied; assessment of circulation, motion, and sensation; length of time off and condition of skin underneath [if reapplication]).			
Applying a Sequential Compression Device			
Assessment			
1.–3. Follow Checklist steps 1–3 of the General Procedure for Applying Bandages and Binders (identify purpose, identify part of body to be supported, assess any previously placed bandage or binder).			
Planning			
4.–7. Follow Checklist steps 4–7 of the General Procedure (plan procedure, wash hands, obtain device, plan times to recheck).			
Implementation			
8.–11. Follow Checklist steps 8–11 of the General Procedure (identify patient, explain procedure, provide for privacy and position, remove soiled or used bandage or binder [if present], and wash hands).			
12. Apply sequential compression device. **a.** Place vinyl sleeve over ankle and calf.			
b. Attach connector on sleeve to correct end of connector tubing.			
c. Attach other end of connector tubing to control unit.			
d. Turn power on; adjust according to facility protocol.			
e. Remove at least twice daily for 20–30 minutes; replace immediately after ambulation or care given.			

(continued)

© 1996 by Lippincott-Raven Publishers

Applying a Sequential Compression Device *(Continued)*	Needs More Practice	Satisfactory	Comments
13.–16. Follow Checklist steps 13–16 of the General Procedure (examine for neatness; check circulation, motion, and sensation; question patient regarding comfort; and wash hands).			
Evaluation			
17. Evaluate as in Checklist step 17 (patient comfort, effectiveness, safety).			
Documentation			
18. Document as in Checklist step 18 (time; type of bandage or binder; where applied; assessment of circulation, motion, and sensation; length of time off and condition of skin underneath (if reapplication).			
Wrapping a Stump			
Assessment			
1.–3. Follow Checklist steps 1–3 of the General Procedure for Applying Bandages and Binders (identify purpose, identify part of body to be supported, assess any previously placed bandage or binder).			
Planning			
4.–7. Follow Checklist steps 4–7 of the General Procedure (plan procedure, wash hands, obtain bandage(s), plan times to recheck).			
Implementation			
8.–11. Follow Checklist steps 8–11 of the General Procedure (identify patient, explain procedure, provide for privacy and position, remove soiled or used bandage or binder [if present], and wash hands).			
12. Wrap the stump according to surgeon's preferred method.			
13.–16. Follow Checklist steps 13–16 of the General Procedure (examine for neatness; check circulation, motion, and sensation; question patient regarding comfort, and wash hands).			

(continued)

© 1996 by Lippincott-Raven Publishers

Wrapping a Stump *(Continued)*	Needs More Practice	Satisfactory	Comments
Evaluation			
17. Evaluate as in Checklist step 17 (patient comfort, effectiveness, safety).			
Documentation			
18. Document as in Checklist step 18 (time; type of bandage or binder; where applied; assessment of circulation, motion, and sensation; length of time off and condition of skin underneath (if reapplication).			
Applying a Stump Stocking			
Assessment			
1.–3. Follow Checklist steps 1–3 of the General Procedure for Applying Bandages and Binders (identify purpose, identify part of body to be supported, assess any previously placed bandage or binder).			
Planning			
4.–7. Follow Checklist steps 4–7 of the General Procedure (plan procedure, wash hands, obtain bandage(s), plan times to recheck).			
Implementation			
8.–11. Follow Checklist steps 8–11 of the General Procedure (identify patient, explain procedure, provide for privacy and position, remove soiled or used bandage or binder [if present], and wash hands).			
12. Apply the stump stocking. **a.** Turn stocking inside out and invert over stump.			
b. Put shorter side of stocking on inner aspect of thigh; longer side, on outer aspect.			
c. Check skin under buckles, if present.			
13.–16. Follow Checklist steps 13–16 of the General Procedure (examine for neatness; check circulation, motion, and sensation; question patient regarding comfort; and wash hands).			

(continued)

© 1996 by Lippincott-Raven Publishers

Applying a **Stump Stocking** *(Continued)*	Needs More Practice	Satisfactory	Comments
Evaluation			
17. Evaluate as in Checklist step 17 (patient comfort, effectiveness, safety).			
Documentation			
18. Document as in Checklist step 18 (time; type of bandage or binder; where applied; assessment of circulation, motion, and sensation; length of time off and condition of skin underneath (if reapplication).			
Applying a Straight Abdominal Binder			
Assessment			
1.–3. Follow Checklist steps 1–3 of the General Procedure for Applying Bandages and Binders (identify purpose, identify part of body to be supported, assess any previously placed bandage or binder).			
Planning			
4.–5. Follow Checklist steps 4 and 5 of the General Procedure (plan procedure and wash your hands).			
6. Measure patient's girth and order appropriate size binder.			
7. Plan for time to recheck patient as in Checklist step 7 of the General Procedure.			
Implementation			
8.–11. Follow Checklist steps 8–11 of the General Procedure (identify patient, explain procedure, provide for privacy and position, remove soiled or used bandage or binder [if present], and wash hands).			
12. Apply the abdominal binder. a. Place patient supine. Ask patient to lift midsection and place binder smoothly underneath, or turn patient side to side to place binder.			
b. Bring ends upward around trunk.			
c. Overlap edges of binder snugly over abdomen.			
d. Fasten using Velcro connectors or pins.			

(continued)

© 1996 by Lippincott-Raven Publishers

Applying a Straight Abdominal Binder *(Continued)*	Needs More Practice	Satisfactory	Comments
13.–16. Follow Checklist steps 13–16 of the General Procedure (examine for neatness; check circulation, motion, and sensation; question patient regarding comfort; and wash hands).			
Evaluation			
17. Evaluate as in Checklist step 17 (patient comfort, effectiveness, safety).			
Documentation			
18. Document as in Checklist step 18 (time; type of bandage or binder; where applied; assessment of circulation, motion, and sensation; length of time off and condition of skin underneath (if reapplication).			
Applying a Stretch Net Binder			
Assessment			
1.–3. Follow Checklist steps 1–3 of the General Procedure for Applying Bandages and Binders (identify purpose, identify part of body to be supported, assess any previously placed bandage or binder).			
Planning			
4.–7. Follow Checklist steps 4–7 of the General Procedure (plan procedure, wash hands, obtain binder, plan times to recheck).			
Implementation			
8.–11. Follow Checklist steps 8–11 of the General Procedure (identify patient, explain procedure, provide for privacy and position, remove soiled or used bandage or binder [if present], and wash hands).			
12. Apply the stretch net binder. **a.** Gather the net in your hands.			
b. Stretch and slip it upward over feet and legs to abdomen or over head to chest or abdomen.			
13.–16. Follow Checklist steps 13–16 of the General Procedure (examine for neatness; check circulation, motion, and sensation; question patient regarding comfort; and wash hands).			

(continued)

© 1996 by Lippincott-Raven Publishers

	Needs More Practice	Satisfactory	Comments
Applying a Stretch Net Binder *(Continued)*			
Evaluation			
17. Evaluate as in Checklist step 17 (patient comfort, effectiveness, safety).			
Documentation			
18. Document as in Checklist step 18 (time; type of bandage or binder; where applied; assessment of circulation, motion, and sensation; length of time off and condition of skin underneath (if reapplication).			
Applying a T-Binder			
Assessment			
1.–3. Follow Checklist steps 1–3 of the General Procedure for Applying Bandages and Binders (identify purpose, identify part of body to be supported, assess any previously placed bandage or binder).			
Planning			
4.–5. Follow Checklist steps 4 and 5 of the General Procedure (plan procedure and wash your hands).			
6. Select the appropriate binder based on the patient's sex.			
7. Plan for times to recheck patient as in Checklist step 7 of the General Procedure.			
Implementation			
8.–11. Follow Checklist steps 8–11 of the General Procedure (identify patient, explain procedure, provide for privacy and position, remove soiled or used bandage or binder [if present], and wash hands).			
12. Apply the T-binder. **a.** Have patient lift midsection or turn patient side to side and place binder smoothly under patient with waistband at waist level and tail(s) downward at midline.			
b. Bring waist ends upward and around patient's abdomen.			

(continued)

© 1996 by Lippincott-Raven Publishers

Applying a T-Binder *(Continued)*	Needs More Practice	Satisfactory	Comments
c. Bring lower tail(s) between patient's legs, over dressings.			
d. Joint tails to waistband and secure with pin(s).			
13.–16. Follow Checklist steps 13–16 of the General Procedure (examine for neatness; check circulation, motion, and sensation; question patient regarding comfort; and wash hands).			
Evaluation			
17. Evaluate as in Checklist step 17 (patient comfort, effectiveness, safety).			
Documentation			
18. Document as in Checklist step 18 (time; type of bandage or binder; where applied; assessment of circulation, motion, and sensation; length of time off and condition of skin underneath (if reapplication).			
Applying an Arm Sling			
Assessment			
1.–3. Follow Checklist steps 1–3 of the General Procedure for Applying Bandages and Binders (identify purpose, identify arm to be supported, assess any previously placed sling).			
Planning			
4.–7. Follow Checklist steps 4–7 of the General Procedure (plan procedure, wash hands, obtain sling, plan times to recheck).			
Implementation			
8.–11. Follow Checklist steps 8–11 of the General Procedure (identify patient, explain procedure, provide for privacy and position, remove soiled or used sling [if present], and wash hands).			
12. Apply sling **a.** Method A: (1) With patient facing you, place end of triangle over shoulder on unaffected side.			

(continued)

© 1996 by Lippincott-Raven Publishers

Applying an Arm Sling *(Continued)*	Needs More Practice	Satisfactory	Comments
(2) Bring long straight side down smoothly under hand of affected side.			
(3) Loop sling up around arm, placing other end of triangle over shoulder of affected side.			
(4) Tie or pin ends to one side, not directly behind neck.			
(5) Pleat or fold sling at elbow and pin.			
(6) Check position—hand should be supported in sling.			
b. Method B: (1) With patient facing you, place sling underneath arms, across body.			
(2) Bring corner at unaffected side to back.			
(3) Bring lower corner on affected side up over affected shoulder to back and tie.			
(4) Pleat or fold sling at elbow and pin.			
(5) Check position—hand should be supported in sling.			
13.–16. Follow Checklist steps 13–16 of the General Procedure (examine for neatness; check circulation, motion, and sensation; question patient regarding comfort; and wash hands).			
Evaluation			
17. Evaluate as in Checklist step 17 (patient comfort, effectiveness, safety).			
Documentation			
18. Document as in Checklist step 18 (time; type of sling; to which arm applied; assessment of circulation, motion, and sensation; length of time off and condition of skin underneath (if reapplication).			

© 1996 by Lippincott-Raven Publishers

? QUIZ

Short-Answer Questions

1. List three reasons for the application of bandages.

   a. _____

   b. _____

   c. _____

2. List five methods for applying bandages.

   a. _____

   b. _____

   c. _____

   d. _____

   e. _____

3. The figure 8 method would most commonly be used to bandage _____

   _____ .

4. Bandages should be applied to extremities in a direction from _____

   to _____ .

5. You are applying a sequential compression device to the legs of a postoperative patient for whom you are providing care. What rationale will you give her for the use of this device?

   _____

   _____

6. A sequential compression device should not be ordered for a patient with what problem?

   _____

7. Abdominal binders are used primarily for what two purposes?

   a. _____

   b. _____

8. Two advantages of stretch net binders to hold dressings in place are _____

9. One disadvantage of using safety pins as fasteners is _____

   _____

10. T-binders are available in two types depending on whether the patient is _____

    or _____ .

Multiple-Choice Questions

_____ 11. The recurrent fold method would be used to bandage

   a. the arm.
   b. the elbow.
   c. a joint.
   d. a fingertip.

© 1996 by Lippincott-Raven Publishers

_____ **12.** The arm sling is not tied behind the neck primarily because it

    a. obstructs the blood flow.
    b. does not hold firmly.
    c. places strain on neck muscles.
    d. compresses nerves.

© 1996 by Lippincott-Raven Publishers

MODULE

APPLYING HEAT AND COLD

MODULE CONTENTS

RATIONALE FOR THE USE OF THIS
  SKILL
NURSING DIAGNOSES
SAFETY
APPLYING HEAT
Physiologic Responses to Heat
Purposes for Applying Heat
APPLYING COLD
Physiologic Responses to Cold
Purposes for Applying Cold
GENERAL PROCEDURE FOR APPLYING
  HEAT OR COLD
  Assessment
  Planning
  Implementation
  Evaluation
  Documentation
DEVICES FOR APPLYING HEAT
Water-Flow Heating Pad With Control Unit
Disposable Instant Hot Pack
Gel-Filled Hot Pack
Hot Water Bags (Bottles)
Electric Heating Pad

Heat Cradle/Heat Lamp
Thermal Blanket (Warming)
Diathermy
DEVICES FOR APPLYING COLD
Ice Collar
Ice Cap
Disposable Instant Cold Pack
Gel-Filled Cold Pack
Thermal Blanket (Cooling)
Baths
SPECIFIC PROCEDURES FOR APPLYING
  HEAT
Applying a Warm, Moist Compress
Administering a Soak
Administering a Sitz Bath
SPECIFIC PROCEDURE FOR APPLYING
  COLD
Administering a Cooling Sponge Bath
USE OF THE THERMAL BLANKET FOR
  WARMING OR COOLING
LONG-TERM CARE
HOME CARE
CRITICAL THINKING EXERCISES

PREREQUISITES

Successful completion of the following modules:

VOLUME 1
Module 1   An Approach to Nursing Skills
Module 2   Basic Infection Control
Module 3   Safety
Module 5   Documentation
Module 6   Introduction to Assessment Skills
Module 14 Bedmaking
Module 18 Hygiene

VOLUME 2
Module 33 Sterile Technique (optional)

© 1996 by Lippincott-Raven Publishers

OVERALL OBJECTIVE

To apply heat and cold appropriately, with emphasis on comfort and safety for patients.

SPECIFIC LEARNING OBJECTIVES

Know Facts and Principles	Apply Facts and Principles	Demonstrate Ability	Evaluate Performance
1. Safety			
State five precautionary measures to use in applying heat and cold.	Given a patient situation in which heat or cold is to be used, state appropriate safety measures.	In the clinical setting, use appropriate safety measures when applying heat or cold.	Evaluate with instructor using Performance Checklist.
List signs and symptoms of harmful responses to applications of heat or cold.			Assess patient's responses at frequent intervals to evaluate effects of therapy.
2. Physiologic response to application of heat			
State three responses of body to application of heat.	Given a patient situation, state rationale for application of heat.		
State four indications for local application of heat.	Given a patient situation, discuss expected responses to application of heat.		
3. Application of dry heat			
State four methods used to apply dry heat.	Given a patient situation, select appropriate method of applying dry heat.	In the clinical setting, choose appropriate method for applying dry heat.	Evaluate choice with instructor.
Describe the general procedure for applying dry heat.	Given a patient situation, discuss rationale for applying dry heat.	In the clinical setting, correctly apply dry heat.	Evaluate with instructor using Performance Checklist.
4. Application of moist heat			
State three methods commonly used to apply moist heat.	Given a patient situation, select appropriate method of applying moist heat.	In the clinical setting, choose appropriate method for applying moist heat.	Evaluate choice with instructor.
Describe procedures for application of warm moist compress, soak, and sitz bath.	Modify individual procedure based on patient situation.	In the clinical setting, correctly apply warm moist compress, soak, and/or sitz bath.	Evaluate own performance with instructor using Performance Checklist.

(continued)

© 1996 by Lippincott-Raven Publishers

S P E C I F I C   L E A R N I N G   O B J E C T I V E S   (c o n t i n u e d)

Know Facts and Principles	Apply Facts and Principles	Demonstrate Ability	Evaluate Performance
5. *Physiologic responses to application of cold*			
State three responses of body to application of cold.	Given a patient situation, state rationale for application of cold.		
State five indications for local application of cold.	Given a patient situation, discuss expected responses to application of cold.		
	Explain effect of cold on already edematous area.		
6. *Application of dry cold*			
Describe general procedure for applying dry cold.	Given a patient situation, discuss rationale for applying dry cold.	In the clinical setting, correctly apply dry cold.	Evaluate with instructor using Performance Checklist.
7. *Application of moist cold*			
State four methods used to apply moist cold.	Given a patient situation, select appropriate method of applying moist cold.	In the clinical setting, choose appropriate method for applying moist cold.	Evaluate choice with instructor.
8. *Procedure for administering a cooling sponge bath*			
Describe procedure for administering a cooling sponge bath.	Given a patient situation, decide whether administering a cooling sponge bath is appropriate.	Correctly administer cooling sponge bath.	Evaluate with instructor using Performance Checklist.
9. *Procedure for the use of the thermal blanket for warming or cooling*			
Describe procedure for using thermal blanket for warming or cooling.	Given a patient situation, determine purpose and whether use is appropriate.	In the clinical setting, correctly apply a thermal blanket for warming or cooling.	Evaluate with instructor.
10. *Documentation*			
State appropriate items to be included in progress notes.	Given a patient situation, simulate appropriate documentation.	In the clinical setting, document appropriately with regard to application of heat and cold.	Evaluate with instructor.

© 1996 by Lippincott-Raven Publishers

LEARNING ACTIVITIES

1. Review the Specific Learning Objectives.
2. Read the section on heat production, heat loss, and hypothermia (in the chapter on cognition and sensory perception) in Ellis and Nowlis, *Nursing: A Human Needs Approach,* or comparable material in another textbook.
3. Look up the module vocabulary terms in the glossary.
4. Read through the module as though you were preparing to teach the contents to another person. Mentally practice the techniques.
5. With a partner in the practice setting:
   a. Prepare a warm, moist compress and apply it to the inner aspect of your partner's forearm, protecting the bed and the "patient" from the moisture. Do this as a clean procedure (using medical asepsis).
   b. Reverse roles, and repeat step a as a *sterile* procedure (using sterile technique).
   c. Evaluate one another's performance.
   d. Prepare an ice collar, cap, or glove and apply and secure it to your partner's knee. Have your partner move around to see whether the pack stays in place.
   e. Reverse roles, and repeat step d.
   f. Evaluate one another's performance.
6. In the clinical setting:
   a. Seek opportunities to observe the use of a water flow heating pad with control unit and a thermal blanket.
   b. Apply hot and cold treatments with supervision.

VOCABULARY

antipyretic	edema	metabolism	vasoconstriction
constriction	inflammation	oxygenation	vasodilation
dilation	intracranial pressure	suppuration	

© 1996 by Lippincott-Raven Publishers

Applying Heat and Cold

Rationale for the Use of This Skill

Applications of heat or cold are frequently ordered and may be carried out in many different ways using a variety of equipment. It is essential that the nurse be aware of the indications and rationale for the application of heat and cold, and of safe and effective methods of application, to carry out the procedures in ways that meet the needs of patients.

Policies regarding the application of heat and cold vary within healthcare settings. A doctor's order is usually required, although in some instances there may be protocols that allow the nurse to apply heat or cold according to specific criteria. In any event, you must know the physiologic responses to and appropriate uses of heat and cold and then follow the policies and procedures in your agency.

Applications of heat and cold are also used in long-term and home care settings. You must be able to teach and supervise others in the use of these applications.[1]

▼ NURSING DIAGNOSES

A nursing diagnosis that is important when applying heat or cold is Risk for Injury. Patients can be injured by an application that is either too hot or too cold or by one that is left in place for too long. Applications of heat or cold may also be ordered when patients have a nursing diagnosis of Pain or Chronic Pain. Nursing diagnoses that may be related to the use of the thermal blanket include Ineffective Thermoregulation, Hyperthermia, and Hypothermia.

SAFETY

To apply heat and cold safely, keep in mind the following precautions:

1. *Patients vary in their ability to tolerate heat and cold.* Factors that affect tolerance include age (very young and elderly persons are more susceptible to negative effects of heat and cold therapies), the presence of circulatory or neurologic deficiencies, the level of consciousness, amount of body fat, and the condition of the skin in the area being treated. The patient's diagnosis is also a factor to be considered, as is the particular type of heat

[1]Rationale for action is emphasized throughout the module by the use of italics.

or cold application. Always assess the patient carefully before you proceed with any treatment.

2. *Temperature receptors in the skin adjust rapidly to mild stimulation.* This adaptability explains why a sensation of either warmth or coolness dissipates in a short time. Explain this phenomenon to the patient, so that the temperature of the treatment will not be increased or decreased to an unsafe level.

3. *Because maximum vasodilation occurs in 20 to 30 minutes,* heat treatments should not be continued beyond that time. *A rebound phenomenon can occur in such cases, causing vasoconstriction and tissue congestion, thereby negating the therapeutic effects of the heat application.* Likewise, vasodilation begins *after the temperature of the skin has been decreased to 60°F (15°C),* again reversing the desired effect of the thermal application. Explain the rebound effect to the patient *to gain cooperation with the plan of care.* Heat and cold treatments are sometimes ordered intermittently (30 minutes on and 30 minutes off) to get a more prolonged effect.

4. *Moisture conducts heat better than air,* so take special care when you apply moist heat or cold, *because injuries are more likely. Because air is a poor conductor,* it is used to insulate certain applications of heat and cold. For example, hot water bottles or ice caps are covered with a cloth before application. The air between the cloth and the bag provides insulation.

5. *The length of time the body is exposed to heat or cold, as well as the size of the skin area being treated, affects the ability of the body to tolerate the treatment.* The shorter the exposure time and the smaller the area being treated, the better the tolerance.

APPLYING HEAT

Physiologic Responses to Heat

When heat is applied to an area of the body, the blood vessels in that area *dilate* (expand), *which increases blood circulation and oxygenation to the injured tissues, improving metabolism.* When heat is applied systemically, as in the application of a hyperthermia blanket, the nurse should assess for increased respiratory rate and hypotension, which occur *because of peripheral vasodilation.*

Purposes for Applying Heat

Heat can be used *to relieve pain from muscle spasms and affected joints.* Heat also reduces swelling (and accompanying discomfort) *by increasing circulation (flu-*

id is more easily absorbed from the affected area). Heat also increases circulation, which helps to *eliminate any toxic waste products* that have accumulated in the area of swelling or edema. Heat relaxes muscles. Finally, heat can promote healing *by increasing oxygenation of the tissues and by promoting suppuration in cases of infection.*

The nurse should be particularly cautious with the use of any heat treatment to a patient with diminished arterial or venous circulation (*the patient could be less aware of discomfort*), with decreased alertness or awareness (*the patient could move or tamper with the treatment*), and to either children or older adults, *who are more sensitive to heat and cold. In all of these situations, the patient is more likely to be injured because of a lack of awareness of any problems.*

APPLYING COLD

Physiologic Responses to Cold

The application of cold *constricts* blood vessels in the affected area. *This slows circulation, which retards the reabsorption of fluid into tissues.* Because of this, the formation of edema may be prevented and inflammation reduced. If edema is already present in an area, the application of cold may slow the resolution of the edema *because of the delayed reabsorption of fluid.*

Purposes for Applying Cold

Cold should be applied immediately after a strain, sprain, or contusion occurs, before edema forms. The anesthetic effect of cold on the tissues occurs *because nerve transmission is reduced,* diminishing pain.

Both frank hemorrhage from an external wound and minimal internal bleeding, such as oozing, may be reduced by the application of cold and the *subsequent constriction of blood vessels.* The application of cold is also recommended as an initial first aid treatment for minor burns. The nurse should use caution when applying cold to patients with circulatory problems *because of the risk of decreasing local circulation to such an extent that tissue damage occurs.* In addition, *because of the anesthetic effect of cold on the tissues,* the patient may be less aware of any tissue damage occurring.

GENERAL PROCEDURE FOR APPLYING HEAT OR COLD

There is a general approach you can use to apply heat or cold. It can be modified as necessary according to the type of device being used.

Assessment

1. Check the order for the specific type of heat or cold treatment ordered.
2. Assess the general condition of the patient, noting especially the age, diagnosis, circulatory status, level of awareness, and amount of body fat. Measure the vital signs *to establish baseline information for comparison.* Assess the local site, noting especially the condition and color of the skin. If the treatment has been given before, check the chart or ask the patient for the patient's response to the preceding treatment.
3. Check the patient's room to see what equipment is already there and the space needed for any temperature treatment device.

Planning

4. Wash your hands *for infection control.*
5. Obtain the heating or cooling device you want to use. Some of the less complex heating and cooling devices are located on the nursing unit; others may be obtained from the central supply department.

Implementation

6. Identify the patient *to be sure you are carrying out the procedure for the correct patient.*
7. Explain to the patient what you plan to do, giving particular attention to the length of time the heat or cold application will be left in place and any condition about which the patient should notify you, such as any discomfort.
8. Provide for the patient's privacy and comfort.
9. Prepare the patient and the patient's unit as appropriate. Expose only the area to be treated, uncovering as little of the rest of the patient's body as possible.
10. Place the heating or cooling device over the area to be treated, molding it to that area as closely as possible. Secure it in place with clean cloth or roller gauze. Place the call light where the patient can reach it easily *to alert the nurse to any discomfort.*
11. Completely cover the heating or cooling device with a soft cloth cover, making sure that the cover is as free of folds and wrinkles as possible. Some disposable hot packs or ice collars come with a special outer covering.
12. Return to the patient in 10 to 15 minutes *to check for therapeutic or adverse effects and to be sure that the heating or cooling device is placed properly.*
13. Remove the heating or cooling device at the end of the ordered time or at a maximum of 30 minutes, if no length of time has been specified.
14. Examine the treated area.
15. Replace any linen or clothing removed earlier

© 1996 by Lippincott-Raven Publishers

and leave the patient comfortable, warm, and dry.

16. Wash your hands.

Evaluation

17. Evaluate using the following criteria:

    a. Signs or symptoms of both desirable and undesirable responses to treatment

    b. Patient comfort

Documentation

18. Document the treatment, including the length of time applied and the patient's response, on the patient's progress record.

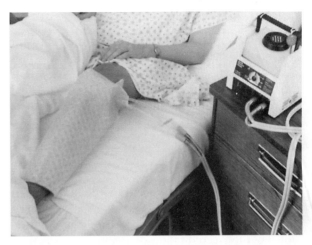

Figure 27–1. Waterflow heating pad with control unit.

DEVICES FOR APPLYING HEAT

The water-flow heating pad with control unit, the disposable heat pack, and the gel-filled hot pack are the most commonly used methods of applying dry heat in healthcare settings today. Heat cradles and heat lamps are used infrequently but will be discussed briefly. *Hot water bottles or bags and electric heating pads are frequently used in home care situations,* so you should be aware of how to safely apply them when giving care in the home setting or when teaching others. The methods and safety factors for these appliances are similar in both the healthcare and home settings.

Water-Flow Heating Pad With Control Unit

An order is usually needed to use these devices to apply heat. The water-flow heating pad consists of a distilled water reservoir control unit with two tubes that deliver temperature-regulated water to channels within a rubberized pad. In newer models, the pad is disposable and has a soft, absorbent material on the inside next to the patient and waterproof material on the outside (Fig. 27–1).

These units have various brand names by a number of manufacturers, such as T-Pump, K-Pad, and Hydroculator. The principles of each are similar. Distilled water is used in the unit to prevent build-up of tap water chemicals. A plastic key is provided with

some sets, which allows the temperature control mechanism to be set. *The key provides safety.* The controls of these units may be set and regulated by nursing personnel, the family, or a care provider. The pad may be secured with a gauze wrap or tape but should not be pinned *because of the danger of puncturing the water channels.* These pads work more effectively if the control mechanism and tubing are level with or higher than the pad, *because overcoming gravity places strain on the motor. Because the unit is electrical,* always check cords and controls to be sure they are in good repair and check plugs for grounding.

Disposable Instant Hot Pack

Disposable instant hot packs are available commercially and are used in a variety of settings. They come in a number of sizes and shapes, including one made especially for use in the perineal area. These packs deliver a specific amount of heat for a specified length of time as indicated by the manufacturer's instructions. *Be certain to read these instructions carefully.* To use a hot pack, strike, shake, or knead the package with your hands, being careful not to puncture or damage the outer covering. This creates a chemical reaction that releases the heat. Disposable hot packs are both safe and convenient when used properly.

Example of Nursing Progress Notes Using Narrative Format.

DATE/TIME	
3/18/99 0945	*Disposable hot pack applied to painful left elbow joint for 30 min. States pain decreased. No adverse effects noted.* ——— *K. Green, RN*

© 1996 by Lippincott-Raven Publishers

Gel-Filled Hot Pack

Gel-filled hot packs are available commercially and are reusable. They come in a variety of sizes and shapes and are flexible, making it convenient to mold them around a body part. Be certain to read the manufacturer's instructions for safe use of these products.

Hot Water Bags (Bottles)

The use of the hot water bag or bottle in acute care settings is uncommon *because of the high risk of burns unless special precautions are taken.* The Joint Commission for the Accreditation of Healthcare Organizations (JCAHO) also advises against their use. However, *because some healthcare agencies still use this as a method for applying dry heat to a localized area, and because the method may be in use in the home care setting,* you should be familiar with some of the principles that are essential to its safe use.

1. Fill the water bag with hot water and set it aside. This is done *to heat the sides of the bag* and to check the bag for leaks. Meanwhile, fill a pitcher with hot water. Using a bath thermometer, measure the temperature of the water; it should never exceed 125°F (51.6°C) for the adult or 115°F (46.1°C) for the very elderly patient, infant, or child. If a bath thermometer is not available, check the temperature of the water against the inner aspect of your wrist or arm. Discard the water in the bag.
2. Fill the bag only one-half to two-thirds full with water from the pitcher. Then fold or twist the bag *to remove any air* before you insert the stopper or fold the bag and clamp it shut. This makes the bag easier to apply *because it will conform to the shape of the surface to which it is applied.*
3. Cover the bag with a cloth before you place it in contact with the skin *to protect the skin.*

Electric Heating Pad

Electric heating pads are commonly used in the home *because they are convenient for applying heat to small areas of the body and because they are relatively inexpensive.* The wires that provide the heat must be covered by rubber or plastic insulation *to ensure safety.* Electric heating pads should never be used in the presence of moisture *because of the danger of electric shock.* Instruct the patient not to lie on top of the heating pad *because heat may accumulate and cause a burn.* In addition, it is essential that you follow the precautions already outlined for using electrical equipment.

Heat Cradle/Heat Lamp

Although heat cradles and heat lamps are infrequently used in healthcare settings, you should be aware of how to use them safely if you encounter them. Be sure that nothing larger than a 25-watt bulb is used with the heat cradle and that the bulb is at least 18 inches away from the patient. A 40- to 60-watt bulb may be used with a heat lamp, but in that case, the bulb should be at least 24 inches from the patient. Always check to be sure that cords are not worn or frayed. Patients should be checked at least every 5 minutes *because it is possible for the patient to move closer to the bulb or to grab the lamp or to strike it accidentally in your absence.*

Thermal Blanket (Warming)

This device has the dual purpose of either heating or cooling the body systemically. The blanket is similar to the water-flow heating pad except that it is of blanket size. The thermal blanket is most commonly used for warming after major surgery or trauma. Elderly patients and infants are among those most at risk for hypothermia. For a more detailed discussion, see the section on use of the thermal blanket to provide cooling, page 662.

Diathermy

Diathermy is a deep heat treatment, usually administered by the physical therapy department as a rehabilitation therapy. It is similar to the principle underlying the microwave in that electrical energy is changed to heat. The nurse on the unit should prepare the patient by allaying any anxiety with assurances that the treatment is neither invasive nor dangerous. *Because metal that is bombarded with diathermy waves becomes intensely hot and can burn the patient,* all rings and watches should be removed before the patient leaves the unit. Patients with metal orthopedic screws or pins should not have diathermy treatments on that extremity. Diathermy also is not appropriate for patients who have older model surgically implanted pacemakers, *because exposure to the electrical waves may lead to malfunction.* New models are not prone to such malfunction.

Compresses, soaks, and sitz baths are commonly used to apply moist heat. A *compress* is a wet dressing that is applied to an area to provide moisture. It may be either hot or cold. A *soak* is used to apply moisture through immersion of a body part. A *sitz bath* is a way of providing heat to the perineal and rectal areas.

© 1996 by Lippincott-Raven Publishers

cold. Except for the hypothermia blanket, the procedure is similar regardless of the device used.

Ice Collar

An ice collar is a long, narrow bag made of rubber, plastic, or some other material that is leakproof. Some are made to be disposable; others are reusable. Some ice collars come with ties attached to make it easier to keep them in place. These devices are designed for use around the neck but can be used for other small areas of the body as well (Fig. 27–2).

To prepare for use, fill the bag one-half to two-thirds full with crushed ice, remove excess air by folding or twisting the bag, and insert the stopper. You can also use a rubber glove to apply dry cold. Partially fill it with ice and close it by tying a knot in the open or cuff end.

When a patient needs to continue cold packs at home on a short-term basis, a heavy plastic bag can be used. Simply place crushed ice or ice cubes and a small amount of water in a bag of the appropriate size, remove excess air and seal with a twist tie. Cover with a light clean cloth and apply. A 16-oz bag of frozen peas or cut corn instead of ice also works well as an emergency cold pack and molds nicely to curved areas.

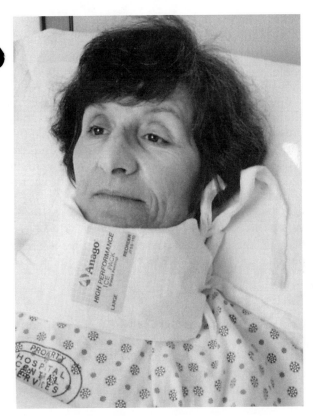

Figure 27–2. The ice collar can be used around the neck as well as for other small areas of the body.

DEVICES FOR APPLYING COLD

Ice collars, ice caps, ice gloves, disposable instant cold packs, gel-filled cold packs, and the hypothermia blanket are all devices for the application of dry

Ice Cap

An ice cap is a larger bag made of rubber, plastic, or some other leakproof material. Ice caps come in a variety of sizes and shapes (one is designed specifi-

Example of Nursing Progress Notes Using SOAP Format.

DATE/TIME	
11/1/99	Altered comfort: left knee pain
1410	S c/o pain left knee.
	O Left knee swollen and painful to touch.
	A Ordered medication not eradicating pain adequately.
	P Secure order for ice pack and apply to left knee for
	30 min to decrease pain.
	J. Sanchez, SN

Example of Nursing Progress Notes Using SOAP Format.

DATE/TIME	
11/1/99	Altered Comfort: left knee pain
1520	S "My leg feels much better."
	O Edema in left knee decreased; Circumference 2.5 cm less than
	yesterday. Moving knee more freely.
	A Ice pack helpful in decreasing edema and left knee pain.
	P Ice pack as nursing action with ordered pain medications to
	relieve edema and discomfort.
	J. Sanchez, SN

© 1996 by Lippincott-Raven Publishers

cally for the head). Other shapes are rectangular and square. These may be disposable or reusable and are prepared for use in the same way as an ice collar.

Disposable Instant Cold Pack

Disposable instant cold packs are used in the same way as disposable instant hot packs. They come in a variety of sizes and shapes, including a shape similar to an ice collar and one made especially for use in the perineal area. These packs deliver a specific amount of cold for a specified length of time, as indicated by the manufacturer's instructions. *Be certain to read these instructions carefully.* To use a cold pack, strike, shake, or knead the package. This creates a chemical reaction that releases the cold. Disposable instant cold packs are both convenient and safe when used properly.

Gel-Filled Cold Pack

Gel-filled cold packs are available commercially and are reusable. They are used in much the same way as are the gel-filled hot packs. Again, you must read the manufacturer's instructions carefully *to ensure safe use of this device.*

Thermal Blanket (Cooling)

When a thermal blanket is being used to provide cooling, it is commonly referred to as a hypothermia blanket. The hypothermia or cooling blanket is usually used for one of two primary purposes. Hypothermia may be induced during surgery *to slow circulation and thus decrease the potential for bleeding or to decrease metabolic activity and thereby reduce oxygen requirements.* The hypothermia blanket is also used to reduce persistent high fevers. Whether of short or long duration, high fevers are often treated with antipyretic medications. These medications may not be appropriate when the patient has a low-grade fever, *because this may be a compensatory mechanism of the body to subdue infection.* A physician's order for giving medication to reduce a fever will stipulate at what level this is to be done, usually 101°F or 102°F (38.3° or 38.8°C).

The insertion and taping of a rectal probe *to assess the patient's temperature while the blanket is operating* is no longer recommended *because of the danger of sphincter damage.* It is better to use a skin sensor or to take the patient's temperature frequently if the blanket is being operated manually. In automatic operation, the patient's temperature is monitored with a probe (skin probe on the nursing unit and esophageal probe in the operating room), and the blanket cools the patient to the desired body temperature and maintains that level (Fig. 27–3).

The nurse should assess for the uncommon but possibly serious complications that can occur when the entire body is mechanically cooled. These include respiratory distress, increased intracranial pressure, and changes in urinary output. When the patient is removed from the blanket, a "rebound" reaction can occur as late as several days afterward. In such a reaction, the patient's temperature "rebounds" against the action of the blanket *because of vasoconstriction,* resulting in a resurgence of fever. When this occurs, the patient may have to be placed back on the blanket at a lower setting for a longer period.

Baths

Cool or tepid water is able to dissipate heat from the body *both by conduction (with heat transported by water around the skin) and by evaporation (the process of water evaporating from the surface of the skin).* Although cool soaks of localized areas of the body are not common,

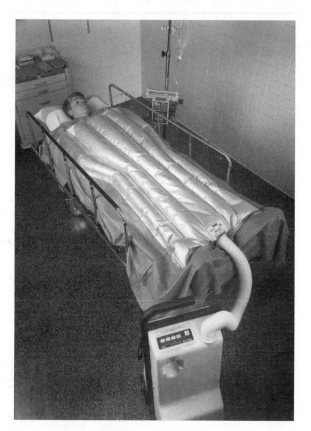

Figure 27–3. Thermal blanket. The mode of operation (manual or automatic) and the desired temperature are set on the control unit attached to the blanket. (Courtesy Cincinnati Sub-Zero.)

© 1996 by Lippincott-Raven Publishers

the patient may have a cool sponge bath *to lower temperature.* Currently, this procedure is performed more for children than for adults. A child may be given a tub bath rather than a sponge bath. In the past, alcohol was added to the bath water *because it evaporates quickly, removing heat rapidly.* This is no longer done in most facilities for a variety of reasons, including the *potentially harmful effect of alcohol fumes and the extreme drying effect of alcohol on the skin.*

SPECIFIC PROCEDURES FOR APPLYING HEAT

Applying a Warm, Moist Compress

Assessment
1.–3. Follow the steps of the General Procedure for Applying Heat or Cold.

Planning
4. Follow the General Procedure.
5. Obtain the material to be used for the compress. Use sterile material (including sterile basin, sterile solution, and sterile gloves) and technique as necessary. A washcloth is commonly used when a small unsterile compress is needed; a towel can be used for a larger area. Premoistened sterile compresses are available commercially. Follow package directions to heat the compress. Obtain a water-flow heating pad or other heating device *to maintain the heat of the compress, if necessary.*

Implementation
6.–9. Follow the steps of the General Procedure.
10. Place a moisture-proof pad under the area to be treated *to protect the bed from moisture.* Assess the area. Drape as necessary.
 a. Moisten the compress in hot water (105°–115°F [40.5°–46.1°C] unless otherwise ordered). In any event, it should not be higher than 115°F (46.1°C). Wring it out, so that it remains moist but does not drip. Apply it to the area to be treated, cover it with plastic, and then cover with further insulation, such as a towel.
 b. Place a water-flow heating pad or other heating device on the outside *to maintain the heat,* if necessary.
 c. Hold the compress in place with ties or a gauze wrap.
11. Cover the area with a cloth and plastic covering so that the heat will be retained.
12. Return to the patient at frequent intervals (at least every 5 minutes) to check for adverse re-

actions and to see that the compress is still in place.
13. Remove the compress after 20 minutes.
14.–16. Follow the steps of the General Procedure.

Evaluation
17. Follow the General Procedure.

Documentation
18. Follow the General Procedure.

Administering a Soak

Assessment
1.–3. Follow the steps of the General Procedure.

Planning
4. Follow the General Procedure.
5. Obtain a basin. If a wound is involved, use sterile material (including sterile basin, sterile solution, and sterile gloves) and technique as necessary.

Implementation
6.–9. Follow the steps of the General Procedure.
10. Fill the basin half full with water, saline, or the medicated solution that has been ordered. The temperature of the water or solution is usually between 105°F (40.5°C) and 115°F (46.1°C), unless otherwise ordered.
11. Place a moisture-proof pad if necessary under the body part being treated. Place the basin on the pad. Slowly place the body part to be treated into the basin, making sure that the rest of the body is in good alignment and that there is no pressure on the part from the edge of the basin. Typically, you will have to pad the edge of the basin with a towel to prevent pressure.
12. Check the patient after the first 5 minutes and at least once during the remainder of the treatment. The duration of a soak is usually 15 or 20 minutes. Remove the body part being soaked from the basin *if the solution cools to the extent that it becomes necessary to remove some of it and add some that has been heated.* Before replacing the body part in the solution, measure the temperature of the solution *to be sure it is not over 115°F (46.1°C).*
13. Remove the body part from the basin and gently pat it dry, using sterile towels or gauze if necessary.
14. Examine the part carefully and reapply a dressing, if indicated.
15.–16. Follow the steps of the General Procedure.

Evaluation
17. Follow the General Procedure.

© 1996 by Lippincott-Raven Publishers

Documentation

18. Follow the General Procedure.

Administering a Sitz Bath

A sitz bath is a method of administering a soak to the pelvic area. Some facilities have special tubs designed for the purpose. Portable chairs and disposable equipment that can be used on a toilet are also available (Figs. 27–4 and 27–5).

Sometimes, a patient is merely placed in a bathtub that has been filled with enough water to reach the umbilicus. This alternative is not recommended *because the blood vessels in the legs also vasodilate, lessening the effect of the treatment to the pelvic area.* Unless otherwise specified, the temperature of the water should be between 105°F (40.5°C) and 115°F (46.1°C), and the treatment should last 15 to 20 minutes.

Assessment

1.–3. Follow the General Procedure.

Planning

4. Follow the General Procedure.
5. Gather the sitz bath equipment. In addition to the equipment for the bath itself, you will need a bath blanket and one or more towels. Place the bath blanket over the patient's shoulders *to pro-*

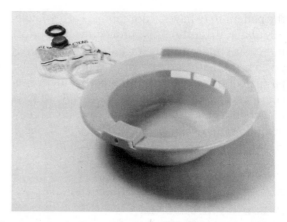

Figure 27–5. The disposable sitz bath basin can be placed on the toilet in a healthcare facility or in the home. (Courtesy Searle Medical Products USA, Inc., Dallas, Texas.)

vide warmth and use the towel *to dry the patient at the end of the treatment.* You may need additional towels *to pad the tub or chair to relieve pressure or to assist with body alignment.*

Implementation

6.–8. Follow the steps of the General Procedure.
9. Assist the patient to the tub room or bathroom. If the room is some distance away, assistive devices may be needed.
10. Fill the tub or chair with enough water to cover the area to be treated. The water should be between 105°F (40.5°C) and 115°F (46.1°C). The disposable sitz bath includes an attached bag that can be filled with water of the desired temperature. It then flows gradually into the basin, displacing the cooler water and maintaining a more constant temperature.
11. Remove the patient's clothing and assess the area to be treated. Assist the patient into the tub or chair, padding as necessary *to minimize pressure and to provide for good body alignment.*
12. Return to the patient frequently during treatment. Monitor blood pressure and pulse after 5 minutes for hypotension, which could lead to dizziness or fainting. *If the patient's condition warrants (first postoperative day, extremely fatigued or weak patient),* stay in the room for the first 5 minutes or for the entire treatment.
13. Assist patient out of tub or chair and dry the entire body.
14. Follow the General Procedure.
15. Help patient to dress and return to room or bed.
16. Follow the General Procedure.

Evaluation

17. Follow the General Procedure.

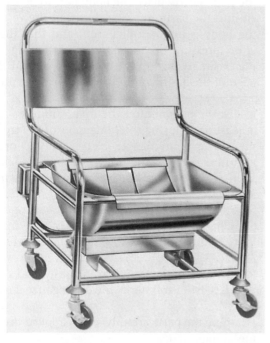

Figure 27–4. Portable sitz bath chair. The patient can receive a sitz bath in own room using this chair. (Courtesy Ille, division of Market Forge.)

© 1996 by Lippincott-Raven Publishers

Documentation

18. Follow the General Procedure.

SPECIFIC PROCEDURES FOR APPLYING COLD

Administering a Cooling Sponge Bath

Occasionally, sponge baths are ordered to help reduce an elevated temperature.

Assessment

1.–3. Follow the steps of the General Procedure.

Planning

4. Follow the General Procedure.

5. Gather the necessary equipment. You will need a basin, several washcloths (at least four), several towels, a bath blanket, and at least two moisture-proof pads to protect the bed.

Implementation

6.–8. Follow the steps of the General Procedure.

9. Close the windows and doors and any bed curtains *to prevent drafts and provide privacy.* Drafts may cause the patient to chill and shiver. Shivering is a heat-producing mechanism and will act against the purpose of the bath.

   a. Remove the spread and blanket, fold them, and place them over the back of a chair for later use.

   b. Position a bath blanket over the patient. Then ask the patient to hold the top of the bath blanket while you pull the top sheet from beneath it. Fold the top sheet and place it over the chair along with the spread and the regular blanket.

   c. Fill the basin with cool water. Temperatures for cooling baths vary from 90°F (32°C) to 65°F (18°C). Some recommend starting with water at 85° to 90°F (29°–32°C) and then cooling it gradually by adding ice chips until the temperature of the water has reached 65°F (18°C). The gradual decrease in the temperature of the water will be more comfortable for the patient and will help to prevent chilling.

10. Wet three washcloths. Wring them out so that they are wet but not dripping, and place them in the axillae and groin. Check them every 5 minutes *to see whether they should be changed.* They will probably warm quickly in these highly vascular areas of the body. In some facilities, cold packs or ice gloves are used instead of the cool washcloths; follow the procedure in your facility.

11. Bathe each extremity for approximately 3 minutes, depending on how the procedure is tolerated. This is done more easily and quickly with two people. Expose only the area(s) of the patient you are bathing. Keep the rest of the body covered with the bath blanket. Pat each extremity dry. *Rubbing the skin will produce warming by increasing cell metabolism.* Have patient turn over. Bathe the back and buttocks for approximately 5 minutes. Again, the length of time will be determined to some extent by how well the patient tolerates the procedure. Dry the back and buttocks. Remove washcloths from the axillae and groin and dry areas.

12. Measure the patient's temperature every 15 minutes *to evaluate the effect of the bath.*

13. Stop the bath before the patient registers a normal temperature *because the body continues to cool even after the bath is finished.* If the patient has not cooled to the desired temperature, you may have to repeat the procedure. Check the patient's temperature, pulse, and respirations again 30 minutes after the procedure to assess for therapeutic and adverse effects.

DATE/TIME	
5/29/99 1945	c/o feeling chilled. Temp. 103.4° orally. Cooling sponge bath given over 20 min. Temp. after bath 100.8°. Resting quietly after treatment. No current evidence of chilling. ———— D. Peters, RN
2015	Temp 100.2° orally. Continues to rest quietly with no evidence of chilling. ———— D. Peters, RN

Example of Nursing Progress Notes Using Narrative Format.

© 1996 by Lippincott-Raven Publishers

14.–16. Follow the steps of the General Procedure.

Evaluation

17. Follow the General Procedure.

Documentation

18. Follow the General Procedure.

Use of the Thermal Blanket for Warming or Cooling

Assessment

1.–3. Follow the steps of the General Procedure.

Planning

4.–5. Follow the steps of the General Procedure.

Implementation

6.–8. Follow the steps of the General Procedure.

9. Remove heavy clothing from the patient. Assess the patient's room for space for the unit and safe electrical outlets.

10. Place a bath blanket over and under the patient to absorb perspiration.

    a. Set the control to the desired setting and turn on the unit for approximately 30 minutes to allow it to reach the desired temperature and to ensure that it is operating properly.

    b. Roll the patient onto the blanket using the technique described in Module 14, Bedmaking, Making the Occupied Bed. A second blanket is sometimes placed on top of the patient to accelerate the warming effects.

    c. If a skin sensor probe is used, carefully place it on the patient's skin and secure it with tape. Otherwise, measure the patient's temperature every 30 minutes until the desired temperature is reached.

11. Cover the patient with top linen over the bath blanket or hyper-/hypothermia blanket.

12. Assess the patient's vital signs and pupil reaction at least every 15 minutes (or more frequently, if indicated) until the temperature has stabilized at the desired level. Monitor skin condition, intake and output, and comfort hourly. Reposition the patient hourly unless contraindicated. Apply extra cover to the arms or feet if the patient complains of discomfort from the cold.

13. Turn off the controls, leaving the patient temporarily on the blanket in case it is necessary to continue the treatment. Monitor the patient's temperature after the blanket has been turned off *because body temperature can continue to rise even after the procedure has been discontinued.*

14. Examine the patient's skin and general condition.

15.–16. Follow the steps of the General Procedure.

Evaluation

17. Follow the General Procedure.

Documentation

18. Follow the General Procedure.

LONG-TERM CARE

In long-term care settings, it is not uncommon for heat or cold to be applied to relieve discomfort. Many older residents may have treated arthritic pain with heat even before they entered the facility and may wish to continue. Depending on the facility's policy, a physician's order may be needed.

The application of heat or cold poses increased risks for older persons because of changes in the skin, circulation, sensation and perception. For example, prolonged exposure to heat or cold may damage the skin. Narrowed blood vessels and decreased cardiac output can intensify or localize heat to a given area because of the body's declining ability to dissipate the heat within the circulatory system. Of particular concern is the resident's decreased awareness of the degree of heat or cold being applied because of the decreased number of skin receptors. Care must be taken to apply heat or cold for only short periods, to assess the resident frequently, and to determine the safety of the procedure.

HOME CARE

Many homes have some type of device available (heating pad, ice packs) for applying heat or cold. All of the risks that exist in healthcare settings also are present in the home. A client of any age can sustain injury if the procedure is misused. Also, clients may fail to seek medical consultation when the "home remedy" of heat or cold application has previously been successful.

Safety must be observed by the client, family members, or home care nurse. Electrical cords and outlets should be in good repair. Heat or ice should never be applied directly to the skin. Above all, conscientious and frequent assessments should be made.

© 1996 by Lippincott-Raven Publishers

CRITICAL THINKING EXERCISES

Your patient, Mr. Simpson, has a reddened intravenous site. The intravenous infusion has been discontinued and the physician has ordered a hot pack to the area. Determine what assessment you will carry out. What physiologic benefits does the application of heat provide?

Identify the hazards that exist in the application of heat and describe nursing actions that can prevent any untoward response. Predict the outcome that you expect and that can be used for your evaluation.

© 1996 by Lippincott-Raven Publishers

PERFORMANCE CHECKLIST

General Procedure for Applying Heat or Cold	Needs More Practice	Satisfactory	Comments
Assessment			
1. Check order.			
2. Assess patient, including general condition, vital signs, local site, and response to previous treatment.			
3. Check patient's room for equipment.			
Planning			
4. Wash your hands.			
5. Obtain appropriate device.			
Implementation			
6. Identify patient.			
7. Explain procedure to patient.			
8. Provide for patient's privacy and comfort.			
9. Prepare patient (expose only area to be treated) and patient's unit.			
10. Place heating or cooling device over body part, molding it to area.			
11. Cover device with soft cloth cover.			
12. Return to patient in 10–15 minutes to assess therapeutic or adverse effects.			
13. Remove heating or cooling device, leaving on no longer than 30 minutes unless ordered.			
14. Examine treated area.			
15. Replace linen or clothing removed; leave patient comfortable.			
16. Wash your hands.			
Evaluation			
17. Evaluate, using the following criteria: a. Signs and symptoms of both desirable and undesirable responses to treatment			
b. Patient comfort			

(continued)

© 1996 by Lippincott-Raven Publishers

General Procedure for Applying Heat or Cold *(Continued)*	Needs More Practice	Satisfactory	Comments
Documentation			
18. Document the treatment, including length of time applied and the patient's response, on the patient's progress record.			
Applying a Warm, Moist Compress			
Assessment			
1.–3. Follow Checklist steps 1–3 of the General Procedure for Applying Heat and Cold (check order, assess patient, check for equipment).			
Planning			
4. Wash your hands as in Checklist step 4 of the General Procedure.			
5. Obtain compress materials (sterile basin, solution, gloves. If commercial package, follow directions.			
Implementation			
6.–9. Follow Checklist steps 6–9 of the General Procedure (identify patient, explain procedure, provide privacy and comfort).			
10. Place moisture-proof pad under area, drape as necessary. **a.** Moisten compress.			
b. Place heating source on outside to maintain heat.			
c. Hold in place with ties or gauze wrap.			
11. Cover area with a cloth and plastic covering so that heat will be retained.			
12. Return to the patient every 5 minutes to check for adverse reactions.			
13. Remove compress after 20 minutes.			
14.–16. Follow Checklist steps 14–16 of the General Procedure (examine treated area, replace any linen or clothing removed, and wash your hands).			
Evaluation			
17. Evaluate as in Checklist step 17 of the General Procedure (signs and symptoms of responses to treatment and patient comfort).			

(continued)

© 1996 by Lippincott-Raven Publishers

Applying a Warm, Moist Compress *(Continued)*	Needs More Practice	Satisfactory	Comments
Documentation			
18. Document as in Checklist step 18 of the General Procedure (on the patient's progress record, document treatment, length of time applied, and patient response).			
Administering a Soak			
Assessment			
1.–3. Follow Checklist steps 1–3 of the General Procedure for Applying Heat or Cold (check order, assess patient, and check for equipment).			
Planning			
4. Wash your hands.			
5. Obtain basin.			
Implementation			
6.–9. Follow Checklist for steps 6–9 of the General Procedure (identify patient, explain procedure, and provide privacy, and prepare patient's unit).			
10. Fill basin half full with water (105°–115°F; 40.5°–46.1°C).			
11. Place basin on moisture-proof pad. Place body part to be treated in basin, checking for body alignment and pressure.			
12. Check patient after first 5 minutes and at least once during remainder of treatment.			
13. Remove body part from basin and dry.			
14. Examine and reapply dressing as needed.			
15.–16. Follow Checklist steps 15 and 16 of the General Procedure (replace any linen or clothing removed and wash your hands).			
Evaluation			
17. Evaluate as in Checklist step 17 of the General Procedure (signs and symptoms of responses to treatment and patient comfort).			

(continued)

© 1996 by Lippincott-Raven Publishers

Administering a Soak *(Continued)*	Needs More Practice	Satisfactory	Comments
Documentation			
18. Document as in Checklist step 18 of the General Procedure (on the patient's progress record, document treatment, length of time applied, and patient response).			
Administering a Sitz Bath			
Assessment			
1.–3. Follow Checklist steps 1–3 of the General Procedure (check order, assess patient, check for equipment).			
Planning			
4. Wash your hands as in Checklist step 4 of the General Procedure.			
5. Gather sitz bath equipment and more than one towel. Place towel over patient's shoulders.			
Implementation			
6.–8. Follow Checklist steps 6–8 of the General Procedure (identify patient, explain procedure, provide privacy and comfort).			
9. Assist patient out of bed or to tub room.			
10. Fill sitz bath device with heated water of 105–115°F or 40.5–46.1°C.			
11. Remove patient's clothing, assess area to be treated.			
12. Monitor patient frequently during treatment. Measure vital signs and stay with patient for the first 5 minutes.			
13. Assist patient out of tub at end of treatment and help dry patient.			
14. Examine the treated area as in Checklist step 14 of the General Procedure.			
15. Help the patient to dress and assist back to bed or to the room.			
16. Wash your hands as in Checklist step 16 of the General Procedure.			

(continued)

© 1996 by Lippincott-Raven Publishers

Administering a Sitz Bath *(Continued)*	Needs More Practice	Satisfactory	Comments
Evaluation			
17. Evaluate as in Checklist step 17 of the General Procedure (signs and symptoms of responses to treatment and patient comfort).			
Documentation			
18. Document as in Checklist step 18 of the General Procedure (on the patient's progress record, document treatment, length of time applied, and patient response).			
Administering a Cooling Sponge Bath			
Assessment			
1.–3. Follow Checklist steps 1–3 of the General Procedure (check order, assess patient, check for equipment).			
Planning			
4. Wash your hands as in Checklist step 4 of the General Procedure.			
5. Gather equipment (basin, washcloths, towels, bath blanket, moisture-proof pads).			
6.–8. Follow Checklist steps 6–8 of the General Procedure (identify patient, explain procedure, provide privacy and comfort).			
9. Close windows, doors, and bed curtains, if present, to prevent air drafts. a. Remove and fold bed linen.			
b. Place bath blanket over patient.			
c. Fill basin with cool water.			
10. Immerse and wring out three washcloths, placing them in axillae and groin for cooling.			
11. Bathe each extremity for 3 minutes. Continue bathing back and buttocks.			
12. Check patient's temperature every 15 minutes.			
13. Discontinue sponging when desired temperature has been reached.			
14.–16. Follow Checklist steps 14–16 of the General Procedure (examine treated area, replace any linen or clothing removed, wash your hands).			

(continued)

© 1996 by Lippincott-Raven Publishers

Administering a Cooling Sponge Bath *(Continued)*	Needs More Practice	Satisfactory	Comments
Evaluation			
17. Evaluate as in Checklist step 17 of the General Procedure (signs and symptoms of responses to treatment and patient comfort).			
Documentation			
18. Document as in Checklist step 18 of the General Procedure (on the patient's progress record, document treatment, length of time applied, and patient response).			
Use of the Thermal Blanket for Cooling or Warming			
Assessment			
1.–3. Follow Checklist steps 1–3 of the General Procedure for Applying Heat or Cold (check order, assess patient, check for equipment).			
Planning			
4.–5. Follow Checklist steps 4 and 5 of the General Procedure (wash your hands and obtain blanket).			
Implementation			
6.–8. Follow Checklist steps 6–8 of the General Procedure (identify patient, explain procedure, provide privacy and comfort).			
9. Remove heavy clothing from patient. Assess room for space for the unit and safe electrical outlets.			
10. Place bath blanket over and under patient. a. Set control and turn on unit.			
b. Roll patient onto temperature control blanket.			
c. Secure sensors to skin with tape, if used.			
11. Cover patient with top linen.			
12. Assess patient's temperature and vital signs every 15 minutes until desirable temperature is reached.			
13. Turn off controls, leaving patient on blanket in case it is necessary to reinstate treatment.			

(continued)

© 1996 by Lippincott-Raven Publishers

Use of the Thermal Blanket for Cooling or Warming *(Continued)*	Needs More Practice	Satisfactory	Comments
14. Examine patient's skin and general condition.			
15.–16. Follow Checklist steps 15 and 16 of the General Procedure (replace linen and wash your hands).			
Evaluation			
17. Evaluate as in Checklist step 17 of the General Procedure (signs and symptoms of responses to treatment and patient comfort).			
Documentation			
18. Document as in Checklist step 18 of the General Procedure (on the patient's progress record, document treatment, length of time applied, and patient response).			

© 1996 by Lippincott-Raven Publishers

? **Q U I Z**

Multiple-Choice Questions

_____ 1. The body's temperature receptors, which register sensations of warmth or coolness, are found in the

    a. skin.
    b. walls of internal organs.
    c. cortex of the brain.
    d. deep muscles.

_____ 2. Which of the following is the *most important* nursing diagnosis to use when applying heat or cold to the patient?

    a. Ineffective Thermoregulation
    b. Ineffective Individual Coping
    c. Risk for Injury
    d. Hyperthermia

_____ 3. Which of the following persons can best tolerate heat or cold with the fewest precautions?

    a. The elderly
    b. Infants
    c. Otherwise healthy adults
    d. Persons with circulatory problems

_____ 4. Heat causes blood vessels to

    a. constrict.
    b. dilate.
    c. become inflamed.
    d. become more elastic.

_____ 5. Heat reduces edema because

    a. it increases diaphoresis.
    b. output is increased.
    c. fluid is more easily absorbed.
    d. it increases the number of blood vessels to the part.

_____ 6. The application of cold can also decrease edema through which of the following actions?

    a. Increasing circulation
    b. Slowing circulation
    c. Narrowing capillaries
    d. Producing "shivering"

_____ 7. The bulb in a heat cradle is generally no larger than

    a. 15 watts.
    b. 25 watts.
    c. 40 watts.
    d. 60 watts.

© 1996 by Lippincott-Raven Publishers

_____   **8.** A sitz bath is generally administered for

    a. 5–10 minutes.
    b. 15–20 minutes.
    c. 30–40 minutes.
    d. an hour.

_____   **9.** During a cooling sponge bath, cool, wet washcloths are placed in which areas of the body to facilitate cooling?

    a. The forehead and back of the neck
    b. The inner elbows and knees
    c. The axillae and chest
    d. The axillae and groin

_____   **10.** Which of the following is a reaction experienced by a person whose body temperature rises after completion of hypothermia blanket therapy?

    a. "Anaphylactic"
    b. "Recurrent"
    c. "Rebound"
    d. "Residual"

© 1996 by Lippincott-Raven Publishers

MODULE

28

ADMINISTERING ENEMAS

MODULE CONTENTS

RATIONALE FOR THE USE OF THIS
   SKILL
NURSING DIAGNOSES
TYPES OF ENEMAS
Cleansing Enema
   The Large-Volume Enema
   The Small-Volume Enema
   The Prepackaged Disposable Enema
Oil-Retention Enema
Return-Flow Enema
Cooling Enema
Rectal Instillation of Medications
GENERAL PROCEDURE FOR
   ADMINISTERING ENEMAS
   Assessment

Planning
Implementation
Evaluation
Documentation
SPECIFIC ENEMA PROCEDURES
Administering a Large-Volume Cleansing
   Enema
Administering a Premixed Packaged
   Enema
Administering a Return-Flow Enema
PEDIATRIC ENEMAS
Administering a Pediatric Enema
LONG-TERM CARE
HOME CARE
CRITICAL THINKING EXERCISES

PREREQUISITES

Successful completion of the following modules:

VOLUME 1
Module 1   An Approach to Nursing Skills
Module 2   Basic Infection Control
Module 3   Safety
Module 5   Documentation
Module 6   Introduction to Assessment Skills
Module 15 Moving the Patient in Bed and Positioning
Module 20 Transfer

© 1996 by Lippincott-Raven Publishers

To administer enemas to adults and children safely and effectively.

S P E C I F I C   L E A R N I N G   O B J E C T I V E S

Know Facts and Principles	Apply Facts and Principles	Demonstrate Ability	Evaluate Performance
1. Types of enemas and indications for use List types of enemas and purpose of each type.	Given a patient situation, identify whether enema is necessary and which type is appropriate.	In the clinical setting, identify purpose of enema ordered for specific patient.	
2. Patient teaching State what patient needs to be taught regarding procedure.	Given a patient situation, plan appropriate teaching.	In the clinical setting, explain procedure to patient.	Evaluate own teaching by assessing patient's knowledge of procedure.
3. Procedure *a. Equipment* Describe equipment used in enema procedure.	Plan procedure. Select appropriate equipment.	In the clinical setting, carry out procedure correctly.	Evaluate own performance with instructor, using Performance Checklist.
b. Temperature Know correct temperature for solution.	Plan variations of technique for the pediatric patient.		
c. Patient position Describe appropriate patient position(s).			
d. Distance to insert tubing State distance tip of device should be inserted.			
e. Lubrication State rationale for use of a lubricant.			
f. Pressure Explain how pressure is controlled. State how appropriate pressure is determined.	Given a patient situation, plan appropriate action to alleviate problems or to stop procedure if necessary.		

(continued)

© 1996 by Lippincott-Raven Publishers

Know Facts and Principles	Apply Facts and Principles	Demonstrate Ability	Evaluate Performance
4. *Observations*			
List observations to make before, during, and after procedure.	Given a patient situation, identify observations that are significant.	In the clinical setting, identify significant observations. Take corrective action if necessary.	Evaluate own performance with clinical instructor.
5. *Documentation*			
State information and observations that need to be documented.	Given a patient situation, record data as though on a progress note.	Document procedure and observations appropriately for clinical facility.	Evaluate with instructor.

© 1996 by Lippincott-Raven Publishers

LEARNING ACTIVITIES

1. Review the Specific Learning Objectives.
2. Read the sections on the intestinal system and on defecation problems (in the chapter on elimination) in Ellis and Nowlis, *Nursing: A Human Needs Approach,* or comparable material in another textbook.
3. Look up the module vocabulary terms in the glossary.
4. Read through the module as though you were preparing to teach the concepts and skills to another person. Mentally practice the procedures.
5. In the practice setting:
   a. Inspect and become familiar with the types of enema equipment available.
   b. Using equipment in the laboratory, go through the entire procedure as you would with a real patient, including communication, without actually giving the enema. Use a manikin, if available, or improvise a substitute.
   c. Have another student check your performance, using the Performance Checklist.
   d. Evaluate your own performance.
   e. Compare your evaluation with your partner's.
   f. Have your partner do the procedure, and evaluate the performance.
   g. Practice documenting information regarding an enema, using forms available in your practice area. If no forms are available, write a progress note on plain paper.
   h. Repeat this section until you have gone through the procedure correctly.
   i. When you feel you have mastered the procedure, have your instructor evaluate your performance.
6. In the clinical setting:
   a. Identify your facility's policy regarding bowel care interventions that may be initiated by nurses.
   b. Consult with your clinical instructor regarding the opportunity to give an enema to a patient or resident.
   c. Have your instructor supervise and evaluate your performance.

VOCABULARY

anal sphincter (external and internal)	distention	hypotonic	reflex contraction
	electrolyte	impaction	sigmoid flexure
	feces	instillation	Sims' position
anorectal	flatus	normal saline	transverse colon
ascending colon	Harris flush	parasites	
descending colon	hypertonic	peristalsis	

© 1996 by Lippincott-Raven Publishers

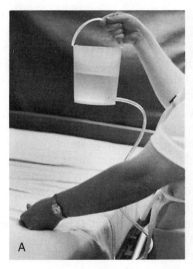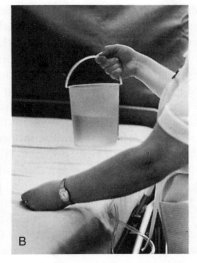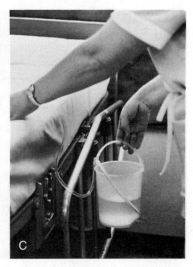

Figure 28–3. Regulating fluid pressure by height of container. **(A)** Moderate pressure; **(B)** Low pressure; **(C)** Negative pressure, for siphoning. (Courtesy Ivan Ellis.)

Rectal Instillation of Medications

Medications can be instilled into the colon *for local or systemic absorption* by means of an enema. There are several reasons for giving medications by rectum using the enema procedure. *Some medications soothe the intestinal mucosa, and others correct electrolyte imbalances or combat infections such as those caused by intestinal parasites.* Some medicated enemas are available in prepackaged form. If not, the medication may be dissolved in 30 to 50 mL solution *so that the volume of fluid will not cause peristalsis and loss of the medication.* The medication is then absorbed through the intestinal wall. It may be necessary to administer a cleansing enema *to clear the colon* before a medicated enema is given.

GENERAL PROCEDURE FOR ADMINISTERING ENEMAS

Assessment

1. Verify the order. You are responsible to check the physician's order for the enema *to be sure the correct type is being administered to the correct patient.*
2. Assess the patient's ability to retain the fluid and to tolerate the activity ordered. In very young, very old, or very debilitated patients, check pulse, respirations, and blood pressure to provide baseline observations for later evaluation of the patient's "tolerance" of the procedure.

Planning

3. Wash your hands *for infection control.*
4. Obtain the appropriate equipment for the type of enema to be given and carry it to the patient's bedside. (See the specific procedures below for the exact equipment needed.)
   a. Be sure the enema solution is at the correct temperature (100°–105°F; 37.7°–40.5°C). *The correct temperature helps to preserve homeostasis by eliminating the body's need to use large amounts of energy to compensate for heat lost into the enema solution.* Also, *warmth stimulates peristalsis and is more comfortable for the patient.*
   b. Use a bath blanket or sheet *to drape the patient,* a waterproof pad *to place under the patient's hips to protect the bed* (these are usually provided in commercial enema kits), and adequate lighting.
   c. Use a lubricant *to facilitate the insertion of the tube and to prevent trauma to anorectal tissue.* A water-soluble lubricant is most commonly used *because it is easy to remove.* A mineral-based lubricant is also acceptable. Some commercial enema kits come with lubricated tips.
   d. Wear clean disposable gloves.
5. Decide whether the patient will use a bedpan, a commode, or the toilet for expelling the enema, and make the necessary arrangements.

Implementation

6. Identify the patient *to be sure you are performing the procedure on the correct patient.*
7. Explain the procedure. Although some persons have had enemas previously or are familiar with them, others have their first experience with an enema in a healthcare facility. Your first task is to determine how much the patient knows about the procedure and how he or she feels about it. Then you can teach the patient

© 1996 by Lippincott-Raven Publishers

what is needed, *particularly what to expect in terms of the body's responses*. Allow time for the patient to express personal feelings regarding the procedure.

8. Prepare the patient. Close the curtains or drapes *to provide privacy*. Raise the bed to a comfortable working height for you. Place the patient in left Sims' position. *This position allows the fluid to flow by gravity and fill the descending colon*. When an extreme, complete cleansing is necessary (for example, before a barium enema), after you have administered 300 to 400 mL, position the patient on the back for the next 300 mL. Then turn the patient to the right side while an additional 300 mL is instilled. *This procedure allows the fluid to fill the transverse and the ascending colon*, but it can be difficult for the patient and is not done routinely.

   Enemas can also be administered with a patient on the right side or on the back for comfort or as indicated by the patient's condition. These positions are successful, but *the patient may experience pressure at the anus with a smaller amount of fluid*.

   Cover the patient with a drape of some kind (such as a bath blanket) so that only the rectal area is exposed. *This lessens the patient's embarrassment and prevents chilling*. Then place a waterproof pad under the patient's hips *to protect the bed*. Occasionally, a patient may ask to have an enema given while sitting on the toilet. This practice is undesirable because *the fluid is instilled against gravity, making it difficult for the patient to retain the fluid and resulting in a less effective cleansing of the bowel*.

   Patients receiving large amounts of solution (750–1,000 mL) usually cannot retain the solution for longer than 5 minutes, so it is comforting for them to have a commode or bedpan readily available.

9. Put on clean gloves.

10. Administer the enema according to the specific procedure below. When the correct amount of fluid has been instilled, clamp the tubing and remove it. By clamping the tubing first, *you prevent the fluid from dripping out of the tube after the tube is removed*.

11. Encourage the patient to retain the fluid as long as possible.

12. Assist the patient onto the bedpan or commode or to the bathroom.

13. If the patient can be left alone, provide a call light and toilet tissue and leave the room. Inform the patient not to flush the toilet. You can place a piece of tape across the flushing handle

as a reminder. Make sure you are close by to help the patient if necessary.

14. After the patient has defecated, assist him or her to a comfortable position. The patient may need help cleaning the anorectal area after receiving an enema. Also, provide an opportunity for handwashing. *Because an enema is typically tiring*, allow the patient to rest, and assist with other comfort measures as indicated.

15. Clean or dispose of the enema equipment. Some disposable equipment may be cleaned and reused for the same patient. Dry the equipment thoroughly *to prevent the growth of microorganisms*, and label it with the date and the patient's name. If nondisposable equipment is used, send it to the appropriate area to be disinfected.

16. Remove gloves and discard.

17. Wash your hands.

Evaluation

18. Observe and evaluate the results. During the procedure, observe the patient's response to the enema, skin color, and respiratory rate. Check the patient's pulse rate before and after the procedure. Also watch for signs of excessive fatigue. *If the patient's response is adverse*, discontinue the procedure and consult the physician.

    When the procedure is completed, evaluate using the following criteria:

    a. Results, such as the quantity of stool (small, moderate, or large) and a description of its color and consistency (particles, soft, hard)

    b. Patient's response, skin color, respirations, pulse rate, and degree of fatigue

Documentation

19. Document on the patient's chart the type of enema administered, the amount of fluid instilled, and the time the enema was given. Also document the results and describe the patient's response to the procedure.

SPECIFIC ENEMA PROCEDURES

For each specific enema procedure discussed, some steps of the General Procedure may be modified. We have included completely the modified steps as well as references to the steps of the General Procedure that remain the same.

Administering a Large-Volume Cleansing Enema

Assessment

1.–2. Follow the steps of the General Procedure for Administering Enemas.

© 1996 by Lippincott-Raven Publishers

Planning

3. Follow the General Procedure.
4. In addition to the equipment listed in step 4 of the General Procedure, also obtain an enema container with tubing (see Fig. 28–1). Rectal tubing is sized using the French method—the larger the number, the larger the diameter of the tubing. Disposable enema sets usually have size 18 to 22 French tips. Examine the tip for irregularities that could damage anorectal tissue.
5. Follow the General Procedure.

Implementation

6.–9. Follow the steps of the General Procedure.
10. Administer the enema.
   a. Fill the container with 500 to 1,000 mL of the ordered solution. *For thorough cleansing, 500 to 1,000 mL fluid is usually needed.* We recommend starting with 1,000 mL; you can always stop instilling fluid before the container is empty. Use solution that is slightly warmer than body temperature (100°–105°F [37.7°–40.5°C] is appropriate). Check the temperature of the solution with a bath thermometer. If a bath thermometer is not available, estimate the temperature by testing it on the inner aspect of your forearm, as you would check the temperature of a baby's formula. It should feel comfortably warm but not hot. *By the time it is instilled through the tubing it will be approximately at body temperature.*
   b. Remove air from the enema tubing by allowing fluid to flow through to the tip and then clamping the tubing. *Instilling air into the bowel increases patient discomfort by causing distention and makes retention of the fluid more difficult.*
   c. Lift the patient's upper buttock to expose the anus. Insert the lubricated enema tip upward toward the umbilicus 3 to 4 inches. *This places it past the internal anal sphincter and well into the rectum, so that the fluid does not put immediate pressure against the sphincter or create as much potential for trauma to the intestinal wall as would further insertion.* It is possible to traumatize the intestinal mucosa severely, especially if the tubing is inserted into the sigmoid flexure or the descending colon. Have the patient breathe through the mouth *to relax the anal sphincter.* Another technique *for relaxing the sphincter* is to touch the enema tip to the sphincter, wait for the reflex contraction to subside, and then insert the tip. If you encounter an obstruction, stop the procedure and report it.
   d. Raise the enema container above the patient's hips and unclamp the tubing. *The higher the enema container is held above the level of the patient's hips, the greater the pressure. Negative pressure is achieved by holding the fluid below the level of the patient's hips* (see Fig. 28–3).

   The pressure created by holding the enema container 12 to 18 inches above the patient's hips is *enough to instill the fluid without being so great as to damage the intestinal mucosa or cause intestinal perforation.* Use low pressure if the patient experiences excessive discomfort or cramping. You may have to use a higher pressure again—briefly—if the fluid is partially blocked by fecal material and does not flow with the usual pressure. *If cramping occurs despite the use of low pressure,* stop the inflow of fluid temporarily *to allow the bowel to accommodate the fluid already given.* If severe cramping does not subside, the enema is usually discontinued.

   If the patient has a large amount of gas, it is sometimes helpful to administer a return-flow enema first *to remove the gas. The patient is better able to retain the enema fluid, and the evacuation will be more effective.*

   Sometimes a patient cannot retain the fluid *because of weakness or lack of control of the anal sphincter.* In such a case, hold the buttocks firmly together around the tubing *to help the patient retain the fluid,* or place a baby-bottle nipple over the tubing and hold it at the sphincter. *If small amounts of fluid drain back constantly,* place the curved side of an emesis basin against the buttocks *to catch the fluid as it drains out.* Sometimes a retention catheter is inserted and the balloon inflated *to help retain fluid or medication in the bowel.* In some instances the patient must be placed on a bedpan *to avoid extreme soiling of the bed, which would distress the patient.*

11.–19. Follow the steps of the General Procedure.

Administering a Premixed Packaged Enema

Assessment

1.–2. Follow the steps of the General Procedure for Administering Enemas.

Planning

3. Follow the General Procedure.
4. In addition to the equipment listed in step 4 of the General Procedure, also obtain the correct premixed packaged enema.
5. Follow the General Procedure.

© 1996 by Lippincott-Raven Publishers

Implementation

6.–9. Follow the steps of the General Procedure.

10. Administer the enema.

    a. Warm the enema by immersing the container in a basin of warm water *to enhance patient comfort and the effectiveness of the enema.*

    b. Remove the cover from the prelubricated tip.

    c. Insert the tip into the patient's rectum, directing it toward the umbilicus. The tips on most commercially prepared enemas are constructed in such a way that they can only be inserted a short distance.

    d. Squeeze the plastic container until all the fluid has been instilled.

    e. Remove the tip from the patient's rectum.

11.–17. Follow the steps of the General Procedure.

Evaluation

18. Follow the General Procedure.

Documentation

19. Follow the General Procedure.

Administering a Return-Flow Enema

Assessment

1.–2. Follow the steps of the General Procedure for Administering Enemas.

Planning

3. Follow the General Procedure.

4. In addition to the equipment listed in step 4 of the General Procedure, also obtain an enema container with tubing.

5. Follow the General Procedure.

Implementation

10. Administer the enema.

    a. Use approximately 500 mL fluid.

    b. Clear the tubing of air.

    c. Lubricate the tip of the tubing if not prelubricated.

    d. Insert the tip into the rectum.

    e. After 200 mL fluid has been instilled, lower the enema container below the level of the patient's bowel and siphon the fluid and gas from the bowel.

    f. Next, raise the container, instill a small volume of fluid again, and then lower the container to siphon the fluid and gas. Repeat these steps until no gas is returned. If the fluid does not return, you may have to move the tip of the tubing slightly *so that it is in contact with the fluid in the bowel.*

    g. Clamp the tubing before removing it from the patient's rectum.

11.–17. Follow the steps of the General Procedure.

Evaluation

18. Assess the patient for excess fatigue, distress, or other adverse symptoms throughout the procedure. Stop the enema if the patient responds adversely. When the procedure is completed, evaluate using the following criteria:

    a. Quantity of gas expelled with fluid

    b. Degree of patient's comfort after procedure

Documentation

19. Follow the General Procedure.

DATE/TIME	
9/2/98	Alteration in Bowel Elimination: Constipation
1330	S "I haven't had a bowel movement since I've been here."
	O Admitted to unit 4 days ago. No documentation of bowel movement, abdomen soft but mildly distended.
	A Patient is constipated.
	P Administer ordered Fleets enema.
	S. Rushmore, NS

Example of Nursing Progress Notes Using SOAP Format.

DATE/TIME	
9/2/98	Complained of absence of bowel movements since admission.
1330	Abdomen soft but mildly distended. No bowel movements noted on records. Fleets enema administered, which resulted in moderate amount of soft, brown stool. Patient stated that she felt more comfortable.
	S. Rushmore, NS

Example of Nursing Progress Notes Using Narrative Format.

© 1996 by Lippincott-Raven Publishers

PEDIATRIC ENEMAS

When an enema is administered to an infant or child, the basic procedure remains unchanged. Some modifications need to be made, however, depending on the patient's age and size.

Administering a Pediatric Enema

Assessment

1.–2. Follow the steps of the General Procedure for Administering Enemas.

Planning

3. Follow the General Procedure.

4. In addition to the equipment listed in step 4 of the General Procedure, obtain a pediatric enema kit or prepackaged enema. If your facility does not stock pediatric enema kits, you can use a small-diameter catheter and a small fluid container. Attaching a size 10 French catheter to a 50-mL catheter-tip syringe with the plunger or bulb removed works satisfactorily. Hold the syringe to administer the fluid by gravity drainage. The short tubing prevents the fluid container from being held too high, *to protect the infant or child from excess pressure.* For a child, a conventional enema administration set with a size 10 to 14 French catheter can be used.

Normal saline is the preferred solution used in children *because tap water, a hypotonic solution, can cause rapid fluid shift and fluid overload, and commercial enemas have potential for serious complications* (Wong, 1993).

5. Follow the General Procedure.

Implementation

6. Follow the General Procedure.

7. Explain the procedure.

Consider the child's age and developmental level in determining an approach to take and how much teaching is appropriate.

For an infant, you will not have to give any explanation, but talk in warm, caring tones during the procedure and handle the infant gently *to alleviate anxiety.*

For a toddler, give explanations simply as you perform each step. *Information given early will only increase anxiety.* Having a parent assist may help *decrease the toddler's fear. Because the toddler will be upset by such an intrusive procedure,* it is often necessary for another person to hold the toddler in order to administer the enema quickly and safely.

8. Prepare the patient.

Position the infant on his or her back for the enema. *This provides easy access to the anus and al-*

lows you to observe the infant throughout the procedure. Place the infant on a pediatric bedpan *to contain the fluid that is expelled around the tubing.* Pad the bedpan and support the infant's back and head with a pillow. One way to keep an infant on a bedpan is to put a towel or diaper under the bedpan, bring the ends of the towel over the legs of the infant, and tuck the towel ends under the legs and the bedpan. You may need to pin the towel ends in place *to hold the infant securely in one position for the procedure.* This will free your hands to manage the equipment.

Position the child who is preschool age or older as you would an adult. Remember that *children, too, are modest, and draping is important.*

9. Follow the General Procedure.

10. Administer the enema.

a. Instill the appropriate volume of fluid, which varies with the child's size and age. *The infant who is not yet toilet trained will not retain fluid.* Therefore, the total volume used may not be in the bowel at one time *because fluid will return around the tubing.* If the child can retain the fluid, watch for any sign given by the child that might indicate discomfort *to prevent excessive pressure.*

No research data are available that accurately identify the exact volume of fluid to be instilled for a certain age or size child. Therefore, general guidelines for the appropriate amount of fluid for certain age groups are given in Table 28–1 (Wong, 1993). Do not hesitate to use less fluid if this action seems appropriate in a particular situation.

b. Insert the tubing a short distance. The objective is to place the tip beyond the internal sphincter without damaging the tender bowel lining. General guidelines for the appropriate distance to insert the tubing for various age groups are given in Table 28–1 (Wong, 1993).

Always insert the tubing slowly and gently *to minimize the possibility of trauma.* Do not use force. If you feel a blockage, stop the insertion and instill a small amount of fluid in the bowel. *The fluid will dilate the bowel and allow insertion of the tubing.*

c. Give the fluid slowly and observe the infant or child closely.

11. Encourage the child to retain the fluid as long as possible. If the child is too young to retain the fluid, hold the buttocks together for 3 to 5 minutes after the fluid has been instilled. For an oil-retention enema, you may wish to tape the patient's buttocks together *to allow the oil to be retained long enough to soften the stool.*

© 1996 by Lippincott-Raven Publishers

Table 28–1. Guidelines for Administration of Enemas to Children

Age	Amount (mL)	Insertion Distance (cm/inches)
Infant	120–240	2.5 (1 inch)
2–4 years	240–360	5.0 (2 inches)
4–10 years	360–480	7.5 (3 inches)
11 years	480–720	10.0 (4 inches)

(Wong, D. (1993). *Whaley & Wong's Essentials of Pediatric Nursing*, (4th ed.). St. Louis: C. V. Mosby, p. 701)

12. Gently massage the patient's abdomen *to aid the evacuation of the fluid.*

14. Provide for cleanliness and comfort. After the fluid has been expelled, clean the infant or child and rediaper the infant. Then hold and comfort the infant or play with the young child *to help alleviate the stress caused by the procedure.* This reassurance is especially important for a toddler, *who does not understand the procedure but is old enough to have strong feelings about body boundaries and who fears any intrusive procedure.*

15.–17. Follow the steps of the General Procedure.

Evaluation

18. Follow the General Procedure.

Documentation

19. Follow the General Procedure.

LONG-TERM CARE

For the elderly residents in a long-term care setting, there may be *increasing intolerance of certain food* that was once enjoyed, which can cause gastric distention and flatulence. Constipation is also a common problem, and *muscular relaxation of the intestinal walls* may add to the difficulty of adequate fecal elimination. Because of this, bowel programs are frequently a part of care plans in these settings. Enemas may be an early part of a bowel program. But typically other parts of the program (such as increased fluids, diet therapy, exercise, and medication) achieve the desired outcome without the frequent use of enemas.

When an enema is a part of the care of an elderly resident, several considerations are important. The nurse should be attentive to providing privacy for the older client, who may be more modest than a person of a younger age. You may need to use a small volume of fluid and give it slowly because the elderly individual often has more difficulty retaining enema fluid. *Because of urgency,* a bedpan, commode, or assistance to the bathroom should be readily available.

The program of daily living should include sufficient exercise, a high-fiber diet, and adequate fluids. These measures will *help prevent periods of constipation and the need for enemas.* Your role as a member of the nursing staff may be to administer enemas or to teach others on the staff.

HOME CARE

Enemas may be taken at home *because of occasional episodes of constipation or on the recommendation of the physician as preparation for a test.* Clients being cared for in the home may also have need for this procedure. As a home care nurse, your responsibility may be include assessing the client and instructing the family. You may help the client by setting up a bowel care program that includes diet and fluid management as well as exercise. Knowing when an enema is appropriate is important. With most persons, enemas should be given only if sufficient exercise, a high-fiber diet, and adequate fluids fail to relieve distention and constipation. The guidelines in the home are the same as those for giving an enema in the hospital or long-term care setting. When the individual needing the enema is an infant or child, you can convert the recommended amounts of fluid to be administered into cups for teaching purposes.

© 1996 by Lippincott-Raven Publishers

CRITICAL THINKING EXERCISES

You are administering a return flow enema to a 70-year-old man who has recently undergone hernia repair surgery. You have repeated the procedure three times with a large amount of flatus returned. Flatus is still being returned, but the patient states he is tired. What observations are appropriate for you to make? Formulate an assessment and identify the nursing interventions you would undertake.

References

Wong, D. (1993). *Whaley & Wong's Essentials of Pediatric Nursing*. (4th ed.). St Louis: C.V. Mosby.

© 1996 by Lippincott-Raven Publishers

✔ **PERFORMANCE CHECKLIST**

General Procedure for Administering Enemas	Needs More Practice	Satisfactory	Comments
Assessment			
1. Verify order.			
2. Check patient's ability to retain fluid and tolerate the activity ordered.			
Planning			
3. Wash your hands.			
4. Gather equipment. a. Solution at correct temperature			
b. Bath blanket or drape and waterproof pad			
c. Lubricant			
d. Clean gloves			
5. Obtain commode or bedpan if needed.			
Implementation			
6. Identify patient.			
7. Explain procedure to patient.			
8. Prepare patient by providing privacy and by positioning and draping patient.			
9. Put on clean gloves.			
10. Administer enema. (Use specific procedure below.)			
11. Encourage patient to retain fluid as long as possible.			
12. Assist patient with bedpan or commode or to bathroom.			
13. Provide toilet tissue and call light.			
14. Help patient to position of comfort.			
15. Clean the equipment or dispose of it.			
16. Remove gloves and discard.			
17. Wash your hands.			

(continued)

© 1996 by Lippincott-Raven Publishers

General Procedure for Administering Enemas *(Continued)*	Needs More Practice	Satisfactory	Comments
Evaluation			
18. Evaluate, using the following criteria: **a.** Quantity and description of feces			
b. Patient's response, skin color, respirations, pulse rate, and degree of fatigue			
Documentation			
19. Document on progress notes the time and type of enema given, fluid instilled, results, and patient's response.			
Administering a Large-Volume Cleansing Enema			
Assessment			
1.–2. Follow Checklist steps 1 and 2 of the General Procedure for Administering Enemas (verify order and patient's ability to retain fluid and tolerate activity).			
Planning			
3. Wash your hands.			
4. Obtain enema container with tubing.			
5. Obtain bedpan or commode if needed.			
Implementation			
6.–9. Follow Checklist steps 6–9 of the General Procedure (identify patient, explain procedure, provide privacy, and put on clean gloves).			
10. Administer the enema. **a.** Use 1,000 mL fluid at 100°–105°F (37.7°–40.5°C).			
b. Clear tubing of air.			
c. Insert lubricated tip of tubing 3–4 inches.			
d. Give fluid with safe pressure (not to exceed 18 inches above patient's hips).			
11.–17. Follow Checklist steps 11–17 of the General Procedure.			
Evaluation			
18. Evaluate, using the following criteria: **a.** Quantity and description of feces			

(continued)

© 1996 by Lippincott-Raven Publishers

Administering a Large-Volume Cleansing Enema *(Continued)*	Needs More Practice	Satisfactory	Comments
b. Patient's response, skin color, respirations, pulse rate, and degree of fatigue			
Documentation			
19. Document on progress notes the time and type of enema given, fluid instilled, results, and patient's response.			
Administering a Premixed Packaged Enema			
Assessment			
1.–2. Follow Checklist steps 1 and 2 of General Procedure for Administering Enemas (verify order and patient's ability to retain fluid and tolerate activity).			
Planning			
3. Wash your hands.			
4. Obtain correct premixed packaged enema and clean gloves.			
5. Obtain commode or bedpan if needed.			
Implementation			
6.–9. Follow Checklist steps 6–9 of the General Procedure (identify patient, explain procedure, provide privacy, and put on clean gloves).			
10. Administer the enema **a.** Warm contents in warm tap water.			
b. Remove cover from prelubricated tip.			
c. Insert tip into rectum.			
d. Squeeze plastic container until all fluid has been instilled.			
e. Remove tip.			
11.–17. Follow Checklist steps 11–17 of the General Procedure.			
Evaluation			
18. Evaluate, using the following criteria: **a.** Quantity and description of feces			
b. Patient's response, skin color, respirations, pulse rate, and degree of fatigue			

(continued)

© 1996 by Lippincott-Raven Publishers

Administering a Premixed Packaged Enema *(Continued)*	Needs More Practice	Satisfactory	Comments
Documentation			
19. Document on progress notes the time and type of enema given, fluid instilled, results, and patient's response.			
Administering a Return-Flow Enema			
Assessment			
1.–2. Follow Checklist steps 1 and 2 of the General Procedure for Administering Enemas (verify order and patient's ability to retain fluid and tolerate activity).			
Planning			
3. Wash your hands.			
4. Obtain enema container with tubing.			
5. Obtain bedpan or commode if needed.			
Implementation			
6.–9. Follow Checklist steps 6–9 of the General Procedure (identify patient, explain procedure, provide privacy, and put on clean gloves).			
10. Administer the enema a. Use 500 mL fluid at 100°–105°F (37.7°–40.5°C).			
b. Clear tubing of air.			
c. Lubricate tip of tubing.			
d. Insert tip into rectum.			
e. After 200 mL fluid has been instilled, lower container below level of bowel.			
f. Alternate instilling and siphoning fluid while gas is returned with fluid.			
g. Clamp tubing before removing it.			
11.–17. Follow Checklist steps 11–17 of the General Procedure.			
Evaluation			
18. Evaluate, using the following criteria: a. Quantity of gas expelled with fluid			
b. Degree of patient's comfort after procedure			

(continued)

© 1996 by Lippincott-Raven Publishers

Administering a Return-Flow Enema (Continued)	Needs More Practice	Satisfactory	Comments
Documentation			
19. Document on the progress notes the time of the return flow, the amount of gas expelled, and the degree of comfort after the procedure.			
Administering a Pediatric Enema			
Assessment			
1.–2. Follow Checklist steps 1 and 2 of the General Procedure for Administering Enemas (verify order and patient's ability to retain fluid and tolerate activity).			
Planning			
3. Wash your hands.			
4. Gather equipment and volume of fluid appropriate to child's age.			
5. Obtain commode or bedpan if appropriate.			
Implementation			
6. Identify patient.			
7. Explain procedure for child's age.			
8. Position child appropriately for age.			
9. Put on clean gloves.			
10. Administer enema. a. Instill appropriate volume of fluid for age.			
b. Gently insert lubricated tip of tubing appropriate depth for age.			
c. Give fluid slowly and observe closely for response to fluid and pressure.			
11. Encourage child to retain fluid as long as possible.			
12. Gently massage abdomen.			
13. Clean child and rediaper infant.			
14. Spend time with child for reassurance.			
15.–17. Follow Checklist steps 15–17 of the General Procedure (clean or dispose of equipment, remove gloves and discard, wash your hands).			

(*continued*)

© 1996 by Lippincott-Raven Publishers

Administering a Pediatric Enema (Continued)	Needs More Practice	Satisfactory	Comments
Evaluation			
18. Evaluate results of enema and child's response.			
Documentation			
19. Record time, type of enema, amount of fluid instilled, results, and child's response.			

© 1996 by Lippincott-Raven Publishers

? QUIZ

Short-Answer Questions

1. List four types of enemas and give the purpose for each type.

Type	Indication for use
a. _____	_____
b. _____	_____
c. _____	_____
d. _____	_____

2. List three reasons enemas upset many persons.

   a. _____

   b. _____

   c. _____

3. List four observations to be made of the patient while administering an enema.

   a. _____

   b. _____

   c. _____

   d. _____

4. How is fluid siphoned out of the bowel when giving a return-flow enema?_____
   _____

5. If a patient complains of severe cramping while an enema is being administered, what action should you take?_____
   _____

6. What are two advantages of prepackaged disposable enemas?

   a. _____

   b. _____

7. List three reasons medications are instilled by rectum.

   a. _____

   b. _____

   c. _____

8. What size tubing should be used to give an enema to a 7-month-old?
   _____

9. What is the maximum volume of fluid that can be used for a cleansing enema for a 4-year-old child? _____

© 1996 by Lippincott-Raven Publishers

10. What two adaptations may be necessary when administering enemas to the person of advanced age?

a. _____

b. _____

© 1996 by Lippincott-Raven Publishers

MODULE

29

TUBE FEEDING

MODULE CONTENTS

RATIONALE FOR THE USE OF THIS
  SKILL
TYPES OF FEEDING TUBES
FORMULAS FOR TUBE FEEDING
ADMINISTERING MEDICATIONS WHEN
  TUBE FEEDING
SCHEDULING A TUBE FEEDING
ADMINISTERING A TUBE FEEDING
PROCEDURE FOR TUBE FEEDING
  Assessment
  Planning
  Implementation
  Evaluation
  Documentation
USE OF A PUMP FOR TUBE FEEDINGS
COMPLICATIONS OF TUBE FEEDING
OPENING AN OCCLUDED FEEDING
  TUBE
CRITICAL THINKING EXERCISES

PREREQUISITES

Successful completion of the following modules:

VOLUME 1
Module 1   An Approach to Nursing Skills
Module 2   Basic Infection Control
Module 3   Safety
Module 5   Documentation
Module 6   Introduction to Assessment Skills
Module 10 Intake and Output

© 1996 by Lippincott-Raven Publishers

OVERALL OBJECTIVE

To safely administer tube feeding, using water and the appropriate formula in the proper amounts.

SPECIFIC LEARNING OBJECTIVES

Know Facts and Principles	Apply Facts and Principles	Demonstrate Ability	Evaluate Performance
1. Formulas Know components of various basic formulas and correct temperature for administration.	State relationship of formula chosen to needs of patient.	In clinical situation, identify formula ordered.	
2. Equipment List items needed to carry out tube feeding.	Select or adapt equipment.	Use equipment in safe, efficient manner.	Using Performance Checklist, review type of equipment with instructor.
3. Safety Name methods for checking placement of tube.	Decide which are the more reliable methods.	Use reliable methods for checking placement of tube correctly in practice.	Evaluate own performance, using Performance Checklist.
4. Psychological support Discuss importance of presenting a *meal* rather than a treatment to patient.	Adapt equipment to improve patient's psychological response.	Maintain attitude that allows patient dignity.	
5. Carrying out tube feeding Outline correct procedure and reasons for each step.	Identify modifications needed for individual patients.	Carry out tube feeding using correct technique.	Evaluate own performance, using Performance Checklist.
6. Documentation State format and items to be recorded, including pertinent observations.	Explain recording format used in specific facility.	Document procedure using proper format and including pertinent observations.	Evaluate own performance, using Performance Checklist.

© 1996 by Lippincott-Raven Publishers

LEARNING ACTIVITIES

1. Review the Specific Learning Objectives.
2. Read the chapter on nutrition in Ellis and Nowlis, *Nursing: A Human Needs Approach,* or a comparable chapter in another textbook.
3. Look up the module vocabulary terms in the glossary.
4. Read through the module as though you were preparing to teach the contents to another person. Mentally practice the procedure.
5. Review the anatomy of the gastrointestinal and respiratory tracts.
6. In the practice setting:
   a. If tube feeding equipment is available, arrange for time to become familiar with the equipment you will need to carry out the procedure.
   b. If a manikin is available, simulate the procedure, using different types of equipment.
   c. Evaluate your performance with a partner or your instructor.
7. In the clinical setting:
   a. Observe the administration of a tube feeding. Was the procedure properly followed?
   b. When you are ready, administer a tube feeding with your instructor's supervision.
   c. Review your performance with your instructor.
   d. Document the procedure and your observations.
   e. Share your documentation with your instructor.

VOCABULARY

aspiration	gag reflex	lumen	percutaneous endo-
comatose	gastric gavage	nasal mucosa	scopic gastrostomy
distention	gastrostomy	nasogastric tube	(PEG) tube
esophagus	jejunum	osmolarity	peristalsis
flatus	lactose	patent	reservoir

© 1996 by Lippincott-Raven Publishers

Tube Feeding

Rationale for the Use of This Skill

The purpose of tube feeding is to enhance the nutritional status of patients who are unable to take adequate amounts of food normally. For example, patients with chronic conditions such as cancer or acquired immune deficiency virus (AIDS) may experience wasting from inadequate nutrition and may need supplements that they are unable to take orally. Unconscious patients need nutrients supplied for them until they regain consciousness. Tube feeding formulas can supply them with a well-balanced and complete diet. It is one of the nurse's primary functions to carefully and efficiently provide feedings through the feeding tube until patients can eat unaided.[1]

TYPES OF FEEDING TUBES

Tube feeding is done by introducing the feeding or formula through a tube directly into the gastrointestinal tract. The tube most commonly used is a nasogastric tube, which is passed through the nose, down the esophagus, and into the stomach.

Standard nasogastric tubes are made of firm, clear plastic and come in three general sizes: adult, pediatric (for small children), and infant. Red rubber nasogastric tubes have generally been replaced with those made of plastic. Tubes are manufactured in a variety of sizes, designated by "French" categories. A number 16 French tube is larger than a number 14 French.

Another type of tube used is the small-diameter silicone rubber tube (Keofeed). These tubes are made of a white, very soft, nonirritating rubber. They are used because they cause less irritation and because the cardiac sphincter at the top of the stomach closes more tightly around them, thus *decreasing the potential for regurgitation of stomach contents around the feeding tube.* Research has shown that one disadvantage of the small-bore tubes is difficulty in aspirating gastrointestinal contents to validate proper placement.

In adults and children, the tube is usually passed through the nostril into the stomach and remains in place for intermittent or continuous feedings. A clean tube should be inserted into the other nostril *when the current tube is 1) no longer patent, 2) irritating the nasal mucosa, or 3) possibly harboring microorganisms. Because there are no clearly defined times,* the decision to change the tube often rests with the nurse.

Some facilities have a policy specifying the interval between tube changes.

For infants, such as those who are premature and who must be fed by a nasogastric tube, you may introduce the tube through the mouth each time a feeding is needed, administer the formula, and remove the tube. A clean tube is used each time.

You will also be caring for patients who are being fed through a tube that has been surgically placed directly through the abdominal wall into the stomach. This surgical procedure is called a *gastrostomy.* The tube used has a much larger lumen than the nasogastric tube, may be sutured into place until healing is complete, and is protected by a light dressing.

A percutaneous endoscopic gastrostomy (PEG) tube is a gastrostomy tube that has been placed through the skin into the stomach using an endoscope to ensure correct placement rather than using an open surgical procedure to place the tube. These tubes may be used for those with long-term feeding needs such as the chronically ill, the comatose patient, or the child with burns of the esophagus.

A jejunostomy tube is used for feedings for some patients. This tube may be inserted in the same way a gastrostomy tube is inserted, but its end is positioned in the jejunum. Because the feeding goes directly into the jejunum, the possibility of regurgitation and aspiration of feedings is almost eliminated. Vomiting may still occur with resultant aspiration.

An esophagostomy tube is surgically inserted into the esophagus. It is usually located above the clavicle to one side of the trachea. It passes beside the trachea into the esophagus that is located posteriorly. The esophagostomy tube is more often used for the ambulatory or home care patient who has a condition of the mouth and throat that makes it impossible to take oral food and fluids. Feedings can be done without the patient removing clothing as is necessary when using a gastrostomy tube.

FORMULAS FOR TUBE FEEDING

Many types of formulas are used for tube feeding, some offering a more balanced diet than others.

Most commercially prepared formulas contain approximately 1 kcal/mL. Some companies also make a high-calorie formula that provides 1.5 or 2 kcal/mL. This high-nutrient content is valuable for those whose caloric needs are so great that too large a volume of the standard formula would have to be administered to provide the desired calories. The high-calorie formula is more likely to cause adverse responses, such as diarrhea and vomiting.

The standard formulas contain all the required ba-

[1]Rationale for action is emphasized throughout the module by the use of italics.

© 1996 by Lippincott-Raven Publishers

sic nutrients. They contain proteins that provide all the essential amino acids and a wide array of vitamins and minerals. Essential fatty acids are included, and most have polyunsaturated fats as opposed to saturated fats. Carbohydrates provide the needed calories. The standard formulas are designed to provide a complete nutritional balance when all dietary calories are derived from the formula.

A variety of specialized formulas are also available. Some contain soluble fiber to assist with bowel function. Some have a specific low lipid content for those who need a dietary restriction on fat. Lactose-free formula is available for the lactose-intolerant person who develops diarrhea and bloating from ingesting foods containing lactose. Formulas that have a low osmolarity are available *because some individuals develop diarrhea from high-osmolarity formula.*

In some settings, a formula prepared by the dietary department may be used. This formula consists of eggs, milk, corn syrup, salt, a blenderized vegetable, fruit juice, and water. Pureed meat and cereal may be added. This formula is carefully designed to provide all needed nutrients. However, it is more likely to become contaminated *because it is not processed in the same way as commercial formula.* Therefore, extra care must be taken in its use. It is also more subject to precipitation and occlusion of the tube than is commercial formula. Its main advantage is its lower cost.

Formulas are also available that contain only substances that require little or no digestion and do not leave residue in the intestine. These are known as elemental feedings. They can be administered into the stomach or directly into the small intestine. They may be used when digestion is impaired or when the bowel must be rested. Commercially canned formulas need not be refrigerated until they are opened. They are then promptly cooled and stored in the refrigerator *to prevent growth of microorganisms.* If the opened refrigerated can is not used within 24 hours, it is discarded. Check the can of formula for an expiration date, and do not administer if outdated. Bockus (1993) lists the characteristics of the more commonly used tube feeding formulas. Additional water is usually needed by the person receiving tube feedings. The amount may be ordered by the physician or may be adjusted by the nurse based on observation of the urine. If the urine remains pale and dilute (of a low specific gravity), then the patient is usually receiving enough water. Dark or concentrated urine usually indicates that the patient needs more water. The water may be given after intermittent feedings to rinse out the tube, after medications are administered, and at prescribed times.

ADMINISTERING MEDICATIONS WHEN TUBE FEEDING

Oral medications can also be given by tube. Ideally, medications should be in liquid form. Consult with the pharmacist and the physician to facilitate obtaining medications that are available in liquid form. However, some medications are not available in liquid form or the liquid form may contain sweeteners or other additives that are contraindicated.

For medications not in liquid form, the following guidelines apply. Gelatin-like medications such as stool softeners can be briefly microwaved in a paper cup on a low setting to liquefy the product. They are cooled and then administered by tube. Products containing psyllium are dissolved in large quantities of water *because they tend to solidify and obstruct the feeding tube.* When psyllium is used for the treatment of diarrhea, the product should be mixed with room temperature formula. Tablets that are not enteric coated must be finely crushed and dissolved in water to be administered. Capsules are opened and the contents dissolved in water. Sometimes the contents do not dissolve well but may be suspended in the water long enough for administration. Enteric-coated tablets and time-release capsules or tablets should not be crushed for administration *because the time of absorption will be changed, resulting in too much drug at one time and not enough at another.*

Flush the tube thoroughly with water after administration of all medications *to avoid obstruction of the tube.* It is best to give medication at the beginning of a feeding *so that if, for any reason, the full amount of formula is not given, the medication will have been administered.* Medications should never be dissolved in the formula *because you cannot ensure that the patient receives the whole dose in a timely manner.*

SCHEDULING A TUBE FEEDING

The physician will determine the type and amount of tube feeding and the intervals at which it is to be administered. The most common method is continuous infusion over a 24-hour period. When long-term use of tube feedings is necessary, a cyclic method is often more convenient for the patient. In this method, the tube feeding is given over 16 hours, and no feeding is administered during the other 8-hour period. For an ambulatory patient, the period without the tube feeding is usually during the daytime to facilitate activity. Bolus feedings in which a prescribed volume is given over 30 to 60 minutes, four to six times a day, are used in some instances.

© 1996 by Lippincott-Raven Publishers

When tube feedings are initiated, it is common practice to begin with a slow rate of administration and gradually increase the rate as the patient exhibits the ability to tolerate the feeding without adverse effects. Table 29–1 is an example of a planned program for initiating feedings using a variety of formulas.

ADMINISTERING A TUBE FEEDING

When administering a tube feeding to any patient, do not hurry or force the feeding; *this can cause distention and discomfort*. In fact, if the patient is alert, you will find that the time for feeding *is an excellent time for communication and assessment*.

Use clean technique when you administer a tube feeding, and remember that this feeding is actually the patient's meal. The formula should be at room temperature but not warm *because milk products with added nutrients can be an ideal medium for the growth of bacteria*. Serving tube feedings at refrigerator temperature can cause cramping. Cold formula also has been found to increase diarrhea. Commercial formulas have been heat sterilized and are considered

safe for administration if they do not hang at room temperature longer than 8 hours.

In some facilities, a blue or green food coloring is added to tube feedings *to make it easier to identify formula contamination of respiratory secretions*. In the past, methylene blue was used for this purpose. This is not advised because methylene blue must be excreted by the kidneys and may increase the chance of renal dysfunction. Excess methylene blue is deposited in the patient's tissues, and patients have been known to develop a bluish coloring of the skin and mucous membranes from it. Blue food coloring is currently used for this purpose, although many experts advise that this is not necessary.

Formula in respiratory secretions can be identified through testing for glucose content of secretions. Normal respiratory secretions do not have high glucose content. Respiratory secretions contaminated with formula have high glucose content. This indicates that the patient is aspirating formula, and the chance of aspiration pneumonia is very high. Follow the procedure in your facility regarding coloring of the formula. When food coloring is added, only a few drops per can of formula is necessary *because the tube feeding needs only a slight touch of color*.

Table 29–1. Feeding Schedule Information

	Osmolite Osmolite HN			Ensure plus HN TwoCal HN Vital HN		
	Step	Strength	Rate mL/hr	Step	Strength	Rate mL/hr
Continuous (infusion over a 24-hr period)	1	Full	50	1	Half	50
	2	Full	75	2	Half	75
	3	Full	100	3	Half	75–100
	4	Full	100–125	4	3 qtr	75–100
				5	Full	75–100
Cyclic (infusion over a 16-hr period)	1	Full	50	1	Half	50
	2	Full	75	2	Half	100
	3	Full	100	3	Half	125–150
	4	Full	125	4	3 qtr	125–150
	5	Full	150	5	Full	125–150
Bolus (A prescribed volume given over 30–60 min 4–6 times/day) Total vol in 24 hr 2,400 mL			mL/fdg			mL/fdg
	1	Full	300–4x/d	1	Half	300–4x/d
	2	Full	400–4x/d	2	Half	400–4x/d
	3	Full	400–5x/d	3	3 qtr	400–4x/d
	4	Full	400–6x/d	4	Full	400–5x/d
				5	Full	400–6x/d

(Courtesy Group Health Cooperative, Seattle, Washington)

© 1996 by Lippincott-Raven Publishers

When tube feedings are first initiated, the formula may be used in a dilute form, and an amount less than the expected caloric needs may be given—for example, equal parts of formula and water. The feedings are then gradually increased in strength and amount. *This practice helps to prevent diarrhea, which can result from the sudden change in consistency and content of the diet.*

PROCEDURE FOR TUBE FEEDING

Assessment

1. Check the physician's order. The type and specific amount of formula and water and the time of the feedings will be noted. This information may be found on both the original order and the medication sheet in some facilities.
2. Read any observations about previous feedings noted in the patient's chart. *This will give you a clearer idea of the patient's tolerance for the procedure.*

Planning

3. Wash your hands *for infection control.*
4. Identify whether the patient is to be fed using the intermittent or continuous method. If the continuous method is to be used, determine if a pump is at the bedside or is available.
5. Gather any equipment you will need. Regardless of the method, you will need a stethoscope *for checking the position of the feeding tube*, the ordered tube feeding formula, clean gloves, and one of the following:
   a. Reservoir tube feeding set
   b. Prefilled tube feeding set
   Feeding sets and tubing for continuous feedings are changed every 24 hours *to protect the patient from bacterial growth in the equipment.* Graham et al. (1993) found that there were no adverse effects for the patient if the feeding set was cleaned properly and changed every 72 hours instead of every 24 hours. Check with the policy of the facility. Label the equipment with date and time *to facilitate appropriate changing of equipment.*

Implementation

6. Identify the patient *to be sure you are carrying out the procedure for the correct patient.*
7. Explain what you are going to do.
8. Place the patient in semi-Fowler's position. *This position will help gravity empty the stomach after feeding and prevent aspiration.*
9. Put on clean gloves.
10. Test for the correct position and patency of the tube and for residual formula.
   a. Because the tube may have become dis-

lodged in the interval between feedings, it is important that you check for position and patency each time before feeding. Research has shown that the most reliable method is to aspirate gastric contents. Use a minimum amount of pressure when aspirating a small-bore tube *to keep it from collapsing.* When done skillfully, this continues to be the most reliable method for checking placement. *This method also is a check for digestion of the previous feeding.* In addition, you may also wish to verify placement by introducing a small amount of air through the tube and listening through a stethoscope for gurgling sounds over the stomach. Metheny (1992) considers the aspiration method as more reliable to verify feeding tube placement than the auscultatory method. The pH of the aspirated contents can also be tested to check for placement. If measured to be acidic (4 or below), the feeding tube is most likely placed correctly in the stomach (Bockus, 1993). This method must be used cautiously *because medications and some medical conditions can alter the gastric pH.*

When initially placed, it is common practice to check small-bore feeding tubes for placement with an x-ray. The position of a feeding tube in continuous use is checked every 8 hours. Although unlikely, it is possible for the tube to shift in position. A tube that is in the esophagus will usually cause aspiration as the formula moves upward as well as downward.

   b. "Checking for residual" refers to aspirating the contents of the stomach *to determine whether there is residual formula from the last feeding.* When feedings are being given on a continuous basis through a pump feeding system, the formula should be consistently moving into the small intestine *so that the residual amount is less than 50 mL.* When there is a large residual, the patient is more likely to have regurgitation of formula through the gastric sphincter into the esophagus and from there it may be aspirated into the lungs, causing aspiration pneumonia. The amount of residual formula in the stomach that indicates that the feeding should be withheld may be indicated in the physician's orders or by facility policy.

   If the aspirated contents contain formula that appears noncurded, or much like the fresh formula, the feeding may be omitted or decreased in amount. In some hospitals, if more than 50 mL undigested formula

© 1996 by Lippincott-Raven Publishers

contents is aspirated, the next feeding is withheld, and the aspirated material is reinstilled through the tube. Gastric contents of any amount should always be returned to the stomach, *so as not to disturb the body's chemical balance.*

11. Depending on the equipment used in your facility, administer a small amount of water first (*to ensure that the tube is patent*), then any medications ordered and, last, the formula. Follow with the remainder of the water, *which rinses formula out of the tubing.*

   a. Reservoir method: In most facilities where a reservoir is used, it is used more than once. Therefore, it must be kept thoroughly cleaned between feedings *so that microorganisms are not harbored in the bag.* The reservoir usually consists of a square-shaped plastic bag with markings calibrated in milliliters. Attached to the reservoir is a drip chamber and tubing (Fig. 29–1).

   (1) Hold the top of the bag open as you instill a portion of the water ordered.

   (2) Open the stopcock until the water has displaced the air left in the tube.

   (3) Attach the tube to the patient's nasogastric tube, and allow the water to enter.

   (4) Clamp before air enters from the bag.

   (5) Pour the formula into the bag and regulate the drip using the stopcock. If the feeding is being delivered by a pump, set the pump appropriately.

   Researchers found that gastrointestinal distress was related to the total volume given and the rate at which it was given. Based on this, the researchers determined that amounts up to 250 mL can be administered at 6 mL/min. For amounts greater than that, 3 mL/min was recommended. Typically, information on the number of drops per milliliter delivered by the equipment is hard to find. It is usually given in the product literature, which may be in the central supply department. Some brands deliver 20 drops/mL. With this equipment, you would give the formula at 60 drops/min to deliver 3 mL/min.

   (6) Before the formula runs completely down the tube, introduce the remainder of the water. *This prevents air from being instilled and rinses the feeding out of the tube.*

   (7) Close the stopcock and detach the reservoir tubing from the nasogastric tube.

   (8) Clamp or plug the nasogastric tube.

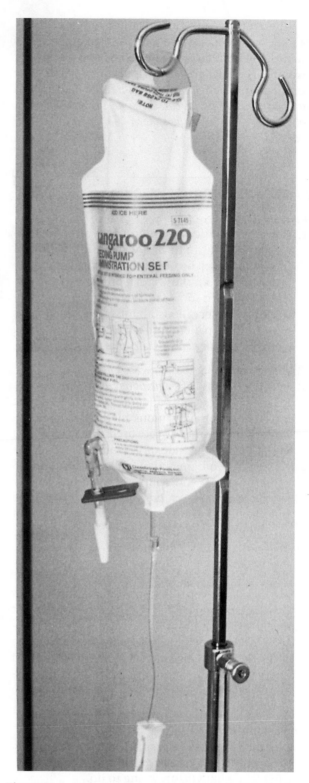

Figure 29–1. In the reservoir method of tube feeding, the formula is in a reservoir container, and the rate of administration is controlled by a roller clamp.

© 1996 by Lippincott-Raven Publishers

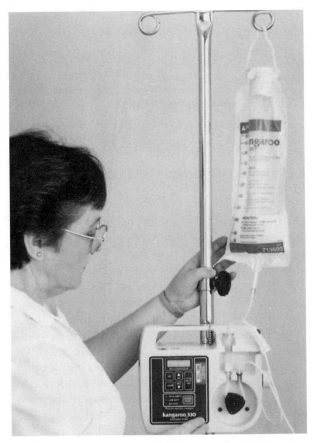

Figure 29–2. A feeding pump controls the rate of administration for the tube feeding.

(9) Clean the bag or bottle thoroughly with water.

Sets that come with a feeding pump that administers a preset volume of formula during a predetermined period (Fig. 29–2) are available.

Because these feedings are frequently given either continuously or over a long period, the formula can grow bacteria. One device has a double pouch *so that ice chips can be placed in the outer section to keep the formula cooled to a safe level.* The formula warms as it drips slowly, so that the patient is not affected.

b. Prefilled tube feeding set: These sets are available commercially and consist of premeasured formula in a plastic container or a minibottle with a drip chamber and tubing (Fig. 29–3).

(1) Remove the sealed screw cap and screw in its place the cap with the drip chamber and tubing.

(2) Hang the bottle on an intravenous pole. Check for placement and residual.

(3) Introduce a small amount of water with an asepto syringe *to ensure that the nasogastric tube is patent.*

(4) Start the flow from the minibottle *to fill the tubing with formula instead of air, so that air is not introduced into the stomach.*

(5) When the formula has filled the tubing, attach the set to the patient's nasogastric tube and begin the feeding.

(6) Follow with water, using the asepto syringe *to flush the formula out of the tubing.*

If this equipment is not available, a small, empty, sterile intravenous bottle and tubing can be successfully adapted for use.

Note: Both methods use gravity flow to move the formula through the tube. If the flow slows or stops, gentle pressure on the asepto bulb or "milking" the tubing may help. If the patient gags during the feeding, stop the procedure.

12. After the feeding, put on clean gloves, disconnect the administration tubing from the patient's feeding tube, clamp the tube tightly or plug it. Discard your gloves.

13. Reposition the patient in low or semi-Fowler's position. If the patient is comatose, the entire patient should be turned so that the head is to

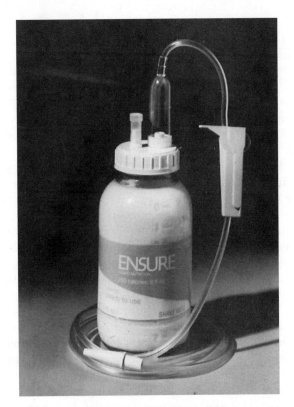

Figure 29–3. A prefilled tube feeding set provides convenience for the patient on continuous infusion. (Courtesy Ross Laboratories, Columbus, Ohio.)

© 1996 by Lippincott-Raven Publishers

DATE/TIME	
6/22/99 1400	GI 350 ml house formula/50 ml water instilled per gastric tube. Feeding retained. —— M. Sumata, SN

Example of Nursing Progress Notes Using Narrative Format.

one side *to prevent aspiration into the lungs if vomiting occurs.*

14. Wash your hands.

Evaluation

15. Return to the patient in approximately 30 minutes *to make sure the feeding has been retained.*

Documentation

16. Document on the medication sheet or progress notes. Your notes should include the date, time, type and amount of formula, amount of water, and patient's response. *Most patients being fed by tube are on intake and output,* so an appropriate entry should be made after each feeding. The total fluid should be entered on the intake and output worksheet.

USE OF A PUMP FOR TUBE FEEDINGS

To deliver tube feedings at a precise rate or through very small-diameter tubes, a rate-controlled pump is sometimes used (see Fig. 29–2). These pumps provide constant positive pressure to the feeding tube. A tubing compatible with the particular pump is used with a reservoir or prefilled tube feeding bag. The procedure is identical to the procedure when a reservoir without a pump is used, except that when the entire setup is complete, the tubing is threaded through the pump according to the directions provided by the manufacturer, and the rate is set on the machine. The machine gives a warning signal if the flow is interrupted or if the tubing runs dry.

Even when feedings are provided continuously, the position of the tube should be rechecked each time additional formula is added to the reservoir. *This prevents unsafe administration of tube feeding in the event the tubing has moved out of correct position.* Rinse the tubing with water after checking for correct position. *This helps to prevent clogging of the tubing and lessens the risk of the growth of microorganisms in the tubing.*

COMPLICATIONS OF TUBE FEEDING

The most common complication of tube feeding is diarrhea. This can be severe enough to compromise nutritional and electrolyte status. Even when it is not severe, skin breakdown and cleanliness become difficult management concerns. Diarrhea can be particularly hazardous for the elderly. Galindo-Ciocon (1993) found that patients on continuous tube feeding experienced more diarrhea than did those on an intermittent tube feeding schedule. High osmolarity, lactose content, too rapid feeding, and too cold a formula (refrigerator temperature) have been identified as possible causes of diarrhea. However, Winslow (1994) presented several research studies that relate tube feeding diarrhea to factors other than the properties of the tube feeding formula. She reports that 79% of cases of diarrhea were not caused by the formula but by prescribed medications. Therefore, when faced with this problem, the nurse should begin by assessing for possible causes. Consultation with the physician may be appropriate. Trial and error is sometimes the only way to find out the specific cause of diarrhea. Table 29–2 lists guidelines for problem-solving.

Researchers have identified dry mouth, sore throat, thirst, and feelings of deprivation as problems experienced by persons on tube feedings. Dry mouth can be improved by frequent mouth care. The use of a small-bore tube helps to prevent sore throat. Throat sprays and gargles cannot be used if the person has an inadequate gag reflex, but they can be of help if the person is alert and has a good cough and gag reflex. Deprivation may be somewhat alleviated by attention to aesthetics and interpersonal relationships.

OPENING AN OCCLUDED FEEDING TUBE

A feeding tube may become occluded with coagulated formula or particles of tablets that were not completely dissolved. To avoid having to remove

© 1996 by Lippincott-Raven Publishers

Table 29–2. Guidelines for Solving Tube Feeding Problems

Complication	Prevention/Treatment
Tube-related	
Aspiration	Check residuals. Evaluate HOB. If ↓ LOC consider jejunostomy. Obtain chest x-ray. Use food coloring in formula if patient is at risk for aspiration.
Obstruction	Irrigate the tube. Always irrigate tube with 30–50 mL water or saline q med. administration. Use elixir forms of drugs. Instillation of a carbonated beverage may be helpful in the event of tube obstruction.
Displacement	Allow sufficient length of tubing to prevent tension or pulling on the tube. Routinely check the position of markings on the tube to determine if slippage has occurred.
Irritation	Esophageal or oropharyngeal—consider smallest diameter tube possible or gastric placement. Nasal or oral—clean and moisten nose, teeth, and oral cavity several times daily and ensure tube is not creating any pressure points.
Gastric distention	Check placement of the tube. If using hypertonic formula, change to one with reduced osmolality.
Metabolic	
Diarrhea	A) Check if patient is receiving medications associated with diarrhea and change the medication if possible. If not, treat with antidiarrheal agent. B) Reduce administration rate, check for impaction, ensure adequate water intake, or use a bulk agent. C) With hyperosmolar formula, reduce strength of formula. D) Check for bacterial contamination of formula or equipment. E) Check serum albumin level. If less than 2.5, may need to change to parenteral route of administration. F) Check for fat malabsorption and change formula. G) Change to a higher-fiber formula. H) Check for presence of menses. Diarrheal episodes often accompany menstruation and usually need no treatment. I) Consider clostridium difficile infection. J) Give Metamucil, 1 tsp qd (flush tube completely with H_2O after Metamucil).
Constipation	A) Give a laxative or enema. B) Use a bulk agent or change to a higher-fiber formula. C) Check for insufficient water given with formula. D) Check if patient is receiving a medication that causes decreased intestinal motility and determine if this can be changed or give stool softeners, additional water, or laxatives, as required. E) Determine if decreased intestinal motility is due to inactivity; increase patient's activity when possible.
Dehydration/↑ Sodium	Correct any abnormal losses, provide increased free water, or adjust formula to decrease the renal solute load.
Glucosuria	Change formula to one of lower CHO content or give insulin. If glucosuria has led to diuresis, provide adequate water replacement.
Azotemia (uremia)	Change formula to one of lower protein content or increase water to aid excretion.
Electrolyte imbalance	Check electrolyte levels for imbalances, determine the cause (ie, concentration of the formula, excessive losses or insufficient excretion, or water depletion or excess), and administer appropriate therapy.

(Courtesy Group Health Cooperative, Seattle, Washington)

and replace a feeding tube, the policy in some facilities allows the nurse to attempt to clear the feeding tube using an enzyme solution. Webber-Jones (1992) suggested instilling a carbonated drink solution through the tube (if this is not contraindicated) before trying the enzyme solution. When used, the enzyme, in liquid form, breaks down the obstructing material and allows it to be flushed out with water. The enzymes used are ones that are broken down by the gastrointestinal system and therefore will not harm the patient. The policy in the institution will prescribe the specific enzyme solution and quantity that may be used. A physician's order may be needed to use this technique.

The enzyme is dissolved in water and then put into the tube with a large syringe that has a tubing

© 1996 by Lippincott-Raven Publishers

DATE/TIME	
2/12/99 0830	D: Patient remains comatose. Left nostril around feeding tube shows mild excoriation.
	A: Obtained order to remove tube and reinsert in right nostril. A&D ointment applied to area.
	R: No crusting around nasogastric tube.
	E. Stowe, RN

Example of Nursing Progress Notes Using Focus Format.

adapter instead of a needle. The enzyme solution is left in place for 10 to 30 minutes to act on the obstruction. The syringe may be used to push and pull the solution in the tube, which may help the enzyme to contact more of the material. When material begins to move in the tube, it is thoroughly flushed with clear water. Carefully flushing the tube with water after feedings and after instilling medications *will help to prevent this problem.*

CRITICAL THINKING EXERCISES

Your 62-year-old male patient experienced a stroke (CVA) 2 weeks ago and has been in a coma. For the last 10 days, he has been on continuous tube feeding and has had copious diarrhea. Identify three possible causes of the diarrhea that relate to tube feeding. What assessment might you carry out to ascertain the cause(s) of the diarrhea? For each possible cause, determine the nursing actions you might take.

Your patient has a small-diameter feeding tube in place. The physician's order is: "Begin tube feeding. One can of complete nutritional formula (Compleat) every 8 hours." You observe that the patient has a low-grade fever and is very diaphoretic. Devise an individualized care plan for this patient.

References

Bockus, S. (1993). When your patient needs tube feedings: Making the right decisions. *Nursing '93, 23*(7), 34–42.

Galindo-Ciocon, D. J. (1993). Tube feeding: Complications among the elderly. *Journal of Gerontological Nursing, 19*(6), 17–22.

Graham, S., McIntyre, M., Chicoine, J., Gerard, B., Laughren, R., Cowley, G., Morrison, J., Aoki, F. Y., & Nicolle, L. E. (Summer 1993). Frequency of changing enteral alimentation bags and tubing, and adverse clinical outcomes in patients in a long term care facility. *Canadian Journal of Infection Control, 8*(2), 41–43.

Meehan, M. (1992). Nursing diagnosis: Potential for aspiration. *RN, 55*(1), 30–34.

Metheny, N. (1992). Effectiveness of the auscultatory method in predicting feeding tube location. *Nursing Research, 41*(3), 41–43.

Webber-Jones, J. (1992). How to declog a feeding tube. *Nursing '92, 22*(4), 62–64.

Winslow, E. H. (1994). Diarrhea not always linked to tube feedings. *American Journal of Nursing, 94*(4), 59–60.

© 1996 by Lippincott-Raven Publishers

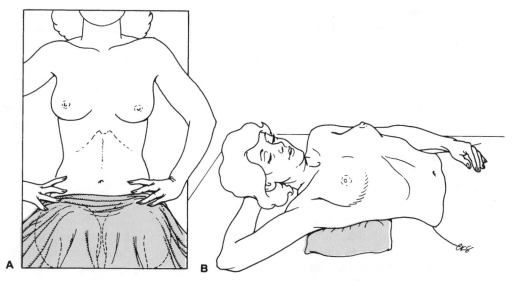

Figure 9–6. Examining the breasts. (**A**) Ask the patient to press hands against hips to bring out dimpling or retraction that might otherwise not be noticed. (**B**) Place a small pillow under the patient's shoulder on the side you are examining and have the patient raise that arm over the head.

by gently compressing the breast tissue against the chest wall. The consistency of breast tissue varies among females, primarily according to age: that of younger women is firm and elastic; that of older women is more stringy and nodular. In addition, be aware of the stage of the menstrual cycle of menstruating females because the breasts can be particularly sensitive at the time of menstruation.

5. Document and report the breast assessment only, the examination of the heart, lungs, and breasts together, or incorporate these findings into a more comprehensive assessment.

Abdomen/Rectum

Inspection of the abdomen, auscultation of bowel sounds, percussion and palpation of the abdomen, palpation of the liver, assessment for ascites, and digital examination of the rectum are grouped together because aspects of these examinations are commonly considered together. Although they may all be done at the same time, they can, of course, be done separately. As indicated, you will use inspection, auscultation, percussion, and palpation when you assess the abdomen and rectum.

Bowel Sounds

Normal bowel sounds, which indicate normal peristaltic activity, are relatively high-pitched and occur every 5 to 15 seconds. They are more frequent im-

mediately before and after eating. The absence of sound or the presence of very soft or infrequent sounds (commonly called *hypo*active bowel sounds) indicates decreased motility, as would occur after abdominal surgery, or with peritonitis or paralytic ileus. Loud, high-pitched rushing sounds (or *hyper*active bowel sounds) indicate increased motility and occur with gastroenteritis, diarrhea, and laxative use.

Vascular Sounds

Bruits are abnormal blowing sounds accompanying each heartbeat or pulse, which are sometimes heard over the aorta, or the renal, iliac, or femoral arteries. They may indicate a narrowed vessel or an aneurysm.

Percussion of the Abdomen

The abdomen is percussed to disclose patterns of tympany and dullness that might give clues to what you can expect to find when palpating. Tympany indicates air in the intestines; dullness occurs when you percuss over a distended· bladder, fluid, or a mass.

Palpation of the Abdomen and Liver

Inspect and auscultate the abdomen before carrying out percussion and palpation *because percussion and palpation can change the bowel sounds.*
    Palpate the abdomen *to evaluate muscle tone and to*

© 1996 by Lippincott-Raven Publishers

check for distension and tenderness. If tenderness is noted, assess for guarding (muscle rigidity). Guarding may occur because the patient is nervous or ticklish, or it may indicate an acute inflammatory process. Palpation of the liver is part of the overall procedure. The normal liver is not palpable. An enlarged nontender liver suggests chronic disease; an enlarged tender liver suggests acute disease.

Ascites

Ascites is a large accumulation of fluid in the peritoneal cavity that can cause respiratory distress because of the pressure of the fluid on the diaphragm. Ascites can be difficult to identify, especially in an obese person. One way to differentiate between obesity and ascites is to test for a fluid wave, which indicates the presence of fluid in the peritoneal cavity. Tap one side of the abdomen. If fluid is present, the impact of the tap will be felt by the other hand placed alongside the opposite abdominal wall.

Ongoing assessment of ascites usually includes serial measurement of abdominal girth *to identify changes that are occurring.* You will need a felt-tip marker and a measuring tape *to carry out this procedure.*

Digital Examination of the Rectum

A digital examination of the rectum is usually performed *when fecal impaction is suspected,* based on the patient's complaint of long-term or abnormal constipation, or the leakage of watery stool in the absence of actual bowel movements.

PROCEDURE FOR ASSESSMENT OF THE ABDOMEN/RECTUM

This procedure includes assessment of bowel and abdominal vascular sounds, percussion and palpation of the abdomen and liver, assessment for ascites, and digital examination of the rectum.

1. Determine the need for assessment of the abdomen or rectum.
2. Obtain a stethoscope to assess the abdomen. If you plan to do a digital examination of the rectum, you will also need clean gloves, a lubricant, and a bedpan.
3. Place the patient in the supine position and arrange the patient's gown or pajama top to cover the chest and expose the abdomen. Fanfold the bed linen down to the symphysis pubis.

4. Inspect the abdomen, noting especially any scars, rashes, or other lesions; contour (flat, rounded, or distended); symmetry; and any visible masses or pulsations.
5. Listen for bowel sounds and vascular sounds.
   a. Lightly place the diaphragm of the warmed stethoscope on the abdomen.
   b. Auscultate all four quadrants in a systematic fashion.
      (1) Place the diaphragm of the stethoscope lightly against the skin of the right lower quadrant.
      (2) Start with the right lower quadrant *because bowel sounds are often most pronounced (and most easily heard) there. Because bowel sounds are irregular,* listen for 4 or 5 minutes before you report absent bowel sounds.
      (3) Move systematically until you have listened to all four quadrants. If no sounds are heard in a quadrant, continue to listen in that quadrant for a minimum of 2 to 5 minutes.
   c. Continuing to use the diaphragm of the stethoscope, but using firmer pressure, listen over the aorta and renal, iliac, and femoral arteries for the presence of bruits. If you hear any bruits, do not palpate over the area where the abnormal sounds were heard.
6. Percuss the abdomen. To make your examination systematic and to clarify your descriptions, mentally divide the abdomen into quadrants. The horizontal line extends across through the umbilicus; the vertical line extends downward from the xiphoid process to the symphysis pubis. The four quadrants are the *right upper quadrant* (RUQ), the *right lower quadrant* (RLQ), the *left lower quadrant* (LLQ), and the *left upper quadrant* (LUQ) (Fig. 9–7). Dullness may indicate the presence of fluid. Tympany in the left upper quadrant may indicate a gastric air bubble.
7. Palpate the abdomen.
   a. Use the pads of your fingers to palpate the abdomen. Your fingernails should extend only to the tips of your fingers. If your fingernails are too long, palpation will be difficult for you to perform without causing discomfort to the patient.
   b. Ask the patient to breathe through the mouth *to enhance relaxation.*
   c. Moving systematically, palpate gently for tone (softness versus rigidity), swelling, and tenderness. Also assess for rebound tenderness (pain elicited when you release your

© 1996 by Lippincott-Raven Publishers

✔ PERFORMANCE CHECKLIST

Procedure for Tube Feeding	Needs More Practice	Satisfactory	Comments
Assessment			
1. Check physician's order for type, amount, and time of feedings.			
2. Read any notations on chart about previous feedings.			
Planning			
3. Wash your hands.			
4. Identify whether intermittent or continuous method is to be used.			
5. Gather equipment needed.			
Implementation			
6. Identify patient.			
7. Explain what you are going to do.			
8. Place patient in semi-Fowler's position.			
9. Put on clean gloves.			
10. Check tube for correct placement and residual formula.			
11. Proceed with instillation.			
12. After the feeding, put on clean gloves, disconnect tubing, and clamp or plug both tubings. Remove gloves.			
13. Reposition patient with head to one side.			
14. Wash your hands.			
Evaluation			
15. Return to patient in approximately 30 minutes to be sure feeding has been retained.			
Documentation			
16. Document procedure in patient's chart or on medication record.			

© 1996 by Lippincott-Raven Publishers

? Q U I Z

Multiple-Choice Questions

_____ **1.** Each milliliter of blended formula normally yields approximately

    a. 1 calorie.
    b. 2 calories.
    c. 5 calories.
    d. 10 calories.

_____ **2.** For administration, the formula should be

    a. hot.
    b. cold.
    c. at room temperature.
    d. at whatever temperature is convenient.

_____ **3.** To prevent gastric distention, you should

    a. feed the patient only every 4 hours.
    b. allow as little air as possible to enter the tube.
    c. rinse the tube well with water after the feeding.
    d. feed rapidly.

_____ **4.** The head of a comatose patient should be turned to the side after feeding to prevent

    a. vomiting.
    b. aspiration.
    c. distention.
    d. indigestion.

_____ **5.** The patient should be checked approximately 30 minutes after feeding for

    a. vomiting.
    b. drowsiness.
    c. anorexia.
    d. diarrhea.

_____ **6.** If the tubing does not appear to be in the stomach when you check it, your first action should be to

    a. give the feeding slowly.
    b. remove the tube immediately.
    c. not give the feeding.
    d. call the physician for a decision.

_____ **7.** If the patient begins to gag while you are tube feeding, you should

    a. stop the feeding for a time.
    b. continue with the feeding as planned.
    c. give additional feeding.
    d. give medication for nausea.

Short-Answer Questions

8. When is plain water given to a patient through a feeding tube?

_____

_____

© 1996 by Lippincott-Raven Publishers

9. How can you check respiratory secretions to determine if the patient has aspirated formula?

_____

_____

10. If there is 150 mL residual tube feeding aspirated, what should be your next step?

_____

_____

11. Research has shown that one of the most common causes of diarrhea for the person who is being fed is/are _____

_____

12. How might an occluded feeding tube be opened?

_____

© 1996 by Lippincott-Raven Publishers

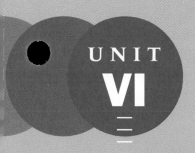

Procedures for Special Situations

MODULE 30
Emergency Resuscitation Procedures

MODULE 31
Postmortem Care

MODULE

30

EMERGENCY RESUSCITATION PROCEDURES

MODULE CONTENTS

RATIONALE FOR THE USE OF THIS
  SKILL
INTRODUCTION
INFECTION TRANSMISSION CONCERNS
  IN CPR
CARDIOPULMONARY RESUSCITATION
PERFORMING ADULT CPR
One-Rescuer CPR
  Airway
  Breathing
  Circulation
Two-Rescuer CPR
  Airway
  Breathing
  Circulation
Monitoring the Patient
Terminating CPR
PERFORMING CPR FOR INFANTS
  AND SMALL CHILDREN

Airway
Breathing
Circulation
CPR in the Healthcare Facility
Documentation
MANAGEMENT OF FOREIGN-BODY
  AIRWAY OBSTRUCTION
Foreign-Body Airway Obstruction: Adults
  Recognition
  Management
Foreign-Body Airway Obstruction: Infants
  and Small Children
  Recognition
  Management
LONG-TERM CARE
HOME CARE
CRITICAL THINKING EXERCISES

PREREQUISITES

Successful completion of the following modules:

VOLUME 1
Module 6 Introduction to Assessment Skills
Module 7 Temperature, Pulse, and Respiration

© 1996 by Lippincott-Raven Publishers

OVERALL OBJECTIVE

To recognize the need for emergency resuscitation procedures and to perform these on adults, children, and infants.[1]

SPECIFIC LEARNING OBJECTIVES

Know Facts and Principles	Apply Facts and Principles	Demonstrate Ability	Evaluate Performance
1. Cardiopulmonary resuscitation (CPR)			
a. Airway			
State usual method for opening airway. State method used in case of cervical injury.	Given a patient situation, identify appropriate method for opening airway.	Open airway on manikin, using both methods described.	Evaluate with instructor and lab partner.
b. Breathing			
Describe usual method for rescue breathing. Describe alternative methods used in special situations.	Given a patient situation, identify appropriate method of rescue breathing.	Demonstrate mouth-to-mouth, mouth-to-nose, and mouth-to-barrier device breathing.	Evaluate effectiveness by checking chest for movement.
c. Circulation			
State where to palpate carotid pulse. State where to apply compression on adults and children. State distance sternum must be moved for effective compression.		Apply compression in appropriate location. Move sternum appropriate distance when doing cardiac compression.	Evaluate by checking for adequate compression on manikin gauge, if available.
d. One rescuer			
State ratio of breaths to compression for one rescuer.		Perform CPR alone on manikin.	Evaluate with instructor, using Performance Checklist.
e. Two rescuers			
State ratio of breaths to compression for two rescuers.		Perform two-person CPR with partner on manikin.	Evaluate with instructor, using Performance Checklist.
f. Age considerations			
State differences in procedure for adults, small children, and infants.		Perform CPR on infant manikin, incorporating techniques that differ from adult procedure.	Evaluate with instructor, using Performance Checklist.

(continued)

---

[1]Material in this module, including Figs. 30–13 and 30–15 through 30–18, conforms to the American Heart Association recommendations as of 1992.

© 1996 by Lippincott-Raven Publishers

S P E C I F I C   L E A R N I N G   O B J E C T I V E S (c o n t i n u e d)

Know Facts and Principles	Apply Facts and Principles	Demonstrate Ability	Evaluate Performance
g. Documentation State two items of particular importance to be observed and documented when CPR is carried out.		Observe and document accurately during real or simulated CPR.	Evaluate own performance with instructor.
2. Foreign-body airway obstruction *a. Recognition* Describe the universal distress signal for choking.	Given a patient situation, state whether you would intervene.	In a simulated situation, demonstrate how to determine that airway obstruction is present.	
b. Management Describe two aspects of attempting to dislodge a foreign-body airway obstruction.	Given a situation (victim conscious or unconscious), state how procedure would be carried out.	Using a manikin, demonstrate correct procedure for dislodgment of foreign body in both upright and supine positions.	Evaluate with your instructor.
c. Age considerations State differences in procedure for infants and small children.		Using an infant manikin, demonstrate correct procedure for dislodgment of foreign body.	Evaluate with your instructor.

© 1996 by Lippincott-Raven Publishers

LEARNING ACTIVITIES

1. Review the Specific Learning Objectives.
2. Read the section on basic life support (in the chapter on circulation) in Ellis and Nowlis, *Nursing: A Human Needs Approach*, or comparable material in another textbook.
3. Look up the module vocabulary terms in the glossary.
4. Read through the module as though you were preparing to teach CPR to another person. Mentally practice the skills.
5. In the laboratory, practice with a Resusci-Annie or similar manikin under your instructor's supervision.
   a. Establish an airway on the adult manikin.
   b. Breathe 12 times per minute into the adult manikin, allowing 1½ to 2 seconds per breath, watching for the rise and fall of the chest wall and allowing for "exhalation."
   c. Practice closed chest massage on the adult manikin at a rate of 80 to 100 compressions per minute, compressing the sternum 1½ to 2 inches each time.
   d. Establish an airway on an infant manikin.
   e. Breathe 20 times per minute into the infant manikin, allowing 1 to 1½ seconds per breath, using only the amount of air needed to cause the chest to rise.
   f. Practice closed chest massage on the infant manikin at a rate of 100 compressions per minute, using only the tips of your index and middle fingers to compress the sternum ½ to 1 inch each time.
6. With a partner, practice CPR on both adult and infant manikins, using the Performance Checklist as a guide. Take turns doing the breathing and the closed chest massage. Have your instructor evaluate your performances.
7. With your partner as observer and evaluator, practice CPR alone on both the adult and infant manikins, using the Performance Checklist as a guide. When you are satisfied with your performance, trade places and have your partner demonstrate CPR on the adult and infant manikins with you observing and evaluating. When you are both satisfied with your performances, have your instructor evaluate them.
8. Working as a pair, simulate the recognition and management of foreign-body airway obstruction on each other or on an adult manikin, using the Performance Checklist as a guide. Practice management of foreign-body airway obstruction on the infant manikin as well. When you are satisfied with your performance, have your instructor evaluate you.

VOCABULARY

airway	defibrillation	sternum	xiphoid process
cardiac arrest	Heimlich maneuver	trachea	ventricular fibrillation
carotid pulse	respiratory arrest	tracheostomy	

© 1996 by Lippincott-Raven Publishers

Emergency Resuscitation Procedures

Rationale for the Use of This Skill

The nurse is expected to carry out emergency resuscitation procedures efficiently, whether on the street, in the home, or in a healthcare facility. The nurse must be able to perform these lifesaving procedures—as a member of a team or alone—on adults, children, and infants. It is good practice to take a refresher course once a year to maintain expertise.[2]

INTRODUCTION

Although these procedures could have been written in such a way as to clearly show the nursing process approach, we chose not to do so for these reasons:

1. Rote memorization is necessary so that you can respond automatically in an emergency situation.
2. National organizations that teach these procedures do not use this format, and it may confuse those who have already been exposed to such courses.

When reviewing the procedures, you may wish to identify for yourself which steps constitute assessment, planning, implementation, and evaluation.

INFECTION TRANSMISSION CONCERNS IN CARDIOPULMONARY RESUSCITATION (CPR)

There is an extremely low likelihood of disease transmission during Cardiopulmonary resuscitation (CPR) practice and during actual performance of mouth-to-mouth resuscitation. However, healthcare providers may choose to give mouth-to-barrier device ventilation during an actual resuscitation (Fig. 30–1). The Centers for Disease Control and Prevention (CDC) (1994) recommends that these devices be available in acute care settings where CPR is likely to occur more frequently, such as hospitals and day surgery centers.

In healthcare settings, gloves will be available for your use during CPR, providing protection in the event you are exposed to body fluids during an

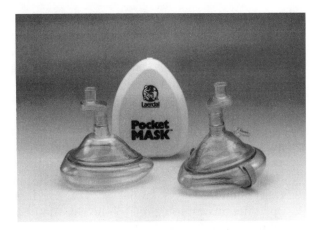

Figure 30–1. Position the barrier device over the patient's mouth and nose, ensure an adequate airseal, and initiate mouth-to-barrier device breathing. The device on the right has an O_2 inlet. (Laerdal™ Pocket Mask™ courtesy Laerdal Medical Corporation, Armonk, New York.)

emergency. It is prudent to carry gloves in your pocket at all times. In other settings you may not or may not have access to gloves. In those situations, use your own best judgment as to how to proceed.

CARDIOPULMONARY RESUSCITATION

CPR is a process of rescue breathing and chest compression that is provided to a person whose heart has stopped beating and who has stopped breathing. No matter where this person is, he or she needs immediate assistance *to restore breathing and circulation. If the delay is longer than 4 minutes, the potential for permanent brain damage is great.* Eventually, you may be involved not only in performing the skill, but in teaching it to other professionals and lay people as well.

PROCEDURE FOR PERFORMING ADULT CPR

Basic CPR is as easy to remember as ABC: Airway, Breathing, and Circulation.

One-Rescuer CPR

Airway

1. Determine unresponsiveness.
   a. When you find a person in a state of collapse, grasp the shoulder firmly, shake, and shout, "Are you all right?"
   b. If you get no response, activate the emergency medical system (EMS) in the healthcare

---

[2]Rationale for action is emphasized throughout the module by the use of italics.

© 1996 by Lippincott-Raven Publishers

facility or, if you are outside the healthcare facility, in your community. *Because most adults with sudden nontraumatic cardiac arrest are found to be in ventricular fibrillation,* a life-threatening cardiac dysrhythmia, survival is highly dependent on early defibrillation, or early system access (American Heart Association, 1992).

2. Position the person flat on the back on a firm, flat surface. If you must roll the person over, try to move the entire body at once, as a single unit, to avoid worsening any injury to the neck, back, or long bones.

3. Open the airway using one of the two methods below.

   a. *Head-tilt/chin-lift maneuver*: Tilt the patient's head back by placing the palm of one hand on the forehead and applying firm backward pressure. Place the fingers of the other hand under the bony part of the lower jaw near the chin, and lift to bring the chin forward. *This will clear the tongue out of the airway.*

   b. *Jaw-thrust maneuver*: *If a patient has been in an accident (an automobile crash, a fall) and you suspect there is a neck injury,* do not open the airway using the chin-lift method. Instead, grasp the angles of the victim's lower jaw and lift with both hands, one on each side, displacing the mandible forward. *Because this maneuver can usually be accomplished without extending the neck,* it is the safest first approach to opening the airway of the child or adult with a possible neck injury (Fig. 30–2). Carefully support the head without tilting it backward or turning it from side to side. If mouth-to-mouth breathing is necessary, you can occlude the nostrils by placing your cheek tightly against them.

Breathing

4. Determine breathlessness. Place your ear close to the patient's mouth and do three things:

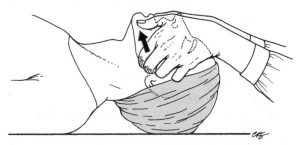

Figure 30–2. Jaw-thrust maneuver. Displacing the mandible is the safest way to open the airway for victims of all ages with suspected neck injury.

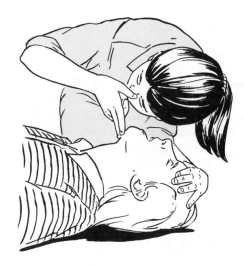

Figure 30–3. Checking for breathing, the airway is kept open by using the head-tilt/chin-lift maneuver.

   a. *Look* at the chest and the stomach for movement.
   b. *Listen* for breathing sounds.
   c. *Feel* for air against your cheek (Fig. 30–3).

5. Sometimes a person begins to breathe spontaneously after an airway has been established. But if you cannot see chest movement, hear breathing sounds, or feel air on your cheek, the patient is not breathing, and you must provide rescue breathing.

   Perform rescue breathing using one of the following methods:

   a. *Mouth-to-mouth breathing*:
      (1) Keeping the airway open by using the head-tilt/chin-lift maneuver, gently pinch the nose closed using the thumb and index finger of the hand on the forehead (Fig. 30–4). *This will prevent air from escaping through the patient's nose.*
      (2) Place your mouth over the patient's mouth, make an airtight seal, and give two initial breaths of 1½ to 2 seconds each. Be sure to allow time for deflation of the patient's lungs between breaths.

   b. *Mouth-to-nose breathing:* If mouth-to-mouth breathing is not desirable or possible (for example, in the presence of vomiting or injury to the mouth or jaw), mouth-to-nose breathing can be done by closing the mouth with one palm and breathing into the nose. The position of the head is the same as for mouth-to-mouth breathing.

   c. *Mouth-to-stoma breathing:* Breathing is possible if the patient has a permanent tracheostomy. In such a case it would not be necessary to tilt the head back to open the airway as you

© 1996 by Lippincott-Raven Publishers

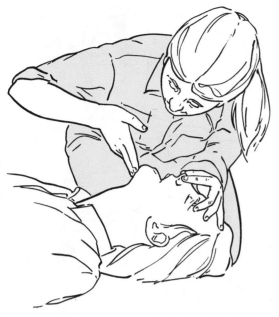

Figure 30-4. To occlude the nostrils, the thumb and index finger of the hand on the forehead gently pinch the nose closed.

would for mouth-to-mouth and mouth-to-nose breathing.

d. *Mouth-to-barrier device:* Two broad categories of barrier devices—mask devices and face shields—currently are available. Mask devices often have a one-way valve *to prevent exhaled air from entering the rescuer's mouth.* Many face shields have no such valve, and air often leaks around the shield. If rescue breathing is necessary and you wish to use a barrier device, position the barrier device over the patient's

mouth and nose, ensure an adequate air seal, and initiate mouth-to-barrier device breathing using slow inspiratory breaths as just described.

6. If after performing rescue breathing you observe the patient's chest rising and falling, showing that air has entered, proceed to step 8 under "Circulation."

7. If, however, you feel resistance when you try to breathe into the patient's mouth and the patient's chest wall does not rise and fall as you breathe, reposition the head and attempt to breathe again. If you still feel resistance, proceed with foreign-body airway obstruction maneuvers, pages 730–732.

Circulation

8. Determine pulselessness. Feel for the carotid pulse by locating the larynx (voice box) and sliding your fingers off into the groove beside it. You should feel for the pulse on your side of the patient (Fig. 30–5) *to avoid compressing the other carotid artery with your thumb.* Adequate time (5–10 seconds) should be allowed, *because the pulse may be slow, irregular, or very weak and rapid.*

   a. *If you locate a pulse,* perform rescue breathing at a rate of 12 breaths/min, rechecking the pulse after each 12 breaths.

   b. *If you cannot locate a pulse,* you will have to provide artificial circulation in addition to rescue breathing.

9. Kneel at the level of the patient's shoulders. *You will then be in a position to perform both rescue breathing and chest compression without moving your knees.* The patient should be on a hard sur-

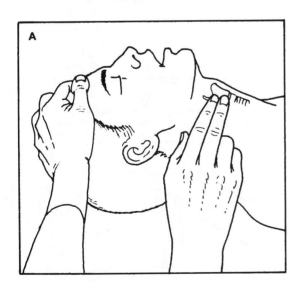
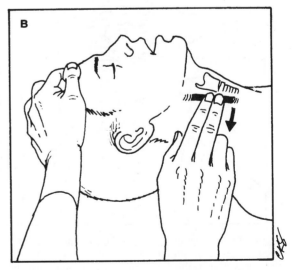

Figure 30-5. To determine pulselessness, feel for the carotid pulse by locating the larynx and sliding your fingers toward yourself into the groove beside it.

© 1996 by Lippincott-Raven Publishers

face to achieve best results. In a healthcare facility, slip a cardiac board under the patient.

10. Position your hands correctly on the patient's chest.

   a. Locate the lower margin of the patient's rib cage on the side nearest you. Run the fingers of the hand nearest the patient's legs up along the rib cage to the indentation where the ribs meet the sternum. Keeping one finger on the indentation, place another immediately above it, on the lower end of the sternum (Fig. 30–6).

   b. Place the heel of your other hand just above that finger, at right angles to the sternum. *This will keep the main force of compression on the sternum and decrease the chance of rib fracture.*

   c. Remove your fingers from the indentation and place that hand on top of the one already in position. Your hands should be parallel and directed away from you (Fig. 30–7). Your fingers may be either extended or interlaced, but they must be kept off the chest *to avoid fracturing a rib* (Fig. 30–8).

11. With your shoulders directly above the patient's chest, compress downward, keeping your arms straight. Move the sternum of an adult 1½ to 2 inches with each compression (Fig. 30–9).

   You must release compression pressure after

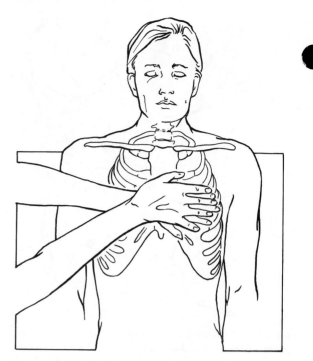

Figure 30–7. Hands in place for chest compression. Your hands should be parallel and directed away from you.

each compression *to allow blood to flow into the heart.* The time allowed for release should equal the time required for compression. Therefore, your motion should be a rhythmical 50% down and 50% back up. Avoid quick, ineffective jabs to the chest *that can increase the possibility of injury*

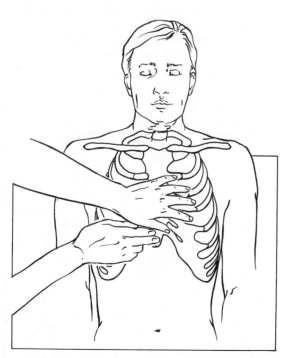

Figure 30–6. To locate the correct hand position for external chest compression, run the fingers of the hand nearest the patient's legs up along the rib cage to the indentation where the ribs meet the sternum. Keeping one finger on the indentation, place another immediately above it and place the heel of your other hand just above that finger.

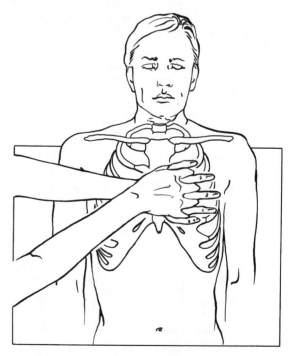

Figure 30–8. Hands in place with fingers interlaced. Fingers must be kept off the chest to avoid fracturing a rib.

© 1996 by Lippincott-Raven Publishers

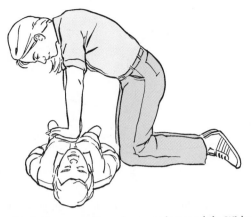

Figure 30–9. Proper position of rescuer for an adult. With your shoulders directly above the patient's chest, compress downward, keeping your arms straight.

and may decrease the amount of blood circulated by each compression. Your hands should not be lifted from the chest or their position changed in any way *so that you do not lose correct hand position.*

12. Provide the proper ratio of compressions to breaths at the appropriate rate. The ratio and rate is 15 compressions to 2 breaths at a rate of 80 to 100 compressions/min (a minimum of 80 compressions per minute to 100 compressions per minute if possible). *You must maintain this rate to compensate for the compressions lost when you take time out to do the breathing.* Move smoothly from one function to the other, keeping a steady rhythm. Say, "One and two and three and . . . " (or any helpful mnemonic) to yourself to maintain the correct rate.

Two-Rescuer CPR

If a second rescuer arrives, he or she activates the EMS system (if this has not already been done by the first rescuer) and does one-rescuer CPR *if the first rescuer has become fatigued.*

Airway
1.–3. Follow the steps of the procedure for one-rescuer CPR.

Breathing
4.–7. Follow the steps of the procedure for one-rescuer CPR.

Circulation
8. Follow the procedure for one-rescuer CPR.
9. Position yourselves on opposite sides of the patient. Rescuer 1 is at the patient's side and compresses chest. Rescuer 2 is at the patient's head and breathes.
10. Rescuer 1 should compress the sternum at a rate of 80 to 100 compressions per minute. Rescuer 2 maintains an open airway, monitors the

carotid pulse *for adequacy of chest compressions,* and ventilates the patient after every fifth compression. A pause should be allowed for the ventilation (1–1½ sec/breath). Rescuer 1 (the compressor) says, "One and two and three and . . . " aloud *to help both rescuers maintain the rate and ratio.*

11. When either of the rescuers tires, Rescuer 1 calls for a change of tasks and completes the ongoing series of five compressions.
12. Rescuer 2 breathes after the fifth compression.
13. Rescuer 1 moves up and checks the carotid pulse for 5 seconds.
14. Rescuer 2 gets in position to compress the sternum and waits.
15. If the carotid pulse is absent, Rescuer 1 ventilates once and says, "Continue CPR." Rescuer 2 restarts the compressions immediately after the breath. If there is a pulse but no breathing, continue appropriate ventilation and monitoring.

Monitoring the Patient

In two-rescuer CPR, Rescuer 2 assumes the responsibility for monitoring the pulse and breathing. Rescuer 2 checks the carotid pulse during compressions *to assess the effectiveness of Rescuer 1's external chest compressions. To determine whether the patient has resumed spontaneous breathing and circulation,* chest compressions must be stopped for 5 seconds at about the end of the first minute and every few minutes thereafter.

Terminating CPR

CPR is terminated when one of the following occurs:

1. Breathing and a spontaneous heartbeat are detected.
2. An advanced life-support team arrives to take over the patient's care.
3. A physician pronounces the patient dead and states that CPR can be discontinued.
4. The rescuer(s) becomes physically exhausted and no replacement(s) is available. This is the most difficult reality for a rescuer to face, but there are limits to one's physical endurance. Fortunately, this does not happen often.

PROCEDURE FOR PERFORMING CPR FOR INFANTS AND SMALL CHILDREN

The procedure used with infants and small children is similar to that used with adults. However, there are some important differences to keep in mind.

© 1996 by Lippincott-Raven Publishers

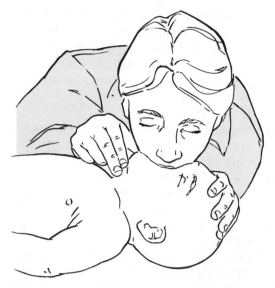

Figure 30–10. To breathe for an infant, cover both the mouth and the nose of the infant with your mouth.

Airway

1. Because the most common cause of arrest in the pediatric age group is primary respiratory arrest or an obstructed airway, assess the patient and provide approximately 1 minute of rescue support before activating EMS (American Heart Association, 1992).
2. Some believe that overextension of the head closes the trachea in small babies. Although there is no proof of this, avoid overextension *because it is unnecessary.*

Breathing

1. Cover both the mouth and the nose of the infant with your mouth (Fig. 30–10). If the patient is a larger child, occlude the nostrils with the fingers of the hand that is maintaining head tilt, and make a mouth-to-mouth seal.
2. For an infant or child, breathe once every 3 seconds, or 20 times per minute. Give two slow breaths (1–1½ sec/breath), pausing between to breathe yourself.
3. *Because the volume of air in an infant's lungs is smaller than that in an adult's,* use only the amount of air needed to cause the chest to rise. Watch carefully—as soon as you see the chest rise and fall, you are using the right volume of air.

Circulation

Because the carotid artery is difficult to locate in an infant's short, chubby neck, the brachial artery is recommended instead. Locate the brachial pulse on the inside of the upper arm, between the elbow and shoulder, by placing your thumb on the outside of the arm and

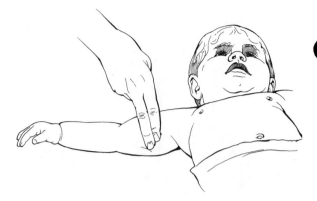

Figure 30–11. The brachial pulse is located on the inside of the upper arm of the infant.

pressing gently with your index and middle fingers (Fig. 30–11).

Because research has suggested that lay rescuers cannot count pulses consistently, you should not emphasize the pulse check when teaching CPR to laypersons. If a layperson finds an infant or child who is not breathing spontaneously, it is likely that the child has a slow heartbeat or is without heartbeat and needs cardiac compressions (American Heart Association, 1992).

Position the child in a horizontal supine position on a hard surface, as you would an adult. For an infant, the hard surface can be the palm of the hand not performing the compressions. The weight of the infant's head and a slight lift of the shoulders then provide head-tilt.

1. *Infants*
   a. Locate an imaginary line between the nipples over the sternum. Place the index finger of the hand farthest from the infant's head just un-

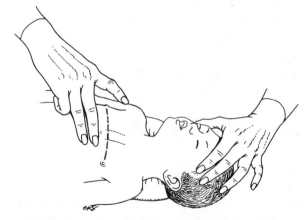

Figure 30–12. To identify finger position for chest compressions in an infant, locate an imaginary line between the nipples. Place the index finger of the hand farthest from the infant's head just under that line where it intersects with the sternum. The correct area for compression is one finger width below this intersection.

© 1996 by Lippincott-Raven Publishers

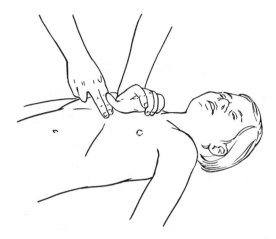

Figure 30–13. Correct hand position for chest compressions in a child. The correct area for compressions is located the same way it is for an adult, and the chest is compressed with the heel of one hand.

der that line where it intersects with the sternum. The correct area for compression is one finger width below this intersection, where your middle and ring fingers are located.

   b. Using two or three fingers, compress the sternum ½ to 1 inch at a rate of at least 100 times per minute (Fig. 30–12).

2. *Small children*

   a. Position your hands correctly; the correct area for compressions is located in the same way as for an adult.

   b. Use the heel of *one* hand to compress the chest 1 to 1½ inches at a rate of 80 to 100 times per minute (Fig. 30–13).

If the child is large or older than approximately 8 years of age, use the method previously described for adults. A good rule of thumb is that the sternum of an infant or child is compressed approximately one-third to one-half the depth of the chest.

For both infants and small children, breathe after every fifth chest compression.

CPR in the Healthcare Facility

Acute healthcare facilities follow a specific procedure whenever resuscitation is necessary.

1. The person who discovers the victim's collapse activates the EMS system and calls for assistance. *To simplify matters and to avoid alarming other patients,* the EMS is activated using a designated code. The code number differs from facility to facility, but code 99 and code 199 are used in many places.

2. The discoverer initiates CPR, following the above procedures.

3. The person who responds to the call for help gathers the emergency equipment (cardiac board, breathing bag, oxygen setup, emergency medications, and so forth) and brings it to where the victim has collapsed.

4. The second person then assists as necessary. This might include placing the cardiac board and participating in two-person CPR.

5. Most facilities designate a team of specially trained personnel (including a physician) to respond to all codes. This team arrives with special life-support equipment, including a defibrillator, emergency drugs, and breathing equipment (such as an Ambu bag), and takes over care completely. Information about Ambu bags and their use in ventilating patients can be found in Module 38, Administering Oxygen (Fig. 38–5). The first persons to reach the victim relinquish care to the team. These persons may stay to assist if that is part of the procedure for the facility, or they may return to their other duties.

6. If sufficient personnel are available, someone should reassure any family members and any patients in the immediate area. Increasingly, it is becoming the role of a registered nurse or a chaplain to assist in addressing the psychosocial needs of families by allowing them to be present in the area where the CPR is taking place. Although not always practical, some believe the emotional benefits to the family outweigh the legal risks for the staff.

Documentation

Certainly, the initiation of CPR is of primary importance. But it is also a nursing responsibility to maintain a record of all resuscitation activities. Include the indication for and time of CPR initiation; the time and nature of all events that take place during resuscitation activities; assessment of the patient before, during, and after CPR; any medications given; the patient's response to all measures; and the time resuscitation activities are stopped. Most facilities have a flow sheet to simplify documentation of this detailed information (Fig. 30–14).

MANAGEMENT OF FOREIGN-BODY AIRWAY OBSTRUCTION

Foreign-body obstruction of the airway usually occurs during eating. Meat is frequently the cause of an obstruction in adults. Other foods and foreign bodies may be the cause in children and some adults. Choking on food may result from elevated

© 1996 by Lippincott-Raven Publishers

CARDIOPULMONARY ARREST RECORD

DATE	TIME OF ARREST	PATIENT DIAGNOSIS		PATIENT INTUBATED
				AT (TIME)
HOW WAS ARREST RECOGNIZED (ASYSTOLE, V TACH., ETC)?				COMPLICATIONS

VENTILATION INITIATED		MOUTH TO MOUTH/MASK	ANESTHESIA BAG AND MASK	
AT (TIME)		☐ YES ☐ NO	☐ YES ☐ NO	
BY WHOM		EXTERNAL CARDIAC MASSAGE INITIATED AT (TIME)	PRECORDIAL THUMP ☐ YES ☐ NO	PATIENT INTUBATED PRIOR TO ARREST ☐ YES ☐ NO	ESTIMATED PERIOD OF APNEA

TIME	VITAL SIGNS	EPINEPH.	ATROPINE	LIDOCAINE	BICARB						IV DRIPS	RATE	DEFIBRILLATION			COMMENTS (LAB RESULTS, LOC, PUPILS, RHYTHM, ETC.)
													PRE-SHOCK RHYTHM	WATT-SEC	RESULTING RHYTHM	

COMMENTS:	PERSONNEL:
PRESUMED CAUSE / NATURE OF ARREST	
TERMINATION OF CPR (TIME / RATIONALE / RESULTS)	SIGNATURE - RECORDER
FAMILY NOTIFIED	SIGNATURE - PHYSICIAN IN CHARGE

Figure 30–14. Cardiopulmonary arrest record. The use of a flow sheet simplifies documentation of resuscitation activities.

blood alcohol level, poorly fitting dentures, or large, inadequately chewed pieces of food.

PROCEDURE FOR FOREIGN-BODY AIRWAY OBSTRUCTION: ADULTS

1. Recognition
   a. A foreign body can cause partial or complete airway obstruction. If the victim's airway is only partially obstructed, some degree of air exchange may be possible. If the air exchange is good, the victim may be able to cough forcefully. You should not interfere in this situation. Encourage the victim to attempt to cough and breathe spontaneously.
   b. If the victim has initial poor air exchange or

© 1996 by Lippincott-Raven Publishers

good air exchange that has deteriorated to poor air exchange (ineffective cough, crowing noises when inhaling, bluish color), manage as though it were complete airway obstruction.

c. Establish that the airway is obstructed. The victim may know the universal distress signal for choking—clutching the neck with the hand(s) (Fig. 30–15). Ask the victim, "Are you choking?" If the answer is an affirmative shake of the head, intervene immediately.

2. Management

The Heimlich maneuver (subdiaphragmatic abdominal thrusts) is recommended by the American Heart Association for relieving foreign-body airway obstruction. Your hands should not be placed on the xiphoid process of the sternum or on the lower margins of the rib cage *to prevent possible damage to internal organs.* Your hands should be below this area but above the navel in the midline.

a. Conscious victim

(1) Stand behind the victim and wrap your arms around his or her waist. Then grasp one fist with your other hand, and place the thumb side of that fist against the victim's abdomen in the midline slightly above the navel as described (Fig. 30–16).

(2) Next, press into the victim's abdomen with a quick upward thrust (Fig. 30–17**A**). Each

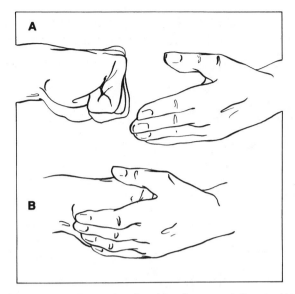

Figure 30–16. Correct hand position for manual thrusts. **(A)** Make a fist with one hand and grasp the fist with your other hand. **(B)** Use the thumb side of the fist for subdiaphragmatic thrusts.

thrust should be a separate and distinct movement. You may need to deliver 6 to 10 thrusts to clear the airway.

(3) Continue until the foreign body is expelled or the victim loses consciousness.

b. Unconscious victim

(1) Position victim on the back.

(2) Kneel astride the victim's thighs.

(3) Place the heel of one hand against the victim's abdomen (as described) with the second hand directly on top of the first. Press into the abdomen with a quick upward thrust (Fig. 30–17**B**). Deliver 6 to 10 abdominal thrusts.

Chest thrusts are recommended *only* when the victim is in the late stages of pregnancy or when the Heimlich maneuver cannot be used effectively on the unconscious, very obese victim. In such cases, place the victim in the supine position and kneel at the victim's side. Using the same hand position as for external cardiac compression, deliver each thrust slowly and distinctly.

(4) Use the finger sweep only in the unconscious patient to attempt to grasp the foreign body and remove it.

(a) With the victim face up, use one hand to open the mouth by grasping the lower jaw and tongue between your thumb and fingers and lifting. This draws the tongue away from the back of the throat and away from any foreign body lodged there.

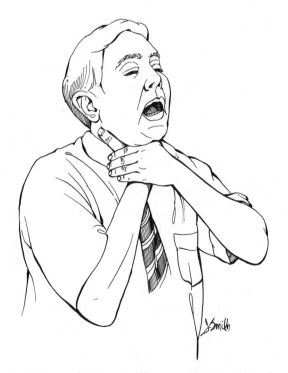

Figure 30–15. The universal distress signal for choking is the victim clutching the neck with his or her hand(s)

© 1996 by Lippincott-Raven Publishers

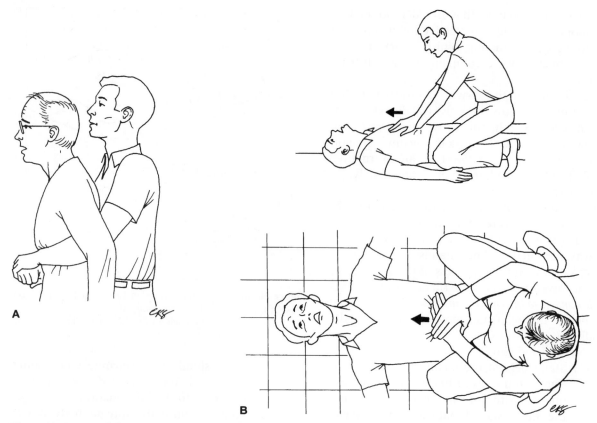

Figure 30–17. Heimlich maneuver. **(A)** Conscious victim—Continue abdominal thrusts until the foreign body is expelled or the victim loses consciousness. **(B)** Unconscious victim—Kneel astride the victim's thighs and do six to ten abdominal thrusts.

(b) Insert the index finger of your other hand along the inside of the victim's cheek, using a hooking action to dislodge any foreign body so it can be removed. Be careful not to push the foreign body further into the airway.

(5) Open the victim's airway and attempt rescue breathing.

(6) Repeat the sequence of Heimlich maneuver, finger sweep, and attempt to ventilate as long as necessary.

If a victim who was initially conscious loses consciousness, the muscles may become more relaxed, allowing for successful intervention.

PROCEDURE FOR FOREIGN-BODY AIRWAY OBSTRUCTION: INFANTS AND SMALL CHILDREN

Although the procedure for relieving foreign-body airway obstruction in infants and small children is similar to that used for adults, there are some important differences to keep in mind.

1. Recognition
   a. Infants
      (1) Airway obstruction may be caused by an object, such as a small toy or a peanut, or by an infection that results in swelling of the airway. It is important to differentiate between the two.
      (2) Seek treatment if the obstruction is caused by an infection. The procedure presented here is not effective in the case of infection and will only delay necessary treatment.
   b. Small children
      (1) If the child has good air exchange, encourage him or her to cough and breathe spontaneously.
      (2) If the child has poor air exchange, manage the situation as though it were complete airway obstruction.
      (3) Establish that the airway is obstructed. Ask the child, "Are you choking?" If answer is yes, intervene immediately.
2. Management
   a. Infants
      (1) Straddle an infant over your arm, with the

© 1996 by Lippincott-Raven Publishers

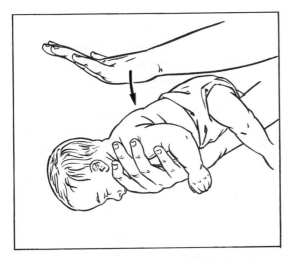

Figure 30–18. For infant back blows, straddle the infant over your arm, support the head by placing a hand around the jaw and chest, and deliver five back blows between the infant's shoulder blades.

head lower than the trunk. Support the head by placing a hand around the jaw and chest (Fig. 30–18).

(2) Deliver five back blows between the infant's shoulder blades.

(3) Place your free hand on the infant's back so that the baby is "sandwiched" between your two hands (one supports the neck, jaw, and chest while the other supports the back). Turn the infant and place him or her on your thigh, with the head lower than the trunk, then deliver five thrusts in the same way as for external chest compressions.

If the infant is too large for this positioning, kneel on the floor and place the child across your thighs, keeping the head lower than the trunk. Now deliver five back blows. Then, supporting the head and back, roll the infant over onto the floor and deliver five chest thrusts (as for external chest compression).

(4) Open the airway, and if breathing is absent, attempt rescue breathing (see Performing CPR for Infants and Small Children [above]).

(5) If the infant's chest does not rise, reposition the head and attempt rescue breathing again.

(6) Repeat the sequence of five back blows, five chest thrusts, and attempt to breathe as long as necessary.

(7) Because a foreign body can easily be pushed further back in the airway and cause increased obstruction, avoid blind finger sweeps in infants and children. If the victim is unconscious, open the mouth by lifting the lower jaw and tongue forward. If you can see the foreign body, remove it with your finger.

b. Small children

(1) Conscious child—standing or sitting

(a) Stand behind the child and wrap your arms around the waist.

(b) Deliver 6 to 10 subdiaphragmatic abdominal thrusts as you would for an adult, but more gently.

(c) Continue until the foreign body is expelled or the child loses consciousness.

(2) Conscious or unconscious child—lying

(a) Position the child on his or her back.

(b) If the child is on the floor, kneel at the feet; if the child is on a table, stand at the feet. The "astride" position used for adults is not recommended for small children but may be used for a large child.

(c) Deliver 6 to 10 subdiaphragmatic abdominal thrusts as you would for an adult, but more gently.

(d) Open the airway, and if breathing is absent, attempt rescue breathing (see Performing CPR for Infants and Small Children [above]).

(e) If the chest does not rise, reposition the child's head and attempt breathing again.

(f) Repeat the sequence of Heimlich maneuver and attempt to breathe as long as necessary.

(g) Avoid blind finger sweeps.

LONG-TERM CARE

Many individuals who live in long-term care facilities have decided not to have CPR carried out when they stop breathing or when their heart stops. You should be aware of the "code status" of every resident for whom you are caring at any time. This will prevent residents from undergoing CPR against their stated wishes or against the orders of the physician. In addition, the outcomes of CPR in very elderly individuals are exceedingly poor, often resulting in an increase in longevity and a decrease in quality of life.

© 1996 by Lippincott-Raven Publishers

HOME CARE

Because the need for resuscitation or the removal of a foreign body commonly occurs outside of healthcare facilities, it is also important for people other than healthcare providers to be able to perform these skills. Although it is desirable that someone in every household be able to perform CPR, it is especially important in situations in which there is an individual(s) who is particularly at risk for cardiac problems. If you are providing care in such a situation, you are responsible to identify the person or persons who might be most able to learn and perform the necessary skills. Also, although everyone is potentially at risk for aspiration of a foreign body, the parents or care providers for infants and small children may be more likely to find it necessary to use the Heimlich maneuver. While providing care in the home or while doing discharge teaching, you have a unique opportunity to identify these needs and to suggest that appropriate individuals attend classes provided in your setting or in the community.

Some states have now enacted legislation that allows those receiving home care to establish "no code" status. This may be done by completing specific documents and wearing a special identification bracelet. These documents provide legal protection to emergency response personnel in following the advance directives of individuals who do not wish to be resuscitated. In states or provinces where this is not a part of legislation, emergency response personnel may be obligated to carry out all resuscitation measures if they are called to the scene. Home care personnel need to be familiar with the relevant legal standards in their community to appropriately respond to and teach clients and families.

CRITICAL THINKING EXERCISES

You are the nurse assigned to care for the family during a code in the Emergency Department. Your facility's policy allows family members to be in the room when CPR is being administered. In this situation, the family of an accident victim has just arrived, and you have been called. The patient has been severely disfigured as the result of the accident he has been in. Explain how you will handle the situation.

References

American Heart Association. (1992). Guidelines for cardiopulmonary resuscitation and emergency cardiac care. *JAMA, 268,* 2171–2302.

Centers for Disease Control and Prevention. (1994). Draft guideline for isolation precautions in hospitals: Part I. Evolution of isolation practices and Part II. Recommendations for isolation precautions in hospitals. *Federal Register,* 59(214), 55552–55570.

© 1996 by Lippincott-Raven Publishers

✔ PERFORMANCE CHECKLIST

One-Rescuer CPR

	Needs More Practice	Satisfactory	Comments
Airway			
1. Determine unresponsiveness. **a.** Shake and shout, "Are you all right?"			
b. If no response, activate the EMS.			
2. Position patient on back on firm surface.			
3. Establish airway using head-tilt/chin-lift maneuver or, if neck injury is suspected, jaw-thrust maneuver.			
Breathing			
4. Determine breathlessness. **a.** Look for chest movement.			
b. Listen for breathing sounds.			
c. Feel for air.			
5. If patient does not begin breathing, perform rescue breathing.			
6. If chest rises and falls, continue with step 8.			
7. If chest does not move and you feel resistance, reposition the head and attempt to breathe again. If you still feel resistance, clear the obstruction and then continue.			
Circulation			
8. Determine pulselessness. Palpate carotid pulse; if absent, begin chest compression.			
9. Kneel beside patient's shoulders.			
10. Position hands correctly on patient's chest.			
11. Compress downward, keeping arms straight and moving sternum 1½–2 inches.			
12. After each 15 chest compressions at a rate of 80–100 compressions/min, breathe twice (1–1½ sec/breath).			
Two-Rescuer CPR			
1.–8. Follow Checklist steps 1–8 for one-rescuer CPR.			

(continued)

© 1996 by Lippincott-Raven Publishers

Two-Rescuer CPR *(Continued)*	Needs More Practice	Satisfactory	Comments
9. Position yourselves on opposite sides of the patient. Have one rescuer breathe while the other compresses chest.			
10. Breather should give one breath between each five chest compressions at a rate of 80–100 compressions/min.			
11. Rescuer 1 calls for change and completes on-going series of five compressions.			
12. Rescuer 2 breathes after the fifth compression.			
13. Rescuer 1 moves up and checks carotid pulse for 5 seconds.			
14. Rescuer 2 gets in position to compress and waits.			
15. If carotid pulse is absent, Rescuer 1 says, "Continue CPR" and ventilates once. Rescuer 2 restarts compressions immediately after the breath.			
CPR for Infants and Small Children			
Airway			
1. Assess and provide 1 minute of rescue support before activating the EMS.			
2. Avoid overextension of the head in infants.			
Breathing			
1. Cover both mouth and nose of infant with your mouth.			
2. Breathe once every 3 seconds for an infant or child.			
3. For infants, use only the amount of air needed to cause the chest to rise.			
Circulation			
1. Infants a. Position two or three fingers one finger width below an imaginary line between the nipples.			
b. Compress the sternum ½–1 inch at a rate of at least 100 times/min.			

(continued)

© 1996 by Lippincott-Raven Publishers

CPR for Infants and Small Children *(Continued)*	Needs More Practice	Satisfactory	Comments
2. Small children **a.** Position hands as for adult.			
b. Use heel of one hand only to compress the chest 1–1½ inches at a rate of 80–100 times/min.			
Foreign-Body Airway Obstruction: Adults			
1. Recognition **a.** If victim has good air exchange, encourage attempts to cough and breathe spontaneously.			
b. If victim has poor air exchange, manage as complete airway obstruction.			
c. Ask victim, "Are you choking?" If answer is affirmative, intervene immediately.			
2. Management **a.** Conscious victim (1) Stand behind victim and wrap your arms around waist.			
(2) Deliver 6 to 10 subdiaphragmatic abdominal thrusts.			
(3) Continue until foreign body expelled or victim loses consciousness.			
b. Unconscious victim (1) Position on back.			
(2) Kneel astride victim's thighs.			
(3) Deliver 6 to 10 subdiaphragmatic abdominal thrusts.			
(4) Use finger sweep to attempt to remove foreign body.			
(5) Open airway and attempt rescue breathing.			
(6) If unable to ventilate, deliver 6 to 10 subdiaphragmatic abdominal thrusts and repeat sequence as long as necessary.			

(continued)

© 1996 by Lippincott-Raven Publishers

Foreign-Body Airway Obstruction: Infants and Small Children	Needs More Practice	Satisfactory	Comments

1. Recognition
  a. Infants
    (1) Differentiate between obstruction by object or by infection causing swelling of airway.			

(2) Seek treatment if infection.			
b. Small children			
(1) If child has good air exchange, encourage attempts to cough and breathe spontaneously.			
(2) If child has poor air exchange, manage as complete airway obstruction.			
(3) Ask child, "Are you choking?" If answer is yes, intervene immediately.			

2. Management
  a. Infants
    (1) Straddle infant over your arm, head lower than trunk.			

(2) Deliver five back blows between infant's shoulder blades.			
(3) Sandwich infant between your hands, turn infant over, and deliver five chest thrusts.			
(4) Open airway, and if breathing is absent, attempt rescue breathing.			
(5) If chest does not rise, reposition head and attempt breathing again.			
(6) Repeat sequence of five back blows, five chest thrusts, and attempt to breathe as long as necessary.			
(7) Blind finger sweeps are not recommended in infants.			

b. Small children
    (1) Conscious child—standing or sitting
      (a) Stand behind child and wrap your arms around waist.			

(b) Deliver 6 to 10 subdiaphragmatic abdominal thrusts.			
(c) Continue until foreign body expelled or child loses consciousness.			

(*continued*)

© 1996 by Lippincott-Raven Publishers

Foreign-Body Airway Obstruction: Infants and Small Children *(Continued)*	Needs More Practice	Satisfactory	Comments
(2) Conscious or unconscious child—lying (a) Position on back.			
(b) If on floor, kneel at child's feet; if on table, stand at child's feet.			
(c) Gently deliver 6 to 10 subdiaphragmatic abdominal thrusts.			
(d) Open airway, and if breathing is absent, attempt rescue breathing.			
(e) If chest does not rise, reposition head and attempt breathing again.			
(f) Repeat sequence of Heimlich maneuver and attempt to breathe as long as necessary.			
(g) Avoid blind finger sweeps in children.			

© 1996 by Lippincott-Raven Publishers

? Q U I Z

Short-Answer Questions

1. What is the first step you should take when you see an adult collapse? Why is the first step different when the patient is an infant or child?_____

   _____

   _____

2. How do you position the victim's head if a neck injury is suspected? _____

   _____

3. How can you quickly locate the carotid pulse?_____

   _____

4. How is the brachial pulse located in an infant? _____

   _____

5. Where should the chest of an adult be compressed? _____

   _____

6. How many chest compressions per minute should be performed in the following situations?

   a. One-rescuer CPR _____

   b. Two-rescuer CPR _____

   c. CPR for an infant _____

   d. CPR for a small child _____

7. What is the ratio of breaths to chest compressions in one-person CPR? _____

   _____

8. What is the ratio of breaths to chest compressions in two-person CPR? _____

   _____

9. What is the universal distress signal for choking?_____

   _____

10. Where is the Heimlich maneuver correctly delivered? _____

11. Under what circumstances is the finger sweep maneuver used?_____

   _____

MODULE

31

POSTMORTEM CARE

MODULE CONTENTS

RATIONALE FOR THE USE OF THIS
SKILL
THE PRESENCE OF FAMILY AND
FRIENDS AT THE TIME OF DEATH
ORGAN OR TISSUE DONATION
ADVANCE DIRECTIVES
DEFINING DEATH
PRONOUNCEMENT OF DEATH
THE DEATH CERTIFICATE
REPORTING A DEATH TO THE MEDICAL
EXAMINER
CHANGES IN THE BODY AFTER DEATH
Rigor Mortis
Algor Mortis

Livor Mortis
Skin Indentation
CARING FOR THE BODY
Assessment
Planning
Implementation
Evaluation
Documentation
DEATH OF AN INFANT
AUTOPSY (POSTMORTEM
EXAMINATION)
LONG-TERM CARE
HOME CARE
CRITICAL THINKING EXERCISES

PREREQUISITES

Successful completion of the following modules:

VOLUME 1
Module 1 An Approach to Nursing Skills
Module 2 Basic Infection Control
Module 5 Documentation

Portions of the following modules may also prove useful:

VOLUME 1
Module 4   Basic Body Mechanics
Module 9   The Nursing Physical Assessment
Module 15 Moving the Patient in Bed and Positioning
Module 18 Hygiene
Module 20 Transfer

© 1996 by Lippincott-Raven Publishers

OVERALL OBJECTIVES

To care for the patient's body after death in a skilled and respectful manner, and to support the family in their pursuit of personal, religious, or cultural practices.

SPECIFIC LEARNING OBJECTIVES

Know Facts and Principles	Apply Facts and Principles	Demonstrate Ability	Evaluate Performance
1. Organ donation			
State benefits of the organ donation system for the patient, the family, and the community.	Given a situation in which donation is desired, discuss ways of initiating the process.	In the clinical setting, explore the policies and accessibility of organ donation.	Evaluate by discussing with other students and faculty in pre-clinical or postclinical conference.
2. Pronouncement of death			
State criteria for pronouncing patient dead.	Given a situation, list nursing actions to determine whether death has occurred.	In the clinical setting and with assistance, determine whether death has occurred.	Evaluate own performance with instructor.
3. Medical examiner's cases			
List instances in which death should be reported to medical examiner.	Given a situation, discuss whether death is reportable.	In the clinical setting, determine whether death should be reported.	Evaluate by reviewing criteria for your locale.
4. Body changes after death			
a. Privacy and the family			
Discuss ways to provide privacy for patient and family.		In the clinical setting, provide privacy and demonstrate concern for patient's family.	Evaluate by discussing with other students and faculty in preclinical or postclinical conference.
b. Positioning			
Describe proper positioning of body after death.	In the practice setting, position body as if in death.	With assistance, administer postmortem care to patient after death, including positioning body, cleaning body, caring for valuables and personal effects, and identifying body.	Evaluate with instructor, using Performance Checklist.
c. Cleaning and preparing			
Outline procedure for cleaning and preparing body.			
d. Care of valuables and personal effects			
State appropriate disposition of valuables and personal effects.	Identify form used for disposition of valuables and effects.		
e. Identification of the body			
Describe methods for body identification.			

(*continued*)

© 1996 by Lippincott-Raven Publishers

SPECIFIC LEARNING OBJECTIVES (continued)

Know Facts and Principles	Apply Facts and Principles	Demonstrate Ability	Evaluate Performance
6. Documentation Identify essential information regarding death that must be included in patient's record.	Given a situation, simulate final progress note on chart.	In the clinical setting, make correct and accurate final entry on patient's record.	Evaluate completeness of documentation with instructor.
7. Death of an infant Discuss ways to approach the family regarding viewing the infant's body.		In the clinical setting observe the interaction of a nurse with a family whose infant has died.	Evaluate by discussing with your fellow students and instructor in preconference or postconference.
8. Autopsy Define autopsy. List reasons for performance of autopsy.	Given a situation, discuss reasons for autopsy.	In the clinical setting, observe an autopsy.	Evaluate by discussing with other students and faculty in preclinical or postclinical conference.

© 1996 by Lippincott-Raven Publishers

LEARNING ACTIVITIES

1. Review the Specific Learning Objectives.
2. Read the section on death care and grief (in the chapter on death and loss) in Ellis and Nowlis, *Nursing: A Human Needs Approach,* or comparable material in another textbook.
3. Look up the module vocabulary terms in the glossary.
4. Read through the module as though you were preparing to teach the concepts and skills to another person.
5. In the practice setting:
   a. Demonstrate the proper positioning of a body by positioning a partner.
   b. Reverse roles and have your partner position you.
   c. Discuss the reasons for positioning with your partner.
   d. With your instructor as facilitator, join in a small group with three or four classmates. Explore together some of your feelings concerning:
      (1) Touching and caring for a patient after death
      (2) Interacting with the deceased patient's family members and friends
      (3) Organ donation
6. In the clinical setting:
   a. Read your facility's procedure and policy manuals regarding caring for the patient after death, the responsibility and process for reporting deaths to a medical examiner, and the organ donation procedure.
   b. Examine the various forms (for release of body, for autopsy) used in your facility.
   c. If an opportunity arises, arrange to observe a staff member discuss organ donation with the family of a dying patient. In postclinical conference, role-play discussing organ donation with a family.
   d. If death occurs, assist the instructor or a staff nurse for your first experience in giving death care.
   e. When a subsequent opportunity arises, give death care with the assistance and evaluation of your instructor.
   f. In postclinical conference, share with your classmates your experiences and feelings related to caring for a patient and his or her family after death.

VOCABULARY

advance directive
algor mortis
autopsy
coroner
deceased
edema
electroencephalogram
forensic medicine
funeral director
funeral home
hyperalimentation
livor mortis
medical examiner
morgue
mortician
mortuary
next-of-kin
organ donor
pathologist
pathology
postmortem examination
repose
resuscitate
rigor mortis
shroud
sphincter
turgor

© 1996 by Lippincott-Raven Publishers

Postmortem Care

Rationale for the Use of This Skill

In addition to the important task of giving comfort and emotional support to bereaved families and friends, the nurse also has the responsibility of caring for patients' bodies after death. Postmortem care is a continuation of the quality of care a nurse gives patients before death. Essential to this task is an attitude of respect. In addition, survivors commonly view a body in the hospital or nursing home, and this makes postmortem care an even more essential task.

To have patients clean and in repose after death not only comforts the bereaved, but is a nursing function that reflects personal involvement with individual patients. Remember, patients are the nurse's responsibility from the time they enter the unit until the time they leave—whether in recovery or in death.

In some facilities, the physical aspects of death care are carried out by nursing assistants. On many units, including the area of critical care, postmortem care is given by nurses as part of the total care concept. The nurse must possess the skills and the sense of dignity necessary to care for a patient's body or to supervise that care.[1]

THE PRESENCE OF FAMILY AND FRIENDS AT THE TIME OF DEATH

The death of a patient in the healthcare facility has become much more personal in that the family and close friends are increasingly included. Before the time of death, the nurse should clearly determine how important it is to those who are significant to the patient that they be physically present at the time of death. If this is important, every effort should be made to have those persons present. Planning to accommodate the family or special friends in a sensitive manner *can offset later feelings of anger and guilt.* It is also important for the patient to have a caring person present. The nurse can openly discuss the situation with the patient, family, or friends during the final stages of an illness. The wishes of those involved can be communicated by noting them on the care plan and by verbally relating them to the healthcare team. The same considerations are important when the dying patient is being cared for at home.

ORGAN OR TISSUE DONATION

The willingness of people to donate their organs after death is increasing. The result of this change is a growing number of persons whose life is prolonged or who gain renewed function of a body part or system through transplantation (Table 31–1). Congress has recently passed legislation that requires hospital personnel to request organ and tissue from families of patients who are appropriate donors (Fig. 31–1).

It is useful to remember that virtually anyone who dies can be considered a potential donor for some type of tissue. Unlike the donors of solid organs (see Table 31–1), tissue donors do not need to be supported on a ventilator after death is declared (unless, of course, they are to be both organ and tissue donors). There is a continuous need for corneas, cadaver skin (used on burns until tissue regeneration occurs), bone, and connective tissue. Be aware of the patient's wishes before death regarding the donation of certain tissues and organs or of the wishes of the family after death. It is also useful to be aware of the views of various religious groups on organ and tissue donation ("Religious views," 1994). *Many families find some consolation in knowing that other persons will benefit from donated organs.* In either case, signed permission is required. Forms are available for this purpose.

To ensure the viability and usefulness of tissues, move promptly when you know that organ donation has been requested by the patient before death or by the family afterward. In most states, even when the patient has indicated a desire to donate organs, the family has to agree after the death for the organs actually to be removed. When death results from an accident and the patient's wishes are not known, the family members can direct a donation of organs. Consult the patient's physician regarding the request to donate organs and the nursing supervisor regarding the appropriate agency to contact.

Most states participate in a system of organ recovery that works on a local and regional basis, and also on a nationwide basis through computer connection to the United Network for Organ Sharing (UNOS), the national organ procurement and transplant network designated by the federal government. When a local group does not have a suitable matching recipient for an organ, the donor information is entered into the UNOS computer. The computer then determines the transplant center with the most urgent need and within the most reasonable distance, and the organ is made available to that center. An exhaustive effort is made to use every suitable organ donated (Organ Recovery Procedure Manual, 1990).

---

[1]Rationale for action is emphasized throughout the module by the use of italics.

© 1996 by Lippincott-Raven Publishers

Table 31–1. One-, Two-, and Three-Year Graft and Patient Survival Rates, by Organ, for U.S. Transplants between October 1, 1987 and December 31, 1992

Organ	N	1-Year Survival (%)	Std. Error	2-Year Survival (%)	Std. Error	3-Year Survival (%)	Std. Error
Kidney							
(Cadaveric)							
Graft	38,599	80.3	0.2	74.5	0.2	68.7	0.3
Patient	38,629	93.2	0.1	90.4	0.2	87.5	0.2
Kidney							
(Living)							
Graft	10,926	91.2	0.3	87.7	0.3	83.7	0.4
Patient	10,931	97.3	0.2	95.9	0.2	94.3	0.3
Liver							
Graft	12,869	68.0	0.4	63.6	0.4	60.5	0.5
Patient	12,869	78.6	0.4	74.9	0.4	72.2	0.5
Pancreas							
Graft	2,312	71.9	0.9	66.9	1.0	62.2	1.1
Patient	2,311	89.5	0.6	85.5	0.8	81.7	0.9
Heart							
Graft	10,131	82.4	0.4	78.3	0.4	74.6	0.5
Patient	10,131	82.4	0.4	78.3	0.4	74.7	0.5
Heart–Lung							
Graft	299	59.1	2.9	51.2	3.0	48.1	3.1
Patient	299	59.1	2.9	51.2	3.0	48.1	3.1
Lung							
Graft	1,271	68.8	1.3	59.7	1.5	50.8	1.9
Patient	1,271	68.8	1.3	59.7	1.5	50.9	1.9

(Source: UNOS Scientific Registry data as of July 29, 1994.)
Notes: N denotes the number of transplants for which a survival time could be determined. The survival rates were computed using the Kaplan-Meier method.

ADVANCE DIRECTIVES

Some patients, based on their own wishes or the decisions made by their families and physicians, are designated "no code" or DNR (do not resuscitate), meaning that no heroic measures will be taken and resuscitation will not be attempted in the event of death. It is of utmost importance that you know the "code status" of each patient under your care. As a nurse, you must understand that "no code" does not mean "no care." When a "no code" patient is in the terminal stages of an illness, you should continue the high quality of care you would give to any patient until the moment of death.

As recent dilemmas in the definition of death for legal and organ retrieval purposes show, confusing situations can arise. To improve clarity in decision-making regarding end-of-life issues, the legislatures of an increasing number of states are enacting laws providing for advance directives. One type, the Natural Death Act, is similar to the "living will," which is informational but not legally binding. A natural death act provides a legally binding mechanism whereby individuals may decline heroic or extraordinary measures to prolong life if more than one physician declares their condition to be terminal and irreversible. Another type, the durable power-of-attorney for healthcare, may be used by individuals to designate a specific person to make decisions regarding end-of-life issues if they are not capable of

© 1996 by Lippincott-Raven Publishers

NOPA Procedure Manual
Consent

Consent for Organ and Tissue Donation

Out of consideration for those in need, and by reason of my relationship to the deceased, I hereby consent to the removal of the following organs or tissue for transplantation or the advancement of medical science and education.

I, _____ , authorize the donation of the following
(full legal name of next of kin)

organs/tissues from _____ .
(full legal name of donor)

Tissues   **Organs**

_____ Eyes   _____ Kidneys

_____ Bone and connective tissue   _____ Heart

_____ Skin grafts   _____ Lungs

_____ Heart for valves   _____ Liver

_____ Additional research tissues   _____ Pancreas

_____ Limitations: _____   _____ Other (specify): _____

I understand that tissue samples may be tested and pertinent diagnostic and medical information will be reviewed to assure medical suitability and that all donors must be tested for transmissible diseases (AIDS, hepatitis, syphilis) before transplantation can occur.

I hereby acknowledge that this consent is voluntarily given and motivated by humanitarian instincts without expectation of reward or compensation. It implies no obligation on the part of the recipient, this facility or its designees. Distribution and determination of use of these gifts will be coordinated by the procurement program in accordance with medical and ethical standards. I understand that copies of the medical record may be made available to the procurement program, and I consent to release this information.

I understand that any additional charges directly associated with the donation will be covered by the procurement agency. Disposition of the body after the removal of organs and tissue will remain the responsibility of the next of kin.

_____
Signature of next of kin   Date/time   Relationship

_____
Address   Phone

_____
City, State, Zip

_____
Signature of person obtaining consent   Date

_____
Witness   Date

_____
Facility City/State

Figure 31–1. Consent for organ and tissue donation.

decision-making. In 1991, the Patient Self-Determination Act became a federal law. This law requires healthcare agencies who participate in Medicare or Medicaid to inform patients, on admission to the agency, of their right to refuse treatment by enacting an advance directive. Familiarize yourself with your responsibilities regarding this law in the setting in which you work.

DEFINING DEATH

A long-standing practical definition of death has been the point at which there is complete cessation of respiration, heartbeat, and blood pressure. *Because peripheral pulses can disappear long before the heart actually stops beating,* check for apical heartbeat using a stethoscope. *The heartbeat is usually the last vital sign to disappear.*

© 1996 by Lippincott-Raven Publishers

When the patient's basic vital functions are being sustained by machines, identifying death is more complex. Death is then determined based on neurologic criteria. The Uniform Determination of Death Act (UDDA), or something similar, is now recognized in all 50 states. "The UDDA defines death as irreversible cessation of circulatory and respiratory functions, *or* irreversible cessation of all functions of the brain, including the brain stem" (Chabalewski & Norris, 1994, p. 29). Neurologic criteria for brain death are still being defined. In addition, many facilities have identified their own criteria for brain death. A complete discussion of this area is beyond the scope of this module. Always follow your facility's policies and procedures.

For patients who do not have DNR orders and for whom you have determined that respiration and heartbeat have stopped, initiate resuscitation according to your facility's procedure (see Module 30, Emergency Resuscitation Procedures). Resuscitation measures continue until the patient recovers vital functions or the physician pronounces the patient dead. Only after death has been pronounced and the option of organ donation is discussed with the family should machines supporting vital functions be turned off.

PRONOUNCEMENT OF DEATH

Once you have identified the cessation of vital function, note the time and call the physician. In most states, only a physician can legally pronounce a patient dead. Nurses can, however, legally determine and pronounce a patient dead in some states. In other states, there are certain specified situations (such as death in a long-term care facility or in a hospice setting when death has been expected for some time and is clearly imminent) in which the nurse may pronounce the patient dead and determine the time of death. The nurse then notifies the physician and completes appropriate records. In these cases, postmortem care is given, and the patient's body is removed from the unit. The death certificate, which is the official record of death, is signed by a physician in all states.

THE DEATH CERTIFICATE

You have no responsibility for filing a death certificate. However, *because you may serve as a resource person for the family,* you should understand the process.

Federal law mandates that a death certificate be completed for each death. After this document is completed by the mortician, it is signed by both the mortician and physician, then filed with the local health department. One to three copies are given to the family for insurance purposes and other legal matters. The family may make additional copies, if necessary.

REPORTING A DEATH TO THE MEDICAL EXAMINER

If any of the circumstances listed in Fig. 31–2 exist, you should call the office of your county's coroner or medical examiner. Other jurisdictions may require you to report deaths that occur under other circumstances, such as deaths involving negligence or damaged or improperly used equipment, deaths occurring less than 24 hours after admission to a hospital, and the death of a prominent or unidentified person (Descheneaux, 1991). When in doubt, call and ask. Give the data required, such as name and address of patient, nearest kin, and the circumstances of death. Typically, the examiner will decide that an autopsy is unnecessary and will simply supply a number to be entered on the patient's record. If the examiner does consider an autopsy necessary, be sure that the patient's body is either held at the facility for examination or transferred to the medical examiner's laboratory.

The person responsible for reporting applicable deaths to the coroner or medical examiner varies from facility to facility. Read the policy manual where you practice to know your role and the specific procedure(s) to be followed.

CHANGES IN THE BODY AFTER DEATH

Several changes occur in the body immediately after death. These include rigor mortis, algor mortis, and livor mortis. If the body is not handled gently, skin indentation may also occur.

Rigor Mortis

Rigor mortis is the stiffening of a dead body *accompanying the depletion of adenosine triphosphate in the muscle fibers.* It occurs rapidly, sometimes within an hour if the patient has died suddenly while being active or exercising. In the chronically ill, bedridden patient, rigor mortis may not take place for some hours. The degree of rigor mortis differs greatly from one patient to another. It begins in the involuntary muscles but initially becomes noticeable in the muscles of the head and neck. It then travels downward

© 1996 by Lippincott-Raven Publishers

Criteria for Reportable Deaths

1. Persons who die suddenly when in apparent good health and without medical attendance within 36 hours preceding death.
   a. Sudden death of an individual with no known natural cause for the death;
   b. Death during an acute or unexplained rapidly fatal illness, for which a reasonable natural cause has not been established;
   c. Deaths of individuals that were not under the care of a physician;
   c. Deaths of persons in nursing homes or other institutions where medical treatment is not provided by a licensed physician.
2. Circumstances indicate death caused entirely OR IN PART, by unnatural or unlawful means.
   a. Drowning, suffocation, smothering, burns, electrocution, lightning, radiation, chemical or thermal injury, starvation, environmental exposure, neglect;
   b. Unexpected deaths during, associated with, or as a result of, diagnostic or therapeutic procedures;
   c. All deaths in the operating room whether due to surgical or anesthetic procedures;
   d. Narcotics or other addictions, other drugs including alcohol or toxic agents, or toxic exposure;
   e. Death thought to be associated with, or resulting from, the decedent's occupation; this includes chronic occupational disease such as asbestosis and black lung;
   f. Death of the mother caused by known or suspected abortion;
   g. Deaths occurring from apparent natural causes during the course of a criminal act, e.g., victim collapses during a robbery;
   h. Deaths that occur within one year following an accident even if the accident is not thought to have contributed to the cause of death;
   i. Death following all injury producing accidents, if recovery was considered incomplete OR if the accident is thought to have contributed to the cause of death, (regardless of the interval between accident and death).
3. Suspicious circumstances.
   a. Deaths resulting from apparent homicide or suicide;
   b. Hanging, gunshot wounds, stabs, cuts, strangulation, etc.;
   c. Alleged rape, carnal knowledge, or sodomy;
   d. Death during the course of, or precipitated by, a criminal act;
   e. Deaths that occur while in jail, prison, in custody of law enforcement, or other nonmedical public institutions.
4. Unknown or obscure causes.
   a. Bodies that are found dead.
   b. Deaths during or following an unexplained coma.
5. Deaths caused by any violence whatsoever, whether the primary cause or any contributory factor in the death.
   a. Injury of any type including falls.
   b. Any deaths due to, or contributed to, by any type of physical trauma.
6. Contagious disease. This category includes only those deaths wherein the diagnosis is undetermined, and a contagious disease which may be a public health hazard is a suspected cause of death.
7. Bodies that are not claimed.
8. Premature and stillborn infants. This category includes only those stillborn or premature infants whose birth was precipitated by maternal injury, criminal or medical negligence, or abortion under unlawful circumstances.
9. All infants under the age of one year and suspected of Sudden Infant Death Syndrome.

Figure 31–2. Medical Examiner's cases, King County, State of Washington.

to the trunk and finally to the lower extremities. Rigor mortis is most evident about 48 hours after death and subsides gradually after about 96 hours (a time lapse in which you are not involved).

Algor Mortis

Algor mortis, or postmortem cooling, is the gradual decrease in body temperature that occurs *as circulation slows and stops.*

Livor Mortis

Livor mortis is the skin discoloration that occurs after blood circulation stops *because of the release of hemoglobin from the red blood cells that are breaking down. Gravity pulls the blood toward the dependent areas of the body after the heart stops pumping,* so that discoloration is most apparent in those areas. Handle the body gently *to prevent excessive discoloration, especially in areas that may be viewed later.*

© 1996 by Lippincott-Raven Publishers

Skin Indentation

Rough handling can also result in skin indentation. *After death, the skin immediately loses its natural turgor and elasticity.* Once this happens, *the lightest pressure can indent the skin,* a condition that is intensified if the patient had edema.

PROCEDURE FOR CARING FOR THE BODY

Assessment

1. Verify that vital functions have ceased. This includes complete absence of respiration, heartbeat, and blood pressure. Pronounce the patient dead if you are permitted to do so. Otherwise, notify the physician. In some facilities, a "house physician" will be designated to pronounce the patient dead. Record both the time of death and the time the patient is pronounced dead.

2. Notify the people and departments listed below. Be sure you have the necessary information at hand when you call. Policies and procedures vary from place to place. Follow the policies in your facility, and check with your supervisor if you are unsure.

   a. The attending physician—In some settings the attending physician is responsible for both pronouncing the patient dead and notifying the next of kin.

   b. The nursing supervisor or other designated supervisory personnel—In some settings the nursing supervisor is responsible for making some of the notification calls: for example, to the medical examiner, when appropriate.

   c. Next of kin or emergency contact person— This responsibility may not be yours to carry out, but it *is* your responsibility to be certain it has been done. In some facilities the notification of the next of kin is always the responsibility of the physician. It is prudent to ask whether the family will be coming in to view the body and collect the belongings as well as the name of the mortuary to be notified.

   d. Admitting or Census Department—This department is usually responsible for giving out information on patients' conditions and should be notified as soon as possible. Calling the mortician may be the responsibility of this department as well.

   e. The appropriate agency if any organ procurement is to take place.

   f. The medical examiner, if appropriate—If you are uncertain whether the circumstances meet the criteria for reportable deaths, call the medical examiner's office for assistance.

   g. The designated mortician if the patient is not a medical examiner's case.

Planning

3. Plan for any special religious or cultural practices desired by the family that may need to take place before you begin the actual "after death" care. Rituals cover a broad spectrum, from the Orthodox Jewish practice of washing the body to the Roman Catholic rite of anointing of the body by a priest. It is useful, of course, for you to be aware of specific preferences before the patient dies.

4. If the patient is not in a private room and it is possible to do so, offer to transport any other patient(s) in the room to another location temporarily. Otherwise, pull the curtains around the unit and close the door *to provide privacy for the family and friends of the deceased patient.*

5. Wash your hands *for infection control.*

6. Gather the equipment. You will need clean gloves (probably at least two pairs), soap, washcloth(s), towel(s), a basin, a clean gown, clean linen as needed for the bed if the patient is to be viewed, clean dressings or ostomy bag if a wound or ostomy is present, two ABDs or other disposable pads, a shroud or sheet, identification tags, and masking tape. In some facilities, it is the practice to place on the room door a sign saying "No visitors—Check at Nurses' Station" *to ensure privacy.* A "morgue pack" may contain some of these items, including the shroud, identification tags, and sign for the door.

Implementation

7. Place the "No visitors—Check at Nurses' Station" sign on the door.

8. Place the body in the supine position with the bed flat. Place the arms at the patient's side. Do not cross the hands *because the underlying hand will become discolored and indented.*

9. Place a low pillow under the head. *This prevents blood from pooling in the face, which can cause discoloration.*

10. Close the patient's eyes. Gently hold your index fingers on the eyelids for a few seconds and *the eyes will remain closed.*

11. Remove the patient's watch and jewelry. Make an itemized list of all the patient's possessions. Regardless of monetary worth, *these items are often important as mementos for the family.* Ask the spouse or closest relative what to do with the patient's wedding band if one is worn. *Some prefer that the band never be removed,* in which case tape it carefully in place. *Others may want to keep the ring,* in which case remove it and give it personally to the family. Always chart the disposi-

© 1996 by Lippincott-Raven Publishers

tion of jewelry and obtain a signature from the family stating that the valuables of the deceased have been received. *These actions prevent the loss of valuables and protect you legally.*

12. Put on clean gloves *to protect yourself from body secretions.*

13. Replace the patient's dentures. *This gives the person's face a more familiar and natural appearance if the patient is to be viewed by loved ones before being taken to the mortuary.* Do not attempt to replace the dentures if you encounter any resistance. *Marks or indentations can be left on the lips, jaw, or face if pressure is exerted.* Place the dentures instead in a labeled container and send them with the body for the mortician to insert. Some mortician and facility procedures specify that dentures not be replaced.

14. Place a small towel under the chin *to support the mouth in a closed position.*

15. Remove intravenous lines, nasogastric tube, urinary catheter, and oxygen equipment. If it is a medical examiner's case or an autopsy is to be performed, and the patient had special indwelling lines or catheters (such as those used to take direct blood pressure readings, to deliver hyperalimentation solutions, or to dialyze the patient), cut the line or catheter approximately 1 inch from the body and tape the end to the skin. These do not interfere with the viewing, and *their insertion sites and functioning may prove important medically or legally in cases of obscure causes of death. Some medical examiners insist that lines be neither cut nor removed,* so check your facility's policy concerning this. (See the following section on Autopsy.)

16. Remove soiled dressings and ostomy bags and replace them with clean ones.

17. Wash the soiled areas of the body. Pat the body dry. *Brisk rubbing may cause undue discoloration of the tissues.*

18. Place ABDs or other disposable pads in the perineal area *to absorb any stool or urine released as the sphincter muscles relax.*

19. Remove and discard gloves.

20. Put a clean gown on the patient.

21. Leave the wrist identification band in place. This is removed only if it is restricting the arm. *It serves as an excellent method of identifying the body.* All pieces of identification should have the patient's name, hospital number, and physician's name. The hospital band contains other data, including the date of admission.

22. Attach a second identification tag to the ankle or great toe. It is prudent to have two pieces of identification attached to the body *in case one becomes detached and lost.* The ankle or great toe is an appropriate area *because any marking on the skin there will not be noticeable when the body is viewed.* The procedure in your facility will indicate where identification tags are to be placed.

23. If the family and friends intend to view the body:
    a. Replace the top linens (top sheet, spread, and pillowcase) *to give the bed a fresh and clean appearance.*
    b. Tidy the unit, disposing of any equipment. If the family is to visit, provide chairs *so that they can sit with the body if they wish.* It is also thoughtful to rearrange any flowers that may be present. Dim the lights. Turn off the ceiling lights and use the bedside lights, *which will soften the features of the deceased for viewing.*

24. After the viewing, leave dentures in the patient's mouth or place them in a denture container. If the body is to be viewed at services later, morticians request that dentures and eyeglasses be sent with the body. Later, if the body is to be cremated, the funeral director usually discards these items with the permission of the family.

25. Place the patient's personal effects in the container used by your facility. Include cards or letters received by the deceased. If possible, give these items to a family member and record the name of the recipient. If this is not possible, send these items to the department specified by your facility for safekeeping.

26. Wrap the body in a shroud or cover it with a clean sheet. In many facilities masking tape is used *to fasten the shroud closed.* Attach the tape gently *to prevent indenting the body.* An identification tag is usually placed on the outside of the shroud. In some facilities there is a special covering for the body of a patient who had been in isolation. In others, a special tag is attached. Adhere to the policy in your facility *to protect all those coming in contact with the body.*

27. Transport the body to the facility morgue or leave it in the room until the mortician arrives. In the latter case, open the windows *to cool the room, thus retarding the deterioration of the tissue.* In many facilities it is customary to close the doors of all other patient rooms before the cart bearing the body passes by, *to prevent distress on the part of other patients and their visitors.*

28. Put away or dispose of equipment, supplies, linen, and garbage appropriately.

29. Wash your hands.

© 1996 by Lippincott-Raven Publishers

DATE/TIME	
2/5/99	*Vital signs ceased. Pronounced dead by Dr. Calhoun.*
3:20 AM	*Postmortem care given. Body viewed by the family.*
	Wedding ring taped in place. Wristwatch and wallet
	given to wife. ———— S. Kelly, SN

Example of Nursing Progress Notes Using Narrative Format.

Evaluation

30. Evaluate using the following criteria:
  a. Body cared for and transported appropriately.
  b. All necessary notifications carried out.
  c. Family was able to carry out rituals, viewing, and spend time with patient as desired.
  d. Possessions handled appropriately.

Documentation

31. Document the postmortem activities, including:
  a. Time of cessation of vital signs.
  b. Persons notified and time of notification.
  c. List and disposition of valuables and personal effects.
  d. Time body removed from unit, destination (facility morgue or funeral home), and by whom removed.
  e. Any other information required by your facility. In some places there is a special form that indicates and includes spaces for all information required (Fig. 31–3.)

DEATH OF AN INFANT

The death of an infant can be an especially sad and sensitive time. If you work in a labor and delivery area, you will need to be aware of your responsibility with regard to baptism in the event of infant death. Make sure the family knows they can see and hold the infant's body. If they wish to see the infant, wrap the child in a receiving blanket and carry the body of the baby as you would a living baby. Encourage the family to hold and examine the infant as desired. They may wish for you to unwrap the baby *if they are not comfortable doing so.* You may wish to provide a nursery crib *if the family is not comfortable holding the baby.* Offer the family the opportunity to be alone *because they may feel inhibited with a nurse in the room.*

AUTOPSY (POSTMORTEM EXAMINATION)

An autopsy is the examination of the body after death. Autopsies may be complete or partial. A complete autopsy consists of an examination of each of the body's organs, including the brain. A partial autopsy consists of an examination of only those organs of interest in determining the cause of death. Autopsies may serve several purposes: to ascertain the exact cause of death (in some cases, this may help the family recover insurance benefits or a legal settlement), to add to scientific knowledge, and to help in statistical data gathering. If an autopsy is done in the hospital at a physician's request, the family is usually not charged. On occasion, the family asks to have an autopsy performed, and a charge is then incurred. Check the specific policies in your facility.

It is the physician's responsibility to secure permission for an autopsy. Standard forms are available (Fig. 31–4); these should be made out in duplicate, with original signatures on each one.

The methods followed for autopsy permission are defined by state law, and again you should know the specifics for your state. A general guideline is to secure the consent of the closest blood relative, although some states have broad guidelines, even allowing telephone permission with two witnesses on the line. For example, the guidelines of Washington State are presented in Fig. 31–5. Your facility may have a policy about staff members' witnessing an autopsy consent. Some facilities discourage the practice, and others do not. Again, check the policy at your facility. It is useful for you to be aware of the views of various religious groups toward autopsy.

In certain deaths, an autopsy is required by law, in which case permission of the next of kin is not needed. County and state laws vary slightly in different areas. Know the law of the jurisdiction in which you practice. Cases requiring an autopsy are

(text continues on page 757)

© 1996 by Lippincott-Raven Publishers

PATIENT EXPIRATION FORM

Date & Time of Death:_____

Attending Physician:_____

Pronounced By:_____M.D._____R.N.

Signature of Persons filling out form:

Nursing:_____Admitting_____

I. NOTIFY IMMEDIATELY (to be completed by Nursing)

A. Attending Physician_____Time_____

B. Patient Care Coordinator_____Time_____

C. Next of Kin_____Phone Number_____
and/or Emergency Notification Person
Relationship to Deceased_____

Who notified next of kin?   Nurse_____Physician_____

D. Admitting Department_____Time_____

II. PREPARATION OF THE BODY (to be completed by Nursing)
Initial when Done _____

A. Observe Religious Protocol _____

B. Close eyes and replace dentures _____
(If unable to do so, wrap, label and tape to body.)
C. Clean and straighten the body _____

D. Remove jewelry Yes _____ No _____
(Rings taped at family's request) _____

E. Remove tubes (*only if NOT an M.E. case or autopsy*) _____

F. Remove gown; wrap in sheet/shroud _____

G. Attach 4 tags   1) Morgue door log _____   2) Foot _____

3) Sheet/Shroud _____   4) Chest (if applicable) _____

III. DISPOSITION OF THE BODY (to be completed by Nursing and Admitting)

A. Medical Examiners Case   Yes_____   No_____

If yes, name of M.E. notified_____

By whom at GHC?_____

Case Number_____

M.E. accepts body?   Yes_____   No_____

Is than an NJA case?   Yes_____   NJA#_____   No_____

B. Autopsy to be performed: Yes_____   No_____

If yes, permit signed: Yes_____   No_____   By Whom_____

Pathology Notified   Yes_____   No_____   Time_____

Autopsy completed   Time_____Date_____

| M.E. = Medical Examiner |
| NJA = Non Jurisdictional Action |

C. Mortuary_____Phone_____

Time and Date notified_____

Morgue Release signed by_____

Date and Time of Release_____

Reception Clerk_____

IV. Circle which one VALUABLES/PERSONAL BELONGINGS (to be completed by Nursing and Admitting)

A. List valuables:_____

_____

_____

_____

_____

B. Released to:_____Date & Time_____

C. No family present, valuables secured by_____

Location_____

V. ORGAN DONOR: Yes_____   No_____

Which organ_____

_____

_____

VI. DOCUMENTATION

A. Patient Expiration Notification form to the Admitting Office as soon as possible with two discharge cards (if applicable).

B. Completed chart taken to Medical Records Department.

WHITE · INPATIENT'S CHART / CANARY · ADMITTING / PINK · NURSING
Patient Expiration Form

Figure 31–3. Patient expiration form.

© 1996 by Lippincott-Raven Publishers

NAME OF DECEASED		ROOM NO.	AGE	PHYSICIAN
HOSPITAL NUMBER		MEDICAL EXAMINER NOTIFIED YES ☐ NO ☐		
DATE & TIME OF EXPIRATION		MEDICAL EXAMINER'S CASE YES ☐ NO ☐		

AUTHORIZATION FOR AUTOPSY

I (WE) REQUEST AND AUTHORIZE THE PHYSICIANS AND SURGEONS IN ATTENDANCE AT THE SWEDISH HOSPITAL

MEDICAL CENTER TO PERFORM A COMPLETE AUTOPSY ON THE REMAINS OF _____
AND I (WE) AUTHORIZE THE REMOVAL AND RETENTION OR USE FOR DIAGNOSTIC, SCIENTIFIC, THERAPEUTIC
PURPOSES AND FOR RESEARCH OR STUDY, OR PRESERVATION FOR USE IN GRAFTS OR TRANSPLANTS UPON
OR FOR LIVING PERSONS, OF SUCH ORGANS, TISSUES, AND PARTS INCLUDING EYES, BRAIN, SPINAL CORD,
AND INNER EAR AS SUCH PHYSICIANS AND SURGEONS DEEM PROPER, AND TO DISPOSE OF ANY OR ALL TISSUES
IN A PROPER AND SUITABLE MANNER.
THIS AUTHORITY IS GRANTED SUBJECT TO THE FOLLOWING RESTRICTIONS:

_____
(IF NO RESTRICTIONS, WRITE "NONE")

I (WE) REPRESENT THAT I AM (WE ARE) THE _____ OF THE DECEASED AND ENTITLED
BY LAW TO CONTROL THE DISPOSITION OF THE REMAINS, BY MAKING THIS CERTIFICATION I (WE) REPRESENT THAT
I AM (WE ARE) AWARE THAT THE SWEDISH HOSPITAL MEDICAL CENTER WILL BE ACTING ON OUR REPRESENTATION
AND IF IN FACT ANY ACTION IS BROUGHT AGAINST SWEDISH HOSPITAL MEDICAL CENTER FOR MAKING AN UN-
AUTHORIZED AUTOPSY, I (WE) PERSONALLY AGREE TO INDEMNIFY SAID SWEDISH HOSPITAL MEDICAL CENTER FOR
ANY LOSS THEY MAY INCUR, INCLUDING THEIR COSTS OF DEFENDING SUCH ACTION FOR UNAUTHORIZED AUTOPSY
PROCEDURE.

WITNESS: _____   SIGNED _____

_____   DATE _____ TIME _____
(If authorization obtained by telephone, two (2) witnesses must sign as having heard telephone conversation.)   PERMIT SIGNED

RELEASE TO FUNERAL DIRECTOR

I (WE) WISH THE REMAINS TO BE RELEASED TO:

_____   _____   _____
NAME OF UNDERTAKING ESTABLISHMENT   CITY   STATE

SIGNED _____

AUTOPSY COMPLETED: _____   MORTICIAN NOTIFIED: _____
DATE   TIME   DATE   TIME

SIGNATURE OF MORTICIAN _____

AUTHORIZATION FOR AUTOPSY

Figure 31–4. Permit for autopsy.

© 1996 by Lippincott-Raven Publishers

Autopsy or postmortem may be performed in any case where authorization has been given by a member of one of the following classes of persons in the following order of priority:

1. The surviving spouse.
2. Any child of the decedent who is eighteen years of age or older.
3. One of the parents of the decedent.
4. Any brother or sister of the decedent.
5. A person who was guardian of the decedent at the time of death.
6. Any other person or agency authorized or under an obligation to dispose of the remains of the decedent. The chief official of any such agency shall designate one or more persons to execute authorizations pursuant to the provisions of this section.

If the person seeking authority to perform an autopsy or postmortem makes reasonable efforts to locate and secure authorization from a competent person in the first or succeeding class and finds no such person available, authorization may be given by any person in the next class.

Figure 31–5. Washington state requirements for autopsy.

called coroner's or medical examiner's cases. The family is not charged for an autopsy that is required by law.

The word *coroner* originates from the word *crown*. (A king would designate an appointee to oversee the disposition of bodies and estates.) A coroner need not be a physician and is either an elected official or a political appointee. A medical examiner is a physician, usually with a special degree in pathology or forensic medicine, and is appointed. Increasingly, counties are moving from having a coroner to having a medical examiner.

Besides investigating unusual circumstances of death, the coroner or medical examiner has jurisdiction over any real property of an unidentified or unclaimed deceased person.

LONG-TERM CARE

Although some individuals are admitted to long-term care facilities for limited periods (for specific reasons such as rehabilitation), many more move to nursing homes with the clear expectation that they will live out the remainder of their lives there. In fact, it is the policy in many nursing homes to ask residents and their families *on admission* to indicate the mortuary they want notified when the resident dies. It is a *legal requirement* for the facility, if it receives Medicare or Medicaid funding, to offer each resident the opportunity to establish an advance directive on admission to the facility. Residents are also requested to indicate their wishes regarding donation of tissues and organs after death. It is especially important that the nurse know whether the resident wishes to be resuscitated, and if so, exactly which components of resuscitation are to be included (CPR, drugs, mechanical ventilation, or a combination of these).

As a resident nears death, considerations regarding the presence and participation of family members are much the same as in an acute care facility. Nurses must be aware of the expressed needs of family and friends to be present at the moment of death so that they can honor those needs, if possible.

Recall that in some states registered nurses employed in long-term care facilities can legally pronounce a resident dead. The death certificate must be signed by a physician.

Staff members in long-term care facilities may have cared for some residents over a long period. For these staff members, the deaths of certain residents feel like deaths of a family member. In some facilities, brief memorial services are held on care units to help staff members work through their feelings of loss.

© 1996 by Lippincott-Raven Publishers

HOME CARE

Increasingly, terminally ill individuals are choosing to die at home. In some cases, family and friends are able to provide much of the required care, with a home care nurse assisting as needed. In other situations, a hospice nurse supervises care, and in still others, caregivers other than family and friends provide most of the care. Depending on the situation, the nurse or the family must know the law regarding what is to be done and who is to be notified when death occurs in the home. As is true in healthcare agencies, an unexpected death in the home is handled differently than is an expected one, perhaps requiring notification of the coroner or medical examiner. It is always prudent to call when unsure.

CRITICAL THINKING EXERCISES

A patient for whom you are caring has just died. The family left the facility about 10 minutes ago, and you know it will take them at least 45 minutes to get home. You do not know whether they will wish to see their loved one again. How will you proceed with caring for the body?

References

Chabalewski, F., & Norris, G. (1994). The gift of life: Talking to families about organ and tissue donation. *AJN, 94*(6), 28–33.

Descheneaux, K. (1991). Death investigations: How you can help. *Nursing 91, 21*(9), 52–55.

Organ Recovery Procedure Manual. (1994). Seattle: Northwest Kidney Center/Northwest Procurement Agency.

Policy and Procedure Manual. (1994). Seattle: Seattle–King County Department of Public Health, Medical Examiner Division.

Staff. (1994, Summer). Religious views on organ and tissue donation. *Procure,* p. 6.

PERFORMANCE CHECKLIST

Procedure for Caring for the Body	Needs More Practice	Satisfactory	Comments
Assessment			
1. Verify that vital functions have ceased and pronounce patient dead if permitted to do so. Otherwise, notify physician and record time of death and time pronounced dead.			
2. Notify the following people/departments: a. The attending physician			
b. The nursing supervisor			
c. Next of kin/emergency contact person			
d. Admitting or Census Department			
e. Appropriate agency for organ procurement			
f. Medical examiner, if appropriate			
g. Designated mortician, if not a medical examiner's case			
Planning			
3. Plan for any special religious/cultural practices desired by family.			
4. Offer to transfer any other patient(s) in room to another location temporarily.			
5. Wash your hands.			
6. Gather equipment.			
Implementation			
7. Place "No visitors—Check at Nurses' Station" sign on door.			
8. Place body in supine position with bed flat.			
9. Place low pillow under head.			
10. Close patient's eyes.			
11. Remove watch and jewelry and make list of all possessions.			
12. Put on clean gloves.			
13. Replace patient's dentures.			
14. Place small towel under chin.			

(continued)

© 1996 by Lippincott-Raven Publishers

Procedure for Caring for the Body *(Continued)*	Needs More Practice	Satisfactory	Comments
15. Remove IVs and other tubes unless autopsy is to take place.			
16. Remove soiled dressings/ostomy bags and replace.			
17. Wash soiled areas of body.			
18. Place ABDs in perineal area.			
19. Remove and discard gloves.			
20. Put clean gown on patient.			
21. Leave wrist identification in place.			
22. Attach second identification tag.			
23. If body is to be viewed: **a.** Replace top linens.			
b. Tidy unit.			
24. Care for dentures and eyeglasses.			
25. Gather personal effects and give to family or provide for safekeeping.			
26. Wrap body and attach identification tag on outside, if facility policy indicates.			
27. Transport body to facility morgue or await arrival of mortician.			
28. Put away or dispose of equipment/supplies.			
29. Wash your hands.			
Evaluation			
30. Evaluate, using the following criteria: **a.** Body cared for and transported appropriately.			
b. All necessary notifications carried out.			
c. Family able to carry out rituals, viewing, and spend time with patient as desired.			
d. Possessions handled appropriately.			
Documentation			
31. Document postmortem activities, including: **a.** Time of cessation of vital signs			
b. Persons notified and time of notification			

(continued)

© 1996 by Lippincott-Raven Publishers

Procedure for Caring for the Body *(Continued)*	Needs More Practice	Satisfactory	Comments
c. List and disposition of valuables and personal effects			
d. Time body removed from unit, destination, and by whom removed			
e. Other information required by facility			

© 1996 by Lippincott-Raven Publishers

? QUIZ

Multiple-Choice Questions

_____ **1.** The last vital sign to disappear is usually the

    a. temperature.
    b. respiration.
    c. heartbeat.
    d. blood pressure.

Short-Answer Questions

2. The benefit derived for families who donate organs of their deceased loved ones is

_____

3. Among the organs currently being used for transplantation are _____

_____

4. It is important to report the availability of a donor promptly after death to ensure

_____

5. Describe the difference between a coroner and a medical examiner.

_____

6. Name five instances in your county when a death must be reported to the coroner or medical examiner.

    a. _____

    b. _____

    c. _____

    d. _____

    e. _____

7. Give three changes in the body after death.

    a. _____

    b. _____

    c. _____

8. List four special considerations you should take when the patient is to be viewed in the hospital room by the family.

    a. _____

    b. _____

    c. _____

    d. _____

9. List two different considerations when the patient is an infant.

    a. _____

    b. _____

© 1996 by Lippincott-Raven Publishers

10. Why should the arms be placed at the patient's side? _____

_____

11. Name four types of treatment equipment that are removed from the body after death.

    a. _____

    b. _____

    c. _____

    d. _____

12. Define autopsy. _____

_____

13. Name three reasons for performing autopsies.

    a. _____

    b. _____

    c. _____

© 1996 by Lippincott-Raven Publishers

GLOSSARY

abduction   The act of drawing away from the median line or center of the body.

accommodation   The adaptation or adjustment of the lens of the eye to permit the retina to focus on images or objects at different distances.

acetone   A colorless volatile solvent; commonly used as a synonym of ketone body; see *ketone body.*

acid   A substance that ionizes in solution to free the hydrogen ion; turns litmus paper pink.

acuity   The degree of seriousness of a person's illness.

acute care   Healthcare provided for a person who has a current problem that is expected to be resolved within a limited period of time.

adduction   The act of drawing toward the median line or center of the body.

adherent   A material that sticks to some other object or surface.

adhesions   Scar tissue that attaches surfaces within the body that are normally separate from one another.

ADLs   Activities of daily living.

advance directive   A legal document in which an individual makes known his or her wishes with regard to healthcare, especially with regard to the use of extraordinary measures at the end of life.

adventitious sounds   Abnormal sounds, as in the lungs.

advocate   A person who speaks on behalf of another.

afebrile   Without fever.

affected   Involved, such as the part of the body involved with pain or disease.

agility   The state of being nimble or of moving with ease.

AIDS (Acquired Immunodeficiency Syndrome)   A viral disease of the immune system causing decreased immune function that can be transmitted through the blood and certain body substances of infected persons.

airway   (1) The passageway by which air circulates in and out of the lungs. (2) A device used, generally when a patient is not fully alert, to prevent the tongue from slipping back and occluding the throat.

algor mortis   The gradual decrease in body temperature that occurs as circulation slows and stops after death.

alkaline   Having characteristics of a base; neutralizes an acid.

alignment   Arrangement of position in a straight line. Used to refer to body parts being positioned so that they are in correct relationship, with no twisting.

alternating pressure mattress   A plastic mattress attached to a motor that alternately inflates and deflates the tubular sections of the mattress, so that the pressure against any one section of the patient's body changes constantly. It is placed over the regular mattress on the bed.

alveoli   Air sacs of the lungs, at the termination of a bronchiole.

AMA   Against medical advice.

ambulate   To walk from place to place.

amoeba   Any of various protozoans of the genus *Amoeba* and related genera, occurring in water, soil, and as internal animal parasites, characteristically having an indefinite, changeable form and moving by means of pseudopodia.

ampule   A small, sterile glass container that usually holds a parenteral medication.

anal sphincter   The two ringlike muscles that close the anal orifice. One is called the *external anal sphincter;* the other, the *internal anal sphincter.* The actions of both sphincters control the evacuation of feces.

anatomic position   A body position in which body parts are in correct relationship to one another and in which correct function is possible.

aneroid manometer   An air pressure gauge that indicates blood pressure by a pointer on a dial.

anorectal   Referring to the distal portion of the digestive tract, including the entire anal canal and the distal 2 cm of the rectum.

anorexia   Loss of appetite.

antecubital space   A depression in the contour of the inner aspect of the elbow.

antiemetic   An agent used to prevent vomiting.

765

© 1996 by Lippincott-Raven Publishers

antineoplastic   An agent that inhibits the growth of abnormal cell tissues or neoplasms.

antipyretic   A medication that lowers body temperature.

apex   The narrow or cone-shaped portion of an organ. In the heart, the point located in the area of the midclavicular line near the fifth left intercostal space; in the lung, the narrower, more pointed, upper end.

apical   Pertaining to the apex.

apical pulse   The heartbeat heard through a stethoscope held over the apex of the heart.

apnea   The absence of respiration.

arrhythmia   Any irregularity in the force or rhythm of the heartbeat.

ascending colon   The portion of the colon on the right side of the abdomen that extends from the junction of the small and large intestine to the first major flexion near the liver.

ascitic fluid   An abnormal accumulation of serous fluid in the abdominal cavity; also called *ascites*.

asepto syringe   A medical instrument that is used to aspirate and instill a fluid. The tip is graduated in size so that it fits into tubings of various sizes; the rounded bulb is used to create suction to fill the barrel and pressure to expel the fluid.

aspirate   To remove gases or fluids by suction.

aspiration   Removal of gases or fluids by suction.

assessment   The process of gathering data and analyzing it to identify patients' problems; the first step in the nursing process.

asymmetry   Difference in form or function on opposite sides of the body.

auscultation   Listening with a stethoscope to the sounds produced by the body.

auscultatory gap   During the measurement of blood pressure, the disappearance of the usual sounds heard over the brachial artery when cuff pressure is high, and their reappearance at a lower level as the pressure is reduced.

autopsy   An examination of the body after death to determine the cause of death and to further scientific investigation.

axilla   The armpit.

bacteria   Single-celled plantlike microorganisms that can cause disease.

ball-and-socket joint   A joint in which a ball-shaped end of a bone rests in a socketlike cavity. Examples are the shoulder and hip.

barrier   (1) Anything that acts to obstruct or prevent passage. (2) A boundary or limit.

base   The broad or wide end of an organ. In the heart, the area located at the second left and right intercostal spaces at the sternal borders; in the lungs, the wide lower end.

base of support   That which makes up the foundation of an object or person and supports the weight.

bath blanket   An absorbent, light-weight cotton blanket used for draping during the bath.

bedboard   A thin board, often hinged for easy use and storage, that is placed underneath a mattress when a firmer sleeping surface is wanted.

bedpan   A metal or plastic receptacle for the excreta of bedridden persons.

bell   On the stethoscope, the cone-shaped head that is most often used for listening to heart sounds.

bilirubin   A yellowish pigment that is derived from the destruction of hemoglobin.

binder   A type of bandage, worn snugly around the trunk or body part, that provides support.

bivalving   The process of using a cast saw to cut a cast in half lengthwise when the cast causes skin problems or undue pressure. The two parts of the cast are then held together by an elastic bandage when the patient is moving.

blood borne   Referring to those microorganisms that are transported by blood and specific body fluids such as semen, vaginal secretions, and spinal fluid.

body language   Conveying thoughts or meanings through the posturing or positioning of the body.

body mechanics   The analysis of the action of forces on the body parts during activity.

Body Substance Precautions   A set of behaviors designed to prevent the transmission of microorganisms that are transported by any body substance such as urine, saliva, and feces.

bone marrow   Soft material that fills the cavities of bones.

bounding pulse   A body pulse that strikes the fingers with excessive strength.

brachial artery   An artery that supplies blood to the shoulder, arm, forearm, and hand.

bradycardia   An abnormally slow heartbeat, usually defined as below 60 beats/min.

bradypnea   Respirations that are regular in rhythm but slower than normal in rate (usually below 16 in the adult). Bradypnea may be normal during sleep.

bronchi   The branches of the trachea that lead directly to the lungs.

bruit   An abnormal sound that results from circulatory turbulence.

cachexia   Extreme wasting of the body.

© 1996 by Lippincott-Raven Publishers

cane A rehabilitative device used as an aid in walking.

canthus The corner at either side of the eye, formed by the meeting of the upper and lower eyelids. *Inner canthus* is the corner next to the nose; *outer canthus* is the corner to the outside of the face.

cardiac arrest The cessation of heart action.

cardiac sphincter A circular muscle between the esophagus and the stomach that opens at the approach of food. The food then moves into the stomach as a result of peristalsis.

caries The decay of bone or tooth.

cariogenic That which contributes to the formation of dental caries.

carotid artery Either of the two major arteries in the neck that carry blood to the head.

carotid pulse The wave of blood felt as it passes through the carotid artery.

cast padding A "waffled" padding, consisting of soft, thin cotton layers between two outer layers of closely woven cotton, used to provide cushioning between the patient's skin and a cast.

catheter A slender flexible tube, of metal, rubber, or plastic, that is inserted into a body channel or cavity to distend or maintain an opening; often used to drain or to instill fluids.

caustic Having the ability to burn, corrode, or dissolve by chemical action.

Celsius A temperature scale, devised by Anders Celsius, that registers the freezing point of water at 0°C and the boiling point at 100°C, under normal atmospheric pressure; also called *centigrade*.

center of gravity A point in an object or person at which gravitational pull functions as if the entire weight of the object or person were at that single point.

centigrade See *Celsius*.

cerebrospinal fluid (CSF) The serumlike fluid that bathes the lateral ventricles of the brain and the cavity of the spinal cord.

cerumen A yellowish waxy secretion of the external ear; earwax.

cervical collar A device worn around the neck that prevents flexion, extension, and rotation of the cervical spine and supports the head. May be constructed of foam rubber or rigid plastic.

cervical traction Traction applied to the cervical spine by the use of weights attached by ropes to either skull tongs or a chin harness.

chart The official, legal record of healthcare.

Cheyne-Stokes A cyclic pattern of respirations that gradually increase in depth followed by respirations that gradually decrease in depth, with a short period of apnea between cycles.

Chux A brand name for a waterproof pad which is placed under the patient to protect bed linens.

circadian rhythm The approximately 24-hour cyclic pattern of rest and activity in humans.

CircOlectric bed A special bed designed to maintain immobilization and provide for turning. The patient is placed between two mattresses on frames and the turn is vertical.

circular bandage A bandage that is wrapped in circular fashion around a body part.

circumcise To surgically remove the prepuce (foreskin) of the penis.

circumduction A circular movement of the eye or of a body part.

Clinitron bed A special bed with a mattress filled with ceramic beads that move constantly when air is blown through them. This eliminates continuous pressure on any one point and minimizes shear while decreasing pain.

clove hitch A knot that consists of two turns, with the second held under the first.

colic Severe paroxysmal abdominal pain in infants, that usually results from the accumulation of gas in the alimentary canal.

comatose Unconscious.

commode A portable toileting device that resembles a chair on wheels. The seat lifts to reveal a recessed pan or container for the collection of urine or feces.

computerized record A mechanism for documenting data regarding a client through the use of a computer file.

concurrent Happening at the same time or place.

condyloid joint A joint in which a knuckle-shaped end of a bone rests in an oval depression. Examples are the wrist, fingers (excluding the thumb), and toes.

confidentiality The right to have personal matters kept private.

consensual When both pupils move and focus together.

consent The right of a competent adult to make his or her own decisions regarding healthcare.

consolidation The process of becoming solid or the condition of being solid; used to describe the lung as it fills with exudate in pneumonia.

contact guard assistance (CGA) Assistance provided to a patient while transferring by remaining in physical contact to provide immediate assistance if needed.

constriction A feeling of pressure or tightness.

contaminate To introduce microorganisms to an object or person.

© 1996 by Lippincott-Raven Publishers

contracture A shortening of a muscle that causes distortion or deformity of a joint.

contraindicate To indicate the inadvisability of an action—for example, in treatment.

convergence Two objects moving toward one another. When both pupils follow a point as it moves closer to the nose and both move medially (toward the nose).

coroner A public officer whose primary function is to investigate by inquest any death thought to be of other than natural causes.

counterbalance Using your weight and the patient's weight as a balance to assist in lifting or moving.

countertraction Exerting pull in opposition to a traction system.

crackles A sound similar to hair strands being rubbed together that is heard upon auscultation of the lungs and indicates moisture in small airways.

cradle A frame shaped like an inverted baby's cradle that is used to protect the lower extremities from the pressure of bed linen or to supply electrical heat.

cradle cap Yellowish oily scales on the scalp of an infant that result from the accumulation of sebaceous secretions.

cranium The portion of the skull that encloses the brain.

critical care Healthcare provided for acute, life-threatening illness.

crutch A staff or support that is used by the disabled as an aid in walking; usually has a cross-piece that fits under the armpit and often is used in pairs.

crutch palsy A weakness or paralysis of the hands caused by damage to the brachial nerve plexus through leaning on the cross-piece of crutches.

culture and sensitivity (C&S) A laboratory test in which a swab or smear is placed in a nutrient medium to observe for growth of microorganisms. If microorganisms do grow, the culture is then tested with various antibiotics to determine whether the microorganisms are sensitive to the effects of these antibiotics. If the microorganism is destroyed, it is termed *sensitive* to the antibiotic. If the microorganism is not destroyed, it is termed *resistant*.

cytology A laboratory test in which cells are examined microscopically.

data Information, especially material that is organized for analysis or used as a basis for decision-making.

deceased Complete cessation of respiration, heartbeat, and blood pressure; dead.

decubitus ulcer An open sore or lesion of superficial tissue caused by pressure, specifically one caused by remaining in a decubitus (lying) position for prolonged time.

defecation The act of expelling the contents of the bowel.

dependent edema See *edema*.

descending colon The portion of the colon on the left side of the abdomen that extends from the major flexion at the spleen to the point where the colon again flexes into the sigmoid portion.

dexterity Skill in the use of the hands or body.

dialysis cannula A surgically inserted tube that provides access to the circulatory system for hemodialysis.

diaphoresis Perspiration, especially copious or medically induced perspiration.

diaphragm (1) A muscular membranous partition that separates the abdominal and thoracic cavities and that functions in respiration. (2) On a stethoscope, the flat, drumlike head that is used most often for listening to blood pressure, the lungs, and bowel sounds.

diarrhea Pathologically excessive evacuation of watery feces.

diastole The normal rhythmically recurring relaxation and dilatation of the heart cavities during which the cavities are filled with blood.

diastolic blood pressure The lowest pressure reached in the arteries during the heart's resting phase.

digital Pertaining to a finger. A digital examination is one carried out with a finger.

dignity Inherent worth.

dilation The condition of being enlarged or stretched.

displacement The act whereby a substance is replaced by another either in weight or in volume.

distal In anatomy, located far from the origin or line of attachment.

distention Bloat and turgidity from pressure within; usually refers to the stomach, bowel, or bladder. May also refer to the dilated blood vessel when filled with blood.

diuresis The increased production and output of urine.

diuretic A drug that increases the production and output of urine.

dorsalis pedis artery An artery located on the top of the foot, used for palpating the pedal pulse.

dorsal recumbent position A position in which the person lies on back with knees bent.

© 1996 by Lippincott-Raven Publishers

dorsiflexion   Bending or moving a part in a backward direction.

double T-binder   A binder with two tails that is used to hold a dressing in place on the perineum of a male patient, so that the testicles are not restricted.

droplet nuclei   Microscopic particles that, when surrounded by moisture, become airborne.

dullness   In percussion, not sharp or intense.

dysphagia   Difficulty in swallowing.

dyspnea   Difficulty in breathing.

edema   An excessive accumulation of serous fluid in the tissues. *Dependent edema* is fluid that has accumulated in the lower areas of the body due to gravity, *periorbital edema* is fluid that has accumulated in the soft tissue around the eyes, and *pretibial edema* is fluid that has accumulated over the tibia.

"egg crate" mattress   A foam mattress which has rounded projections and indentations resembling an egg crate. Used to diminish pressure on tissues.

elastic bandage   A bandage constructed of a heavy, stretchable material. The elastic bandage is usually applied to an extremity, providing pressure. ACE bandage is one brand name for this type of bandage.

elastic net binder   A binder of stretchable, large-mesh material used to hold dressings in place. Elastic net binders are available in a variety of sizes.

electroencephalogram (EEG)   A record of brain waves measured on the electroencephalograph.

electrolyte   A substance that dissociates into ions in solution; in the body, electrolytes are critically important chemicals.

epigastrium   The upper middle region of the abdomen.

esophagus   The portion of the gastrointestinal tract that extends from the pharynx, through the chest, to the stomach.

ethical   Pertaining to or dealing with principles of right and wrong.

ethnic   Characteristic of a religious, racial, national, or cultural group.

eupnea   Normal, unlabored respirations.

evaluation   The process of determining the outcomes of a course of action.

eversion   Turned in an outward direction.

exception   A situation that does not conform to normal rules.

excoriate   To chafe or wear off the skin.

excoriation   An area of the skin that has become reddened, inflamed, and abraded.

excretion   The process of eliminating waste matter, such as feces, urine, or sweat.

expectorate   To eject from the mouth; spit.

extension   The act of straightening or extending a limb.

external disaster   A disaster occurring in the community which may affect the medical facility.

external rotation   Moving a body part outward on an axis.

exudate   Fluid drainage from cells.

face shield   A barrier that protects the face from splashed fluids.

Fahrenheit   A temperature scale that registers the freezing point of water at 32°F and the boiling point at 212°F, under normal atmospheric pressure.

fanfold   To fold or gather in accordion fashion; for example, the top linen of a bed toward the bottom or one side.

febrile   Having an elevated body temperature.

feces   Waste excreted from the bowels.

femoral artery   Either of the two large arteries that carry blood to the lower abdomen, the pelvis, and the lower extremities.

fever   Abnormally high body temperature.

fiberglass cast   A "light" cast, made of fiberglass, that is impermeable to water.

figure-8 bandage   A bandage that is wrapped around a body part in a figure-8 configuration.

fixation   Holding an object in a fixed position. Used to refer to holding broken bones in a correctly aligned position for healing.

flaccid   Lacking firmness; soft and limp; flabby.

flatness   In percussion, a short high-pitched sound without resonance or vibration.

flatus   Gas generated in the stomach or intestines and expelled through the anus.

flexion   Bending of a joint.

flow sheet   A schematic representation of a sequence of operations or events.

"Focus" charting   A style of charting in which narrative notes are organized by entering "Data," "Action," and "Response."

fontanel   Any of the soft membranous intervals between the incompletely ossified cranial bones of fetuses and infants.

footboard   A board or small raised platform against which the feet are supported or rested.

footdrop   The abnormal permanent plantar flexion of the foot that results from paralysis or injury to the flexor muscles.

footrest   A canvas sling or padded bar at the distal end of a leg cast used to support the foot.

© 1996 by Lippincott-Raven Publishers

forensic medicine   The legal aspects of medical practice.

foreskin   The loose fold of skin that covers the glans of the penis; the prepuce.

Foster bed   A special frame used to maintain immobilization and provide for turning. The patient is placed between two mattresses on frames and the turn is lateral.

Fowler's position   A position in which the patient is in bed on his or her back with the head elevated approximately 60° (also called *mid-Fowler's position*). Traditionally, knees were also elevated, but this is seldom done today. The degree of elevation of the head can vary: in *semi-Fowler's position* (*low Fowler's position*) the head is at a 30° angle from the horizontal; in *high Fowler's position,* the head is as close to 90° as possible.

fracture pan   A container of metal or plastic with a lower edge, or lip, than a conventional bedpan; used for purposes of excretion by bedridden patients, especially those with fractured hips or in casts.

friction   The rubbing of one object or surface against another.

funeral director   A licensed person who is responsible for a body from the time of death until ultimate disposition; *mortician.*

funeral home   A place where the deceased are prepared for burial or cremation; mortuary.

gait   A way of moving on foot; a particular fashion of walking, running, or the like.

gait belt   A strong, webbing belt with a safety release buckle used to provide support for a patient during transfer and ambulation. Sometimes called a transfer and ambulation belt or simply transfer belt.

gastric gavage   Introducing a feeding by tube into the stomach.

gastric secretions   Enzymes produced by the glands of the lining of the stomach which digest certain components in food. Examples are hydrochloric acid and pepsin.

gastrocolic reflex   The emptying of the colon resulting from the filling of the stomach.

gastrostomy   A surgical opening into the stomach; usually for feeding by tube.

gauze bandage   A bandage of a soft, meshlike material. This type of bandage is usually used to wrap a part of the body and may or may not be stretchable. Kling is one of the brand names for a stretchable gauze bandage.

genital area   The body area that contains the reproductive organs.

girth   The distance around a body part, usually referring to the abdomen.

gliding joint   A joint in which a bone glides over the surface of another. The foot and vertebrae of the spine have gliding joints.

glucose   A dextrose sugar.

goggles   A barrier to protect the eyes from splashed fluids.

gooseneck lamp   An adjustable lamp with a slender flexible shaft.

graphic   Represented by a graph; often used to refer to the record of temperature, pulse, and respiration.

gravida   A pregnant woman; used with numerals to designate the number of pregnancies a woman has had regardless of outcome.

gravity   The force exerted by the earth on any object, tending to pull the object toward the center of the earth.

"green" cast   A cast that is still damp or not thoroughly hardened.

guaiac   A natural resin that is used as a reagent to test for blood in specimens.

gurgles   A bubbling sound of moisture in large airways heard upon auscultation of the lungs.

hairline fracture   A simple fracture of a bone that is not displaced. Shows on x-rays as a "hairline" image.

Harris flush   A term used to refer to a return-flow enema.

healthcare system   All those individuals, organizations, and agencies that provide health services and health financing considered as a whole.

health status   A person's level of ability in meeting his or her own needs.

Heimlich maneuver   An emergency procedure (also called subdiaphragmatic abdominal thrusts) devised for relieving foreign body airway obstruction.

Hematest   A brand name for a product that is used to test for the presence of blood in fecal specimens; commonly used to refer to the test itself.

hematuria   The presence of blood in the urine.

hinge joint   A joint in which the convex end of one bone rests on the concave surface of another. Examples are the elbow, knee, and ankle.

Homan's sign   A pain in the dorsal calf when the foot is forcibly flexed that can indicate thrombophlebitis.

horizontal   Parallel to or in the plane of the horizon.

humerus   The long bone of the upper part of the arm, extending from the shoulder to the elbow.

© 1996 by Lippincott-Raven Publishers

hydraulic Moved or operated by a fluid, especially water under pressure.

hydrometer An instrument that is used to determine specific gravity.

hyperalimentation The intravenous introduction of nutrients into a large vein, usually the subclavian.

hyperextension Extension of the joint beyond the straight position.

hypertonic Having a higher osmotic pressure than body fluid.

hypostatic pneumonia Pneumonia caused by lack of movement.

hypotonic Having a lower osmotic pressure than body fluid.

hypovolemic shock A state of shock that is caused by an abnormally low volume of body plasma.

iliac crest The highest portion of the broad rim of the hipbone.

immunosuppression The suppression of the body's natural immune system by drugs or disease.

impaction Compressed material in a confined space; for example, hardened feces in the bowel.

implementation The carrying out of a plan of action.

increased intracranial pressure A state in which there is a higher than normal pressure within the cranium.

incubate To warm so as to promote development and reproduction of microorganisms.

inflammation Localized heat, redness, swelling, and pain as a result of irritation, injury, or infection.

infused Put into or introduced.

infusion The introduction of a solution into a vessel; commonly, the introduction of a solution into a vein.

ingested See *ingestion*.

ingestion The taking in of food, liquids, or other substances by swallowing.

inspection A careful, critical visual examination.

instillation The process of pouring in drop by drop; commonly used to indicate a slow process of introducing fluid.

integument Skin.

intercostal space The space between the ribs.

interdigital Between the fingers (digits).

intermittent Stopping and starting at intervals.

internal disaster A disaster occurring within the medical facility.

internal girdle Those muscles of the abdomen, back, and hips that provide support to the abdominal contents and the pelvis.

internal rotation Moving a body part inward on an axis.

intracranial pressure The pressure maintained within the enclosed skull or cranium. When greater than normal, the term **increased intracranial pressure** is used.

intravenous infusion The introduction of a solution into a vein.

invasive Any procedure that involves the insertion or placement of a device through the skin or into a body orifice or cavity.

inversion Turning in an inward direction.

isometric exercises Contracting and relaxing the muscles voluntarily without obvious movement of the part.

isolation To set apart from the environment so that organisms cannot be readily transferred from one person to another.

isotonic exercises Exercises performed by the tightening and relaxing of various muscles without moving a body part.

isotope A radioactive substance used for diagnosis and treatment.

jejunum The second portion of the small intestine that extends from the duodenum to the ileum.

ketone body A substance synthesized by the liver as a step in the combustion of fats. May be present in increased amounts in abnormal situations, such as uncontrolled diabetes mellitus.

Kling bandage A brand name that is commonly used as a synonym for a loosely knit, lightweight, stretch roller bandage.

Korotkoff sounds The characteristic sounds, produced by the pressure of blood entering the artery during systole, that are heard on auscultation of an artery after it has been occluded.

Kussmaul's respirations Deep rapid respirations, often seen in states of acidosis or renal failure.

kyphosis An exaggerated posterior curvature of the thoracic spine. Produces a "humped" back.

labia The lips or folds of tissue that surround the female perineum.

lactase An enzyme secreted by the intestine which is necessary for the digestion of lactose (sugar found in milk).

lancet A small, sharp device for piercing the tissue.

legibility Able to be read or deciphered.

lesion A wound or injury in which tissue is damaged.

Levin tube A slender rubber or plastic tube that

© 1996 by Lippincott-Raven Publishers

is usually used for decompression of the stomach.

lithotomy position A position in which a person lies on back with legs flexed and spread apart.

litmus paper White paper that is impregnated with litmus and is used as an acid-base indicator.

livor biopsy The excision of microscopic liver tissue for examination.

livor mortis The skin discoloration that occurs after blood circulation stops due to the release of hemoglobin from the red blood cells that are breaking down.

LOB (loss of balance) An abbreviation used to expedite documentation related to activity. Used to indicate the presence or absence of loss of balance during standing, transfer or ambulation.

logrolling Turning a patient so that the entire body turns at one time with no twisting.

lumbar puncture (LP) The insertion of a needle into the spinal canal for purposes of withdrawing spinal fluid or instilling contrast dye materials; also called a *spinal tap.*

lumbosacral Pertaining to the lumbar and sacral regions of the spinal column.

lumen The inner, open space of a needle, tube, or vessel.

macerate To soften by prolonged contact with moisture.

macular A skin rash consisting of separate, circular flat reddened spots.

malleable Capable of being shaped or formed.

malnutrition A condition in which a person has less than the body's requirements of essential nutrients.

manometer An instrument that measures the pressure of liquids and gases.

medical asepsis The technique designed to prevent the spread of microorganisms from one person (or area) to another.

medical examiner An appointed public official, usually a forensic pathologist, whose function it is to investigate deaths that result from traumatic causes (homicide, suicide, accident) and sudden natural deaths in the absence of medical attention.

meniscus The curved upper surface of a liquid column.

mental practice A technique of reviewing a manual activity in the mind while "feeling" and "seeing" oneself performing each step correctly.

metabolism The complex of physical and chemical processes concerned with the disposition of the nutrients absorbed into the blood following digestion.

microorganism An animal or plant of microscopic size, especially a bacterium or protozoa.

midclavicular line An imaginary line running vertically through the midway point of the clavicle or collarbone.

military (24-hour) clock A system for noting time in which time is recorded as part of a 24-hour cycle, beginning at midnight. Hours before 10:00 AM are noted with a zero before the hour; minutes after the hour are noted immediately after the numbers for the hour. For example, 15 minutes after 1:00 AM would be recorded as 0115; the hours after noon are numbered 13, 14, and so on, so 15 minutes after 1:00 PM would be 1315.

minibottle A small container for intravenous infusion solutions.

minimum data set (MDS) A standardized data collection form that is required in nursing homes by government regulation.

mitered corner A method of folding a sheet or blanket to achieve a smooth squared covering over the corner of the mattress.

morgue A place in a healthcare facility where the bodies of deceased patients are temporarily held pending release to a mortician, coroner (medical examiner), or other authorized person.

mortician A funeral director and embalmer who is responsible for the care and disposition of a deceased person.

mortuary A place where the deceased are prepared for burial or cremation.

nares The openings in the nasal cavities; the nostrils.

narrative charting The traditional style of recording data on a patient's chart in a time-sequenced story-like form.

nasal mucosa The mucous membrane lining of the nose.

nasal speculum An instrument that is used to dilate the nostrils for purposes of inspecting or treating the nasal passages.

nasogastric tube A long, slender rubber or plastic tube that is introduced through the nose and esophagus into the stomach, for purposes of feeding or aspiration.

net binder A tube made of netlike material that is used to secure dressings to the body.

neurosensory Sensory function which is innervated by the nervous system, relating to seeing, hearing, smelling, tasting, and feeling.

next-of-kin The closest relative of a person.

NPO Nothing by mouth.

normal saline A solution of sodium chloride

© 1996 by Lippincott-Raven Publishers

with the same osmolality of tonicity as body fluid, usually given as 0.9 percent.

nosocomial An infection considered to have been acquired in a healthcare institution.

nursing diagnosis (1) The intellectual processes of sorting and classifying data collected, recognizing patterns and discrepancies, comparing these with norms, and identifying patient responses to health problems that are amenable to nursing intervention. (2) Also the end statement of the nursing process, which includes a statement of the problem and its etiology.

nursing history The initial data gathered through interview by the nurse.

nursing process A thoughtful, deliberate use of a problem-solving approach to nursing.

nystagmus Involuntary (vertical or horizontal) rapid, rhythmic movement of the eyeball.

objective Based on observable phenomena.

occiput The posterior, inferior portion of the cranium.

occult Hidden.

ombudsman An official designated to act as an advocate for a member of the public in disputes with a health care agency.

ophthalmoscope An instrument that consists of a light and a disc with an opening through which the interior of the eye is examined.

opposition Positioned opposite one another; for example, the thumb to the fingers.

organ donor A deceased person who donates organs for transplantation through a personal predeath bequest or through the bequest of the family after death.

orthopnea A state in which a person has difficulty breathing in the recumbent position and is relieved by sitting upright or standing.

orthostatic hypotension A sudden drop in blood pressure that is caused by a change in position, from lying to sitting or standing; may cause dizziness, fainting, and falling. Also called *postural hypotension*.

osmolarity The number of osmotically active particles in a unit of fluid.

otoscope An instrument, for inspecting the ears, consisting of a light and a cone.

ova The female reproductive cells of animals; eggs. Microscopic examination of stool is often done to identify the ova of intestinal parasites.

oximetry A technique for determining blood oxygen saturation by measuring the amount of light transmitted through a translucent part of the skin such as the ear lobe or fingertip.

oxygen saturation A measurement of the oxygen content of the blood compared to the oxygen capacity of the blood expressed as a percentage. Calculated by dividing the oxygen content by the oxygen capacity.

oxygenation Treating, combining, or infusing with oxygen.

palpation Examining or exploring by touch.

para Used with numerals to designate the number of pregnancies a woman has had in which a viable fetus (over 20 weeks' gestation or 500 g weight) is produced.

paracentesis The insertion of a trocar into the abdominal cavity for the removal of excess fluid.

paralysis Loss or impairment of the ability to move or have sensation in a bodily part as a result of injury to or disease of its nerve supply.

parasite Any organism that grows, feeds, and is sheltered on or in a host organism while contributing nothing to the host's survival.

parenteral fluid Fluid given directly into tissues or blood vessels.

password A code that provides an individual with access to computerized files.

patellar tendon A continuation of the quadriceps tendon that leads from the patella to the tibia.

patent Open.

pathogenic organism A microorganism that causes disease.

pathologist A specialist in pathology.

pathology The study of structural and functional changes caused by a disease process.

pavilion Related buildings forming a complex.

pectoralis muscles Four muscles of the chest.

pedal pulse A pulse wave that can be felt over the arteries of the feet.

percussion (1) A process of striking a finger held against the body surface with a fingertip of the opposite hand and listening to the resulting sound as part of assessment. (2) The striking of a hand on the chest wall to produce a vibration or shock that loosens secretions retained in the lungs.

perineum The portion of the body in the pelvic area that is occupied by urogenital passages and the rectum.

periorbital edema Edema around the eyes or the orbits.

periphery The outermost part or region.

peristalsis Wavelike muscular contractions that propel contained matter along the alimentary canal.

petaling Forming adhesive or moleskin "petals" by cutting strips into pointed or rounded ends and tucking around the rough edges of a cast in such a way that the skin is protected.

© 1996 by Lippincott-Raven Publishers

pH A measure of the acidity or alkalinity of a solution; 7.0 is neutral, and numbers below that indicate an acid solution and numbers above it indicate an alkaline solution, in a range of 1 to 14.

piggyback An intravenous infusion setup in which a second container is attached to the tubing of the primary container through a short tubing.

pinwheel A wheel-like instrument with sharp points that is used to test peripheral sensation of the body.

pivotal joint A joint in which the axis or protuberance rests in the atlas or cavity of another. The neck is an example of a pivotal joint.

planning The second step in the nursing process, in which information is reviewed and synthesized in order to form goals and a plan of action.

plantar flexion Bending the foot so that the toes point downward.

plaster of Paris cast A cast made of calcium sulfate, which, when combined with water, forms gypsum producing a light but rigid and durable structure.

popliteal artery The major artery that extends from the femoral artery down behind the knee.

popliteal space The hollow area behind the knee joint.

postmortem examination See *autopsy.*

postural hypotension A sudden drop in blood pressure that is caused by a change in position, from lying to sitting or standing; may cause dizziness, fainting, and falling; also called *orthostatic hypotension.*

preformed water The water content of ingested foods.

pressure ulcer Erosion of the skin, commonly over bony prominences, caused by excessive pressure. Sometimes called a decubitus ulcer.

pretibial edema Fluid accumulated in the tissue over the tibia.

prism glasses Glasses that direct the vision upward and then horizontally so that a patient in the supine position can see television or read books.

privacy The right to have matters of a personal nature not shared with anyone who does not have a need to know them.

problem-oriented medical record (POR or POMR) A system of keeping medical records that is organized according to the patient's problems.

proctoscope An instrument that dilates the anus to allow inspection or treatment of the lower intestine.

profuse Plentiful, overflowing, copious.

pronation Turning the palm or inner surface of the hand or forearm downward.

prone position A position in which the patient is lying on the abdomen with the head turned to one side.

protein An organic compound that contains amino acids as its basic structural unit.

protuberance An area of the body that protrudes above the usual surface, such as a distended abdomen or enlargement over a joint.

proximal Near the center part of the body or a point of attachment, or origin.

ptosis Paralytic drooping of the upper eyelid caused by nerve failure.

pulley A grooved wheel that allows free movement of a rope.

pulmonary embolus Obstruction of the pulmonary artery or one of its branches by an embolus.

pulse deficit The difference in rate between apical and radial pulses.

pulse pressure The difference between systolic and diastolic blood pressure readings.

pureed Strained, as in food.

PWB (partial weight bearing) An abbreviation used to expediate documentation related to activity. Used when the patient can bear only partial weight on the affected lower extremity.

pyrexia Fever.

quad cane A cane with a four-legged base for stability.

quadriplegia Paralysis of all four extremities.

radial artery The artery that descends from the brachial artery along the radius of the arm.

radial deviation Bending the hand on the wrist in the direction of the thumb (toward the radius).

radiolucent A surface through which x-rays can be taken.

rales Abnormal or pathologic respiratory sounds heard on auscultation; also called "crackles."

reagent A substance that is used in a chemical reaction to detect, measure, examine, or produce other substances.

rebound tenderness The pain or discomfort that is experienced when pressure is quickly withdrawn from an area.

recumbent The lying down position.

recurrent bandage A bandage that is wrapped in such a way that it recurs, or folds over, on itself.

referral A specific plan for directing a patient or client to other health care resources.

reflex contraction An involuntary response of muscle contraction.

© 1996 by Lippincott-Raven Publishers

reflex hammer   A small rubber-headed hammer that is used to test body reflexes; also called a *percussion hammer.*

reflux   The return of fluid substance backward through a valve that is not working correctly. For example, esophageal reflux refers to stomach contents moving into the esophagus; ureteral reflux refers to urine moving from the bladder into the ureters.

regurgitate   To vomit.

remittent   Increasing and decreasing in measurement.

renal calculi   Kidney stones.

reservoir   A container used to hold a fluid for continuous administration, such as in tube feeding.

resonance   In percussion, a vibrating sound that is produced in the normal chest.

respiratory arrest   The sudden cessation of breathing.

respite   An interval of rest or relief.

resuscitate   To revive or restore to life.

retraction   An abnormal pulling in of soft tissue of the chest on inspiration; commonly seen in the supraclavicular, intercostal, and substernal areas.

reverse spiral   A bandage that is applied, usually on a limb, in a circular fashion with a reverse fold.

rhonchi   Coarse rattling sounds that are produced by secretions in the bronchial tubes; also called "gurgles."

rigor mortis   Muscle stiffening after death.

roller bandage   Bandaging material that has been rolled to provide for easier application; commonly used to refer to rolls of gauze.

rotation   A circular movement around a fixed axis.

Roto-Rest bed   An electrically operated special bed that turns side to side continuously. Cervical, thoracic, and rectal areas can be cared for through posterior hatches.

saddle joint   A joint in which two bones rest together in convex-concave position. The thumb is an example of a saddle joint.

sanction   Authoritative permission or approval.

sanctions   Specific disapproval by a formal group.

SBA (standby assist)   An abbreviation used to expedite documentation related to activity. Used when the patient needs someone present during activity (especially transfer and ambulation) for assessment and possible assistance even if that individual usually does not need to provide actual support.

scalpel   A sharp surgical knife.

scoliosis   An abnormal lateral curvature of the spine.

scultetus binder   A heavy fabric binder that is held to the body by the interwrapping of cloth tails in an oblique fashion across the abdomen.

self-care   The ability to manage one's own life in such a way as to meet one's own needs.

self-determination   See *consent.*

semi-Fowler's position   See *Fowler's position.*

sequential compression device   An electronic device used to provide intermittent compression over the lower leg and/or thigh to promote venous return and prevent deep vein thrombosis and pulmonary embolism. Amounts of pressure may be adjusted on an attached control unit.

shock   A state of massive physiologic reaction to bodily illness or trauma, usually characterized by marked loss of blood pressure and the depression of vital processes and resulting in insufficient blood supply to vital tissue.

shroud   A cloth used to wrap a dead body.

side-lying position   A position in which the patient is on the side with the head supported on a low pillow.

sigmoid flexure   The distal portion of the colon, which appears as an S-shaped curve preceding the rectum.

sigmoidoscope   A tubular instrument with a light that is used to dilate the anus for inspection and treatment of the sigmoid.

Sims' position   A side-lying position with the top leg flexed forward.

skull tongs   Device inserted into each side of patient's cranium as an attachment for the application of traction.

smegma   A thick whitish substance, composed of epithelial cells and mucus, which is found around external genitalia.

Snellen chart   A chart printed with black letters in gradually decreasing sizes, used in testing vision.

SOAP   An acronym for a format used to record progress notes: *S*ubjective data, *O*bjective data, *A*ssessment, *P*lans.

sordes   Accumulation of dried secretions and bacteria in the mouth caused by not eating, mouth-breathing, and inadequate oral hygiene.

specific gravity   A measurement of the concentration of urine. Overhydration leads to a low specific-gravity figure; dehydration results in a high figure.

sphincter   A circular muscle that controls an internal or external orifice.

© 1996 by Lippincott-Raven Publishers

sphygmomanometer An instrument that measures blood pressure in the arteries.

spiral bandage A bandage that is applied, usually on a limb, in a circular ascending fashion.

spreader bar A bar that extends across the traction frame to allow traction pull to be aligned as needed.

stab wound A direct scalpel puncture into skin or membrane.

stereotype A presumed form or pattern that is attributed to a group and generalized to an individual.

sternum A long flat bone that forms the midventral support of most of the ribs; the breastbone.

stertorous Respirations having a heavy snoring sound.

stethoscope An instrument that is used for listening to sounds produced in the body; also see *bell* and *diaphragm.*

stockinette A soft, stretchy, ribbed material that comes in a tube shape of different circumferences. When pulled over a body part, it provides a smooth surface and protection from the inner surface of a cast.

stopcock A valve that regulates a flow of liquid through a tube.

straight abdominal binder A large cloth that is placed snugly around the lower part of the trunk to give support or to secure a dressing.

Stryker turning frame A special frame used to maintain immobilization and provide for turning. The patient is placed between two canvas suspension frames and the turn is lateral.

stylet A slender pointed instrument; a surgical probe that fits inside a hollow tubular instrument.

subjective Personal; in assessment, refers to information from the patient's viewpoint.

subungual Beneath the fingernails.

supine Position in which the person is lying flat on the back.

supination Turning or placing the hand and forearm so that the palm is upward.

supporting muscles The broad muscles of the body (back, abdomen and legs) that facilitate effective body mechanics.

suprasternal notch The notched bone formation that occurs at the uppermost end of the sternum.

suppuration The formation or discharge of pus.

sutures The thread, gut, or wire used to stitch tissues.

symmetry The equal configuration of opposite sides.

symphysis pubis The area at the front center of the pelvis, where the pubic bones from either side fuse into one bone.

symptom A perception of illness reported by the individual experiencing it.

synovial fluid A secretion of the synovial sac surrounding a joint. This clear fluid acts as a lubricating agent for the movement of the joint.

systole The rhythmic contraction of the heart, especially of the ventricles, by which blood is driven through the aorta and pulmonary artery after each dilation, or diastole.

systolic blood pressure The highest pressure reached in the arteries, created by the contraction of the ventricles of the heart.

tachycardia An abnormally rapid heartbeat, usually defined as above 100 beats/min, in the adult.

tachypnea Very rapid respirations.

T-binder A binder with a single tail that is used to hold a dressing in place on the perineum of a female patient.

technical proficiency Skill in the performance of tasks.

temporal artery One of the two three-branched arteries that lie at the temple of the head.

tepid Lukewarm.

thermistor A resistor made of semiconductors that has resistance that varies rapidly and predictably with temperature; able to measure extremely small temperature changes.

thoracentesis The insertion of a trocar into the pleural space of the chest for the removal of air or fluid.

thready pulse A weak, faint pulse.

thrombophlebitis Inflammation of the veins.

toe pleat A method of folding top bed linen to provide extra room for the feet.

tolerance In activity, the capacity to endure.

torsion The act or condition of being twisted or turned; the stress caused when one end of an object is twisted in one direction and the other end is held motionless or twisted in the opposite direction.

torso The trunk of the human body.

trachea A thin-walled tube of cartilaginous and membranous tissue that descends from the larynx to the bronchi, carrying air to the lungs.

tracheostomy A surgically devised opening into the trachea from the surface of the neck.

traction Applying a pulling force to bones. Usually used to reduce bone fractures.

transverse colon The portion of the colon across the top of the abdomen from the hepatic flexure to the splenic flexure.

trapeze A short, horizontal bar suspended from

© 1996 by Lippincott-Raven Publishers

a frame over the top of a bed. It is used by the patient to facilitate moving in bed and transfer.

tremor An involuntary trembling motion of the body.

Trendelenburg position A position in which the head is lower than the feet with the body on an inclined plane.

triage A process for assessing the level of care needed for a group of patients, often in an emergency situation.

trocar A sharp-pointed surgical instrument that is used with a cannula to puncture a body cavity for fluid aspiration.

trochanter The bony processes below the head of the femur; often used to refer to the greater trochanter, which is on the lateral aspect of the femur.

trochanter roll A roll made from a sheet, bath towel, or pad that is placed firmly beside the hip to stabilize the hip joint and prevent the leg from rotating outward.

tube feeding (1) The process of providing nutrients through a tube directly into the gastrointestinal tract for the person who is unable to eat a regular diet; (2) the liquid formula of nutrients instilled through a tube for the patient who is unable to eat a regular diet.

tuning fork A small two-pronged instrument that, when struck, produces a sound of fixed pitch; used to test auditory acuity.

turgor Normal tissue fullness in relationship to superficial body fluids.

twist support A strong plaster bar between two casted extremities or between a casted extremity and the body cast, formed by twisting a wetted plaster roll during the application of a cast.

tympanic Referring to the drum-like covering of the middle ear or to drum-like sounds heard on auscultation.

tympany In percussion, a low-pitched, drum-like sound.

ulnar deviation Bending the hand on the wrist in the direction of the fifth, or small finger.

Universal Precautions A set of behaviors designed to prevent the transmission of blood borne microorganisms by being used on all clients at all times.

urethral meatus The opening of the urethra onto the surface of the body through which urine is passed.

urinal A receptacle for urine that is used by bedridden patients.

urinalysis The chemical analysis of urine, which commonly includes color, clarity, pH, specific gravity, and checks for the presence of glucose, RBCs, casts, and WBCs.

urination The act of excreting urine.

urine refractometer A microscope-like instrument that refracts a beam of light through a drop of urine to give a reading of glucose content. Often used by nurses on the nursing unit.

urinometer An instrument that is used to determine the specific gravity of urine.

uvula The small, conical fleshy mass of tissue that is suspended from the center of the soft palate above the back of the tongue.

vaginal speculum An instrument that is used to dilate the vagina for purposes of inspecting or treating the vaginal passages or to obtain a specimen for a diagnostic test.

vasoconstriction A decrease in the lumen of blood vessels created by contraction of smooth muscle in the vessel wall.

vasodilation An increase in the lumen of blood vessels created by the relaxation of smooth muscle in the vessel wall.

venipuncture The act of piercing the vein with a needle.

venous Of or pertaining to a vein or veins.

venous pressure The pressure of blood in the veins; often measured in the superior vena cava. This measurement, called *central venous pressure* (CVP) is normally between 4 and 10 cm water.

venous thrombosis Formation of a blood clot inside of a vein.

ventricular fibrillation A cardiac arrhythmia characterized by rapid contractions of the ventricular muscle fibers without coordinated ventricular contraction. A frequent cause of cardiac arrest.

vesicant Any agent that can cause blistering or necrosis, the sloughing of tissue.

vibration A rapid, rhythmic "to and fro" motion.

void To empty any body cavity. Most commonly the emptying of urine from the bladder through the urethra; to urinate.

vulva The external female genitalia, including the labia majora, the labia minora, the clitoris, and the vestibule of the vagina.

walker A rehabilitative device that is used by a disabled person for support while standing or walking.

walking heel A metal or plastic implant embedded in the heel of a plaster or fiberglass leg cast to facilitate walking.

water balance A state of the body in which the fluid intake is in equilibrium with the fluid output.

© 1996 by Lippincott-Raven Publishers

water bed   A special water-filled mattress used to distribute pressure evenly over the body.

WBT (weight bear as tolerated)   An abbreviation used to expedite documentation related to activity. Used when the patient is permitted to bear as much weight as is comfortable on the affected lower extremity.

weight-bearing   The side on which the weight of the body can be placed while standing; *partial weight-bearing* indicates that an individual cannot stand solely on the affected limb and must have other means of support also.

wheezes   Hoarse whistling sounds, produced by breathing, that are considered abnormal.

"whiplash"   Injury of the neck or cervical spine due to a sudden whiplike motion of the body.

windowing   The procedure of cutting an opening in a cast to allow for observation, care of the skin underneath, and relief of pressure.

xiphoid process   The lower tip of the sternum.

© 1996 by Lippincott-Raven Publishers

ANSWERS TO QUIZZES

Module 1 An Approach to Nursing Skills

1. **a.** Right to self determination/consent
   b. Right to information upon which to base decisions
   c. Right to privacy/confidentiality
   d. Right to safe care
   e. Right to personal dignity
   f. Right to individualized care
   g. Right to assistance toward independence
   h. Right to criticize and obtain changes in care
2. Any one of the following: calling patient by preferred name; helping person to be physically clean and attractive; always pulling drapes and closing doors for privacy
3. **a.** Assessment
   b. Nursing Diagnosis
   c. Planning
   d. Implementation
   e. Evaluation
4. Gathering data, analyzing data, and identifying the problems present
5. **a.** Correct technique
   b. Organization
   c. Dexterity
   d. Speed
6. Past practice and sound deductive reasoning from known facts
7. To identify the outcomes of nursing action
8. Imagine yourself performing the actions in the procedure while "feeling" and "seeing" yourself doing the movements and skills described.

Module 2 Basic Infection Control

1. d
2. d
3. d
4. b
5. d
6. c
7. **a.** Microorganisms move through space on air currents.
   b. Microorganisms are transferred from one surface to another whenever objects touch.
   c. Microorganisms are transferred by gravity whenever one item is held above another.
   d. Microorganisms move slowly on dry surfaces but very quickly through moisture.
   e. Blood-borne microorganisms may enter the body through mucous membranes.
   f. Needle stick injuries are more likely to occur when needles are handled or broken.
   g. Feces contain large quantities of microorganisms that are difficult to eradicate with routine handwashing.

Module 3 Safety

1. **a.** The facility is complex and unfamiliar.
   b. Space is often limited.
   c. A variety of equipment is used.
2. **a.** Good body mechanics
   b. Walking, not running
   c. Keeping to the right in hallways
   d. Turning corners and opening doors carefully
   e. Using stretchers properly
   f. Using brakes on beds, wheelchairs and stretchers
   g. Using elevators correctly
3. Side rails or restraints used cautiously; bed in low position; patient positioned so that extremities are free; protection from sharp objects, with special attention to eyes and air passages.
4. Prevention of aspiration of materials or fumes.
5. To protect the patient and the staff.
6. Any three of the following: falls, contractures, pressure sores, dehydration, chronic constipation, functional incontinence, loss of bone mass and muscle tone, loss of ability to move around independently.
7. Safe areas for exercise
   Alarm systems
8. Wrist; mitt
9. Belt; vest
10. Risk for injury related to confusion
11. Cigarettes not for sale in facilities; designated smoking "No smoking" policies on the premises; placing patients in rooms according to smoking habits.

© 1996 by Lippincott-Raven Publishers

12. **a.** Be familiar with code procedure.
    b. Remove patients from immediate vicinity of fire.
    c. Initiate code.
    d. Return to unit if you did not call code.
    e. Never use elevators.
    f. Return patients to rooms and close doors.
    g. Calm patients.
    h. Follow directions of person in charge.
    i. Stand in hallway.
    j. Evacuate according to procedure if necessary.
    k. Remain calm.
    l. Wait for directions at all clear signal.
13. To be knowledgeable, report as designated and perform skills as predetermined by plans.
14. **a.** To document an event.
    b. To serve as a record for insurance and legal purposes.
    c. To identify need to modify or rectify a policy or procedure.
15. **a.** Most residents are elderly.
    b. Many have mobility problems.
    c. Some have impairment of neurosensory function.
16. **a.** Assess the home environment for safety.
    b. Make suggestions for improving environment for safety.

Module 4   Basic Body Mechanics

1. T
2. T
3. F
4. F
5. T
6. F
7. These muscles may become tired or injury to the back may occur.
8. It is easier to move an object on a level surface than to move it up a slanted surface against the force of gravity.
9. Enlarging the base of support in the direction of the force to be applied increases the amount of force that can be applied.
10. It takes less energy to hold an object close to the body than at a distance from the body; it is also easier to move an object that is close.

Module 5   Documentation

1. b
2. c
3. a

4. **a.** Source-oriented method
    b. Problem-oriented record
5. (Name two of three)
    a. Narrative format
    b. SOAP format
    c. Focus notes
6. So that others may check the original data and make their own inferences
7. Upset
8. Line through incorrect information and write "Error 175 ml SJ"
    or
    "wrong amount SJ"
    "clear yellow urine 175 ml"
9. The hospital
10. Patients have a right to the information contained in the record. Usually there is a procedure to follow in the facility.

Module 6   Introduction to Assessment Skills

1. a
2. c
3. b
4. e
5. S
6. O
7. S
8. O
9. O
10. Any five of the following: color, odor, size, shape, symmetry, movement
11. **a.** What is being done
    b. Why it is being done
    c. What the patient can do to make it easier for himself or herself and the nurse

Module 7   Temperature, Pulse, and Respiration

1. 37°C; 98.6°F
2. Any four of the following: time of day; age; presence of infection; environment; exercise; emotions; metabolism
3. Prevent injury to the mucosa
4. 8 minutes; 3 minutes; 9 minutes; only seconds; only seconds.
5. 3, 2, 1
6. 50, 100
7. Any four of the following: exercise; application of heat or cold; medications; emotions; blood loss
8. **a.** Radial
    b. Carotid
    c. Temporal

© 1996 by Lippincott-Raven Publishers

9. 16; 20
10. Any four of those listed in answer 7, as well as disorders of the respiratory tract

Module 8 Blood Pressure

1. c
2. c
3. b
4. d
5. a
6. b
7. 140/80/70
8. Because low-pitched sounds are more easily heard with the bell head than with the diaphragm
9. a. The disappearance of the usual sounds heard over the brachial artery when cuff pressure is high and their reappearance at a lower level when the cuff pressure is reduced
b. By pumping the hand bulb on the blood pressure cuff to a point 30 mm of mercury beyond the point at which you last felt a pulse

Module 9 The Nursing Physical Assessment

1. a. Size
b. Shape
c. Equality of pupils
2. In a position above 45°
3. 4 and 10 cm
4. Around the eyes
5. Because the breasts may be particularly sensitive at the time of menstruation
6. Because palpation and percussion can change the bowel sounds that might be heard
7. Fifth intercostal space near the nipple line (the apex)
8. Any one of the following: bronchial obstruction; chronic lung disease; shallow breathing
9. Pneumonia
10. If the scratchy sound correlates with the rate and rhythm of the heartbeat, not the respirations, it is a pericardial friction rub.

Module 10 Intake and Output

1. a
2. c
3. c
4. b
5. a

6. c
7. c
8. a
9. b
10. b
11. a
12. d

Module 11 Collecting Specimens and Performing Common Laboratory Tests

1. Assess the patient for signs or symptoms of problems that would relate to abnormality. Notify the physician as appropriate.
2. Procedure manual or laboratory manual of the facility.
3. Getting the right amount of specimen in the right container, from the right patient, and tested in the right way.
4. Whenever there is any possibility of contacting a body substance.
5. Put the specimen container in a plastic bag.
6. T
7. F
8. F
9. F
10. F

Module 12 Assisting with Diagnostic and Therapeutic Procedures

1. a. Meeting the physical and psychologic needs of the patient
b. Gathering necessary equipment and assisting the physician
2. Dyspnea, pallor, sudden pain, cough, or diaphoresis
3. Reduce bleeding at the site
4. a. Privacy
b. Set up and clean table
c. Obtain equipment
d. Provide lighting
5. F
6. T
7. T
8. d
9. c
10. a

Module 13 Admission, Transfer, and Discharge

1. b
2. a
3. c

© 1996 by Lippincott-Raven Publishers

4. c
5. d
6. d
7. d
8. d
9. b
10. A discharge planner
11. Elevated temperature
12. It is an extension of care and makes the transition more effective.
13. **a.** Share information that is needed, identifying needs.
   b. Answer questions the patient and family might have concerning the new environment.

Module 14   Bedmaking

1. Clean and wrinkle-free; provides comfort
2. Conserves energy
3. The postop bed is in high position for easy transfer and the linen is fanfolded so the patient can be easily covered to prevent chilling.
4. Use side rails appropriately to protect the patient from falling.
5. Decreases the effectiveness of the mattress
6. b
7. d
8. a
9. c
10. b
11. 6,8,5,2,1,4,7,3

Module 15   Moving the Patient in Bed and Positioning

1. So as not to be working against the gravitational pull.
2. **a.** Promotes physical progress
   b. Adds to the patient's self-esteem
3. Dislocation of the shoulder
4. The patient's trunk
5. **a.** For the patient's comfort and safety
   b. To make sure there is no undue pressure on parts
6. **a.** To prevent pressure sores
   b. To prevent joint contractures
   c. To improve muscle tone and circulation
7. Trochanter roll
8. Flexed
9. **a.** Feet in space between mattress and footboard
   b. Roll placed under ankles
10. Develop a teaching plan and teach the proper

method of moving and positioning residents or affected family members.
11. b
12. b
13. c

Module 16   Feeding Adult Patients

1. (in any order)
   a. Environment
   b. Emotions
   c. Physical disability
   d. Dentures
2. (in any order)
   a. Hot or cold temperature foods
   b. Cooked vegetables
   c. Pureed fruits
   d   Thickened liquids
3. (in any order)
   a. Water, tea, or coffee
   b. Tough, stringy foods
   c. Sticky foods
   d. Apple juice or other juices
4. c
5. b
6. a
7. F
8. F
9. T
10. F

Module 17   Assisting with Elimination and Perineal Care

1. **a.** Basic infection control principles
   b. Psychologic comfort principles
   c. Principles related to normal bowel function
2. **a.** Bedpan
   b. Urinal
   c. Fracture pan
   d. Emesis basin
3. **a.** Pad the pan.
   b. Warm it.
4. **a.** Lifting the buttocks
   b. Rolling onto the pan
5. **a.** Getting the patient out of the bed
   b. Ambulating the patient
6. Any five of the following: amount; color; consistency; odor; blood; mucus; foreign matter
7. **a.** Postpartum patients
   b. Surgical patients
   c. Patients with catheters in place
8. Refer to Performance Checklist.
9. For aesthetic purposes
10. On the nursing care plan

© 1996 by Lippincott-Raven Publishers

11. To prevent contamination of the urinary meatus with microbes from the rectal area

Module 18   Hygiene

1. c
2. b
3. d
4. In sterile saline or special soaking solution
5. **a.** Place a drop of saline or lens solution in the eye.
   b. Place one finger on the upper lid and one on the lower lid.
   c. Raise the upper lid and gently push in on the lower lid at the lower margin of the lens to pop it out.
6. To avoid scratching the lenses
7. Remove the battery and place in a safe, dry place.
8. Toileting. Hands and face washed. Teeth brushed. Bed checked for dry and clean.
9. Toileting. Hands and face washed. Teeth brushed. Bed straightened. Clean pillowcase and gown as needed. Back rubbed.
10. F
11. T
12. T
13. F
14. T
15. F
16. T
17. T
18. T

Module 19   Basic Infant Care

1. The thickest part is placed where the greatest absorbency is needed, and the infant has free movement of legs.
2. Urine or feces on the skin contributes to a variety of skin problems.
3. Close them and put them out of reach of the infant.
4. Diaper rash is a reddened rash throughout the diaper area. Scald is a solid red, burn-type area.
5. Place a small amount in your hand and smooth it over the infant's skin rather than "sprinkling" it on, because it acts as an irritant to the respiratory tract.
6. Shake some on the inner aspect of your wrist.
7. Hold the bottle so that the nipple is filled with fluid, not air.
8. Because once infants have tasted the naturally sweet fruit, they will prefer to continue eating it and will not want to finish the plain food

9. It will not slip and become tighter, cutting off circulation.
10. Any three of the following: avoid chilling; keep one hand on the infant; check water for correct temperature; place basin on a safe surface; put side rail or crib net in place when finished
11. Apply a non-water soluble ointment to the diaper area. Wash thoroughly after each stool and reapply ointment.
12. Lying on the right side.

Module 20   Transfer

1. Any four of the following: maintains and restores muscle tone; stimulates respiration; stimulates circulation; improves elimination; improves psychologic well-being
2. Any two of the following
   a. They give the patient a sense of security.
   b. They prevent slipping.
   c. They prevent foot injury.
   d. They protect against contaminated floors.
3. Ease patient back onto bed or chair of origin or gently to the floor.
4. Chair must be placed on left side; extra support may be needed; right leg must be braced with nurse's leg or knee while pivoting
5. To provide a firm handhold and support for the nurse when transferring the patient
6. **a.** Bed to chair: one-person maximal assist
   b. Bed to chair: two-person maximal assist
7. To prevent dizziness
8. Any two of the following: patient's body alignment; patient's comfort; safety for the patient; safety and proper body mechanics for the nurse(s) involved
9. Any three of the following: pain; fatigue; pulse and respiration rate; blood pressure changes; dizziness
10. When moving the supine patient between bed and stretcher.
11. Injury to the care providers and dropping the patient.

Module 21   Ambulation: Simple Assisted and Using Cane, Walker, or Crutches

1. Any four of the following: maintains muscle tone; restores muscle tone; stimulates respiratory system; stimulates circulatory system; improves psychologic well-being; facilitates elimination
2. Falls

© 1996 by Lippincott-Raven Publishers

3. They give better support, are less likely to slip, and usually stay on better.
4. A transfer and ambulation belt; a cane; a walker; or crutches
5. Crutches should extend from the floor, about 6 inches out from the foot, to the side of the chest 2 inches under the axilla.
6. Four-point gait.
7. Push up from arms of the chair (or the bed).
8. Opposite the weak leg
9. Hold both in one hand.
10. Three-point gait
11. Crutches, weak leg, strong leg
12. Any three of the following: stairs, narrow doors, rugs, furniture placement, inadequate lighting.

Module 22   Range-of-Motion Exercises

1. **a.** To maintain joint mobility
   b. To prevent lengthy rehabilitation
2. **a.** When increasing the level of energy expended or the level of circulation is potentially hazardous
   b. When joints are swollen or inflamed or there is injury near the joint
3. Flexors
4. Elbow, knee, and ankle
5. Thumb
6. Gliding
7. Active
8. Supination
9. Abduction
10. b
11. c
12. c

Module 23   Caring for Patients with Casts and Braces

1. Plaster of Paris; plastic
2. Hard; inexpensive
3. Easy to apply; rigid and durable
4. Serious skin breakdown or infection after casting
5. Folded down stockinette; petaling
6. Motion; sensation; pain
7. Cotton padding, plastic, and metal
8. The weight and confinement of the brace may disturb balance.
9. d
10. b
11. b
12. c
13. b

Module 24   Applying and Maintaining Traction

1. Skin traction is applied to the muscles or skin through the use of tapes, belts, or halters. Skeletal traction is applied to the skeletal frame or bones through wires, pins, or tongs that are surgically inserted through or into the bone.
2. Footboard; plantar flexion
3. Any four of the following: constipation; respiratory complications; boredom; anorexia; skin breakdown; thrombophlebitis
4. (1) a
   (2) d, f
   (3) d
   (4) h
   (5) c
   (6) e, g
   (7) e
5. d
6. c

Module 25   Special Mattresses and Therapeutic Frames and Beds

1. **a.** To prevent or treat pressure sores
   b. To keep patient immobile so healing can take place
2. Circulation of air
3. The Stryker frame turns laterally while the CircOlectric turns vertically.
4. Do not put the special sheets in with the general laundry; do not use pins which can puncture the mattress covering; remove watches because they can be damaged by the dispersement of microscopic particles.
5. Unplug the bed to provide a firm surface.
6. b
7. a
8. b
9. b
10. c

Module 26   Applying Bandages and Binders

1. **a.** To provide support
   b. To protect wounds
   c. To protect and hold underlying dressings
2. **a.** Circular
   b. Spiral
   c. Reverse spiral
   d. Figure 8
   e. Recurrent fold
3. A joint
4. Distal; proximal

© 1996 by Lippincott-Raven Publishers

5. To promote venous return and prevent deep vein thrombosis and pulmonary embolism.
6. Severe arterial disease of the lower extremities.
7. **a.** To hold layer dressings in place
   b. For support
8. Stretch net bandages are easy to wash, provide air circulation, and are comfortable for the patient.
9. Safety pins have hard surfaces and may cause tissue damage if the patient rests on them.
10. Male; female
11. d
12. c

Module 27   Applying Heat and Cold

1. a
2. c
3. c
4. b
5. c
6. b
7. b
8. b
9. d
10. c

Module 28   Administering Enemas

1. Any four of the following: *cleansing*—to remove fecal material and clean the bowel; *medicated*—to allow medication to be absorbed; *oil-retention*—to soften fecal material; *cooling*—for extremely elevated temperature; *return-flow*—to remove gas
2. **a.** Embarrassment
   b. Modesty
   c. Fear of discomfort
3. **a.** Color
   b. Respiratory rate
   c. Pulse
   d. Signs of excess fatigue
4. By lowering the fluid container below the level of the bowel
5. Slow the flow rate of fluid. If cramping still continues, stop the procedure until cramps subside.
6. **a.** Can be given more rapidly
   b. Cause less distention and discomfort
7. **a.** Soothe the intestinal mucosa
   b. Combat infections
   c. Correct electrolyte imbalances
8. Size 10 French
9. 300 ml

10. **a.** Being meticulous about providing privacy
    b. Giving less solution more slowly

Module 29   Tube Feeding

1. a
2. c
3. b
4. b
5. a
6. c
7. a
8. After each feeding or medication administration. To provide fluids required by the patient or ordered by the physician.
9. Test the secretions for glucose content. Secretions containing formula will have a high glucose content.
10. Withhold the feeding. Check the policy manual or the physician's orders to determine the amount of residual allowable before resuming feeding.
11. Medications, lactose intolerance, cold formula, sudden change in consistency of diet.
12. Introducing a carbonated beverage if not contraindicated or instilling an enzyme solution to digest and dissolve the obstruction.

Module 30   Emergency Resuscitation Procedures

1. Shake the person and say loudly, "Are you all right?"
2. Because the most common cause of arrest in the pediatric age group is primary respiratory arrest or an obstructed airway, the procedure is to assess the patient and provide approximately one minute of rescue support before activating EMS.
3. Flat, with the neck straight
4. Locate the larynx (voice box), and slide your fingers toward yourself to the hollow beside it.
5. By placing your thumb on the outside of the infant's upper arm and pressing gently with your index and middle fingers on the inside of the upper arm
6. 1-1/2 inches above the xiphoid process
7. **a.** 80–100/min
   b. 80–100/min
   c. At least 100/min
   d. 80–100/min
8. 2 breaths to each 15 chest compressions
9. 1 breath to each 5 chest compressions
10. Clutching the neck in the area of the larynx between the thumb and index finger

© 1996 by Lippincott-Raven Publishers

11. In the midline, below the xiphoid process of the sternum but above the navel
12. Only in the unconscious patient to attempt to grasp a foreign body and remove it

Module 31   Postmortem Care

1. c
2. The realization of offering an extension of life to another
3. Kidneys, hearts, skin, corneas, pituitaries, and bones
4. Viability and usefulness of tissues
5. Coroner is elected or appointed, not necessarily a physician. Medical examiner is an appointed physician, usually holding a special degree in pathology.
6. See your county's requirements.
7. Any three of the following: rigor mortis; livor mortis; skin indentation; algor mortis
8. Any four of the following: clean the patient; place the patient in repose; straighten the unit; soften the lights; rearrange flowers; provide chairs
9. Any two of the following: make sure the family knows they can see and hold the infant; wrap the infant in a receiving blanket and carry as you would a living baby; provide a nursery crib if the family is not comfortable holding the baby; offer the family the opportunity to be alone.
10. To prevent discoloration and indentation of the underlying hand if folded over the chest
11. a. IVs
    b. Nasogastric tubes
    c. Urinary catheters
    d. Oxygen equipment
12. An examination of the body after death
13. a. To determine cause of death
    b. To gather scientific knowledge
    c. To add to statistical data

© 1996 by Lippincott-Raven Publishers

INDEX

Page numbers followed by *f* indicate illustrations;
t following a page number indicates tabular material.

A

Abbreviations, 81, 82*t*, 83*t*
  for hygiene procedures, 396*t*
Abdomen
  assessment of, 167–170, 175
    performance checklist, 183–184, 186
    procedure for, 168–170, 169*f*
    quadrants of, 168, 169*f*
Abdominal binder(s), 632
  application of, 632–633, 632*f*
    performance checklist, 645–646
Abdominal bruit, listening for, 168
Abdominal thrusts, for foreign-body
    airway obstruction, 731–732, 731*f*, 732*f*
    performance checklist, 737, 738–739
AccuChek bG, 229
Ace bandage, 624
Acetest, 216*t*
  drug interference with, 225*t*
  procedure for using, 227
    performance checklist, 240
Acetone, testing urine for, 227–228
    performance checklist, 240–241
Achilles reflex, 176, 177*f*
Acquired immunodeficiency syndrome
    (AIDS), 20
Active low air loss bed, 605, 606*f*, 608*t*–611*t*
Activity, assessment of, 114, 119
Activity Intolerance (nursing diagnosis), 126
Activity(-ies) of daily living (ADL),
    flow sheet for, 395*f*
Addressing patient, patient's dignity
    and, 8
ADL (activities of daily living), flow
    sheet for, 395*f*
Admission, 277–285
  delegating tasks at, 291
  documentation at, 284–285, 285*f*–287*f*
  to long-term care, 291
  nurse's responsibilities at, 282–285
  performance checklist, 293
  placement of patients at, 282
  quiz, 297–298
  rationale for skill, 282
Advance directives, 748–749

Advocate, patient, 9
Against medical advice (AMA) depar-
    ture, 289
AIDS (acquired immunodeficiency
    syndrome), 20
Air-fluidized bed, 605–606, 606*f*, 608*t*–611*t*
Air mattress(es), 602, 602*f*
Airway
  of dependent patient, protection of, 42
  obstruction of, by foreign body. *See*
    Foreign-body airway obstruc-
    tion
  opening of
    in CPR, 724, 724*f*
    for infant, 728
Albustix, 216*t*
Alcohol, in cooling sponge bath, 663
Aldomet (methyldopa), interference
    by, in urine glucose testing, 225*t*
Algor mortis, 751
Alternating pressure mattress(es), 602
AMA (against medical advice) depar-
    ture, 289
Ambulation, 489–519
  general procedure for, 492–493
    performance checklist, 507–508
  in home care, 505, 505*f*
  in long-term care, 505
  nursing diagnoses related to, 492
  performance checklist, 507–517
  quiz, 519
  rationale for skill, 492
  simple assisted, 493–494, 493*f*
    performance checklist, 508–509
  using cane, 494–495, 494*f*–496*f*
    performance checklist, 509–510
  using crutches. *See* Crutchwalking
  using walker, 495–496, 497*f*
    performance checklist, 510–512
Ambulation belt, 461, 493, 493*f*
AM care, 409
  in long-term care facility, 410
Analysis
  in nursing process, 10
  recording of, in nursing record, 76
Anderson frame, 314, 314*f*
Aneroid manometer, 145, 145*f*

Anesthetic bed, procedure for making,
    310–311, 310*f*
  performance checklist, 319–320
Ankle(s), assessment of, 175
  performance checklist, 187
Ankle joint, 526*t*
  bandage application to, 627–628
    performance checklist, 640–641
  range-of-motion exercise for,
    531–533, 535*f*
    performance checklist, 540
Ankle restraint(s), 44, 45*f*
Ankle roll, 335
Anterior spinal hyperextension brace,
    560, 561*f*
Antiembolic stockings. *See* Elastic
    stockings
Apical pulse, 132, 132*f*
Apical-radial pulse, 132
  performance checklist, 138
  procedure for, 134
Appliance(s), electrical
  oxygen and, 41
  safety in using, 39, 39*f*
Arm(s)
  assessment of, 172
    performance checklist, 185
  joints of, 526*t*
Arm cast(s), 554, 555*f*
Arm sling(s), 632
  application of, 633–635, 635*f*, 636*f*
    performance checklist, 648–649
Arthritis, range-of-motion exercise for
    patient with, 537
Artificial tears, 407
Ascites, 168
  assessment for, 169
    performance checklist, 183–184
  removal of. *See* Paracentesis
Ascorbic acid, interference by, in urine
    glucose testing, 225*t*
Asepsis, 19
Aspiration (event), of tube feeding for-
    mula, detection of, 706
Aspiration (procedure)
  bone marrow, assisting with, 255*t*, 261, 272–273
  for verifying feeding tube place-
    ment, 707

© 1996 by Lippincott-Raven Publishers

Assessment, 103–298
  baseline, at admission, 283–284, 285f, 286f
  data on, in nursing record, 76
  at discharge, 291
  in elderly patient, 117–118, 117f
  functional, 114
  in home care, 118
  human needs approach to, 114–116, 119–120
  in long-term care, 117–118
  methods of, 109–113
  in nursing process, 10
  physical, 114–116, 119–120, 155–191
    "3-minute head-to-toe," 179, 188–189
    "15-minute head-to-toe," 178–179, 188
    basic techniques for, 111–112, 113f
    comprehensive, 171–178, 173f–175f, 177f, 178f
    performance checklist, 181–189
    quiz, 191
    rationale for skill, 160
  psychosocial, 116, 120
  quiz, 121
  rationale for skill, 109
Athletic shoes, to prevent footdrop, 314, 336
Auscultation, 112
Auscultatory gap, 146
Autopsy, 754–757, 756f, 757f
Axillary temperature, 130
  procedure for measuring, 134
    performance checklist, 137

B
Babinski reflex, 176, 177f
Baby powder, 436
Back, assessment of, 174, 175f
  performance checklist, 186
Back blows, for foreign-body airway obstruction in infant, 733, 733f
Back rub, 401–402, 401f, 402f
  performance checklist, 418–419
Balanced suspension traction, 586–587, 587f
Ball-and-socket joint(s), 525
Bandage(s), 619–652
  application of
    assessment after, 623–624, 625f
    general procedure for, 623–624
    methods for, 624–627, 626f, 627f
    performance checklist, 639–645
    specific procedures for, 627–630
  in home care, 637
  in long-term care, 635–637
  quiz, 651–652
  rationale for skill, 623
  types of, 624
Bath(s)
  bed. *See* Bedbath(s)

for cooling, 662–663
  performance checklist, 673–674
  procedure for, 665–666
in home care, 410
for infant, 438–439, 438f, 439f
  performance checklist, 447–448
in long-term care, 410
performance checklist, 414–417
procedures for, 396–401, 397f–399f
sitz, 660
  performance checklist, 672–673
  procedure for, 664–665, 664f
tub, 399–400
  performance checklist, 416
Bath blanket(s), 396
Bathing/Hygiene Self-Care Deficit (nursing diagnosis), 394
Bathroom, safety in, 40
Bed(s). *See also* Bedmaking
  accessories for, 313–315, 313f, 314f
  brakes on, 38
  closed, 308
  moving patient in. *See* Moving patient in bed
  open, 308, 309f
  positioning in. *See under* Positioning
  position of, safety considerations in, 42
  therapeutic, 597–601, 602–612, 608t–611t
    in home care, 612
    in long-term care, 612
    performance checklist, 613
    procedure for using, 607–612
    quiz, 615–616
    rationale for skill, 601
  traction, 579–580, 579f
  transfer from. *See under* Transfer technique(s)
Bedbath(s)
  complete, 396–399, 397f–399f
    performance checklist, 414–415
  for infant, 438–439, 438f, 439f
  partial, 399
  self, 399
Bedboard(s), 313
Bed cradle(s), 314–315, 314f
Bedmaking, 301–324
  body mechanics in, 305–306, 305f
    performance checklist, 317
  in home care, 315
  infection control in, 305
    performance checklist, 317
  in long-term care, 315
  nursing diagnoses related to, 305
  for occupied bed, 311–313, 312f
    performance checklist, 320–322
  performance checklist, 317–322
  for postop (anesthetic, surgical) bed, 310–311, 310f
    performance checklist, 319–320
  quiz, 323–324
  rationale for skill, 305
  with special mattresses, 314, 601, 602

for unoccupied bed, 306–309, 307f, 309f
  performance checklist, 317–319
Bedpan(s), 375–376, 375f, 376f
  assisting with, 377–379, 378f
  performance checklist, 385–386
Beliefs, patient's, assessment of, 116, 120
Belt(s), transfer, 461, 493, 493f
Belt restraint(s), 43, 44f
Benemid (probenecid), interference by, in urine glucose testing, 225t
Biceps reflex, 176, 177f
Bili-Labstix, 216t
Binder(s), 619–624, 632–652
  application of
    general procedure for, 623–624
    performance checklist, 639–640, 645–649
    specific procedures for, 632–635
  in home care, 637
  in long-term care, 635–637
  quiz, 651–652
  rationale for skill, 623
  types of, 632
Biodyne bed, 605
Biopsy
  bone marrow, assisting with, 255t, 261, 272–273
  liver, assisting with, 254t, 259–260, 270–272
Bivalving, 554–556, 556f
Blackbird chart, 173
Blanket(s)
  bath, 396
  thermal. *See* Thermal blanket
Bleach, as germicide, 21, 23
Blink reflex, 176
Blood
  collecting specimen of, 218t, 220
  glucose in. *See* Blood glucose
  occult
    testing urine for, 228
    test products for, 216t
  in stool, testing for, 230–231, 243–245
Blood-borne infection(s), preventing spread of, 20–22, 20t
Blood glucose, testing for, 229–230
  performance checklist, 242–243
  products used in, 216t
Blood pressure, 141–153. *See also* Vital signs
  diastolic, 148
  measurement of
    alternative techniques for, 148–149, 149f
    equipment for, 144–145, 145f
    in home care, 149
    in long-term care, 149
    performance checklist, 151–152
    procedure for, 145–148, 145f
    rationale for skill, 144
    at thigh, 148
  norms and variables for, 144
  nursing diagnoses related to, 144

© 1996 by Lippincott-Raven Publishers

quiz, 153
recording of, 147*f*, 148
systolic, 148
Blood specimen, collection of, 218*t*, 220
Body mechanics, 59–69
in bedmaking, 305–306, 305*f*
performance checklist, 317
in home care, 64–65
importance of, 37
in long-term care, 64
nursing diagnoses related to, 62
performance checklist, 67
principles of, 62–64, 63*f*, 64*f*
quiz, 69
rationale for skill, 62
Body Substance Precautions, 20
Body temperature. *See* Temperature
Body weight
at admission, 283
daily, in fluid balance monitoring, 197
loss of, significance of, 114
Bolster(s), for wheelchair, 46
Bone marrow aspiration, assisting with, 255*t*, 261
performance checklist, 272–273
Bone marrow biopsy, assisting with, 255*t*, 261
performance checklist, 272–273
Boston brace, 560, 561*f*
Boston scoliosis brace, 560, 560*f*
Bottle-feeding, 439–441, 440*f*, 441*f*
performance checklist, 449
Bowel sounds, 167
procedure for assessing, 168
performance checklist, 183
Brace(s), 545–550, 558–562
assisting with application of, 570–571
procedure for, 562
cast with, 561, 561*f*
emotional support for patient with, 563
in home care, 563
in long-term care, 563
nursing diagnoses related to, 550
purposes of, 558
quiz, 573
rationale for skill, 550
types of, 559–562, 559*f*–562*f*
Brachial pulse, 131
in infant, 728, 728*f*
Brachioradial reflex, 176
Bradycardia, 130
Brakes, 38
Breast(s), assessment of, 166–167, 167*f*
performance checklist, 182–183
Breathing. *See* Respiration(s)
rescue. *See* Cardiopulmonary resuscitation; Rescue breathing
Breath sounds, 164
Bruit(s), 167
abdominal, listening for, 168
Bryant's traction, 583, 583*f*

Bucket lift, 464–465, 465*f*
Buck's traction, 581–582, 582*f*
Burping, after infant feeding, 440, 441*f*

C

Calcium sulfate cast. *See* Plaster of Paris cast(s)
Cancer metabolite(s), interference by, in urine glucose testing, 225*t*
Candida infection, of infant skin, 436, 437
Cane(s)
ambulation using, 494–495, 494*f*–496*f*
performance checklist, 509–510
quad, 494, 494*f*
Capillary refill time, 170
Cardiopulmonary resuscitation (CPR), 723–729
for adult, 723–727, 724*f*–727*f*
performance checklist, 735–736
documentation of, 729, 730*f*
in healthcare facility, 729
for infant or child, 727–729, 728*f*, 729*f*
performance checklist, 736–737
infection transmission concerns in, 21–22, 23, 723, 723*f*, 725
monitoring patient during, 727
one-rescuer, 723–727, 724*f*–727*f*
performance checklist, 735
performance checklist, 735–737
termination of, 727
two-rescuer, 727
performance checklist, 735–736
Care
individualized, patient's right to, 8–9
safe, patient's right to, 8
Care plan, as temporary record, 74
Carotid pulse, 131, 131*f*, 725, 725*f*
Cast(s), 545–558
adaptations of, 554–556, 556*f*
assisting with application of, 551–554
performance checklist, 565–569
brace with, 561, 561*f*
change of, 554
continuing care of patient with, 557–558
performance checklist, 570
edging of, 557, 558*f*
emotional support for patient with, 563
in home care, 563
immediate care of patient with, 556–557
performance checklist, 569
in long-term care, 563
materials for, 550–551
nursing diagnoses related to, 550
quiz, 573
rationale for skill, 550
types of, 554, 555*f*
Catheter(s). *See* Urinary catheter(s)

Caustic substances, safety in handling, 40
cc (cubic centimeter), 198
Centers for Disease Control and Prevention (CDC), 37
Centimeter, cubic (cc), 198
Cephalosporin(s), interference by, in urine glucose testing, 225*t*
Cervical collar, 559–560, 559*f*
Cervical halter traction, 584–585, 585*f*
Chair(s)
positioning in, 338, 338*f*
performance checklist, 353
shower, 400
transfer to. *See under* Transfer technique(s)
Chart(s), 74–75. *See also* Documentation; Record(s)
legal standards for, 77–79, 78*f*
maintaining confidentiality of, 7–8
Charting. *See also* Documentation
by exception, 91, 92*f*, 93*f*
focus, 91–94, 94*f*
narrative, 83, 87*f*, 88*f*
"Checking for residual," 707–708
Chemical dot thermometer, 129, 129*f*
Chemical restraint(s), 43
Chemstrip bG, 216*t*
Chest, assessment of, 174–175
performance checklist, 186
Chest compression. *See also* Cardiopulmonary resuscitation
for adult, 725–727, 726*f*, 727*f*
performance checklist, 735
for infant or child, 728–729, 729*f*
performance checklist, 736–737
Chest diameters, 164
Chest restraint(s), for infant, 443
Chest thrusts, for foreign-body airway obstruction, 731
Cheyne-Stokes respirations, 133
Child(ren). *See also* Infant(s)
cardiopulmonary resuscitation for, 727–729, 728*f*, 729*f*
performance checklist, 736–737
dependent, safety for, 42
enema administration to, 689–690, 690*t*
performance checklist, 697–698
foreign-body airway obstruction in, 732–733, 733*f*
performance checklist, 738–739
protecting from electrical shock, 39, 42
rights of, as patient, 6
Chloral hydrate, interference by, in urine glucose testing, 225*t*
Chloramphenicol (Chloromycetin), interference by, in urine glucose testing, 225*t*
Choking, universal distress signal for, 731, 731*f*
Circle bed, 603, 604*f*, 608*t*–611*t*
Circular bandage, 624, 626*f*

© 1996 by Lippincott-Raven Publishers

Circulation, assessment of, 114, 119, 170–171, 170f, 171f. *See also* Circulation, motion, and sensation (CMS) check(s)
in cardiopulmonary resuscitation, 725, 725f, 728, 728f
Circulation, motion, and sensation (CMS) check(s)
for patient with bandage or binder, 623–624
documentation of, 625f
for patient with cast, 556, 557
"Clean catch" urine specimen, 217t
Cleaning, of contaminated surfaces
in Standard Precautions, 23
in Universal Precautions, 21
Cleansing enema(s), 683–684, 684f
procedure for, 686–688
performance checklist, 694–696
Clean technique, 19
Clinistix, 216t
procedure for using, 226–227
performance checklist, 239
Clinitest, 216t
drug interference with, 225t
procedure for using, 226
performance checklist, 238–239
Clinitron bed, 606, 606f
Clock, 24-hour (military), 78–79, 79t
Closed bed, 308
Clove hitch, 45, 46f
CMS check(s). *See* Circulation, motion, and sensation (CMS) check(s)
"Code status," 748
in home care, 734
in long-term care, 733, 757
Cold
application of, 653–657
devices for, 661–663
general procedure for, 658–659
in home care, 666
in long-term care, 666
nursing diagnoses related to, 657
performance checklist, 669–670, 673–675
purposes for, 658
quiz, 677–678
rationale for skill, 657
safety in, 657
specific procedures for, 665–666
physiologic responses to, 658
Cold pack(s), 662
Colonoscopy, assisting with, 255t, 262–263, 262f
performance checklist, 273–274
Comatose patient. *See* Unconscious patient(s)
Combistix, 216t
Commode(s), 376–377, 377f
assisting with, 380
performance checklist, 386–387
Competence, technical, 11–12
Compress(es), 660
warm, moist
performance checklist, 670–671
procedure for application of, 663

Computerized record(s), 75, 75f. *See also* Documentation; Record(s)
access to, 75, 79
errors in, 77
in home care, 96
legal standards for, 77
in long-term care, 96
signature on, 78
time notation on, 79
Condyloid joint(s), 526
Confidentiality
of computerized records, 75, 79
patient's right to, 7–8
Consciousness, assessment of, 115, 119
Consent
for diagnostic or therapeutic procedures, 252
patient's right to give, 6–7
Contact lens(es), care of, 407–408
performance checklist, 425–427
Continuous passive motion (CPM) device, 527–528
Contracture(s), 525
Cooling bath, 662–663
procedure for, 665–666
performance checklist, 673–674
Cooling enema, 684
Cord care, 439
Corneal reflex, 176
Coroner, 757
reporting death to, 750, 751f
Corridor(s). *See* Hallway(s)
CPM (continuous passive motion) device, 527–528
CPR. *See* Cardiopulmonary resuscitation
Crackles, 164
Cradle(s)
bed, 314–315, 314f
heat, 660
Cradle cap, 438
Cranial nerve(s), assessment of, 176
Crib dome(s), 443, 443f
Crib net(s), 443
Crutch(es). *See also* Crutchwalking
adjustment of, for size, 497–498, 497f
Crutchfield tongs, 587
Crutch palsy, 497
Crutchwalking, 496–504
assisting with, 499–502
performance checklist, 512–514
down stairs, 504, 504f
performance checklist, 516–517
gaits for, 498–499, 498f–501f
performance checklist, 513
up stairs, 502–503, 502f, 503f
performance checklist, 514–516
Cubic centimeter (cc), 198
Cultural identity, assessment of, 116, 120
Culture(s)
procedure for obtaining, 231–232, 232f
performance checklist, 245–246
urine, 232

Culturette, 231
Cushion, wedge, 46, 47f

D

Data
objective, 172
in SOAP notation, 85
subjective, in SOAP notation, 85
Data base, in permanent record, 76
Data gathering. *See* Assessment
Death. *See also* Postmortem care
caring for body after, 752–754
performance checklist, 759–761
changes in body after, 750–752
definitions of, 749–750
of infant, 754
presence of family and friends at time of, 747
pronouncement of, 750
reporting of, to medical examiner, 750, 751f
Death certificate, 750
Decision-making, patient's rights in, 6–7
Decreased Cardiac Output (collaborative diagnosis), 126
Dehydration
assessment for, 114, 119
due to diuretic therapy, 203
Dentures, care of, 404–405
in long-term care facility, 410
performance checklist, 421–422
Dependent patient(s). *See also* Unconscious patient(s)
safety for, 41–42
performance checklist, 53
Developmental stage, assessment of, 116, 120
Dexterity, in technical competence, 11
Dextrostix, 216t
Diagnosis(es), nursing, 10, 116–117
Diagnostic procedure(s)
assisting with, 249–275
performance checklist, 265–274
procedure for, 252–253
quiz, 275
rationale for skill, 252
nursing diagnoses related to, 252
Diaper(s)
folding, 435, 436f
types of, 435
Diapering, 435–438
performance checklist, 447
procedure for, 437–438, 437f, 438f
Diaper rash, 436
Diarrhea, due to tube feeding, 710, 711t
Diastix, 216t
testing for glucose with, 226–227
performance checklist, 239
testing for ketones with, 227
performance checklist, 240
Diathermy, 660
Dignity, patient's right to, 8

© 1996 by Lippincott-Raven Publishers

Disaster(s), 49–50
Disaster drill(s), 50
Discharge, 277–282, 289–291
    delegating tasks at, 291
    documentation at, 290f, 291
    to home care, 291
    from long-term care, 291
    nurse's responsibilities at, 289–291
    performance checklist, 294–295
    planning for, 282, 284f
        progress notes on, 89f, 90
    quiz, 297–298
    rationale for skill, 282
    teaching at, 289–291, 290f
Diuretic(s), dehydration due to, 203
DNR (do not resuscitate). *See* "Code
        status"
Documentation, 71–101. *See also*
        Chart(s); Computerized
        record(s); Record(s)
    abbreviations used in, 81, 82t, 83t
    at admission, 284–285, 285f–287f
    charting by exception in, 91, 92f, 93f
    at discharge, 290f, 291
    focus charting in, 91–94, 94f
    forms used in, 81–83
    in home care, 96
    legal standards for, 77–79, 78f
    in long-term care, 95–96
    mechanics of, 77–95
    narrative notes in, 83, 87f, 88f
    in nursing process, 10–11
    performance checklist, 99
    practice situations for, 96–98
    procedure for, 94–95
    progress notes in, 83–94, 87f–94f
    quiz, 101
    rationale for skill, 74
    terminology used in, 79–81, 80t–81t,
        84t–85t
    at transfer, 287, 288f
"Do not resuscitate." *See* "Code status"
L-Dopa, interference by, in urine glu-
        cose testing, 225t
Doppler stethoscope
    blood pressure measurement using,
        148–149, 149f
    pulse assessment using, 135
        performance checklist, 138
Dorsalis pedis pulse, 131–132, 132f
    procedure for assessing, 134
Dorsal recumbent position, 339, 339f
    performance checklist, 353
Double-voided urine specimen, collec-
        tion of, 225–226
Drainage, descriptive terms used for,
        80t
Droplet nuclei, spread of microorgan-
        isms on, 19
Drug(s). *See* Medication(s)
Dry mouth, due to tube feeding, 710
Dullness (sound quality), 112
Durable power-of-attorney for health-
        care, 748–749
Dysphagia, 361–362, 361t, 362f
Dyspnea, 133

E

Ear(s), assessment of, 173, 174f
    performance checklist, 186
Ear canal, temperature measured at,
        128–129, 129f, 130
    procedure for, 134
Eating. *See also* Feeding; Nutrition
    factors affecting, 360–362
Edema, assessment for, 170–171, 170f
"Egg crate" mattress(es), 601
Elastic bandage(s), 624
Elastic net binder(s). *See* Stretch net
        binder(s)
Elastic stockings
    application of, 628–629, 629f
        performance checklist, 641–642
    in home care, 637
    in long-term care, 637
Elbow joint, 526t
    range-of-motion exercise for, 529,
        531f
        performance checklist, 540
Elbow restraint(s), 44, 45f
    for infant, 443
Elderly patient(s)
    assessment in, 117–118, 117f
    normal body temperature in, 126
    pulse assessment in, 130, 132
Electrical appliance(s)
    oxygen and, 41
    safety in using, 39, 39f
Electrolyte balance, assessment of,
        114, 119
Electronic blood pressure recording
        device(s), 148
    for home use, 149
Electronic thermometer(s), 128, 128f
    performance checklist, 137
    procedure for using, 134
Elemental feeding(s), 705
Elevator(s), safety in using, 38, 39f
Elimination
    assessment of, 114, 119
    assisting with, 371–390
        comfort considerations in, 377
        equipment for, 375–377,
            375f–377f
        in home care, 383
        infection control in, 375
        in long-term care, 382
        nursing diagnoses associated with,
            375
        performance checklist, 385–387
        procedures for, 377–380, 378f
        quiz, 389–390
        rationale for skill, 375
Emergency resuscitation, 719–741. *See
        also* Cardiopulmonary resuscita-
        tion; Foreign-body airway ob-
        struction
    in home care, 734
    in long-term care, 733
    performance checklist, 735–739
    quiz, 741
    rationale for skill, 723
Emesis basin, for voiding, 376, 376f

Enema(s), 679–700
    equipment for, 684f
    in home care, 690
    in long-term care, 690
    nursing diagnoses related to, 683
    performance checklist, 693–698
    procedure for, 685–688, 685f
        for child, 689–690, 690t
    quiz, 699–700
    rationale for skill, 683
    types of, 683–685, 684f
Error(s), in documentation, 77
Esophagostomy tube, 704
Ethics, patient rights supported by,
        8–9
Ethnic identity, assessment of, 116,
        120
Evacuation, in case of fire, 49
Evaluation
    data on, in nursing record, 77
    in nursing process, 10
    by patient, 9
Examination. *See* Assessment, physical
Exception, charting by, 91, 92f, 93f
Exercises. *See* Range-of-motion (ROM)
        exercises
External fixation device(s), 588, 588f
Eye(s). *See also* Pupil(s)
    assessment of, 172–173, 173f
        performance checklist, 185–186
    care of, 406–409
        for infant, 438
        performance checklist, 424–427
    of dependent patient, protection of,
        42
Eyeglasses, care of, 408–409
    performance checklist, 427
Eyewear, protective
    in Standard Precautions, 23
    in Universal Precautions, 21

F

Face, assessment of, 172
    performance checklist, 185
Face shield(s)
    in Standard Precautions, 23
    in Universal Precautions, 21
Fall(s), 460
Family
    involvement of, progress notes on,
        90, 90f
    presence of, at time of death, 747
Fanfolding, 308, 309f
Feces. *See* Stool
Feeding, 357–370
    in home care, 366
    for infant, 439–442, 440f–442f
        performance checklist, 449–450
    in long-term care, 365
    nursing diagnoses related to, 360
    performance checklist, 367–368
    procedure for, 362–365, 364f
    psychosocial considerations in,
        360–361

© 1996 by Lippincott-Raven Publishers

Feeding (*continued*)
  quiz, 369–370
  rationale for skill, 360
  tube. *See* Tube feeding
  utensils for, 364f
Feeding tube(s)
  occluded, procedure for opening,
    710–712
  types of, 704
  verifying placement of, 707
Feet. *See* Foot
Femoral pulse, 131
Fiberglass cast(s), 551
  assisting with application of, 554
    performance checklist, 568–569
Figure-8 bandage, 624, 626–627,
    627f
Finger(s)
  assessment of, 172
    performance checklist, 185
  joints of, 526t
  range-of-motion exercise for, 531,
    533t
    performance checklist, 540
Fingernails
  nurse's
    care of, 25, 42
    cleaning of, 24
  patient's, care of, 399
Finger sweep, for foreign-body airway
    obstruction, 731–732
Fire, 48–49
  performance checklist, 55
Fire drill(s), 50
Fire extinguisher(s), 49
Fixation device(s), external, 588,
    588f
Flatness (sound quality), 112
Flexicair static low air loss bed, 605
Flexicare active low air loss bed, 606f
Flooring, 39, 40
Flossing, 403, 403f
Flow sheet(s), 82–83, 86f
  for cardiopulmonary resuscitation,
    729, 730f
  for charting by exception, 91, 92f,
    93f
  for hygiene, 395f
  in permanent record, 76
  procedure for using, 95
  for range-of-motion exercise, 536f,
    537
  signature on, 78
  time notation on, 79
  for transfers, 461, 471f
FluidAir bed, 606
Fluid balance. *See also* Dehydration
  assessment of, 114, 119
Foam rubber mattress pad(s), 601
Focus charting, 91–94, 94f
Food coloring, in tube feeding formu-
    la, 706
Foot (feet)
  assessment of, 175
    performance checklist, 187

joints of, 526t
  range-of-motion exercise for, 533,
    535f
    performance checklist, 540–541
"Football" hold, 438, 438f
Footboard(s), 313–314, 313f, 336f
Footdrop, 314, 336
Forearm, joints of, 526t
Foreign-body airway obstruction,
    729–733
  in adult, 730–732, 731f, 732f
    performance checklist, 737
  in infant or child, 732–733, 733f
    performance checklist, 738–739
Foster turning frame, 603
Four-point gait, 499, 501f
  performance checklist, 513
Fowler's position, 338–339, 338f
  high, 339, 339f
    performance checklist, 353
  performance checklist, 353
Fracture pan, 376, 376f, 378f. *See also*
    Bedpan(s)
Frame(s), therapeutic, 597–601,
    602–612, 608t–611t
  in home care, 612
  in long-term care, 612
    performance checklist, 613
  procedure for using, 607–612
  quiz, 615–616
  rationale for skill, 601
Friction rub(s), 164
Functional assessment, 114
Furniture, 41

G

Gait belt, 461, 493, 493f
Gait pattern(s)
  for cane walking, 494, 496f
  for crutchwalking, 498–499,
    498f–501f
    performance checklist, 513
  for walker use, 496
Gardner-Wells tongs, 587
Gastric secretion specimen, collection
    of, 219t, 221
Gastrointestinal disorder(s), with trac-
    tion, 581
Gastrostomy tube, 704
Gauze bandage(s), 624
General observation, as source of data
    for assessment, 111
Genitalia, assessment of, 176
  performance checklist, 187
Genupectoral position, 340, 340f
  performance checklist, 354
Glasses, care of, 408–409
  performance checklist, 427
Gliding joint(s), 527
Gloves
  in Standard Precautions, 22–23
  in Universal Precautions, 20–21
Glucometer, 229
Glucoscan II, 229

Glucose
  in blood. *See* Blood glucose
  in urine, testing for, 224–227, 225t,
    238–239
Glucostix, 216t
Gown(s)
  in Standard Precautions, 23
  in Universal Precautions, 21
Guaiac testing, 231
  performance checklist, 244
Guarding, 168
Gurgles, 164

H

Hair
  nurse's, 25
  patient's, care of, 405–406, 406f,
    422–424
Hallway(s), safety in, 38, 40, 40f
  performance checklist, 53
Halo traction, 588, 588f
Hand(s)
  assessment of, 172
    performance checklist, 185
  joints of, 526t
  range-of-motion exercise for, 531,
    533t
    performance checklist, 540
Hand lotion, 24
Handroll(s), 335, 336f
Hand vein emptying time, 171
Handwashing, 23–24
  performance checklist, 28
  procedure for, 24, 25f
  rationale for skill, 20
  in Standard Precautions, 23
  in Universal Precautions, 21
Hanging arm cast, 554, 555f
Harris flush. *See* Return-flow enema
"Hat," for urine collection, 198, 198f
Hazardous materials, safety in han-
    dling, 40
Head, assessment of, 172–174, 173f,
    174f
  performance checklist, 185–186
Head-tilt/chin-lift maneuver, in car-
    diopulmonary resuscitation,
    724, 724f
"Head-to-toe" assessment
  3-minute, 179
    performance checklist, 188–189
  15-minute, 178–179
    performance checklist, 188
Hearing, assessment of, 173, 174f
Hearing aid(s), care of, 409
  performance checklist, 427
Heart, assessment of, 161–164, 163f,
    175
  performance checklist, 181, 186
  procedure for, 163–164
Heart sounds, 161–164, 163f
Heat
  application of, 653–658
    devices for, 659–660

© 1996 by Lippincott-Raven Publishers

general procedure for, 658–659
in home care, 666
in long-term care, 666
nursing diagnoses related to, 657
performance checklist, 669–673, 674–675
purposes for, 657–658
quiz, 677–678
rationale for skill, 657
safety in, 657
specific procedures for, 663–665
physiologic responses to, 657
Heat cradle, 660
Heating pad(s)
electric, 660
water-flow, 659, 659*f*
Heat lamp, 660
Heimlich maneuver, 731–732, 731*f*, 732*f*
performance checklist, 737, 738–739
Hema-chek, 216*t*
Hema-combistix, 216*t*
Hemastix, 216*t*
procedure for using, 228
Hematest, 216*t*
procedure for using, 230
performance checklist, 244
Hematuria, testing for, 228
Hemoccult, 216*t*
procedure for using, 230–231
performance checklist, 244
Hepatitis B, 20
High air loss bed, static, 605–606, 606*f*, 608*t*–611*t*
Hinge joint(s), 526
Hip joint, 526*t*
range-of-motion exercise for, 531, 534*f*
performance checklist, 540
Hip spica cast, 554, 555*f*
HIV (human immunodeficiency virus), 20
Home care
ambulation in, 505, 505*f*
application of heat and cold in, 666
assessment in, 118
assisting with elimination in, 383
bandages and binders in, 637
bedmaking in, 315
blood pressure measurement in, 149
body mechanics in, 64–65
casts and braces in, 563
documentation in, 96
emergency resuscitation in, 734
enemas in, 690
feeding in, 366
hygiene in, 410
of infant, 444–445
intake and output measurement in, 204
laboratory tests in, 233
moving patient in bed in, 341
positioning in, 341
postmortem care in, 757–758
range-of-motion exercises in, 537
referral for, 289

safety in, 52
special mattresses and beds in, 612
temperature, pulse, and respiration assessment in, 136
transfer techniques in, 471
transition to and from, 291
Home health aide(s), 410
Horizontal lift, 470–471, 470*f*
performance checklist, 484–485
Horizontal slide, 469–470, 470*f*
performance checklist, 482–484
Hot pack(s)
disposable instant, 659
gel-filled, 660
Hot water bag(s), 660
Human immunodeficiency virus (HIV), 20
Human needs approach to assessment, 114–116, 119–120
Humerus traction, 581, 582*f*
Hydration. *See also* Dehydration
assessment of, 114, 119
Hydroculator (water-flow heating pad), 659
Hydrometer, urine, urine specific gravity measurement using, 223–224, 223*f*, 236–237
Hygiene, 391–430
documentation of, 394–395, 395*f*, 396*t*
general procedure for, 394–395
performance checklist, 413
in home care, 410
infection control in, 394
in long-term care, 410
for nurse, 25
performance checklist, 28
nursing diagnoses related to, 394
performance checklist, 413–427
quiz, 429–430
rationale for skill, 394
specific procedures for, 395–409. *See also specific procedures, e.g.* Bath(s)
Hypertension, 144
Hyperthermia (nursing diagnosis), 126
Hypotension, 144
Hypothermia (nursing diagnosis), 126
Hypothermia blanket, 662, 662*f*
procedure for use of, 666
performance checklist, 674–675

I

Ice cap, 661–662
Ice collar, 661, 661*f*
Ictotest, 216*t*
Immobile patient(s), positioning for, 41
Impaired Physical Mobility (nursing diagnosis), 460
Implementation, in nursing process, 10
Incident report(s), 50, 51*f*
Incontinent patient(s)
perineal care for, 380–382
special mattress use with, 601

Independence, patient's right to assistance toward, 9
Individualized care, patient's right to, 8–9
Ineffective Breathing Pattern (nursing diagnosis), 126
Ineffective Thermoregulation (nursing diagnosis), 126
Infant(s). *See also* Child(ren)
bathing of, 438–439, 438*f*, 439*f*
performance checklist, 447–448
cardiopulmonary resuscitation for, 727–729, 728*f*, 729*f*
performance checklist, 736–737
care of, 431–453
at home, 444–445
performance checklist, 447–452
quiz, 453
rationale for skill, 435
collection of urine specimen from, 198, 199*f*, 218*t*
death of, 754
diapering of, 435–438, 436*f*–438*f*
performance checklist, 447
feeding of, 439–442, 440*f*–442*f*
performance checklist, 449–450
foreign-body airway obstruction in, 732–733, 733*f*
performance checklist, 738–739
holding of, 438, 438*f*
measuring urine output of, 198, 199*f*
pulse assessment in, 135
performance checklist, 138
respiration assessment in, 135
safety for, 442–444, 443*f*, 444*f*
performance checklist, 450–452
Infection control, 15–30
in assisting with elimination, 375
in bedmaking, 305
performance checklist, 317
for blood-borne infections, 20–22, 20*t*
in cardiopulmonary resuscitation, 723, 723*f*, 725
in hygiene, 394
nursing diagnoses related to, 19
principles of, 19–25
quiz, 29–30
rationale for skill, 19
Inflated mattress(es), 602
Information
in medical record
access to, 75, 79
patient's right to, 79
patient's right to, 7
Informed consent. *See* Consent
INH (isoniazid), interference by, in urine glucose testing, 225*t*
Inspection, in physical assessment, 111
Intake and output measurement (I&O), 193–209
assessment for initiating, 197
devices used for, 198, 198*f*, 199*f*
in home care, 204
items measured in, 198

Intake and output measurement (I&O)
    (*continued*)
  in long-term care, 203
  nursing diagnoses related to, 197
  patient participation in, 199
  performance checklist, 205
  procedure for, 199–203
  quiz, 207–209
  rationale for skill, 197
  recording, 199, 200f–202f
  units used in, 198–199
Interim note, 90, 91f
Intervention(s), data on, in nursing
    record, 77
Interview
  at admission, 284
  as source of data for assessment,
    110–111
I&O. *See* Intake and output measure-
    ment
Isoniazid (INH), interference by, in
    urine glucose testing, 225t

J

Jacket restraint(s), 43
Jaw-thrust maneuver, in cardiopul-
    monary resuscitation, 724, 724f
Jejunostomy tube, 704
Jewelry, nurse's, 25
Joint(s), types of, 525–527, 526t

K

Keane Mobility bed, 607
Keflex (cephalexin), interference by,
    in urine glucose testing, 225t
Keflin (cephalothin sodium), interfer-
    ence by, in urine glucose test-
    ing, 225t
Keofeed tube, 704
Keto-diastix, 216t
Ketone bodies, testing urine for,
    227–228
  performance checklist, 240–241
Ketostix, procedure for using, 227
  performance checklist, 240
KinAir bed, 605
Kling bandage, 624
Knee brace(s), 561–562, 562f
Knee-chest position, 340, 340f
  performance checklist, 354
Knee joint, 526t
  range-of-motion exercise for, 531,
    534f
  performance checklist, 540
Knee restraint(s), 44
Knot(s)
  traction, 580, 580f
  for use with safety devices, 45,
    46f
Korotkoff's sounds, 147–148
K-Pad (water-flow heating pad), 659

L

Laboratory test(s), 211–247
  at admission, 283–284
  drug interference in, 225t
  equipment for, 215, 216t
  in home care, 233
  in long-term care, 233
  performance checklist, 235–246
  procedure for, 221–223
  quiz, 247
  rationale for skill, 215
  reference file for, 221f
  requisition slip for, 222f
Labstix, 216t
Lap-board, 46
Law
  documentation and, 77–79, 78f
  patient rights supported by, 6–8
  on restraint use, 43, 47
Leg(s)
  assessment of, 175
    performance checklist, 186
  bandage application to, 627–628
    performance checklist, 640–641
Leg brace(s), 561–562, 562f
Leg cast(s), 554, 555f
Levodopa, interference by, in urine
    glucose testing, 225t
Lighting, 38, 40
Linen, soiled, handling of
  in Standard Precautions, 23
  in Universal Precautions, 21
Listening to patient, patient's dignity
    and, 8
Literature review, 110
Lithotomy position, 339–340, 339f
  performance checklist, 354
Liver, palpation of, 168
  performance checklist, 183
  procedure for, 169, 169f
Liver biopsy, assisting with, 254t,
    259–260
  performance checklist, 270–272
Living will, 748
Livor mortis, 751
Logrolling, 334, 334f
  performance checklist, 349
Long-term care
  admission, transfer, and discharge
    in, 291
  ambulation in, 505
  application of heat and cold in, 666
  assessment in, 117–118
  assisting with elimination in, 382
  bandages and binders in, 635–637
  bedmaking in, 315
  blood pressure measurement in,
    149
  body mechanics in, 64
  casts and braces in, 563
  documentation in, 95–96
  emergency resuscitation in, 733
  enemas in, 690
  feeding in, 365
  hygiene in, 410

  intake and output measurement in,
    203
  laboratory tests in, 233
  moving patient in bed in, 340–341
  positioning in, 340–341
  postmortem care in, 757
  range-of-motion exercises in, 537
  restraint use in, 43, 45
  safety in, 50
  special mattresses and beds in, 612
  specimen collection in, 233
  temperature, pulse, and respiration
    assessment in, 136
  transfer techniques in, 471
Loridine (cephaloridine), interference
    by, in urine glucose testing, 225t
Lotion, for hands, 24
Low air loss bed
  active, 605, 606f, 608t–611t
  static, 604–605, 605f, 608t–611t
Lumbar puncture. *See* Spinal tap
Lung(s), assessment of, 164–165, 165f,
    166f
  performance checklist, 181–182

M

Manometer(s)
  aneroid, 145, 145f
  mercury, 144–145, 145f
Mask(s)
  in Standard Precautions, 23
  in Universal Precautions, 21
Mask device(s), for cardiopulmonary
    resuscitation, 723f, 725
Mattress(es), special, 597–602
  bedmaking with, 314, 601, 602
  in home care, 612
  in long-term care, 612
  performance checklist, 613
  procedure for using, 607–612
  quiz, 615–616
  rationale for skill, 601
MDS (minimum data set), 96, 118
Mechanical lift(s), 467–469, 468f
  in long-term care, 471
  performance checklist, 481–482
Medical asepsis, 19
Medical examiner, 757
  reporting death to, 750, 751f
Medical progress notes, 76
Medication(s)
  administration of, through feeding
    tube, 705
  at bedside, safety in storage of, 41
  hazards associated with, 42
  interference by, in urine glucose
    testing, 225t
  rectal instillation of, by enema, 685
Mediscus bed, 605, 605f
MegaAir bed, 605
Mega Tilt and Turn bed, 607
Mental attitude of patient, documenta-
    tion of, 81t

© 1996 by Lippincott-Raven Publishers

Mental health, assessment of, 116, 120
Mental practice, 12
Mercury manometer, 144–145, 145*f*
Metaxalone (Skelaxin), interference by, in urine glucose testing, 225*t*
Methyldopa (Aldomet), interference by, in urine glucose testing, 225*t*
Methylene blue, in tube feeding formula, 706
Microorganism(s), spread of, 19–20
Military clock, 78–79, 79*t*
Milliliter (mL), 198–199
Minimum Data Set (MDS), 96, 118
Minor(s), rights of, as patient, 6
Mitt restraint(s), 44–45, 45*f*
mL (milliliter), 198–199
Mouth, assessment of, 173–174
  performance checklist, 186
Mouth care. *See* Oral care
Mouth-to–barrier device breathing, 723, 723*f*, 725
Mouth-to-mouth breathing, 724, 725*f*
Mouth-to-nose breathing, 724
Mouth-to-stoma breathing, 724–725
Mouthwash, 402
Moving patient in bed, 325–335
  general procedure for, 329
  in home care, 341
  in long-term care, 340–341
  nursing diagnoses related to, 329
  performance checklist, 343–349
  quiz, 355–356
  rationale for skill, 329
  specific procedures for, 330–335, 330*f*–335*f*
Moving patient out of bed. *See* Transfer technique(s)
Multistix, 216*t*
Mummying, 443–444, 444*f*
  performance checklist, 451–452

N

Nail care
  for nurse, 24, 25, 42
  for patient, 399
Nail polish, 25, 42
Name, patient's, use of, 8
NANDA (North American Nursing Diagnosis Association), 117
Narrative notes, 83, 87*f*, 88*f*
Nasogastric (NG) tube(s), 704
  specimen collection from, 219*t*, 221
National Institute for Occupational Safety and Health, 37
Natural Death Act, 748
Neck
  assessment of, 172
    performance checklist, 185
  joints of, 526*t*
  range-of-motion exercise for, 528–529, 529*f*
    performance checklist, 539

Neck vein(s), assessment of, 171, 171*f*
  performance checklist, 184–185
Needle(s). *See* Sharp(s)
Net binder(s). *See* Stretch net binder(s)
"Neuro signs," pupillary assessment in, 160
Newborn(s). *See also* Infant(s)
  pulse assessment in, 135
    performance checklist, 138
NG (nasogastric) tube(s), 704
  specimen collection from, 219*t*, 221
NIOSH (National Institute for Occupational Safety and Health), 37
"No code." *See* "Code status"
North American Nursing Diagnosis Association (NANDA), 117
Nose, assessment of, 173, 173*f*
  performance checklist, 186
"Nurse server," 40
Nursing care plan, as temporary record, 74
Nursing diagnosis(es), 10, 116–117
Nursing practice, research base for, 9
Nursing process, 9–11
Nursing progress notes, 76, 87*f*. *See also* Progress notes
Nursing record. *See also* Chart(s); Documentation; Record(s)
  content of, 76–77
Nutrition. *See also* Feeding
  assessment of, 114, 119
  descriptive terms used for, 80*t*
Nystagmus, 161

O

Obesity bed, 603
Objective data, 172
  in SOAP notation, 85
Observation, general, as source of data for assessment, 111
Occult blood, testing for
  products used in, 216*t*
  in urine, 228
Occupational Safety and Health Administration (OSHA), 37
  hazardous substances regulations of, 40
  infection control regulations of, 20
Oil-retention enema, 684, 684*f*
  for child, 689
Ombudsman, 9
Open bed, 308, 309*f*
Ophthalmoscope, 173*f*
Oral care, 402–405, 403*f*
  performance checklist, 419–422
  for unconscious patient, 403–404
    performance checklist, 420–421
Oral temperature, 129, 129*f*
  performance checklist, 137
  procedure for measuring, 133–134
Oral thermometer(s), 127, 128*f*
  electronic, 128, 128*f*

  procedure for using, 134
  procedure for using, 133–134
Order(s), physician's
  at admission, 283
  for discharge, 289
  for restraints, 47
  for transfer, 285
Organ donation, 747, 748*t*, 749*f*
Organization, in technical competence, 11
Orientation, for new patient, 283
Orthopneic position, 339, 339*f*
  performance checklist, 353
Orthostatic hypotension, 144
OSHA. *See* Occupational Safety and Health Administration
Output, measurement of, 198. *See also* Intake and output measurement
Oxygen, safety in use of, 41
Oxygenation, assessment of, 115, 119

P

Palpation
  blood pressure measurement by, 148
  in physical assessment, 111–112
Papanicolaou test, 176
Paracentesis, assisting with, 254*t*, 256–257
  performance checklist, 267–269
Paragon bed, 607
Paraldehyde, interference by, in urine glucose testing, 225*t*
Patient advocate, 9
Patient record(s). *See* Chart(s); Documentation; Record(s)
Patient rights, 6–9
Patient room(s), safety in, 40–41
  performance checklist, 53
Patient Self-Determination Act (1991), 749
Patient's property
  at admission, 284, 287*f*
  at discharge, 291
  at transfer, 286–287
Patient teaching, at discharge, 289–291, 290*f*
Pearson attachment, 586
Pedal pulse(s), 131–132, 132*f*
  performance checklist, 138
  procedure for assessing, 134
PEG (percutaneous endoscopic gastrostomy) tube, 704
Pelvic sling traction, 584, 584*f*
Pelvic traction, 583–584, 584*f*
Percussion, 112, 113*f*
Percutaneous endoscopic gastrostomy (PEG) tube, 704
Pericardial friction rub, 164
Perineal care (pericare), 371–390
  in home care, 383
  for infant, 438–439
  in long-term care, 382

© 1996 by Lippincott-Raven Publishers

Perineal care (pericare) (*continued*)
  nursing diagnoses related to, 375
  performance checklist, 387–388
  procedure for, 380–382, 381*f*
  quiz, 389–390
  rationale for skill, 375
Periorbital edema, 170
PERL, 161
PERLA, 161
PERRLA, 161
Personal hygiene. *See* Hygiene
Personal property. *See* Patient's property
Petals, cast edging using, 557, 558*f*
Phenistix, 216*t*
pH of urine, testing for, 228–229
  performance checklist, 241–242
Physical assessment. *See under* Assessment
Physical practice, 12
Physician's order. *See* Order(s)
Pivotal joint(s), 525
Planning
  in nursing process, 10
  recording of, in nursing record, 76–77
Plantar flexion, prevention of
  devices for, 313–314, 313*f*, 336
  in prone position, 338
Plaster of Paris cast(s), 550–551
  assisting with application of, 553–554
    performance checklist, 566–568
Pleural friction rub, 164
PM care, 409
  in long-term care facility, 410
POMR. *See* Problem-oriented record
Popliteal pulse, 131, 131*f*
POR. *See* Problem-oriented record
Poseys. *See* Restraint(s); Safety device(s)
Positioning, 325–329, 335–340
  in bed, 335–338, 337*f*
    aids for, 335, 336*f*
    general procedure for, 329
    performance checklist, 350–352
  in chair, 338, 338*f*
    performance checklist, 353
  in home care, 341
  in long-term care, 340–341
  nursing diagnoses related to, 329
  quiz, 355–356
  rationale for skill, 329
  therapeutic, 338–340, 338*f*–341*f*
    performance checklist, 353–354
  for unconscious or immobile patient, 41
Posterior tibial pulse, 132, 132*f*
Postmortem care, 743–764. *See also* Death
  documentation of, 754, 755*f*
  in home care, 757–758
  in long-term care facility, 757
  performance checklist, 759–761
  procedure for, 752–754
  quiz, 763–764
  rationale for skill, 747

Postmortem examination, 754–757, 756*f*, 757*f*
Postop bed, procedure for making, 310–311, 310*f*
  performance checklist, 319–320
Postural hypotension, 144
Power-of-attorney for healthcare, durable, 748–749
Practice
  mental, 12
  physical, 12
Pretibial edema, palpation for, 170–171, 170*f*
Privacy, patient's right to, 7–8
  records and, 79
Probenecid (Benemid), interference by, in urine glucose testing, 225*t*
Problem(s), temporary, progress notes on, 86, 89*f*
Problem list, in permanent record, 76
Problem-oriented record (POMR, POR), 76
  flow sheets in, 83
  progress notes in, 83–91, 88*f*, 89*f*
Proctoscopy, assisting with, 255*t*, 262–263
  performance checklist, 273–274
Progress notes, 83–94, 87*f*–94*f*
  medical, 76
  narrative, 83, 87*f*, 88*f*
  nursing, 76, 87*f*
  in permanent record, 76
  in problem-oriented record, 83–91, 88*f*, 89*f*
  procedure for using, 95
  SOAP notation for, 85–91, 88*f*, 89*f*
  time notation on, 79
Prone position, 337–338, 337*f*
  performance checklist, 352
Property, personal. *See* Patient's property
Protective device(s). *See* Restraint(s); Safety device(s)
Psychosocial assessment, 116, 120
Psyllium-containing product(s), administration of, through feeding tube, 705
Pulley(s), traction, 580
Pull sheet, moving patient using, 334–335, 335*f*
Pulmonair 40 bed, 605
Pulse, 130–132. *See also* Temperature, pulse, and respiration; Vital signs
  assessment of
    in cardiopulmonary resuscitation, 725, 725*f*, 728, 728*f*
    locations for, 130–132, 130*f*–132*f*
    performance checklist, 138
    procedure for, 134–135
    normal rates for, 130, 130*t*
    nursing diagnoses related to, 126
Pulse deficit, 132
Pump(s), tube feeding using, 709*f*, 710
Pupil(s), assessment of, 160–161, 161*f*

documentation of, 161, 162*f*
  performance checklist, 181
Pyridium, interference by, in urine glucose testing, 225*t*

Q
Quad cane, 494, 494*f*
Quadriceps reflex, 176, 177*f*
Quality assurance, 50
"Quick release" knot, 45, 46*f*

R
Radial pulse, 130–131, 131*f*
  performance checklist, 138
  procedure for assessing, 134
Rales, 164
Range-of-motion (ROM) exercises, 521–543
  active, 527
  active-assistive, 527
  continuous passive, 527–528
  contraindications to, 525
  documentation of, 536*f*, 537
  goals of, 525
  in home care, 537
  joints needing, 527
  in long-term care, 537
  nursing diagnoses related to, 525
  passive, 527
  performance checklist, 539–541
  procedure for, 528–537, 529*f*–535*f*
  quiz, 543
  rationale for skill, 525
  sequence of, 528
  time of, 528
  types of, 527–528
RAPs (Resident Assessment Protocols), 96, 118
Record(s). *See also* Chart(s); Computerized record(s); Documentation
  content of, 75–77
    systems for organizing, 75–76
  as source of data for assessment, 109
  temporary, 74
  types of, 74–75
Rectal instillation of medication, by enema, 685
Rectal temperature, 129–130
  performance checklist, 137
  procedure for measuring, 134
Rectal thermometer, 127, 128*f*
  procedure for using, 134
Rectum
  assessment of, 176–177
    performance checklist, 187–188
  digital examination of, 168
    performance checklist, 184
    procedure for, 169–170
Recurrent fold bandage, 624, 627, 627*f*, 628*f*
Referral(s), to community agencies, 289

© 1996 by Lippincott-Raven Publishers

Reflex(es), assessment of, 175–176, 177*f*
  performance checklist, 187
Refractometer, urine, urine specific gravity measurement using, 224, 224*f*, 237–238
Religious belief, assessment of, 116, 120
Rescue breathing. *See also* Cardiopulmonary resuscitation
  for adult, 724–725, 724*f*, 725*f*
    performance checklist, 735
  for infant or child, 728, 728*f*
    performance checklist, 736
Research, as base for nursing practice, 9
Reservoir method, for tube feeding, 708–709, 708*f*
Resident Assessment Protocols (RAPs), 96, 118
Resonance, 112
Respiration(s), 132–133. *See also* Temperature, pulse, and respiration; Vital signs
  normal rates for, 130*t*, 133
  nursing diagnoses related to, 126
  of patient in traction, 580
  procedure for assessing, 135
    performance checklist, 138
Respiratory secretion(s), identification of tube feeding formula in, 706
Rest, assessment of, 115, 120
Restcue bed, 605
Restraint(s), 42–45, 44*f*–46*f*. *See also* Safety device(s)
  chemical, 43
  for infant, 442–444, 444*f*
    performance checklist, 450–452
  knots used with, 45, 46*f*
  law regarding, 43, 47
  nursing diagnoses related to, 43
  physician's orders for, 47
  procedure for applying, 46–48
    for infant, 442–443, 444*f*
    performance checklist, 54–55
Resuscitation. *See* Cardiopulmonary resuscitation; Emergency resuscitation; Foreign-body airway obstruction
Return-flow enema, 684, 685*f*
  procedure for, 688
    performance checklist, 696–697
Reverse-spiral bandage, 624, 626, 627*f*
Rhonchi, 164
Rights of patient, 6–9
Rigor mortis, 750–751
Risk for Infection (nursing diagnosis), 19
Roller gauze, 624
ROM. *See* Range-of-motion (ROM) exercises
Room(s). *See* Patient room(s)
Rope(s), for traction, 580, 580*f*
Rotation bed, 606–607, 606*f*, 608*t*–611*t*

RotoRest bed, 606*f*, 607
Russell's traction, 582–583, 583*f*

S

Saddle joint(s), 527
Safe care, patient's right to, 8
Safety, 31–58
  agencies concerned with, 37
  assessment of, 115, 119
  for dependent patient, 41–42
    performance checklist, 53–54
  in home care, 52
  for infant, 442–444, 443*f*, 444*f*
    performance checklist, 450–452
  in institutions, 37–41
    performance checklist, 53
  in long-term care, 50
  in patient room, 40–41
    performance checklist, 53
  performance checklist, 53–55
  quiz, 57–58
  rationale for skill, 37
  staff behaviors important to, 37–38
    performance checklist, 53
  in transfers, 460
  in working spaces, halls, and corridors, 38–40
    performance checklist, 53
Safety belt, 46
Safety device(s), 42–48, 44*f*–47*f*. *See also* Restraint(s)
  hazards of using, 43
  for infant, 442–444, 443*f*, 444*f*
    performance checklist, 450–452
  nonrestraint, 45–46, 47*f*
  nursing diagnoses related to, 43
  procedure for applying, 46–48
    for infant, 442–443, 444*f*
    performance checklist, 54–55
Saliva, infection transmission in, 21–22, 23
Sandbag(s), in positioning, 336*f*
Scald, 436
Scale(s), for weighing patient, 283
Scoliosis, assessment for, 174, 175*f*
Scoliosis brace, Boston, 560, 560*f*
Secretion(s)
  descriptive terms used for, 80*t*
  gastric, collection of specimen of, 219*t*, 221
  respiratory, identification of tube feeding formula in, 706
Self-care, patient's right to assistance toward, 9
Self-determination, patient's right to, 6–7
Semi-Fowler's position, 339
  performance checklist, 353
Sensation
  assessment of, 115, 119. *See also* Circulation, motion, and sensation (CMS) check(s)
  skin, assessment of, 176, 178*t*
Sequential compression device, 630*f*

application of, 629–630
  performance checklist, 642–643
Sexuality, assessment of, 116, 120
Shampooing, 406, 406*f*
  for infant, 438
  performance checklist, 423–424
Sharp(s), disposal of, 39, 40*f*
  in Standard Precautions, 23
  in Universal Precautions, 21
Shaving, 399
Sheepskin pad(s), 601
Shoe(s), athletic, to prevent footdrop, 314, 336
Shoulder joint, 526*t*
  range-of-motion exercise for, 529, 530*f*
    performance checklist, 539
Shoulder spica cast, 554, 555*f*
Shower, procedure for, 400–401
  performance checklist, 417
Shower chair, 400
Side-arm traction, 581, 582*f*
Side-lying position, 336–337, 337*f*
  performance checklist, 351
Side rails, 42
Sigmoidoscopy, assisting with, 255*t*, 262–263, 262*f*
  performance checklist, 273–274
Signature, in documentation, 78
Sims' position, 340, 340*f*
  performance checklist, 354
Sitz bath, 660
  procedure for, 664–665, 664*f*
    performance checklist, 672–673
Skelaxin (metaxalone), interference by, in urine glucose testing, 225*t*
Skeletal traction. *See under* Traction
Skin
  changes in, after death, 752
  descriptive terms used for, 80*t*
Skin integrity
  assessment of, 115–116, 120
  bedmaking and, 305
Skin problem(s)
  with diapers, 436–437
  with traction, 580
Skin sensation, assessment of, 176, 178*f*
Skin traction. *See under* Traction
Skull tongs traction, 587–588, 587*f*
Skytron bed, 606
Sleep, assessment of, 115, 120
Sleep Pattern Disturbance (nursing diagnosis), 126
Slider board, 469–470, 470*f*
  performance checklist, 482–484
Sling(s), 632
  application of, 633–635, 635*f*, 636*f*
    performance checklist, 648–649
SMI 3000 bed, 605
SMI 5000 bed, 606
Smoking, 48
Snellen chart, 172–173
Soak(s), 660
  procedure for, 663–664
    performance checklist, 671–672

© 1996 by Lippincott-Raven Publishers

SOAP notation, 85–91, 88f, 89f

Social identity, assessment of, 116, 120

Soiled linen, handling of
in Standard Precautions, 23
in Universal Precautions, 21

Sordes, 403

Sore throat, due to tube feeding, 710

Source-oriented record, 75–76
flow sheets in, 82

Specific gravity, urine, 223–224, 223f, 224f
performance checklist, 237–238

Specimen(s)
blood, collection of, 218t, 220
collection of, 211–247, 217t–219t
in long-term care, 233
performance checklist, 235–246
procedure for, 221–223
quiz, 247
rationale for skill, 215
gastric secretion, collection of, 219t, 221
handling of
in Standard Precautions, 23
in Universal Precautions, 21
labeling of, 222
sputum, collection of, 219t, 220–221
stool, collection of, 219t, 220
urine. *See* Urine specimen(s)

Speculum, vaginal, 176

Speech therapy, for dysphagic patient, 361

Speed, in technical competence, 11

Sphygmomanometer(s), 144–145, 145f

Spica cast(s), 554, 555f

Spinal hyperextension brace, anterior, 560, 561f

Spinal tap, assisting with, 254t, 258–259, 258f
performance checklist, 269–270

Spine
joints of, 526t
range-of-motion exercise for, 533–536, 535f
performance checklist, 541

Spiral bandage, 624, 626f

Splint(s). *See* Brace(s)

Sponge bath(s). *See also* Bedbath(s)
cooling, 663
performance checklist, 673–674
procedure for, 665–666

Sputum specimen, collection of, 219t, 220–221

Square knot, 45

Stairs
crutchwalking down, 504, 504f
performance checklist, 516–517
crutchwalking up, 502–503, 502f, 503f
performance checklist, 514–516

Standard Precautions, 20, 22–23, 22t
performance checklist, 27

Static high air loss bed, 605–606, 606f, 608t–611t

Static low air loss bed, 604–605, 605f, 608t–611t

Static steep Fowler's position bed, 603

Stethoscope(s), 112
in blood pressure measurement, 145
ultrasound. *See* Doppler stethoscope

Stockinette, in casting, 551, 552f

Stocking(s)
elastic (antiembolic). *See* Elastic stockings
stump
application of, 630, 631f
performance checklist, 644–645

Stool
descriptive terms used for, 80t
testing for blood in, 230–231
performance checklist, 243–245

Stool specimen, collection of, 219t, 220

Stretcher(s), safety in using, 38

Stretch net binder(s), 632
application of, 633, 633f
performance checklist, 646–647

Stryker turning frame, 603, 604f, 608t–611t

Stump
bandage application to, 630, 631f
performance checklist, 643–644
stocking application to, 630, 631f
performance checklist, 644–645

Subdiaphragmatic abdominal thrusts, for foreign-body airway obstruction, 731–732, 731f, 732f
performance checklist, 737, 738–739

Subjective data, in SOAP notation, 85

Sulfonamide(s), interference by, in urine glucose testing, 225t

Supine position, 335–336, 337f
performance checklist, 350

Surgical asepsis, 19

Surgical bed, procedure for making, 310–311, 310f
performance checklist, 319–320

Swaddling, 443–444, 444f
performance checklist, 451–452

Swing-through gait, 498, 499f

Symptom assessment, 110

Synovial fluid, 525

Synovial membrane, 525

T

Tachycardia, 130

T-binder(s), 632
application of, 633, 634f
performance checklist, 647–648

Teaching, at discharge, 289–291, 290f

Tears, artificial, 407

Technical competence, 11–12

Technique, in technical competence, 11

Teeth. *See also* Dentures
care of, 402–403, 403f

Temperature, 126–130. *See also* Temperature, pulse, and respiration; Vital signs
measurement of, 133–134
performance checklist, 137–138
sites for, 129–130, 129f
normal, 126
nursing diagnoses related to, 126

Temperature, pulse, and respiration (TPR), 123–139. *See also* Pulse; Respiration(s); Temperature; Vital signs
documentation of, 135, 135f
performance checklist, 138
in home care, 136
in long-term care, 136
procedure for measuring, 133–136
performance checklist, 137–138
quiz, 139
rationale for skill, 126

Temporal pulse, 131, 131f

Temporary problem(s), progress notes on, 86, 89f

Terminology, used in documentation, 79–81, 80t–81t, 84t–85t

Test(s). *See* Laboratory test(s); *specific tests*

Testape
drug interference with, 225t
procedure for using, 226–227
performance checklist, 239

Tetracycline(s), interference by, in urine glucose testing, 225t

Therapeutic agent(s). *See* Medication(s)

Therapeutic bed(s). *See under* Bed(s)

Therapeutic frame(s). *See* Frame(s), therapeutic

Therapeutic procedure(s)
assisting with, 249–275
performance checklist, 265–274
procedure for, 252–253
quiz, 275
rationale for skill, 252
nursing diagnoses related to, 252

TheraPulse bed, 605

Thermal blanket, 662f
for cooling, 662
procedure for use of, 666
performance checklist, 674–675
for warming, 660

Thermometer(s)
electronic. *See* Electronic thermometer(s)
types of, 127–129, 128f, 129f

Thermometer sheath, 128

Thomas splint, 586, 587

Thoracentesis, assisting with, 253–256, 254t
performance checklist, 266–267

Thoracic-lumbosacral spine body jacket, 559f, 560

Thorax, assessment of, 161–167
performance checklist, 186
procedure for, 174–175, 175f

© 1996 by Lippincott-Raven Publishers

Three-point gait, 498, 498*f*
  performance checklist, 513
Three-point-plus-one gait, 498–499,
    500*f*
  performance checklist, 513
Thumb
  joints of, 526*t*
  range-of-motion exercise for, 531,
    533*t*
  performance checklist, 540
Tilt and Turn bed, 607
Time, notations of, in documentation,
    78–79, 79*t*
Tissue donation, 747, 749*f*
Toe(s)
  assessment of, 175
  performance checklist, 187
  joints of, 526*t*
  range-of-motion exercise for, 533,
    535*f*
  performance checklist, 541
Toenails, patient's, care of, 399
Tooth (teeth). *See also* Dentures
  care of, 402–403, 403*f*
Torso support, 46
TPR. *See* Temperature, pulse, and res-
    piration; Vital signs
T-Pump (water-flow heating pad),
    659
Tracheostomy, cardiopulmonary resus-
    citation for patient with,
    724–725
Traction, 575–595
  equipment and setup for, 579–580,
    579*f*, 580*f*
  nursing diagnoses related to, 579
  performance checklist, 591–593
  quiz, 595
  rationale for skill, 579
  skeletal, 586–589
    performance checklist, 592–593
    procedure for maintaining,
      588–589
    types of, 586–588, 587*f*, 588*f*
  skin, 581–586
    performance checklist, 591–592
    procedure for applying, 585–586
    types of, 581–585, 582*f*–585*f*
  special problems for patient in,
    580–581
Traction bed, 579–580, 579*f*
Transfer (within or between institu-
    tions), 277–298
  delegating tasks at, 291
  documentation of, 287, 288*f*
  to long-term care, 291
  nurse's responsibilities at, 285–289
  performance checklist, 294
  quiz, 297–298
  rationale for skill, 282
Transfer belt, 461, 493, 493*f*
Transfer board, 469–470, 470*f*
  performance checklist, 482–484
Transfer technique(s), 457–487
  bed-to-chair

mechanical, 467–469, 468*f*,
    481–482
  one-person maximal assist,
    462–463, 462*f*, 474–475
  one-person minimal assist, 463,
    463*f*
  two-person lift, 465, 465*f*,
    478–479
  two-person maximal assist,
    463–464, 464*f*, 475–476
  chair-to-chair, two-person lift,
    464–465, 477–478
  documentation of, 461, 471*f*
  general procedures for, 460–461
  performance checklist, 473–474
  in home care, 471
  horizontal lift, 470–471, 470*f*
  performance checklist, 484–485
  in long-term care, 471
  mechanical, 467–469, 468*f*
    in long-term care, 471
    performance checklist, 481–482
  nursing diagnoses related to, 460
  performance checklist, 473–485
  quiz, 487
  rationale for skill, 460
  safety in, 460
  six-point seated, 465–467, 466*f*
    performance checklist, 479–481
  using transfer board, 469–470, 470*f*
    performance checklist, 482–484
Transplantation, organ or tissue dona-
    tion for, 747, 748*t*, 749*f*
Transportation, for transferred patient,
    287–289
Trendelenburg position, 340, 340*f*
  performance checklist, 354
Triage, in disaster, 49
Triceps reflex, 176, 177*f*
Trochanter roll, 335, 336*f*
Tub bath(s), 399–400
  performance checklist, 416
Tube feeding, 701–716
  administering medications with, 705
  complications of, 710, 711*t*
  equipment for, 704
  formulas for, 704–705
  performance checklist, 713
  prefilled set for, 709, 709*f*
  procedure for, 706–710, 708*f*, 709*f*
  pump use with, 709*f*, 710
  quiz, 715–716
  rationale for skill, 704
  reservoir method for, 708–709, 708*f*
  scheduling of, 705–706, 706*t*
Tuning fork, 173, 174*f*
Turning frame, 603, 604*f*, 608*t*–611*t*
Turning patient in bed, 332–335,
    333*f*–335*f*
  performance checklist, 347–349
"Turning record," 74
Turn sheet, moving patient using,
    334–335, 335*f*
24-hour clock, 78–79, 79*t*
Twist support, 551, 552*f*

Tympanic thermometer, 128–129, 129*f*
  performance checklist, 137
  procedure for using, 134
Tympany, 112

U
UDDA (Uniform Determination of
    Death Act), 750
Ultrasound stethoscope. *See* Doppler
    stethoscope
Umbilical cord stump, care of, 439
Unconscious patient(s)
  oral care for, 403–404
    performance checklist, 420–421
  positioning for, 41
  protecting eyes of, 42
  rights of, 7
Uniform Determination of Death Act
    (UDDA), 750
Universal distress signal, for choking,
    731, 731*f*
Universal Precautions for Blood and
    Body Fluids, 20–22, 20*t*
Urinal(s), 376, 376*f*
  assisting with, 379–380
    performance checklist, 385–386
Urinary catheter(s)
  perineal care for patient with,
    380–382
  specimen collection from, 216, 217*t*,
    220*f*
Urine
  descriptive terms used for, 80*t*
  specimens of. *See* Urine specimen(s)
  tests on. *See* Urine test(s)
Urine culture(s), 232
Urine hydrometer, urine specific gravi-
    ty measurement using,
    223–224, 223*f*
  performance checklist, 236–237
Urine refractometer, urine specific
    gravity measurement using,
    224, 224*f*
  performance checklist, 237–238
Urine specific gravity, 223–224, 223*f*,
    224*f*
  performance checklist, 237–238
Urine specimen(s)
  "clean catch," 217*t*
  collection of, 215–216, 217*t*–218*t*,
    220*f*
    for culture, 232
    for glucose test, 225–226
    from infant, 198, 199*f*, 218*t*
  double-voided, collection of,
    225–226
  tests on. *See* Urine test(s)
  24-hour, 216
Urine test(s)
  for glucose, 224–227, 225*t*
    performance checklist, 238–239
  for ketone bodies, 227–228
    performance checklist, 240–241

© 1996 by Lippincott-Raven Publishers

Urine test(s) (*continued*)
  for occult blood, 228
  for pH, 228–229
    performance checklist, 241–242
  products used for, 216*t*
  for specific gravity, 223–224, 223*f*,
    224*f*
    performance checklist, 236–238
  using multipurpose strip products,
    228–229
Urinometer, urine specific gravity
    measurement using, 223–224,
    223*f*
  performance checklist, 236–237
Uristix, 216*t*
  procedure for using, 227
    performance checklist, 240

V

Vaginal speculum, 176
Values, patient's, assessment of, 116,
  120
Vascular sounds, 167

Venous pressure, estimation of, 171,
  171*f*
Ventilation system, in infection con-
  trol, 19
Vest restraint(s), 43, 44*f*
Visual acuity, assessment of, 172–173
Vital signs. *See also* Blood pressure;
    Pulse; Respiration(s); Tempera-
    ture; Temperature, pulse, and
    respiration
  disappearance of, at death, 749
  form for recording, 126, 127*f*
  times for taking, 126
"Vital signs list," 74
Vitamin C (ascorbic acid), interference
    by, in urine glucose testing,
    225*t*
Vitamin K, before liver biopsy, 259

W

Walker(s), ambulation using, 495–496,
  497*f*
  performance checklist, 510–512

Walking. *See* Ambulation
Waste, infective, disposal of
  in Standard Precautions, 23
  in Universal Precautions, 21
Water-filled mattress(es), 602
Water-flow heating pad, 659,
  659*f*
Wedge cushion, 46, 47*f*
Weight(s)
  body. *See* Body weight
  for traction, 580
Weight loss, significance of, 114
Wheelchair(s)
  safety in using, 38, 39*f*
  transfer to. *See* Transfer
    technique(s), bed-to-chair
Wheezes, 164
William's position, for pelvic traction,
  584
Windowing, 556
Wrist joint, 526*t*
  range-of-motion exercise for,
    529–531, 532*f*
    performance checklist, 540
Wrist restraint(s), 44, 45*f*

© 1996 by Lippincott-Raven Publishers